Child Maltreatment

Contemporary Issues in Research and Policy

Volume 9

Series Editors
Jill E. Korbin, Ph.D., Professor of Anthropology, Associate Dean, College of Arts and Sciences, Director, Schubert Center for Child Studies, Crawford Hall, 7th Floor, 10900 Euclid Avenue, Cleveland, OH 44106-7068, USA
jill.korbin@case.edu

Richard D. Krugman, MD, Distinguished Professor of Pediatrics, University of Colorado School of Medicine, 13123 E 16th Avenue Box B-390, Aurora, CO 80045, USA
richard.krugman@ucdenver.edu

This series provides a high-quality, cutting edge, and comprehensive source offering the current best knowledge on child maltreatment from multidisciplinary and multicultural perspectives. It consists of a core handbook that is followed by two or three edited volumes of original contributions per year. The core handbook will present a comprehensive view of the field. Each chapter will summarize current knowledge and suggest future directions in a specific area. It will also highlight controversial and contested issues in that area, thus moving the field forward. The handbook will be updated every five years. The edited volumes will focus on critical issues in the field from basic biology and neuroscience to practice and policy. Both the handbook and edited volumes will involve creative thinking about moving the field forward and will not be a recitation of past research. Both will also take multidisciplinary, multicultural and mixed methods approaches.

More information about this series at http://www.springer.com/series/8863

Bob Lonne • Deb Scott • Daryl Higgins
Todd I. Herrenkohl
Editors

Re-Visioning Public Health Approaches for Protecting Children

Springer

Editors
Bob Lonne
School of Health
University of New England
Armidale, NSW, Australia

Deb Scott
Senior Research Fellow
Monash University
Victoria, VIC, Australia

Daryl Higgins
Institute of Child Protection Studies
Australian Catholic University
Melbourne, VIC, Australia

Todd I. Herrenkohl
Marion Elizabeth Blue Professor
of Child and Family
University of Michigan School
of Social Work
Ann Arbor, MI, USA

ISSN 2211-9701 ISSN 2211-971X (electronic)
Child Maltreatment
ISBN 978-3-030-05857-9 ISBN 978-3-030-05858-6 (eBook)
https://doi.org/10.1007/978-3-030-05858-6

Library of Congress Control Number: 2019933899

This Springer imprint is published by the registered company Springer Nature Switzerland AG.
The registered company address is: Gewerbestrasse 11, 6330 Cham, Switzerland

Acknowledgments

This book comes on the back of the work of many who have strived to ensure that our protective systems achieve what we intend them to do – to prevent harm from occurring in the first place; and to liberate children from situations of abuse and neglect, uphold their rights, and assist them and their families to rebuild their relationships and connections. We are indebted to the child welfare community worldwide who have all worked so hard to make a positive difference in children's lives. We are deeply thankful for those who work tirelessly on behalf of vulnerable families.

We also offer our deepest and most sincere thanks to our authors who so masterfully capture both the challenges and opportunities that exist in child welfare at this very moment. We appreciate the effort each author has put toward this endeavor and particularly for producing such high-quality work under the pressures of tight timelines. Without you, we would not have this book!

We also extend our gratitude to Atiqur Rahman for his invaluable assistance in preparing the manuscript and to the series editors, Jill Korbin and Dick Krugman, for their vision and encouragement. Our thanks also extend to the team at Springer for their forbearance when we struggled to meet some of the timelines to which we had initially agreed.

On a personal note, we give thanks to our families and loved ones without whose support this book would not have been possible. They also share in this publication and its contributions to making the world a better place.

If this book can make a valuable contribution to our collective efforts to reduce child abuse and neglect, the work and dedication of all who are mentioned will all be worthwhile. In a globalized world that has witnessed inequality rise substantially, and where "wicked problems" abound, this book is a timely reminder of the importance of continually re-visioning the models we use to build our communities into strong, safe, and relationally connected places that prosper. Our children and families deserve nothing less.

Your colleagues in prevention,
Bob, Debbie, Daryl, and Todd

Acknowledgements

Introduction

Intervening early to prevent maltreatment is essential. Community action to preclude harm to children is foundational to changing the social conditions and institutional arrangements that are associated with increased likelihood of child maltreatment. Preventing child maltreatment starts with understanding the factors that elevate and mitigate the risk for dysfunction in the home – factors we characterize as social determinants of health – as well as broader community risks (particularly poverty, intergenerational cycles of disadvantage, and the unique challenges experienced by Indigenous communities in westernized countries with a history of colonial dispossession and dislocation) and risks within institutions, even those set up to serve and provide care for children and young people.

But the unique contribution of a public health approach is how to introduce preventive frameworks and embed supports across government portfolios, across diverse service delivery platforms, and, most importantly, providing these interventions at a whole-of-population level, not just to a narrow group of high-risk families. They also need to be embedded within new models of "business-as-usual" particularly for those key universal service delivery platforms, like health, education, and early childhood development services. Currently, prevention tends to be delivered via short-term pilot initiatives.

Across the parts in which the various chapters in this book are grouped, we uncover the key concepts of what needs to be incorporated within population-level strategies. We cover the challenges of contemporary child welfare systems, including the successes and key limitations. We outline the key elements of a population-based public health approach, explore and give examples of implementation issues and limitations, and suggest some of the challenges ahead.

As much as research has helped to uncover many such factors, most protective systems have found themselves unable to do more than respond in times of crisis. Prevention is simply not part of the operating model that existing child welfare systems routinely employ. Advocates of public health approaches to protecting children, our colleagues, have for a long while been publicly calling for an emphasis upon prevention rather than solely relying upon reactive responses to situations where maltreatment has already occurred. Yet, change has been slow – far slower than most advocates would prefer. We write this book with the hope that it will draw even more attention to the need and rationale for public health prevention.

The idea for this book came from our own collective frustrations at what we perceived to be very slow progress in transitioning from a reliance upon narrow, forensically oriented child protection approaches to more holistic, community-mobilizing ones. We embraced the need for integrated organizational collaborations to bring necessary help and assistance to vulnerable families struggling to get by in very difficult circumstances.

Despite the benefits in system reform, in our view, however, there were many significant impediments to achieving a truly preventative response to the problem of child maltreatment. Other areas of social harm have achieved significant reductions in harm due to the conceptualization of the issue as a "public health" problem and implementation of population-level responses, for example, road trauma, tobacco-related cancers, and dental health. Issues remain in the conceptualization of public health approaches, their implementation into contemporary child protection systems, and building interagency relations that will facilitate the provision of integrated services, not to mention the flow of information that enables effective primary, secondary, and tertiary responses.

Our hope is that this book provides a platform of knowledge and ideas upon which system reform can provide the web of care for children and families and struggling communities.

The book aims to alert the reader to the multifaceted, critical considerations relevant to building systems that have effective communication, coordination, and collaboration. The book highlights strategies that empower community-based services and mobilize community members to provide accessible support and practical help to vulnerable children, struggling families, and impoverished communities. Hence, the book outlines ways to think about and deliver social and material support that addresses the social inequalities and structural factors associated with an elevated risk of child abuse and neglect. The book promotes approaches that are:

- Humane and compassionate responses to service users
- Population-based, multidisciplinary, and based on the best research evidence and practice wisdom
- Built upon the successes and address the limitations of contemporary child protection interventions, such as the overrepresentation of marginalized groups
- Critical of the dominant ideological, political, and institutional interests that hinder socially just outcomes for vulnerable groups, particularly Indigenous peoples

We do not seek to portray a single or "ideal" way to develop a contextually appropriate preventative system. Rather, we hope to have captured the complexity inherent in addressing the variety of ideological, institutional, and historical issues in protecting children and to intervene early and effectively to prevent harm. We provide a succinct appraisal concerning the prescient issues confronting child protection and offer new insights and different perspectives regarding conceptualizations of public health approaches and how these can shape various ways to deliver services and "make child protection everyone's business." The book grapples with managing system change and the complexities of operationalizing the principles of public health approaches within diverse political, policy, practice, cultural, and community contexts.

In Part I, the book succinctly outlines the checkered history of child welfare/protection and problematizes the systemic, policy, and practice failings that have occurred over time, concluding that despite our best intentions and efforts, contemporary approaches to child protection have significant limitations and unintended consequences for children, parents, families, and communities.

Part II then examines the increased attention focused upon public health approaches to prevent maltreatment and provide earlier interventions to assist vulnerable and struggling families and communities. This is followed by an in-depth and broadly scoped description and critical appraisal of various conceptualizations of public health approaches to reducing the incidence and prevalence of child maltreatment and addressing their underlying ideological foundations and political considerations. A variety of perspectives are provided for how maltreatment can be prevented at societal and community levels.

Part III examines various jurisdictions' systemic reforms and program/practice developments that operationalize early intervention and prevention approaches. The dynamic processes inherent in systemic change are explored, particularly regarding service approaches and information needs. Also covered in detail are the issues that can arise and that influence the implementation of public health approaches. Case studies are used to highlight:

- How particular political, social, cultural, and institutional contexts affect how programs and services are structured and delivered
- Discourses that are used to reshape service user experiences of the interventions used and community perceptions of child maltreatment and approaches to address it
- The pitfalls and successes of systems that are in transition to become better at prevention

In seeking this, we have been steadfast in our conviction that public health approaches offer many advantages over risk-dominated child protection ones.

In Part IV, the book closes by identifying some emerging issues and critical trends that appear likely to affect efforts to prevent and reduce child maltreatment and its social harms. We have not shied away from facing up to the significant challenges and limitations that are part of an emphasis upon early intervention strategies, evidence-based services, and programs and addressing underlying inequities and inequalities that are core to public health models. System reform is usually a long and hard road, with setbacks as well as rewards. It requires our unremitting efforts, our intellect, values-based insights, perseverance, and vitality.

The safety and well-being of all children demands nothing less.

Contents

About the Contributors

Rhonda Barraclough is the executive director of ALIGN Association of Community Services in Edmonton Alberta. ALIGN is a membership organization of the agencies that contract to Children Services to provide support and care to children and families involved in the child intervention system. Rhonda has worked as a social worker in the child welfare field for over 30 years. Her career began as a child care worker in a mental health facility for youth and then moved on to child protection work in both British Columbia and Alberta. She has worked for both government and non-government agencies throughout her career. Rhonda is a registered social worker in Alberta and holds a Bachelor of Social Work and a Masters of Education focusing on adult education and social policy.

J. Bart Klika is the chief research and strategy officer in the national organization Prevent Child Abuse America. His research examines the causes and consequences associated with child abuse and neglect in an effort to prevent its occurrence. On multiple occasions, Dr. Klika served as a research consultant for the Centers for Disease Control and Prevention (CDC), examining issues related to the prevention of child abuse and neglect. In 2011, he was selected for the inaugural cohort of fellows for the Doris Duke Fellowship for the Promotion of Child Well-Being, a national fellowship providing support and mentorship for doctoral students seeking innovations in the prevention of child abuse and neglect. Dr. Klika is on the national Board of Directors for APSAC and is the chair of the APSAC prevention committee. Recently, Dr. Klika served as the senior editor for *The APSAC Handbook on Child Maltreatment* (4th Ed.).

Joni Brodziak is the executive director of the Policy, Practice and Program Development for child intervention (protection) in the Ministry of Children's Services, Alberta, Canada. This branch is responsible for overall program and operational policy related to Child Intervention Service Delivery, which includes Alberta's Child Intervention Practice Framework and other policy, program, and practice development targeted at improving how services are delivered to vulnerable children and their families. Joni has been in the field of child protection for

24 years, working in various roles in the field, starting out in direct service delivery as a frontline child welfare investigator and caseworker in 1993, and then leading a variety of large-scale initiatives before taking on her current role in 2012.

Donald C. Bross is professor emeritus of Pediatrics at the University of Colorado School of Medicine and its Kempe Center for the Prevention and Treatment of Child Abuse and Neglect. He is published on the reporting of child abuse, termination of the parent-child legal relationship, neglect of children before birth, medical and mental health-care neglect, and reporting of sexually transmitted infections. He has served as coeditor in chief of *Child Abuse & Neglect: The International Journal*, executive director of the National Association of Counsel for Children, and legal advisor for ISPCAN. Continuing interests include legislation to address children's health, researching the etiology and prevention of unintentional injury, improving the well-being of children in substitute care, evaluating the effects of child protective services, and developing the discipline of pediatric law, policy, and ethics. In 2018 he helped establish the Chair in Pediatric Law, Policy and Ethics at the University of Colorado School of Medicine, within its Center for Bioethics and Humanities. His most recent award is the Thomas Jefferson Award of the University of Colorado for his contributions to the welfare of children.

Helen Buckley is a fellow emeritus in the School of Social Work and Social Policy, Trinity College Dublin. Prior to her retirement, she was an associate professor and lectured in child protection to undergraduates and postgraduates at the university. She researched and published extensively in the area of child protection, with particular interest in systems, interagency collaboration, service user participation, and the use of evidence in practice. She is the chair of the Irish National Review Panel which reviews serious incidents including the deaths of children in care and a member of the Adoption Authority of Ireland. She recently completed a project commissioned by the Department of Children and Youth Affairs on the development of a profile of children at risk of significant harm.

Paul Bywaters is professor of Social Work at the University of Huddersfield and emeritus professor at Coventry University. He has practiced, taught, and researched in social work since 1970. He co-founded the international Social Work and Health Inequalities Network and co-wrote the International Federation of Social Workers' policy on health. In the last 5 years, he has been leading a series of Child Welfare Inequalities research projects (www.coventry.ac.uk/cwip) funded by the Nuffield Foundation and the Joseph Rowntree Foundation at the head of a team drawn from seven universities across the United Kingdom.

John Canavan is associate director of the UNESCO Child and Family Research Centre at NUI, Galway, in Ireland where he manages the center's extensive work program. He has over 25 years' experience in applied social policy research, working in State and academic settings in the evaluation of social intervention programs. He is particularly interested in prevention, early intervention, and family support and in Child Welfare and Protection contexts. John is principal investigator on a large-scale research study focused on embedded prevention within Ireland's Child Protection and Welfare system. He has published extensively on family support and is coauthor of the 2016 book *Understanding Family Support: Policy, Practice and Theory* with Pat Dolan and John Pinkerton. John teaches at undergraduate, MA, and PhD levels at NUI, Galway.

Martin Chabot is a data analyst at McGill University's Centre for Research on Children and Families and works under the supervision of the Canada Research Chair in Social Services for Vulnerable Children. Mr. Chabot is responsible for the extraction of clinical-administrative data from collaborating child welfare organizations and is involved in the production and analysis of sub-datasets based on project specifications.

Chien-Jen Chiang is currently a doctoral student at Washington University in St. Louis. After getting a MSW in the United States, he worked as a child protective services worker in the United States and Taiwan for more than 10 years. During his services as a supervisor in the child welfare system, he was invited to work with Taiwanese Government in implementing the Structured Decision Making Model in Taiwan. His interests in understanding the effectiveness of this and other similar reforms in child welfare led to his return to study for his PhD. Mr. Chiang's research interests include child neglect and understanding the effectiveness of screening and services for families involved in the child welfare system.

Graham Clifford is professor emeritus at the Institute of Social Work, Norwegian University of Science and Technology, in Trondheim. He was leader at the Regional Centre for Child Welfare Service Development from 1993 to 1997 and at the Centre for Child Psychiatry Research from 1997 to 2006. He was senior lecturer at the Institute for Social Work (1975–1993) and professor at the University College in Trondheim (Social Work) from 2011 to 2014. He studied at Emmanuel College Cambridge (1966–1969) and Trinity College Oxford, 1970–1971. He was awarded the Dr. Philos Degree at the University of Trondheim (1989). His research and publications are in the fields of elderly care and child psychiatric services and child welfare.

Deborah Daro is a senior research fellow at Chapin Hall at the University of Chicago. Dr. Daro's current research and written work focuses on developing effective early intervention systems to support all new parents and examining the impacts of reforms that embed individualized, targeted home-based interventions within universal efforts to alter normative standards and enhance community context. Reflecting her strong commitment to developing leadership in the area of child maltreatment prevention, she designed and directs the *Doris Duke Fellowships for the Promotion of Child Well-Being*. Dr. Daro has served as president of the American Professional Society on the Abuse of Children and as treasurer and executive council member of the International Society for the Prevention of Child Abuse and

Neglect. Dr. Daro holds a PhD in Social Welfare and a master's degree in City and Regional Planning from the University of California at Berkeley.

Ashleigh Delaye is a research associate at McGill University's Centre for Research on Children and Families and works under the supervision of the Canada Research Chair in Social Services for Vulnerable Children. Ms. Delaye's research focuses on social spending and the availability and accessibility of community services for children and families, federal responsibility for First Nations child welfare, and the relationship between poverty and neglect. Ms. Delaye synthesized the literature and contributed input into the manuscript.

Carmel Devaney is lecturer and course director of the master's degree in Family Support Studies in the UNESCO Child and Family Research Centre at NUI Galway. Carmel has a longstanding interest in and commitment to supporting and protecting children and young people within their family context. Carmel is principal investigator on a number of research projects under the Partnership, Prevention and Family Support Programme for Tusla, the Child and Family Agency. Carmel has recently conducted research on the feasibility of a longitudinal study on children in care/leaving care in Ireland. In recent years, Carmel has been lead researcher on a broader range of research projects for Tusla and has designed and delivered a number of family support training initiatives for managers and practitioners. Carmel has also worked for many years in children and family services as both a practitioner and manager. Carmel's recent publications and conference presentations are in the area of family support, child welfare and protection, and well-being.

Ida Drury is a senior instructor at the Kempe Center for the Prevention and Treatment of Child Abuse and Neglect. She serves multiple research and evaluation projects and consults nationally related to child welfare systems and practice. She also serves the Colorado Child Welfare Training System on the evaluation team.

Ida has over 15 years of experience in the human services field, most of which has been in a public child welfare setting. Before joining the Kempe Center, Ida was an analyst and CAPTA administrator for the Colorado Department of Human Services. Before that, she was project director for the Colorado Consortium on Differential Response, where she led a research and implementation project on differential response in Colorado. Her early career was on the front line as a child welfare caseworker.

Ms. Drury earned her Bachelor of Arts and Social Work at Wartburg College in Waverly, Iowa. She received a Master of Social Work at St. Ambrose University in Davenport, Iowa. She looks forward to defending her doctoral dissertation, focused on emotional labor, at the School of Public Affairs at the University of Colorado Denver in 2018.

Deb Duthie is a Wakka Wakka Warumungu woman with family ties to Cherbourg, Queensland, and Tennant Creek, Northern Territory, Australia. She is a senior lecturer in the School of Public Health and Social Work at the Queensland University of Technology (QUT), Brisbane. She was formerly a senior lecturer and academic advisor at QUT's Oodgeroo Unit (Indigenous Student Support). Deb co-developed, coordinated, and lectured in QUT's first Indigenous Knowledges Minor, covering Indigenous politics, cultural safety, representations of Indigenous peoples, and Indigenous research ethics and protocols. Deb successfully coordinated the *Cherbourg-QUT Project*, whereby transdisciplinary student teams collaborate with industry partners on Aboriginal community-initiated projects using a participatory action research framework.

Deb has 10 years' experience working in the domestic and family violence sector and with families experiencing homelessness. In 2012 she completed her PhD – *Reinvigorating the Domestic Violence Sector: Systemically Addressing Power, Conflict and Practitioner Turnover in the Domestic Violence Sector*. She was awarded the QUT Vice Chancellor's Excellence Award for the Cherbourg-QUT Project (2014), the Australian Award for University Teaching (2016), the David Gardiner Teacher of the Year Award (2018), and the Australian Technology Network Learning and Teaching Excellence Award (2018) for her work in teaching Indigenous Knowledges and Studies.

Marcus Erooga is an independent safeguarding consultant and a visiting research fellow at the Centre for Applied Childhood, Youth and Family Research, University of Huddersfield, UK. He spent the majority of his employed career in various roles, including assistant director, relating to child sexual abuse and sexual offending at the NSPCC (National Society for the Prevention of Cruelty to Children. He is a past editor in chief and current associate editor of the *Journal of Sexual Aggression* and past chair of NOTA (the National Organisation for the Treatment of Abusers). In 2016 he gave evidence as an expert witness on "grooming and entrapment" to the Australian Royal Commission into Institutional Responses to Child Sexual Abuse and was co-principal investigator (with Keith Kaufman) of a comprehensive literature review of child sexual abuse in organizations for the Australian Royal Commission. Marcus is author of a number of some 50 publications on child abuse and sex offender-related issues including 5 edited books, including *Protecting Children and Adults from Abuse After Savile: What Organizations and Institutions Need to Do* (JKP, 2018).

Tonino Esposito is an assistant professor at the University of Montreal and adjunct professor at McGill University and recipient of a Tier II Canada Research Chair in Social Services for Vulnerable Children. Dr. Esposito is the lead researcher for province-wide longitudinal studies on children's service trajectories in the Quebec child welfare system and principal investigator on Insight Development Grants on neighborhood socioeconomic disadvantages and child protection service outcomes. The work for this chapter was also supported by Dr. Esposito's Canada Research Chair (SSHRC # 950-230680) and the Social Sciences and Humanities Research Council (SSHRC # 430-2104-00299).

Barbara Fallon is an associate professor and associate dean of Research at the Factor-Inwentash Faculty of Social Work. Dr. Fallon is a Canada Research Chair in Child Welfare and the Factor-Inwentash chair in Child Welfare and the principal investigator for the Ontario Child Abuse and Neglect Data System (OCANDS) and the Ontario Incidence Study (OIS) of Reported Child Abuse and Neglect. Dr. Fallon contributed input into the manuscript.

Agatha Faulkner is experienced in the field of public health research and has worked for organizations such as Cancer Council Victoria, Turning Point Alcohol and Drug Centre, Deakin University, and Monash University. Her experience covers the areas of alcohol and drugs in adolescent and adult populations, family and domestic violence, mental health, and suicide. Recent projects have included a collaboration with the NSW Ombudsman examining the role of alcohol and drugs in child maltreatment and neglect deaths, and currently Agatha works within the Coronial Division (Tasmania) developing and implementing the Tasmanian Suicide Register.

Tamara Fuller is director of the Children and Family Research Center and research associate professor at the School of Social Work at the University of Illinois at Urbana-Champaign. Dr. Fuller has spent her career working with families involved with the public child welfare system, first as a clinical psychologist and later as a researcher examining the effects of child welfare policy and practice on children's safety, health, and well-being. During her career, she has evaluated the effectiveness of numerous child welfare programs, including family-centered services, safety and risk assessment tools, child death review teams, post-adoption and post-reunification services, and, most recently, differential response in child protective services. Within this program of research, there has been emphasis on examining predictors of maltreatment and maltreatment recurrence. Most recently, Dr. Fuller has used her expertise to developing predictive analytic tools that allow child welfare workers to target services to families at highest risk.

Mel Gray is professor of Social Work in the School of Humanities and Social Science at the University of Newcastle in New South Wales, Australia. Her wide-ranging research interests include social work ethics, social policy and social development, knowledge production, research use, and evidence-based practice in social work and the human services. Theory and knowledge for practice, including culturally relevant knowledge along with the influence of global forces, such as neoliberalism, on local welfare and development are constant themes in her research. She also coauthored *Working Ethically in Child Protection* (Routledge 2016) with Bob Lonne, Maria Harries, and Brid Featherstone.

Kassidy Green is a third year Bachelor of Social Work student at MacEwan University. She currently works as an intern with the Policy, Practice and Program Development for child intervention in the Ministry of Children's Services, Alberta, Canada. In this role, she has the opportunity to participate in the development of a wide variety of practice initiatives and approaches, which contributes to her professional growth and academic abilities. Kassidy has had experience with community outreach through her position as a caseworker for the Edmonton Castle Downs Constituency Office, is a volunteer on her university campus, and has a passion for social justice and advocacy work.

Maria Harries is a senior honorary research fellow at the Social Policy and Practice Research Consortium (SPPRC) in the School of Population and Global Health at The University of Western Australia and adjunct professor in the School of Occupational Therapy, Social Work and Speech Pathology at Curtin University, Western Australia. She has a 50-year career in clinical practice, teaching, research, and senior leadership in organizations and on boards of governance. She has conducted numerous case practice reviews, inquiries, and systems evaluations and has been engaged in the redesign of child and family services in a number of jurisdictions. Her focus has been on mental health and the well-being of children and families and ethical practices. She has taught and consulted extensively on ethics in governance and clinical practice.

Todd I. Herrenkohl is professor and Marion Elizabeth Blue Professor of Child and Family at the University of Michigan School of Social Work. Formerly, he was professor and co-director of the 3DL Partnership at the School of Social Work, University of Washington. His scholarship focuses on the correlates and consequences of child maltreatment, risk and resiliency, and positive youth development. His funded studies and publications examine health-risk behaviors in children exposed to adversity, protective factors that buffer against early risk exposure, and prevention. An international scholar, Dr. Herrenkohl works with policymakers, school and child welfare professionals, and community partners to increase the visibility, application, and sustainability of evidence-based programs and practices in prevention, social emotional learning, and trauma-responsive care.

Daryl Higgins is the director of the Institute of Child Protection Studies, Australian Catholic University. He is located at the St. Patrick's (Melbourne) Campus. He was formerly the deputy director at the Australian Institute of Family Studies, where he has led innovative knowledge translation/exchange functions that have increased access to the evidence base for policymakers and practitioners working to protect children and promote family and community well-being. His work has focused in articulating the public health approach to safe family environments and strategies for building child-safe organizational environments. Engagement between the research, policy, and practice communities – in order to understand and improve the circumstances of children, young people, and their families – has been his passion for more than 25 years. As an academic and a senior commonwealth public servant, Daryl has contributed to more than 230 publications and over 440 presentations and media engagements. He has provided advice to key influential bodies on child protection, family policy, and population-level public health approaches to child safety and well-being, in Australia and internationally.

Melissa Jonson-Reid is the Ralph and Muriel Pumphrey Professor of Social Work at the Brown School at Washington University. Prior to academia, she practiced both as a social worker in a domestic violence counseling organization and as a program administrator in public schools in California operating programs like Foster Youth Services and related services for vulnerable youth. As a researcher, a major focus of her work is understanding how responses to childhood abuse and neglect can be improved to support healthy behavioral, educational, and health outcomes. A large part of this work has involved using multi-agency longitudinal administrative data to identify targets of opportunity to leverage existing resources and/or evaluate policy and program efforts. Her work also includes evaluating approaches to maltreatment prevention building on existing home visitation platforms, consultation and evaluation with medical homes for youth in care, and school-linked services.

Melissa Kaltner is a principal research officer in the Department of Family and Community Services, New South Wales, Australia, where she leads a state-wide program of permanency and adoption research. After completion of her psychology honors qualifications, Melissa worked in frontline child protection roles. During this time in the field, she observed inconsistencies in practice that inspired a lifelong passion for developing evidence-based practice in child protection. Melissa is an adjunct senior lecturer at the University of New England and has led programs of applied out-of-home care research for the past 14 years. In 2015, she was awarded a prestigious Winston Churchill Fellowship to explore the role of adoption in creating stability for children unable to live safely with their birth families. Melissa is passionate about using evidence to inform practice in child protection to improve outcomes for children in care.

Cara Karter is a research and evaluation specialist at After School Matters. Her work currently includes leading data collection and reporting for special initiatives involving program model innovations, community policing, and STEM makerspaces. In this role, she is also responsible for conducting program quality observations and creating research briefs and presentations for internal and external stakeholders. Prior to joining After School Matters, Cara worked as a project assistant at Chapin Hall where she provided research assistance, project support, and communications expertise on a variety of projects in order to deliver timely and actionable information to policymakers, funders, and practitioners. Ms. Karter is an active member in the Society for Community Research and Action and the Chicagoland Evaluation Association for which she currently serves as communications chair. Ms. Karter obtained a Bachelor of Science in Social and Economic Development Policy and a Certificate in Leadership Studies from the Illinois Institute of Technology.

Keith Kaufman is a clinical/community psychologist and a professor of Psychology at Portland State University in Portland, Oregon. He is a member of the National Sexual Violence Resource Center's advisory board, the National Coalition to Prevent Child Sexual Abuse and Exploitation, Boys & Girls Clubs of America's National Safety Task Force, and Big Brothers Big Sisters Nation Safety Committee. He is past president of ATSA and recently received that organization's Significant Lifetime Achievement Award. Dr. Kaufman has provided assessment and treatment to both child sexual abuse victims and juvenile sexual offenders as well as their families. He has authored two books, a variety of book chapters, and numerous research articles addressing sexual violence and sexual violence prevention. His most recent edited book is *The Prevention of Sexual Violence: A Practitioner's Sourcebook* (NEARI Press, 2010). Dr. Kaufman is currently working on a $1 million US Department of Justice grant to develop a Campus Situational Prevention Approach to address campus sexual assault.

Joanne Klevens is an epidemiologist in the Division of Violence Prevention at the Centers for Disease Control and Prevention (CDC) in Atlanta. At the CDC, she has conducted research on the effectiveness of interventions to prevent child maltreatment, partner violence, and youth violence. Before joining the CDC, Dr. Klevens worked as a researcher and consultant in violence prevention in Colombia. Her research in Colombia focused on the etiology and prevention of child maltreatment and youth violence. She received her PhD in Epidemiology from the University of North Carolina in Chapel Hill, her MPH from the Hebrew University in Jerusalem, and her MD from the National University in Bogotá.

Bente Heggem Kojan is associate professor of Social Work in the Department of Social Work, Norwegian University of Science and Technology. Her particular fields of expertise are child protection, social inequality, and social justice. Her research focus is on children and families' life situations and their encounters from being involved in child welfare. She has worked as a practitioner within child protection and other areas of social work for many years.

Bob Lonne Professor Lonne has a distinguished professional, management, research, and academic career, with a primary focus on protecting children from maltreatment and developing earlier intervention and prevention strategies. He coauthored the Routledge publications *Reforming Child Protection* (2009) and the follow-up *Working Ethically in Child Protection* (2016) which have influenced debate and critical analysis worldwide of the processes and outcomes of the social and institutional arrangements used to prevent maltreatment and support struggling families. He has a longstanding commitment to the area of child protection and its service delivery and workforce issues and has authored and presented extensively on related issues in social work and the human services. Professor Lonne has participated and contributed to policy forums at the state and federal levels, and internationally, and is recognized by Inquiries as an expert witness in relation to child protection systems. He has been a passionate advocate for earlier intervention and prevention strategies, highlighting how current approaches fail many children and contribute to poor life outcomes for children in state care. Professor Lonne was the national president of the Australian Association of Social Workers from 2005 to 2011.

Bruce MacLaurin is an assistant professor at the Faculty of Social Work, University of Calgary, Alberta, Canada. He was the co-investigator on the three cycles of the Canadian Incidence Study of Reported Child Abuse and Neglect, as well as the principal investigator for provincial studies in BC, Alberta, Saskatchewan, and NWT. His research and publishing has focused on child maltreatment, child welfare, outcomes, foster care, youth at risk, and street-involved youth. He has collaborated with provincial and territorial governments on a variety of government initiatives including front-end services, ongoing services, kinship care, and outcome-based service delivery. Bruce served as an expert panel member for a Legislation Review in the Northwest Territories, the Office of the Child and Youth Advocate in Alberta, the Ministerial Panel on Child Fatalities in Alberta (Phase 1), Ministerial Panel on Child Intervention (Phase 2), and the Auditor General of Canada Review of the Northwest Territories Child Welfare Services.

Edgar Marthinsen is professor of Social Work at the Norwegian University of Science and Technology (NTNU) in Trondheim, Norway. His research interests lie in the history of social work and its relation to the social sciences and politics. His applied research concerns development of research-supported knowledge strategies. Marthinsen have a long history of empirical research on social work practice in the field of child protection and workfare and has written extensively on practice research in Norway. He has edited and contributed to a range of publications. He is coediting a special issue of the *Egyptian Journal of Social Work* (EJSW) on the impact of neoliberal thinking on social work (out 2019). He contributed to Harrikari, Rauhala, and Vironkannas (2014) *Social Change and Social Work: The Changing Societal Conditions of Social Work in Time and Place*. He coedited *Practice Research in Nordic Social Work: Knowledge Production in Transition* (2012) with Ilse Julkunen. He currently teaches at NTNU and is deputy head of the Department for Research at the Department of Social Work.

Ben Mathews is a professor in the School of Law and director of the Childhood Adversity Research Program at Queensland University of Technology in Brisbane, Australia. He has published 15 government reports, 70 refereed papers, and over 20 law reform submissions on issues concerning child maltreatment and the law. His research expertise is in the prevention, detection, and response to child abuse and neglect by legal and social systems, within a framework of law, public health, and children's rights. Specific interests include child sexual abuse, institutional liability, statutes of limitation, and mandatory reporting laws. His multidisciplinary and empirical research centers on the analysis of the impact of law, policy, education and skill development in lived experience, and the study of law and policy as an agent of change. He has advised multiple governments on law reform. He was a professorial fellow to Australia's Royal Commission into Institutional Responses to Child Sexual Abuse, served on the WHO Guideline Development Group on Health Sector Responses to Child Sexual Abuse, and is an adjunct professor at Johns Hopkins University, Bloomberg School of Public Health.

Morag McArthur has over 30 years of research experience in social work, public policy, and child welfare and has worked to bridge the gap between research, policy, and practice. She was the foundation director of the Institute of Child Protection Studies at Australian Catholic University from 2005 to 2016. She has worked on a range of research projects aimed specifically at improving policy and practice that affects children, young people, and their families. Her one key area of expertise is the development of innovative and participatory methodologies which include children and young people.

Caroline McGregor is professor at the School of Political Science and Sociology with lead responsibility for the discipline of social work. She is director of the Masters in Social Work and also a senior research fellow at the UNESCO Child and Family Research Centre. Formerly Dr. Caroline Skehill from Queen's University, her current project work is focused on outcomes for young people leaving care, public awareness of child protection and welfare, family support services and policy, and the interface between child protection and family support practices in child welfare. Caroline also has experience of research and publication in relation to child protection practice and policy, history of the present methodologies, socio-legal studies, and young people in and leaving care.

Lisa Merkel-Holguin assistant research professor at the Kempe Center at the University of Colorado and director of the National Center on Family Group Decision Making, has over 25 years of experience in identifying, developing, and implementing innovative reforms into child welfare systems, particularly in areas of child safety and permanency. Two of the most prominent reforms are family group decision-making and differential response, both which humanize the child welfare system and give professionals the opportunity to build helping relationships with the families who involuntarily make it into this system. With her expertise in implementation and capacity building, she has supported the installation of numerous evidence-based and evidence-informed innovations in child welfare agencies in over 40 States and a number of Canadian provinces. As a principal investigator and senior research analyst, she has led numerous impactful evaluations studying the impacts of different types of family meetings, child abuse prevention programs, and differential response.

Marilyn Metzler is the senior analyst for Health Equity in the Division of Violence Prevention at the Centers for Disease Control and Prevention/Karna, where she leads efforts to integrate a health equity approach across research, surveillance, and program activities. She has coauthored multiple publications, including *Adverse Childhood Experiences and Life Opportunities: Shifting the Narrative* (available via open access), and is a member of the HHS Reentry/Criminal Justice and Children of Incarcerated Parents work groups and the Healthy People 2020 Social Determinants of Health work group. Marilyn is a registered nurse with a BA in

Philosophy from Smith College in Northampton, MA, and an MPH from Morehouse School of Medicine in Atlanta, GA. Prior to arriving at CDC in 1999, Marilyn was the regional coordinator for Community Health Education at the Dartmouth-Hitchcock Medical System in Lebanon, NH.

Tim Moore is deputy director at the Australian Centre for Child Protection at the University of South Australia. Since 2005, Tim has worked with peers to explore the ways that children and young people understand and experience their worlds, their relationships, and the challenges that they and their families encounter. Drawing from experience as a youth worker, Tim has conducted studies on young caring, homelessness, parental drug and alcohol issues, youth justice, and child protection – particularly focusing on how to best respond to children and young people facing adversity. His most recent research has focused on children's perceptions of safety and how institutions can protect children from child sexual abuse and other forms of harm.

Melissa O'Donnell is a National Health and Medical Research fellow at the Telethon Kids Institute, University of Western Australia. Melissa has a master's degree in Psychology and a PhD in Pediatrics and Child Health. Melissa utilizes linked government data from the Western Australian Departments of Health, Child Protection, Education, Justice and Disability Services to investigate outcomes and risk and protective factors for children who have experienced abuse and neglect and external causes of injury. Dr. Melissa O'Donnell collaborates with government agencies to inform policy-relevant research to improve children's outcomes through prevention and early intervention. Her work has contributed to national and state policy and practice in the area of child protection and family support.

Nigel Parton is professor in Applied Childhood Studies at the University of Huddersfield, England. He has been writing and researching about child protection and child welfare for 40 years and now works on a part-time basis. He has held visiting professorships at the University of Tampere (Finland), La Trobe University (Australia), and the University of Edinburgh (Scotland) and been a Senior Hallsworth Fellow at the University of Manchester (England) and a Kempe-Haruv Fellow at the Kempe Centre, University of Colorado (USA). He is the author of over 100 articles and chapters and the author, coauthor, and editor of 25 books, including *The Politics of Child Abuse* (1985); *Governing the Family: Child Care, Child Protection and the State* (1991); *Safeguarding Childhood: Early Intervention and Surveillance in a Late Modern Society* (2006); and *The Politics of Child Protection: Current Developments and Future Directions* (2014). He coedited the journal *Children & Society* from 1995 to 2005 and chaired the Editorial Board from 2006 to 2012. He is currently a member of the Editorial Board and International Advisory Board of ten international journals and is editor in chief of the open access journal *Social Sciences* (www.mdpi.com/journal/socsci).

Antonia Quadara is a senior research fellow at the Australian Institute of Family Studies where she manages the Institute's sexual violence research program. This program examines issues related to child sexual abuse, child and adolescent problem sexual behaviors, adult sexual assault, public health approaches to prevention, and perpetration and sexual offending. Her areas of research interest include the dynamics and intersections between different types of sexual violence, service and systems responses to victim/survivors, criminal justice responses to sexual offences, feminist frameworks sexuality and sexual violence, and prevention and public policy. Antonia has a strong background in qualitative research methods, stakeholder engagement and consultation, and extensive experience in the writing, development, and production of publications and resources for policy and service sectors involved in responding to sexual violence. Before beginning at the Australian Institute of Family Studies, she was a lecturer and researcher in the Department of Criminology (University of Melbourne).

Dominic Richardson has a PhD in Social Policy and is an alumnus of the University of York, United Kingdom. Presently, Dominic is a senior education specialist at UNICEF, Office of Research, Innocenti, where he leads research on issues of equity in education and the relationships between schooling, school outcomes, and child well-being. His present projects include Time to Teach, a study of the determinants of teacher absenteeism in Sub-Saharan Africa, Sports for Development evidence on learning and social inclusion, and violence in schools. Dominic previously worked with OECD Social Policy Division on child well-being, evaluating family policies, and studies of extreme poverty and vulnerability. Dominic has led or coauthored several reports on comparative child and family well-being including *How's Life for Children?* in OECD's 2015 How's Life? and OECD's *Doing Better for Children* and *Doing Better for Families* as well as UNICEF Innocenti Report Cards 7, 9, and 14. Dominic recently coordinated a global project on families, family policies, and the SDGs, which was published in May 2018.

Carol W. Runyan is professor at the Colorado School of Public Health and director of the Program for Injury Prevention, Education and Research. Dr. Runyan graduated from Macalester College, received an MPH from the University of Minnesota and PhD from the University of North Carolina where she was a predoctoral fellow in child and family policy, and then completed a postdoctoral fellowship at Johns Hopkins University. She co-founded the University of North Carolina Injury Prevention Research Center and served as director for 22 years while on the faculty at UNC's Gillings School of Global Public Health. She has conducted research on child and adolescent injury, occupational injury, and suicide prevention and been a leader in continuing education for injury prevention. Honored by the US Centers for Disease Control and Prevention as one of the 20 most influential leaders in the field in 20 years, she also received a Distinguished Career Award from the American Public Health Association.

Desmond K. Runyan is the Jack and Viki Thompson Professor of Pediatrics at the University of Colorado, professor of Epidemiology in the Colorado School of Public Health, and executive director of the Kempe Center. Runyan completed medical school and pediatrics training at the University of Minnesota. He became a Robert Wood Johnson Clinical Scholar and completed a doctorate in Public Health at the University of North Carolina. Runyan then joined the faculty of the University of North Carolina's departments of pediatrics and of social medicine. He moved to Colorado in 2011. His research has addressed the identification and consequences of child abuse and neglect and the epidemiology of child abuse internationally. He designed longest multi-site prospective study of the consequences of child abuse; LONGSCAN is now more than 28 years in duration. Runyan helped design and conduct the first US study examining the incidence and consequences of abusive head trauma and led the development of a set of tools being used to assess child abuse epidemiology in more than 50 countries.

Erica Russ lectures and coordinates field education in Social Work at the University of New England, Australia. Prior to moving into academia, Erica had extensive industry experience in Social Work focusing on child, youth, family, and early childhood services holding significant experience and expertise in child protection, out-of-home care, and adoption as her main fields of practice. During her career in child protection, Erica worked across direct practice, service development, program management, operational and strategic policy, and management including holding senior positions in a statutory child protection agency. Erica has sat on university committees and review boards as an industry and academic representative. Erica has extensive experience in the development and delivery of industry training in the areas of child protection, out-of-home care, staff well-being, and vicarious trauma. She has a particular interest in child protection workforce issues with these being the topic of her doctoral thesis.

Matthew Sanders is a professor of Clinical Psychology and director of the Parenting and Family Support Centre at The University of Queensland. He is the founder of the internationally recognized Triple P-Positive Parenting Program, which is now run in 28 countries around the world in 20 languages. 75,000 practitioners have been trained to deliver Triple P. He has published extensively in the area of parenting, family psychology, and the prevention of behavioral and emotional problems in children. He is a fellow of the Academy of Social Sciences in Australia, Australian Psychological Society, New Zealand Psychological Society, Australian Association of Cognitive Behaviour Therapy, and the Academy of Experimental Criminology. He is an honorary professor in the School of Psychological Sciences at the University of Manchester, Glasgow Caledonian University, and the Faculty of Education at the University of Auckland. He has been a consultant to the Council of Europe on positive parenting and is a former Queenslander of the Year.

Leanne Schubert is an artist and social worker in private practice and affiliate of the University of Newcastle in New South Wales, Australia. She has worked as a research associate with coauthor Mel Gray for several years and has published numerous articles on the relationship between social work and art, community practice, knowledge production, and domestic and family violence and how these are influenced by the contemporary sociopolitical context.

Debbie Scott is a multidisciplinary researcher with nursing and public health background. Her early work as a nurse and public health injury prevention professional has led to a unique perspective to approaches in child protection and child well-being. Debbie has contributed to more than 100 peer-reviewed papers, manuscripts, and government reports and is an experienced speaker, presenting at local, national, and international conferences – including a number of keynote and invited papers. Debbie was the manager of the Queensland Injury Surveillance Unit, using surveillance data to inform policy on product safety, driver licensing for adolescents, and toddler drownings, for example. She has extensive experience in the linkage of larger administrative datasets and health classifications, participating in the development of ICD-11 for child maltreatment coding of health data. She has worked in a number of academic and government settings. Her current work as a senior research fellow for Monash University, Australia, and Strategic Lead for Population Health at Turning Point, Australia, is focused on the intersection of child protection, family violence, mental health, and alcohol and drugs.

Aileen Shaw is the manager of Strategic Development at the UNESCO Child and Family Research Centre in NUI Galway. She has extensive experience in research management, fundraising, and nonprofit practice. In 2015, she completed a PhD study on philanthropic investment in children and youth in Ireland. Her current research interests include commissioning, nonprofit management, and international foundation funding in the child and youth sector. Within the philanthropic field, Aileen has previously worked as research and development director at the National Network of Grantmakers in San Diego, California. She has also acted as a fundraising and communications consultant for several community-based, advocacy organizations in the United States and Ireland.

Kim Spicer is the senior manager of Outcomes and Practice in the Child and Youth Services Division within the Ministry of Human Services, Alberta, Canada. She has worked within the Ministry of Human Services in Child Intervention since 1998 and has provided direct client services as well as provided oversite to staff, policy, and program development in various leadership positions over her career. Kim has been involved in the development and implementation of many child intervention initiatives throughout her career and is passionate about supporting child intervention staff to have the tools they need to support families through enhancing family capacity.

Sharon Steinhauer works for *University nuhelot'įne thaiyots'į nistameyimâkanak Blue Quills* as program lead for social work education since 1998. Blue Quills is a former Indian Residential School now owned and operated by seven First Nations communities in northeast Alberta, Canada. Blue Quills has established programs that students of all cultures describe as transformative, influenced significantly by immersion in Indigenous knowledge, traditional ceremonies, and the relational practice of engaging in circles to build common ground.

Sharon's work with children and families has become more focused in recent years in both training and research activities. A shift occurs when child intervention practitioners understand the colonial and residential school impacts and they stop judging families. The legacy of unresolved historic and intergenerational trauma has resulted in high rates of children in government care and families struggling to recover with little or no societal understanding of their needs or the resources to support them.

Vincent Steinhauer is president of *University nuhelot'įne thaiyots'į nistameyimâkanak Blue Quills* since 2012. He is the third generation of Indigenous resurgence since Blue Quills was taken over from the Canadian government following decades as a Residential School where Indigenous children were placed when they were forcibly removed from their families.

With Vincent's leadership, the school has transformed from a community college to an internationally accredited university. Vincent served as a co-chair of the redesign of Children's Services for the province of Alberta from 1997 to 2000 and also sat as public member on the board of governors for two terms with the Alberta College of Social Workers. Vincent holds two degrees from the University of Alberta and is completing a Doctoral Degree in Indigenous Governance in spring 2018.

Vincent travels on the red road of the *newo iyiniwak* and carries ceremonial bundles for the children. He is a family man from Saddle Lake Cree Nation.

Heather Taussig is a professor and the associate dean for Research at the University of Denver's Graduate School of Social Work. She is also an adjunct professor at the Kempe Center for the Prevention and Treatment of Child Abuse and Neglect at the University of Colorado. Dr. Taussig's research focuses on developing and testing prevention programming for vulnerable youth, primarily maltreated children with child welfare involvement. She developed and directs the *Fostering Healthy Futures* program, an evidence-based mentoring program for children in foster care. She also conducts longitudinal research on risk and protective factors, child welfare outcomes, and policy issues related to child maltreatment and foster care. Dr. Taussig currently serves on the Research Board of the National Mentoring Resource Center, funded by the Office of Juvenile Justice and Delinquency Prevention. She served on Colorado Governor Ritter's Task Force on Foster Care and Permanence and continues to participate in several community collaboratives. Dr. Taussig is an awardee for her work on child abuse and neglect from the International Society for the Prevention of Child Abuse and Neglect.

Nico Trocmé is the director of the School of Social Work and the Philip Fisher Chair in Social Work at McGill University. Dr. Trocmé is the principal investigator for the Canadian Incidence Study (CIS) of Reported Child Abuse and Neglect (1993, 1998, 2003, and 2008) and the lead researcher for a research capacity development and knowledge mobilization initiative involving child welfare and Aboriginal service provider agencies in Quebec. The work for this chapter was supported by the Social Sciences and Humanities Research Council (SSHRC # 895-2011-1015).

Catherine Twinn has been an Alberta lawyer since 1980. In 2011–2013, she initiated and led a large-scale collective impact community and systems' engagement process to reduce the number of Aboriginal children in the child welfare system, utilizing the "Braid Strategy." Childhood trauma – adverse childhood experiences (ACEs) – substantially increases risks for a range of later-in-life negative outcomes including interactions with systems that are not trauma-informed. She is one of the first Peer Support volunteers for the Alberta Lawyers' Assistance Society. She is a trustee for a number of Indigenous Trusts, so Indian Act reserve communities can decolonize and redistribute power and responsibility into good governance bodies fulfilling fiduciary and justice principles.

Kerryann Walsh is a professor in the Faculty of Education at Queensland University of Technology. Kerryann conducts strategic and applied research on child protection, including leading projects for the Australian Royal Commission into Institutional Responses to Child Sexual Abuse. Over the past 10 years, her research has been concerned with generating empirically validated principles for child maltreatment prevention and response and ensuring the uptake of these principles in legislation, policy, and practice. With colleagues, she has researched and published in the areas of school-based child sexual abuse prevention programs, family violence prevention, professionals' reporting of child abuse and neglect, and training interventions for mandatory reporters. This work has been taken up in policy deliberations by Australian governments, has influenced law reform, and has been a catalyst for changes to education policy and practice.

Lindsey Weiler is an assistant professor of Family Social Science and affiliate faculty with the Institute for Translational Research in Children's Mental Health at the University of Minnesota. Dr. Weiler earned her doctoral degree in Applied Developmental Science from Colorado State University where she co-developed and researched the impact of Campus Connections, a multi-level, multicomponent youth mentoring program facilitated by couple and family therapists on at-risk adolescents. Her research focuses on developing, testing, and optimizing preventive interventions for high-risk families. The goal of this research is to identify effective strategies for fostering healthy development among vulnerable populations (e.g., children in foster care, justice-involved families). Her work seeks to leverage adult-youth relationships and the alliance between parents and other caring adults to promote positive outcomes.

Sasha Williams is currently practicing as a solicitor in children law at Jones Myers Solicitors in Leeds, UK. Her qualifications include a Law Degree (LSE), an MSc in Applied Social Studies/DipSW (Oxon) qualifying her to practice social work, a PGDip in Psychology (Open University), and an MSc in Social Research (University of Leeds). She is a member of the Law Society and the British Psychological Society and was until recently registered with the HCPC. Most recently Sasha received ESRC funding to conduct a PhD at the University of Huddersfield exploring how laypeople construct child neglect (main supervisor Nigel Parton). Before returning to legal practice in 2017, Sasha taught pre- and post-qualifying social work students at BSc and MSc level at the University of Huddersfield, and her research has formed the basis of lectures, seminars, advanced children practitioner workshops, publications, and national and international conference presentations.

Marc Winokur director of the Social Work Research Center, joined the School of Social Work Faculty at Colorado State University (CSU) in fall 2004. Dr. Winokur received his PhD in Education and Human Resource Studies with a specialization in Research Methods and Program Evaluation from CSU. Dr. Winokur has 14 years of applied research experience in child welfare that has influenced policies, practices, and procedures at the international, federal, state, and county levels. Dr. Winokur has conducted randomized controlled trials on differential response and home visitation programs and systematic reviews on kinship care and juvenile sexual offender treatment outcomes. Dr. Winokur also has conducted evaluations on foster care, adoption, family preservation services, child maltreatment prevention, child welfare caseworker retention, and family treatment drug courts. Additional research interests include family engagement practices, trauma-informed interventions, child well-being measures, and risk and safety assessment in child protective services.

Tania Withington is the manager of the Children's Health Queensland Hospital and Health Service, Child and Youth Mental Health Service, and Eating Disorder Program. She is a visiting fellow at the Queensland University of Technology in the School of Public Health and Social Work. Dr. Withington is a reviewer for the international journal of *Child Abuse & Neglect*. She is an accredited mental health social worker with the Australian Association of Social Work. Dr. Withington's research interests lie in child and adolescent mental health, child protection (specifically out-of-home care), and relational interventions including evidenced-based models of family therapy. Dr. Withington has published a number of journal and conference papers in these areas. Dr. Withington has a specific interest in garnering and utilizing the perspectives of service users to inform systemic responses to the felt need aiming to achieve best possible outcomes for individuals and families. She continues to work clinically with children and families in a mental health context.

Amy Conley Wright is associate professor of Social Work and director of the Institute of Open Adoption Studies at University of Sydney, where her focus is applied research on open adoption practice and building the evidence about children and their best interests. She is also honorary senior fellow at Early Start Research Institute, University of Wollongong, and was formerly assistant professor of Child and Adolescent Development at San Francisco State University. Her teaching, research, and practice experiences are in the areas of child advocacy, child protection, child and family policy, family support, and child maltreatment prevention. Recent publications include *Six Steps to Successful Child Advocacy: Changing the World for Children* (Sage Publications, 2013) and *Social Investment and Social Welfare: International and Critical Perspectives* (Edward Elgar Press, 2017). She has served as a board member and provided consulting on child and family services for government and non-governmental organizations.

Judith Zatkin is a fifth year doctoral student at Portland State University in Portland, Oregon. Broadly, she is interested in organizational-, community-, and institutional-level approaches to sexual violence prevention. Her work includes working with community and youth-serving organizations on sexual violence prevention interventions, understanding community perceptions of sexual violence perpetration and myths about sexual offending, and understanding perpetration patterns of those who sexually offend. Judith utilizes qualitative and quantitative methodologies to conduct this work.

Part I
The Policy and Program History of Child Protection

Chapter 1
The Successes and Limitations of Contemporary Approaches to Child Protection

Daryl Higgins, Bob Lonne, Todd I. Herrenkohl, and Debbie Scott

1.1 Introduction

While most children live in safe and supportive environments, governments and non-government family support services are aware that too many children are becoming known to statutory child protection services, and the social and financial costs are rapidly escalating. This has led some to a shift in thinking away from solely concentrating on statutory responses to 'risk of harm' reports towards a broader public health approach to protecting children, reducing the likelihood of children coming to the attention of statutory authorities.

In this book, the various authors contribute to a narrative that argues for the adoption of a public health approach to safety and wellbeing of children as a solution to the difficulties experienced by contemporary child protection statutory systems. Public health interventions begin with prevention-focused actions that are taken at a whole-of population level, often through already existing universal service delivery platforms where contact with families occurs (i.e., health, education and child care

D. Higgins (✉)
Institute of Child Protection Studies, Australian Catholic University, Melbourne, VIC, Australia
e-mail: daryl.higgins@acu.edu.au

B. Lonne
School of Health, University of New England, Armidale, NSW, Australia
e-mail: blonne@une.edu.au

T. I. Herrenkohl
School of Social Work, University of Michigan, Ann Arbor, MI, USA
e-mail: tih@umich.edu

D. Scott
Monash University, Richmond, VIC, Australia
e-mail: debbie.scott@monash.edu

B. Lonne et al. (eds.), *Re-Visioning Public Health Approaches for Protecting Children*, Child Maltreatment 9, https://doi.org/10.1007/978-3-030-05858-6_1

services), complemented by community-based actions and population-wide strategies. The latter includes information about child safety, awareness raising actions, regulations and controls, and provision of training, resources and supports—for professionals working with families, as well as direct provision of parenting skills and other supports for families themselves (see Herrenkohl et al. 2015). Why are public health approaches needed? What is the problem that this is trying to fix?

1.2 Overview of Child Protection Systems

Statutory child protection services are overwhelmed, have over-grown their intended purpose, and many would argue that they are at real risk of failing to deliver well enough on the aims they have espoused. But not all systems are the same. Analysts often describe two 'orientations' to child protection systems: the "child protection" orientation (e.g., Australia, Canada, UK, USA) and the "family service" orientation (e.g., Belgium, Sweden, Denmark) (Price-Robertson et al. 2014). A third, informal community care systems, found in countries where formal protective systems are limited, utilizes familial, community and cultural networks (Cameron and Freymond 2006). The child protection orientation has been widely criticized as inadequate, and even dangerous, for a range of reasons (see Higgins 2011; Higgins and Katz 2008; Lonne et al. 2009), including:

- Growth and cost of maintaining the tertiary response system is unsustainable (including many children coming into care early in life and remaining in care for the duration of their childhood);
- Poor response to individuals experiencing vulnerability (many referrals unable to be substantiated, and many not even investigated);
- Activities are largely forensically oriented, with little or no capacity to support families in responding to the safety concerns and the needs of their child(ren) (i.e., limited prevention or treatment-focused interventions to address the needs, and service system fragmentation), with complicated systems of referral, outsourcing and networking to try and link families with support services (despite the design and implementation of differential response pathways for provision of family support—see Chap. 12 in this volume);
- A paucity of evaluated program and system responses;
- Minimal use of population-level data to inform policy and practice development and responses;
- Processes not aligned to best practice in hearing from children and young people their safety concerns and what is needed for them to feel and be safe at home;
- Behavior of workers driven by the legislative framework that underpins the tertiary system's enabling legislation;
- Poor recognition of cumulative effects of low-intensity maltreatment or neglect (Bromfield et al. 2007), the likely overlapping experience of multiple forms of

abuse/victimization (Price-Robertson et al. 2013), and difficulties in finding evidence to substantiate some sub-types of harm (e.g., child sexual abuse);
- The reactive nature of service reform (driven typically by public enquiries or media);
- Negative perceptions from families of their potential—or actual—involvement in statutory services;
- Disconnection between the known drivers of increased demand (poorly treated parental mental health and substance misuse and broader family violence) and the supports needed to prevent and/or address parental problems;
- Gross overrepresentation of marginalized groups, particularly Indigenous peoples;
- Poor morale, burnout and turnover of statutory workers;
- Difficulty in recruiting and retaining foster and kinship carers, the costs of residential care, and problems of placement instability; and
- Dealing with the structural drivers of poverty and neglect.

Systems (and the rise of departments to govern those systems) have evolved significantly since their inception (Krugman 2017; Tomison 2001), including a gradual move toward rights-based practice and public health approaches. Notwithstanding, child protection remains substantially driven by discourses of 'child rescue', with removal of children embraced as a primary method of ensuring protection. As Higgins outlined elsewhere:

> In the 20th century, child protection systems began in the not-for-profit and advocacy sectors, with rapid expansion from the 1960s. They then evolved into state/territory statutory systems for responding to children who could not remain safely in the care of their parent(s) … With the shift towards governments taking responsibility for responding to those children who have been harmed or are at serious risk of harm, a network of intersecting systems has developed to detect child maltreatment, intervene to keep children safe, and respond to their needs. However, these systems have grown beyond what anyone could have imagined back in the 1970s and early 1980s, when communities were just starting to become aware of the serious harms that some children face while supposedly in the care of their parents. Since then, there has been a growing expectation that governments – on behalf of the community – have a responsibility to intervene in private family life to protect the wellbeing of these vulnerable and damaged children (Higgins 2011, p. 5).

Despite the evolution of—and the growth in demand for—statutory systems, there is little evidence that the often-intrusive nature of the investigations and interventions is successful. One common criticizm is the lack of any real interventions after an investigation (US DHHS 2009). There are no studies (and of course, designing an appropriate methodology would be incredibly difficult) to demonstrate positive outcomes of statutory involvement, compared with other types of intervention. As Price-Robertson et al. (2014) noted:

> As these models represent country-level systems that are embedded in complex cultural, social and historical contexts, it is not possible to determine whether these different approaches are 'evidence-based', 'promising' or 'untested' (p. 4).

When children are removed into alternative/out-of-home care, research consistently shows high levels of behavioural and emotional difficulties—which could be due to the trauma of abuse, or to the failure of the statutory responses to adequately respond to their needs. In a rare study looking at follow-up of a US cohort study of high-risk children known as LONGSCAN, Campbell et al. (2010) compared those who experienced a Child Protection Service investigation with those who did not. They found that: "investigation for suspected child maltreatment is not associated with relative improvements in common, modifiable risk factors suggests that we may be missing an opportunity for secondary prevention of maltreatment and maltreatment consequences" (p. 943). Despite being investigated by a statutory service, the problems that these families encountered remained—poor social support, family dysfunction, poverty, low maternal education, and child behavior problems—and were no different from families who were *not* investigated (Campbell et al. 2010). And many families who come to the attention of protective authorities feel deeply stigmatized by their experiences (see Chaps. 2 and 12 in this volume).

1.2.1 Re-referrals and Unmet/Poorly Met Needs of Families Experiencing Vulnerability

One of the most significant challenges of statutory systems is the 'churn': the fact that the same families, and indeed often the same children are 're-referred' (i.e., are notified to a statutory service (often through mandatory reporting mechanisms), when they have already been recently notified (and the risk of harm either substantiated or not). Various terms are used worldwide to describe children and families that are repeatedly involved with children protection systems. These terms include: 'chronic', 'recurrent' (USA and Canada), 're-substantiation' (Australia) and 're-registration' (UK). Australian child protection inquiries into system failures have identified the needs of this core group of families and children as unaddressed by ongoing investigations (Cummins et al. 2012).

In a sense, data on re-referrals are one of the best measures of system failure. A rise in new referrals could be a good thing (reflecting greater community awareness of the safety needs of children, etc., and the success of mandatory reporting and other procedural requirements of other professionals coming into contact with children). However, for children who have already encountered the statutory system, coming back to the attention of the system suggests something was inadequate about the initial contact or support services offered. Re-referrals could be due to a range of factors, including: poor screening and risk assessment tools or processes, misidentification of risk, inadequate resourcing to investigate or respond to risk of harm, or the failure of the interventions themselves to either bring about—or sustain—change to the child's circumstances.

Due to different legislative definitions, service systems and reporting requirements, and data collection methods/intervals, it is impossible to compare re-referral data between jurisdictions. However, the available re-referral data do provide a snapshot of how services might be failing to meet the needs of children at risk and families experiencing vulnerability. For example, the Australian Government Productivity Commission (2017) reports on percentages of children who were reported to a jurisdiction's statutory child protection service, but the risk of harm was not substantiated, and who during the year and who were then also the subject to a subsequent referral which was substantiated within 3 months (ranging from 3.1–9.3% across the 7 states/territories) or within 12 months (9.7–24.5%).

Bentley et al. (2017) found moderately high levels of re-referrals in the UK, though they varied between jurisdictions, and over time. For example, in Northern Ireland, the percentage of children already known to a statutory child protection service subsequently becoming re-registered has been trending upwards from a low of 15% in 2010/11 to 22% in 2015/16. Similarly, based on data from the US National Child Abuse and Neglect Data System, Fluke et al. (2008) estimated that within 24 months, 22% of children were re-reported, and 7% were re-reported with substantiation.

Taking a longer-term perspective, the intergenerational involvement of families in the statutory child protection system demonstrates the same challenges and failures of statutory systems: adults who as children received a statutory intervention or service (including removal and placement in out-of-home care) are more likely to as adults have their own children come to the attention of statutory services. There is a strong connection between structural disadvantage/situational vulnerability and children's risk—with existing responses largely inadequate to prevent intergenerational transmission of disadvantage and risk.

In Chaps. 2 and 3 in this volume, the authors explore further the unintended consequences, poor outcomes, or misalignment with the needs of children and their families experiencing vulnerability and in need of support, and Chap. 20 examines the intergenerational trauma that many Indigenous families and communities experience from ongoing child protection involvement and the removal of children.

1.2.2 Successes in Statutory Child Protection Services

Despite the litany of failures summarized above (and explored more fully in Part I of this book), and the almost constant reviews and inquiries into statutory child protection services in most jurisdictions, it is ironic that these perceived failures are due in part to its successes in creating demand. Improvements in risk assessment (such as actuarial assessment tools, that replace, or support expert clinical judgement), along with introduction of mandatory reporting, and expansion to cover different groups of professionals (or indeed, all citizens in some jurisdictions) and different types of harm, and lowering of the threshold for intervention has been successful in closing gaps between which children experiencing vulnerability could fall, and bringing children at risk to the attention of statutory authorities.

Over the decades, child protection services have evolved from a response to rare, severe events—such as sexual abuse, and the severe physical abuse identified by Kempe and colleagues—to the variety of risks and adverse environments to which children are exposed. This also means grappling with the reality that children are often exposed to multiple forms of harm, as the growing body of research on multi-type maltreatment and polyvictimization demonstrates (Price-Robertson et al. 2013). New risk-assessment processes have been needed to address the issue not only of exposure to multiple types of harm, but also the cumulative effects of 'lower-intensity' events, particularly neglect and emotional abuse (Bromfield et al. 2007; Bromfield and Higgins 2005; Bromfield and Miller 2012).

But the downside is that widening the net hasn't necessarily been accompanied by the sophisticated capability to respond to the wider nature of harm types and, in particular, mandatory reporting has been criticized for creating a culture of 'report' rather than 'respond/manage'—increasing the workload of statutory services, and ironically meaning that risk-averse agencies that might otherwise have provided services seeing it as the responsibility of the statutory system to respond (Melton 2005). The challenge is that only a relatively small proportion of concerns notified to statutory services are substantiated (but more concerning is the relatively large proportion that are not even investigated) and that investigations of neglect, in particular, often entail maltreatment thresholds and determinations of risk that are fraught (Lonne 2015).

When the referral and risks assessments work well, the greatest success of modern statutory systems has been its ability to respond to large numbers of children who need protection from high-risk environments, using court-endorsed care and protection orders. Improvements in placement options have led to an emphasis in many jurisdictions on placement with kin. For example, in Australia, the number of children living with a kinship carer (49%) exceeds those placed with foster carers (39%; AIHW 2017).

1.3 Marginal Reform: Reform at the Margins

Notwithstanding these successes, the criticizms remain; the log of inquiries internationally continues to grow, and there is no evidence in sight of full implementation of alternate systems based on a fundamental re-think of how we keep children safe in families and communities. Rather, the drivers of reform are often public inquiries into tragedies and scandals that result in increased emphasis upon risk and proceduralizm (Lonne and Parton 2014). Despite systemic reform processes, public health approaches have remained as a secondary response to investigation and removal options, and whilst this trend is slow it is occurring in many nations (SPERU 2016). Bold systemic reform, as outlined in Part III, is difficult. Apart from institutional intransigence in some jurisdictions, there is systemic fragility and fatigue evident in some countries due to the continual reform processes.

Nonetheless the need for reform and alternate strategies is evidenced by the fact that many jurisdictions now think about small-scale trials and limited services to prevent, or tailor supports for those at higher risk. For example, in Victoria (Australia), the Cradle to Kinder program targets young mothers in a number of 'high-risk' categories which internal departmental data showed were statistically more likely to experience vulnerability and risk having children removed in the child protection system (Scott et al. 2016b). It focuses on building trusting relationships between parents and support workers, and using that positive relationship to provide practical inputs and supports for improving parenting capacity and skill; empowering parents to plan for the future, and transition to independence (particularly for those young parents who themselves were—or are currently—in case), and addressing practical life skills that support effective parenting and family life (Scott et al. 2016b). The program evaluation of the first 2 years of operation found that the strengths-based, longer-term flexible program largely met its objective:

> It provided intensive and long-term support that made progress on addressing underlying issues such as mental illness, unemployment and unsustainable housing that contributed to the risk of families entering the child protection system (Scott et al. 2016b p. 18).

Emerging evidence suggests that earlier intervention and prevention approaches work; however, too often they are not implemented at scale (i.e., they remain short-term of geographically limited trials), or implemented early enough to prevent risks escalating.

1.3.1 The Rationale for a Public Health Approach

The evidence is mounting that statutory systems, particularly in Anglophone western countries with a 'child protection' orientation have not delivered well enough the aims it espoused. Munro (2011) found the UK child protection system to be over-bureaucratized, compliance-focused, defensive, and inconsistent with good social work child-centred practice. Similarly, statutory systems in Australia have been criticized as "ill-designed to respond to the nature and scope of the contemporary problem of child maltreatment" (Bromfield et al. 2014).

Some of the key challenges that a public health approach to child protection would need to address include:

- Dealing better with poverty and neglect—though there has been progress made with some jurisdictions acknowledging cumulative harm—but again, in terms of meeting threshold for intervention, not in terms of prevention;
- Intergenerational issues (parents with a care history are at greater risk of child protection involvement and subsequent removal of their children);
- The disconnection of statutory child protection services from other supports/ community resources (with problems such as both duplication and gaps, stigma associated with accessing services, client access and/or disengagement);
- The stigma associated with child protection and social care interventions that are seen to be deficit-focused, coercive, and intrusive;
- Poor engagement with services—either because of their lack of availability, or the fact that families have to be 'reported' to child protection in order to get referred to the services they need to address the issues underlying the parenting

capability concerns (particularly mental health, substance misuse and family violence);
- The changing social constructions of children and community expectations;
- Instability in care (frequent placement breakdowns resulting in children having multiple carers throughout their childhood);
- The complex link between domestic and family violence and child protection, and the risk of 'mother blaming' in child protection responses to situations of family violence;
- Addressing both maltreatment that has occurred, and concerns about future;
- Overrepresentation of Indigenous/Aboriginal children—particularly in countries with a colonial history like Australia, New Zealand and Canada;
- A far stronger role and involvement for citizens in ground-up, community-based initiatives that mobilize informal helping networks and resources; and
- Integrated service systems and collaborative organizational approaches.

1.3.2 The Problems of Demand, and the Mismatch Between Incidence of Reported Maltreatment and Underlying Prevalence

One of the best sources of information on the size of the problem and the rise in demand for child protection services, is those countries where there are prevalence or incidence studies—however, they differ dramatically in their methodology, and whether they focus on prevalence of abuse per se, or of service involvement. Nevertheless, it is clear that despite rising notifications of suspected maltreatment that most maltreated children do not come to the attention of authorities. This provides a strong case for an expanded involvement of community members in prevention and support initiatives.

The Canadian Incidence Study of Reported Child Abuse and Neglect (CIS) examines the incidence of reported child maltreatment and the characteristics of the children and families investigated by child welfare authorities. In the most recent data released, 2008, there was an estimated 235,842 child-maltreatment-related investigations conducted in Canada (representing a rate of 39.16 investigations per 1000 children), but only 36% of the investigations were substantiated (14.19 investigations per 1000 children), and 22% of substantiated cases (an estimated 18,510 investigations) involved children of Aboriginal heritage.

In the USA, one data source is the National Incidence Study of Child Abuse and Neglect (NIS), which estimates the numbers of abused and neglected children in the United States who come to the attention of community professionals. The most recent NIS-4 was published in 2010 (Sedlak et al. 2010). Although there was an overall decrease in the incidence of maltreatment since the NIS–3 (1996), an estimated 1,256,600 children experienced maltreatment during the NIS–4 study year (2005–2006), with neglect the largest proportion (61%). In contrast, the other source of data, the National Child Abuse and Neglect Data System (NCANDS)—a voluntary annual collection of maltreatment data from child protective services agencies in each state—shows a rise of 9% in children who received a child protective services investigation response or alternative response from 2011 (3,081,000) to 2015 (3,358,000) and a 3.8% increase in those who were victims from 2011 (658,000) to 2015 (683,000). Again, the rise in referrals (where someone has safety/wellbeing concerns) is rising faster than the rate of actual victimization (US DHHS 2017).

According to the National Society for the Prevention of Cruelty to Children (NSPCC), in the UK, the number of children subject to child protection plans or on child protection registers increased from 50,565 in 2011/12 to 58,239 in 2015/16 (Bentley et al. 2017). Of particular concern, they estimated that in 2011 for every child on a child protection plan or register, another eight were experiencing maltreatment but not getting the support they need. Bilson and Martin's (2017) study found 1 in 5 children in England were referred before the age of five to Children's Services with 1 in 19 investigated.

During 2015–16 in Australia (AIHW 2017), 162,175 (30.2 per 1000) Australian children received child protection services (investigation, care and protection order, or living in an out-of-home care placement). Indigenous children were over-represented and were seven times as likely as non-Indigenous children to have received child protection services. The projection for the state of Victoria is that 1 in 4 children born in 2011 will be notified to the Child Protection Service by the time they end adolescence (Cummins et al. 2012). Similarly, as early as 2007, the NSW statutory child protection service predicted in its annual report that one in every five children in NSW would be reported to the Department at some point before age 18 (Department of Community Services 2007). The work of Bilson et al. (2015, 2017) in Western Australia shows higher rates for children's notification to child protection authorities, with truly alarming rates for Aboriginal children.

Herrenkohl et al. (2016) noted that the pattern of rising notifications is highly concerning, as it is likely to "surpass all reasonable case load expectations and budgetary affordances" (p. 363); but this problem may be its own saviour, providing the economic rationale for moving to a system that more strongly emphases prevention and addressing the known risk factors for child maltreatment is the inevitable solution.

Despite the massive growth in demand for statutory child protection services in the past 2–3 decades, there is still a disconnection between the level of concerns that come to the attention of statutory authorities, and what population surveys show about the risks. Ironically, services that were established to deal with severe cases of physical abuse and sexual abuse, where sexual abuse is now the smallest proportion of harm types—so not only is the system potentially not fit for purpose for those cases of sexual abuse that do come to its attention. However, it is not sensitive enough, given that sexual abuse is the most frequent type of harm that young adults report. For example, research using retrospective self-report show around 20% of females and 5–10% of males recall an experience of childhood sexual abuse (Finkelhor et al. 2014) whereas in the US National Incidence Study 4 incidence was estimated at 1.8 children per 1000, capturing a much smaller percentage than retrospective reports of adults would suggest.

The rise in demand for child protection services—most notably in countries with a 'statutory child protection' rather than a family support orientation to their system—needs to be analyzed from a systems perspective (Bromfield et al. 2014; Munro 2011). Tertiary systems (focused around detection, investigation and child removal) were established to respond to low incidence, serious risks to children—from severe physical abuse, such as multiple fractures and bleeding on the brain. But over decades (and often resulting from inquiries into failures of the system), the scope of what constitutes child abuse and neglect has substantially broadened, expanded notions of risk, and lowering the threshold for statutory intervention. For example, exposure to domestic violence—often coded as 'psychological abuse' and neglect, are now the most frequent harm types that statutory systems have to deal with. This has happened at the same time as (and perhaps due to) changing societal understandings of parenting. Given these changes and system outcomes it appears legitimate to challenge the logic behind the widespread application of forensic investigation as the primary 'service' for identifying and preventing child abuse and neglect.

The broadened scope of child protection services has been gradual, and occurred without a fundamental reappraisal of the assumptions on which child protection services were established (Bromfield et al. 2014). The failure to fundamentally rethink the approach to child protection would be analogous to the health sector having continued to rely on intrusive and expensive hospital treatment as its primary response to smoking—despite the accumulating discoveries of smoking-related diseases. Learning from community-level interventions in the field of injury prevention is likely to assist (Scott et al. 2016a). Development of an evidence base around successful models is critical, though difficult. However, this has to be balanced with the need for jurisdictions to determine the framework and programs that address its own particular social, cultural, economic, political and institutional context.

Public health interventions need to focus on equipping universal services to work with families to prevent known risks for child maltreatment emerging and to be alert for, and able to address, the safety needs of children. These interventions can include:

- Broad availability of evidence-based parenting programs and supports (not just to high-risk families already known to child protection services), and with a range of intensity and back-up supports for parents who may need it (see: https://aifs.gov.au/cfca/expert-panel-project/research-evaluation-and-expert-panel-project-resources#choosing_delivering);
- Public information campaigns to promote information about positive parenting practices, and where to go for further information and supports—though further evaluation is needed of what constitutes an effective campaign (Horsfall et al. 2010); and
- Targeted referrals for intensive family support for those where more support is needed (i.e., progressive universalism).

1.4 Conclusions: The Public Health Approach as the Way Forward

Speaking of the Australian context—though of course there are parallels in many developed countries—Scott (2015) noted:

> The history of child welfare is paved with the pain of children and parents; the Stolen Generations, the Forgotten Australians, the British child migrants, and those affected by forced adoption policies. Why is it always a generation later that we begin to hear of that? Perhaps placement instability is the greatest harm to which children are currently being exposed (p. 17).

In her critique of the system, Scott (2015) identified the central element of the public health approach—population-level interventions—as the key to solving the problem of an overwhelmed system unable to respond to the complex problems of families coming to the attention of statutory authorities:

> Complex social problems cannot be solved solely by services or the reconfiguration of service systems. They require population-based measures that tackle the key risk and protective factors associated with child and family wellbeing. The common risk factors and the common protective factors cut across a range of problems, from low birth weight to school failure, to child abuse and neglect, to juvenile crime (p. 20).

In noting the need for and the shift towards provision of prevention-focused family support, Tomison (2001) argued that the future of child protection in many ways would look similar to the past—with many of the current approaches having been tried a number of times over the last 150 years and look likely to be re-applied in the next few decades:

> Should the preventative approach prove successful, there is likely to be a gradual shift away from the government-run child protection response. Much like the ideal system proposed by proponents of the current "family support" child protection models, only a small number of families—families that health surveillance, early intervention and family support services are unable to help—will receive the statutory child protection response. In many ways such a system could look much like it did before the rise of statutory child protection agencies in the 1970s. Such a utopian system may also lead to greater attention being placed on addressing the structural forces impacting on families (p. 56).

Tomison's (2001) forecast has proved correct in terms of widespread acknowledgement of the need for prevention. However, his ideal of a 'smaller, leaner' statutory service has not yet been realized. As mentioned earlier, the continued rise in notifications to statutory services and their lack of capacity to respond effectively is one of the greatest challenges and criticizms of the status quo. We argue that this is because the reform agenda has largely been placed in the hands of those running the statutory service, rather than finding effective mechanisms to share responsibility for those running primary care, universal services that have the capacity to engage all families and truly embed child abuse prevention efforts across a range of portfolio areas. In this book, we outline not only the 'why' but also the steps that are needed for moving responsibility for child protection out of the statutory service system, and into the community, addressing the 'structural forces impacting on families', supported by whole-of-government thinking and responsibility.

According to a public health model, primary, secondary and tertiary services are all critical elements in the child welfare and protection system. However, a well-balanced system has primary services as the largest component of the service system, with secondary and tertiary services comprising progressively smaller components of the service system. The greatest investment should be in primary prevention services, as they reach the largest number of families and have the greatest likelihood of preventing progression along the service continuum and sparing children and families from the harmful consequences of abuse and neglect.

If successfully implemented, primary prevention services will shift the "risk profile" positively for the entire community, meaning that fewer children and families will need more intensive secondary or tertiary services. "Progressive universalism" refers to having the capacity within a universal service delivery platform (such as a school) to ramp up the intensity or nature of services to meet the needs of those for whom a standard service is not enough (e.g., a school-based hub where family support workers and other professionals using evidence-based programs to equip parents with better parenting skills, or address their vulnerabilities, such as substance misuse or mental illness). Further detail on the public health approach, are provided in Part II.

As argued by Higgins and Katz (2008):

> It is not sufficient to simply 'bolt on' preventive programs to the current child protection processes. Rather it is important to completely rethink the role and function of the child protection system within the wider range of policies and programs aimed at promoting the wellbeing of children (p. 43).

In Part II of this book, the authors of the various chapters provide an outline of how public health approaches to prevention of child abuse can be conceptualized and implemented. While many public health advocates focus on the most prevalent forms of harm driving statutory responses (i.e., neglect, emotional abuse, and exposure to family violence), given the mismatch between low rates of sexual abuse reported to statutory authorities and the frequency with which population surveys identify sexual victimization, we also need to consider the unique responses that are needed for preventing child sexual abuse at a population level (see Chap. 10 in this volume) and safeguarding children in all youth-serving organizations and community settings (see Chap. 11 in this volume). Policy and program limitations and incongruences are identified and critiqued in Chap. 14.

Achieving a reduction in contact with statutory child protection systems for any child will only occur if the characteristics of children's environments associated with maltreatment (i.e., structural determinants, such as poverty and housing; parenting skills, and factors that affect parents' capacity such as poorly treated mental health, substance misuse and family/community violence) are systematically addressed at the population level. However, as will be examined in Part III, the implementation and operationalization of an integrated public health system to prevent child maltreatment is replete with challenges and difficulties, particularly concerning inter-organizational communication collaboration. Nevertheless, significant advances are being made and in Part III initiatives across a number of countries are examined. What is apparent is that broad scale system reforms are a "slow train coming" in many jurisdictions but that there are emerging signs of their successes on a number of fronts. In Part IV a looking forward occurs with regard to trends and desirable directions, such as embedding children's rights, attending to the structural issues underpinning much maltreatment, and developing organizational and community-based initiatives within social, political and policy environments that appear to be increasingly adopting nationalist/populist orientations.

A public health approach emphasizes promotion of safe and caring environments for all children, rather than concentrating on high-risk situations, whereas child protection is driven by ideologies that focus on parental and community failures and largely ignore systemic associations with poverty and social marginalization. This requires a shift in focus to prevention activities, and where they can best be deployed, and who has responsibility for this deployment. Protecting children is not just the work of statutory services: It is part of everyone's business who works and is engaged with children and their families (Higgins 2015). In this book, we explain how equipping and supporting child abuse prevention activities through existing service delivery mechanisms where families are already engaged—including perinatal and early childhood, health and education services. The public health approach can improve outcomes for children and families—both those involved in the child protection system and those at risk of involvement in those systems. In doing so we argue that such approaches are likely to result in a less punitive and stigmatizing protective system which is more social and fiscally sustainable than merely relying upon contemporary approaches to child protection.

References

AIHW. (2017). *Child protection Australia 2015–16.* Canberra: Australian Institute of Health and Welfare (AIHW). Retrieved from https://www.aihw.gov.au/reports/child-protection/child-protection-australia-2015-16/report-editions

Australian Government Productivity Commission. (2017). *Report on Government Services 2017.* Canberra: Author. Retrieved from http://www.pc.gov.au/research/ongoing/report-on-government-services/2017

Bentley, H., O'Hagan, O., Brown, A., Vasco, N., Lynch, C., Peppiate, J., Webber, M., Ball, R., Miller, P., Byrne, A., Hafizi, M., & Letendrie, F. (2017). *How safe are our children? The most comprehensive overview of child protection in the UK 2017.* London: National Society for the Prevention of Cruelty to Children. Retrieved from: https://www.nspcc.org.uk/globalassets/documents/research-reports/how-safe-children-2017-report.pdf

Bilson, A., & Martin, K. (2017). Referrals and child protection in England: One in five children referred to Children's Services and one in nineteen investigated before the age of five. *The British Journal of Social Work, 47*(3), 793–811. https://doi.org/10.1093/bjsw/bcw054.

Bilson, A., Cant, R., Harries, M., & Thorpe, D. (2015). A longitudinal study of children reported to the child protection department in western Australia. *British Journal of Social Work, 45*(3), 771–791.

Bilson, A., Cant, R., Harries, M., & Thorpe, D. (2017). Accounting for the increase of children in care in Western Australia: What can a client information system tell us? *Child Abuse and Neglect, 72*, 291–300.

Bromfield, L. M., & Higgins, D. J. (2005). Chronic and isolated maltreatment in a child protection sample. *Family Matters, 70,* 38–45. Retrieved from https://aifs.gov.au/publications/family-matters/issue-70/chronic-and-isolated-maltreatment-child-protection-sample

Bromfield, L. M. & Miller, R. (2012). *Cumulative harm: Best interests case practice model specialist practice resource*. Melbourne: Victorian Government Department of Human Services in collaboration with the Australian Institute of Family Studies. Retrieved from http://www.cpmanual.vic.gov.au/our-approach/best-interests-case-practice-model/cumulative-harm

Bromfield, L. M., Gillingham, P., & Higgins, D. J. (2007). Cumulative harm and chronic child maltreatment. *Developing Practice: The Child, Youth and Family Work Journal, 19*, 34–42.

Bromfield, L., Arney, F., & Higgins, D. (2014). Contemporary issues in child protection intake, referral and family support. In A. Hayes, & D. Higgins (Eds.), *Families, policy and the law: Selected essays on contemporary issues for Australia* (pp. 121–129). Melbourne: Australian Institute of Family Studies. Retrieved from https://aifs.gov.au/publications/families-policy-and-law/13-contemporary-issues-child-protection-intake-referral-and

Cameron, G., & Freymond, N. (2006). Understanding international comparisons of child protection, family service and community caring systems of child and family welfare. In N. Freymond & G. Cameron (Eds.), *Towards positive systems of child and family welfare: International comparisons of child protection, family service, and community caring systems* (pp. 3–27). Toronto: University of Toronto Press.

Campbell, K. A., Cook, L. J., LaFleur, B. J., & Keenan, H. T. (2010). Household, family, and child risk factors after an investigation for suspected child maltreatment: A missed opportunity for prevention. *Archives of Pediatrics & Adolescent Medicine, 164*(10), 943–949. https://doi.org/10.1001/archpediatrics.2010.166.

Cummins, P., Scott, D., & Scales, B. (2012). *Report of the protecting Victoria's vulnerable children inquiry*. Melbourne: Department of Premier and Cabinet.

NSW Department of Community Services. (2007). *Annual Report 2006/07*. Ashfield, NSW: Author. Available at: http://www.community.nsw.gov.au/DOCSwr/_assets/annual_report07/documents/annual_report06_07.pdf.

Finkelhor, D., Shattuck, A., Turner, H., & Hamby, S. (2014). Trends in children's exposure to violence, 2003–2011. *JAMA Pediatrics, 168*(6), 540–546. https://doi.org/10.1001/jamapediatrics.2013.5296.

Fluke, J. D., Shusterman, G. R., Hollinshead, D. M., & Yuan, Y. T. (2008). Longitudinal analysis of repeated child abuse reporting and victimization: Multistate analysis of associated factors. *Child Maltreatment, 13*(1), 76–88. https://doi.org/10.1177/1077559507311517.

Herrenkohl, T. I., Higgins, D. J., Merrick, M. T., & Leeb, R. T. (2015). Positioning a public health framework at the intersection of child maltreatment and intimate partner violence. *Child Abuse & Neglect [Directions], 48*, 22–28.. Retrieved from. https://doi.org/10.1016/j.chiabu.2015.04.013.

Herrenkohl, T. I., Leeb, R. L., & Higgins, D. (2016). The public health model of child maltreatment prevention. *Trauma, Violence, and Abuse, 17*(4), 363–336.

Higgins, D. J. (2011). Protecting children: Evolving systems. *Family Matters, 89*, 5–10. Retrieved from http://www.aifs.gov.au/institute/pubs/fm2011/fm89/index.html.

Higgins, D. J. (2015). A public health approach to enhancing safe and supportive family environments for children. *Family Matters, 96*, 39–52. Retrieved from https://aifs.gov.au/publications/family-matters/issue-96/public-health-approach-enhancing-safe-and-supportive-family-environments-children.

Higgins, D., & Katz, I. (2008). Enhancing service systems for protecting children: Promoting child wellbeing and child protection reform in Australia. *Family Matters, 80*, 43–50. Available at: https://aifs.gov.au/publications/familymatters/issue-80/enhancing-service-systems-protecting-children.

Horsfall, B., Bromfield, L., & McDonald, M. (2010). *Are social marketing campaigns effective in preventing child abuse and neglect?* (NCPC Issues No. 32). Melbourne: National Child Protection Clearinghouse, Australian Institute of Family Studies. Retrieved from https://aifs.gov.au/cfca/publications/are-social-marketing-campaigns-effective-preventing-child

Krugman, R. D. (2017). The more we learn, the less we know: A brief history of the field of child abuse and neglect. In J. B. Klika & J. R. Conte (Eds.), *The APSAC handbook on child maltreatment* (4th ed.). Thousand Oaks: Sage.

Lonne, B. (2015). Mandatory reporting and the difficulties in identifying and responding to risk of severe neglect: A response requiring a rethink. In B. Mathews & D. Bross (Eds.), *Mandatory reporting laws and the identification of severe child abuse and neglect* (pp. 245–273). New York: Springer.

Lonne, B., & Parton, N. (2014). Portrayals of child abuse scandals in the media in Australia and England: Impacts on practice, policy and systems. *Child Abuse & Neglect, 38*, 822–836. https://doi.org/10.1016/j.chiabu.2014.04.020.

Lonne, B., Parton, N., Thomson, J., & Harries, M. (2009). *Reforming child protection*. London: Routledge.

Melton, G. B. (2005). Mandated reporting: a policy without reason. *Child Abuse & Neglect, 29*(1), 9–18.

Munro, E., (2011). *Munro review of child protection: Final report – A child-centred system*. UK Department for Education. Retrieved from https://www.gov.uk/government/publications/munro-review-of-child-protection-final-report-a-child-centred-system

Price-Robertson, R., Higgins, D., & Vassallo, S. (2013). Multi-type maltreatment and polyvictimisation: A comparison of two research frameworks. *Family Matters, 93*, 84–98. Retrieved from www.aifs.gov.au/institute/pubs/fm2013/fm93/fm93h.html.

Price-Robertson, R., Bromfield, L., & Lamont, A. (2014). *International approaches to child protection: What can Australia learn?* (CFCA Paper no. 23). Melbourne: Australian Institute of Family. *Studies.*. Retrieved from https://aifs.gov.au/cfca/publications/international-approaches-child-protection.

Scott, D. (2015). Children in Australia: Harms and hopes. *Family Matters, 96*, 14–22. Retrieved from https://aifs.gov.au/publications/family-matters/issue-96/children-australia.

Scott, D. A., Lonne, B., & Higgins, D. (2016a). Public health models for preventing child maltreatment: Applications from the field of injury prevention. *Trauma Violence & Abuse [Special Edition on Public Health Approaches to Child Maltreatment Prevention], 17*(4), 408–419. https://doi.org/10.1177/1524838016658877.

Scott, D., Rushton, S., Fong, M., & Higgins, D. (2016b). *Cradle to Kinder: Evaluation of early implementation findings from the Victorian Cradle to Kinder Program 2013–15*. A report to the Victorian Department of Health and Human Services. Melbourne: Australian Institute of Family Studies. Summary report available [click on "Related Resources"]: Retrieved from http://providers.dhhs.vic.gov.au/family-and-parenting-support

Sedlak, A. J., Mettenburg, J., Basena, M., Petta, I., McPherson, K., Greene, A., & Li, S. (2010). *Fourth national incidence study of child abuse and neglect (NIS–4): Report to congress, executive summary*. Washington, DC: US Department of Health and Human Services, Administration for Children and Families. Retrieved from https://www.acf.hhs.gov/sites/default/files/opre/nis4_report_exec_summ_pdf_jan2010.pdf

SPERU (Social Policy Evaluation and Research Unit). (2016). *Modernising Child Protection in New Zealand: Learning from system reforms in other jurisdictions*. Wellington: SPERU.

Tomison, A. (2001). A history of child protection: Back to the future? *Family Matters, 60*, 47–57. Retrieved from https://aifs.gov.au/publications/family-matters/issue-60/history-child-protection.

US Department of Health and Human Services (US DHHS). (2009). *Child maltreatment 2007*. Washington, DC: US Government Printing Office, Administration of Children, Youth and Families.

US Department of Health and Human Services (US DHHS). (2017). *Child maltreatment 2015*. Washington, DC: US Department of Health and Human Services, Administration for Children and Families. Retrieved from http://www.acf.hhs.gov/programs/cb/research-data-technology/statistics-research/child-maltreatment.

Chapter 2
Stakeholder's Experiences of the Forensic Child Protection Paradigm

Helen Buckley, Morag McArthur, Tim Moore, Erica Russ, and Tania Withington

2.1 Introduction

Research over the past two decades has identified the perceptions of service users, mainly parents, engaged with the child protection system (Buckley 2017; Buckley et al. 2011a; De Boer and Coady 2007). This chapter extends this understanding to consider the experiences within the prevailing child protection discourse of all key stakeholders including families, children, foster carers and child protection practitioners. It will demonstrate that despite an overall positive aspiration to promote the welfare of children, the current approach fails to respond to the diverse needs and difficulties of the population and inadvertently alienates many of those who need assistance to prevent further escalation of their difficulties.

The first part of the chapter outlines the type of system required to promote children's safety and well-being and demonstrates the conflicting values underpin-

H. Buckley (✉)
School of Social Work and Social Policy, Trinity College Dublin, Dublin, Ireland
e-mail: hbuckley@tcd.ie

M. McArthur
Institute of Child Protection Studies, Australian Catholic University, Canberra, ACT, Australia
e-mail: morag.mcarthur@acu.edu.au

T. Moore
Australian Centre for Child Protection, University of South Australia, Adelaide, SA, Australia
e-mail: tim.moore@unisa.edu.au

E. Russ
School of Health, University of New England, Armidale, NSW, Australia
e-mail: eruss@une.edu.au

T. Withington
Children's Health Queensland, Hospital and Health Service, Child and Youth Mental Health Service, Queensland Health, Brisbane, QLD, Australia

B. Lonne et al. (eds.), *Re-Visioning Public Health Approaches for Protecting Children*, Child Maltreatment 9, https://doi.org/10.1007/978-3-030-05858-6_2

ning child protection processes that operate in most of the English speaking world. It then examines the way that children and young people experience services that are set up to help them, and their ideal view of how child protection would work best for them. Children that live in care are exceptionally dependent on the quality of social care and social work. Therefore, we examine the interface between current child protection practice and the out-of-home care (OOHC) system, exploring ideas about how the quality of care can be enhanced within a different policy framework.

Without question, a relationship-based approach is key to effective practice and the achievement of this is dependent on a stable and positively disposed workforce that can work collaboratively to gain trust and motivate families in the interests of their children's welfare. In Anglophone countries, the adversarial nature of statutory child care, highlighted by court processes, is known to challenge the ability of child protection staff to operate according to the principles of their profession, hence the high rate of disillusionment and turnover in statutory social work in particular. The chapter concludes by considering the aspects of the current system that are the most detrimental to good practice and by outlining how a public health model would, by addressing each of the domains discussed here, better meet the needs of children and families.

2.2 Child Protection Systems and Their Impact on Key Stakeholders

Child protection is widely recognised as a complex area of practice in the world of human services. As our knowledge about the needs of children and families has developed, our understanding about the key elements of a well-functioning system has also started to take shape. Bronfenbrenner's (1979) well used ecological systems model provides a useful framework to illustrate the intersecting layers that comprise the world of children and families, and it can be applied to the development of a child protection orientation that fits with what we have learned over the decades.

We know from research that children's well-being depends on their physical, emotional and psychological health, their caregiver's physical and mental health, and intellectual capacity to care for them, unfettered by factors such as addiction or poverty. We are also aware that many parents suffer multiple disadvantages that seriously impact on their ability to care adequately for their children. Services are required to support families and children in the short or long term, and possibly with alternative forms of care, and should be delivered by a well-resourced, coordinated workforce in a manner that facilitates empowerment and partnership, not dependency and fear. The services sector requires support by a community that promotes cohesion, collective responsibility and healthy development, within a society that prioritises equality, addresses economic stress, promotes well-being and embeds cultural norms that are inclusive and protective of children. This model aligns with a public health approach, where problems are identified at a societal level, risk factors are identified at societal and community levels, and interventions are proportionately made by community and statutory services. However, as this chapter will demonstrate, these elements are relatively easy to identify, but can be very complex to implement in a system where variables include contradictory political approaches and are often determined by influences that are quite remote from the issues that need to be resolved.

The nature of child maltreatment and children's problems tends to present differently within our more recent perspectives. While 25 years ago, the most prevalent types of child harm coming to the attention of child protection agencies were physical and sexual abuse (Gibbons et al. 1995; Thorpe 1994), more recently reports are primarily about neglect and emotional abuse, connected with family issues such as deficient parenting skills, an inability to manage children's behaviour and interpersonal conflict particularly domestic violence (Doidge et al. 2017; Hood et al. 2016a). These often chronic difficulties are connected with a range of social, health and structural factors such as substance abuse, family violence, intellectual disability, mental illness, homelessness and deprivation. The increasing visibility of these trends has demonstrated the need for an approach that is informed, therapeutic and ecological in its orientation (Lonne 2013).

Critics of the current system have called for a rebalancing of services towards the prevention of child maltreatment through building stronger communities (Melton 2014), increasing access to early childhood and other support services especially for vulnerable families who experience a range of problems (Lonne et al. 2009; Winkworth and McArthur 2007) and when families do come to the attention of the child protection system more responsive and participatory approaches to decision making such as Family Group Conferencing (Bijleveld et al. 2015; Connolly and Masson 2014). Government departments have not been indifferent to calls for reform and have taken the evidence of the dysfunctionality of the system seriously.

Initiatives in the USA, Canada, Australia and New Zealand to develop differential responses (Healy et al. 2016), and in the UK and Ireland to refocus services towards early intervention and family support (Tusla 2017) represent attempts to provide more appropriate and accessible responses to the difficulties of children and their families. The notion of a public health approach gained particular currency during the early 2000s (Scott et al. 2010). Reflected in attempts to reform child protection systems, glimmers of public health approaches have been implemented which aim to shift efforts and thinking away from tertiary child protection (which respond to concerns about high-risk families) to a broader approach to protecting all children (Bromfield et al. 2014; Higgins and Katz 2008). However, as this chapter will show, the aspiration towards a public health approach is greatly challenged by a number of what might be described as interlinked forces. First, it will examine the way that children and young people experience services.

2.3 Children and Young People's Perceptions of the Child Protection System

Since the mid-1980s, researchers and policy-makers have stressed the importance of seeking children and young people's views about their experiences in the child protection system (Magnussen and Skivenes 2015; Matthews 2016; Thomas 2011). It has been argued that the more children and young people feel that their input influences outcomes, the more likely that they are to positively engage in their case planning, to feel confident and competent (Halsey et al. 2006), and to feel as though they are understood and important (Matthews 2016). Although progress has been made, children and young people are still considered the least powerful and influential stakeholders within the system and much needs to be done to respond to their needs and wishes (Bijleveld et al. 2015; Cossar et al. 2016; Leeson 2007).

Studies have consistently found that young people who have been in care often have poorer outcomes than children who have not been in care in relation to their health and well-being (Richardson and Joughin 2000), their education (Harker et al. 2003) and their future opportunities. They are more likely to fall pregnant (Harker et al. 2003) to offend and be engaged in the youth justice system (Morrison and Shepherd 2015; Pinto and Woolgar 2015; Schofield et al. 2015) and become homeless after transitioning from care (Morrison and Shepherd 2015). This is most pressing for those living in residential care (Moore et al. 2016). Although the outcomes are often poor, a growing number of studies have shown that with appropriate support young people in care can develop resilience and do well (Honey et al. 2011; Richardson and Joughin 2000). Young people have called for better services and supports that foster protective factors and meet their immediate and long-term needs (Richardson and Joughin 2000).

2.3.1 *How Children Experience the System*

Studies report a lack of understanding that children and young people have about why they entered the system, how long they will be in care and living away from their families, what decisions have been made about them and their families and what they can expect from those charged with the responsibility of supporting during their time in care (Dillon et al. 2016; Moore et al. 2016; Pinto and Woolgar 2015). Many expressed great confusion, dissatisfaction and anger when they are not provided with adequate information (Dillon et al. 2016; Pinto and Woolgar 2015):

> I was that angry that I wanted to hit someone … but I didn't. I just stayed in my room until I calmed down …there's nothing wrong with my family … and there was really no reason for them to get involved. Liam (Dillon et al. 2016, p. 75).

Studies have also stressed the difficulties they experience whilst in care, particularly as a result of the instability of placements (Moore et al. 2016). Some described a sense of rejection, perceiving themselves to be unwanted and lacking the trust or confidence to forge new relationships (Anglin 2014; Moss 2009). Research has highlighted the grief that children experience, while others relate the destructive behaviours to expressions of their broken attachments.

As research shows, while some children have tended to idealise their experiences prior to their placement in care, some have judged their current lives on an expectation that things should be better for them post-placement (Moore et al. 2016, 2017). They wanted to feel like they belong, that they are physically and emotionally safe, that they feel part of their communities and that they are 'looked after' (Wood and Selwyn 2017).

In a number of studies, children and young people have noted the pejorative way that being labelled a 'foster kid', a 'residential youth' or a 'looked after child' plays out and the lack of expectations that many in the child protection system have of them and their potential (Harker et al. 2003; Mannay et al. 2017). They have stressed the importance of being hopeful and optimistic about children in the system rather than assuming that because they are in care they will do poorly socially, academically and emotionally (Harker et al. 2003; Honey et al. 2011). Young people in one particular study stressed that the child protection system needs to be realistic but work with children and young people to have ideals and meet them. The impacts can be long-lasting and continue after young people leave care (Hyde et al. 2017).

2.3.2 What Children and Young People Want While in the System and Those Who Support Them

Overwhelmingly, children and young people have stressed the importance of having a trusted adult who supports them through their journey in the child protection system (Holtan 2008; Jobe and Gorin 2013; Munro 2001). Good workers are often described as those who are non-judgmental, good listeners, demonstrate warmth and empathy, who value and advocate for children, are respectful, reliable, and available and to whom children and young people can confide. Young people point out that having someone who believes in you and is optimistic about your future has also been valued (Cooley et al. 2015), as is having someone to protect from abuse and harm (Moore et al. 2016) These relationships are often compromised as a result of high staff turnover, competing caseloads and, increasingly, practices that are wary of fostering dependence between staff and clients (Featherstone and Evans 2004).

Children and young people have also stressed the importance of maintaining and enhancing relationships with siblings and birth families, and of providing families supports so that family restoration might be achieved (Featherstone and Evans 2004). Many recognised that this is not always possible but believe that considerable effort should still be invested (Aldgate and McIntosh 2006; Holtan 2008).

2.4 Experiences of Parents as Service Users in the Child Protection System

The children whose experiences were reported above are the sons and daughters of families whose situations had been the subject of intervention at an earlier stage. As research has shown, within the current paradigm, services were not always considered helpful. Child protection systems that are primarily focused on child abuse and neglect see parents investigated and children assessed as harmed or potentially harmed often resulting in intimidating actions supported by an adversarial children's court (Kojan and Lonne 2012). Ironically, despite ambitions to provide a user friendly, relationship based, suite of options for vulnerable families, services have become tightly regulated and heavily bureaucratised in ways that are alienating rather than attractive to service users either seeking assistance for finding themselves the subject of reports (Featherstone et al. 2012). Models of risk assessment are used to deal with escalating numbers of referrals which directs limited resources to those cases in which children are considered at high risk of harm, often because they come from families that are experiencing multiple problems.

Families experience these processes as frightening, intimidating and frustrating. In an Australian study, Harris (2012) demonstrated that the use of assessment frameworks which were designed to be child centred and participatory paradoxically made parents feel mistrusted, humiliated and coerced because of their emphasis on compliance. Although the majority of reports made to child protection systems concern family problems (rather than child maltreatment), services appear to be unable to deal with issues concerning interpersonal relationships, and the emotional impact on children of parental separation in violent or acrimonious circumstances, leaving parents anxious and discouraged (Buckley et al. 2011b). A recent UK study that explored the experiences of parents of the child protection system concluded it was "uncaring, inflexible and for some, harmful to both parents and their children" (Smithson and Gibson 2017, p. 565). All of the above studies reported that parents had some positive experiences, almost all aligned with the quality of the alliance they had formed with workers and the degree of trust achieved. Yet, as Featherstone et al. (2012) and others have pointed out, the type of systems that rely on standard business processes and auditable 'bytes' of work can undermine the possibilities for developing quality relationships.

Mandatory reporting laws in the US, Canada and Australia have seen a steady increase in reports which force child protection systems to apply extremely rigorous entry criteria. This gives rise to a 'revolving door' process whereby vast numbers are reported to the system and are quickly eliminated, in the meantime causing stress and confusion to families. Families seeking help are frustrated by the high thresholds used by services to filter out referrals considered not serious enough. As a mother who participated in an Irish study asserted "You'd need a knife in your child's back in order to get attention" (Buckley et al. 2011a, p 106). Paradoxically, new public service management with its emphasis on quality and accountability may have enhanced the ability of managers and policy makers to measure performance, but has bypassed the stakeholders whose needs it was set up to meet (Hood et al. 2016b).

2.5 Experiences of Foster Carers

Parents as service users include those who take over the care of children on behalf of the state. The impact of the conflictual culture of child protection is also experienced by foster carers. Multiple research projects have found that foster carers depend on quality relationships to maintain placements and to meet the challenges often encountered in looking after children subject to maltreatment (Oke et al. 2013; Withington et al. 2017). The characteristics that define quality relationships are difficult to audit within the current system, which relies on observable measureable evidence. Incongruently, while carers report child-focused outcomes including engagement in genuine relationships and healthy adult functioning as meaningful OOHC outcomes, child protection systems commonly measure success or failure by an individual child's stability in placement. Quality relationships are identified by carers as critical to OOHC placement success, including those with the child, child protection caseworker, child protection system and broader community.

These relationships do not exist in isolation from one another. The carer-child relationship must be supported by the carer-child protection caseworker or system relationship from the beginning of the placement for the best chance at success. Carers consistently report that successful placements require appropriate establishment processes, including preparation of the carer prior to a child being placed in their care, ensuring that the individual carer has the appropriate training to meet the identified child's needs, ensuring the carer is provided with enough information about the child to ensure the child and caring family will be a good fit, and an opportunity to ensure the carer and child are a good match in terms of expectations, personality and interactional style (Butler and Charles 1999; Gilbertson and Barber 2003). These processes are dependent upon practical, supportive and respectful relationships between carers and child protection workers and child protection policies promoting collaborative practice and carer autonomy in child-focused decision making.

Conversely, carers report a primary reason for placement disruption is poor quality relationships between a carer and the child protection worker or agency. A carer's perception that the child protection system is not supportive or responsive or is not providing information, support and resources required to support a placement, can undermine a placement as well as influence a carers willingness to remain in the OOHC system (Khoo and Skoog 2014; Withington et al. 2016). Carers report that placements are undermined by poor relationships with child protection workers, poor communication and a lack of shared information by the child protection worker, and ongoing conflictual relationships with foster care support agencies (Brown and Bednar 2006; Rostill-Brookes et al. 2011). Carers report that a lack of timely responsiveness to individual placement needs, and the exclusion of the carer from decision making about the child by child protection workers, contributes to OOHC placement disruption. Furthermore, where the relationship between carer and child protection worker was perceived as non-functional, carers report an inability to seek assistance for fear of being judged negatively by the case worker and broader child protection system (Rostill-Brookes et al. 2011; Withington et al. 2016).

Investing in building and supporting quality relationships between carers and child protection caseworkers or systems contributes to the likelihood of quality carer-child relationships, and ultimately a sustainable OOHC placement. The key components identified by carers as facilitating quality carer-child relationships include how well a child integrates into the carer family and how likeable the carer perceives the child to be (Leathers 2006; Sinclair and Wilson 2003). Carers report a higher level of commitment to the child and the OOHC placement, even in the face of adversity, where they felt the child was genuinely appreciative of the foster parent, the child perceived the carer as warm and loving, and the carer felt an emotional connection with the child (Butler and Charles 1999; Oke et al. 2013). Where a genuine carer-child relationship was identified, carers have reported themselves as persistent and loving towards the child even in the face of confronting harmful behaviours (Withington et al. 2016).

Carers also report a number of factors related to the carer-child relationship that can undermine an OOHC placement. A placement is at risk of disruption where: a carer is subject to ongoing verbal abuse and threats; the child is unable to comply with the rules and expectations of the care placement the child's behaviour places themselves or others in danger; and where the carer feels ill-prepared for the child's complex health or behavioural needs (Brown and Bednar 2006; Gilbertson and Barber 2003; Strijker et al. 2003). Further placement disruption risk is present where it is evident that the child does not want to be in the placement or is socially withdrawn (or the carer is less able to form a relationship). These challenges are exacerbated where a carer feels unsupported by child protection services, and is isolated from broader community support and resources.

The experience of carers in OOHC offers strong support to re-locating child protection services to a public health framework. This framework would create the opportunity to develop policy and practice across primary, secondary and tertiary level services with the ultimate goal of reducing negative social outcomes for all members of the community across the lifespan. Cross-service level child-focused outcomes at individual, family, community and systems could be used to develop and evaluate services enhancing likelihood of positive outcomes for all children with no distinction in expectations for children from maltreatment backgrounds. A public health framework would enable resource allocation to supports and services aiming to enhance healthy relationships across both continuums. For OOHC carers a public health framework would likely result in stronger connections, clearer expectations, and consistent communication between carers and the child protection system as well as clearly defined roles with common expectations between all key players in the system. Additionally, as carers sit at the tertiary level of care targeted services aiming to reduce the long-term impact of maltreatment on children would be readily available including services that value and support long-term placement and aim for children in OOHC to achieve at the same level as their broader community peers.

2.6 Practitioners' Experiences

As with children, families and carers, current approaches to child protection in systems in Anglophone countries affect workers and the workforce generally with forensic, adversarial, and managerialist approaches common. These systems are challenging contexts for workers, given high public expectations, workload pressures, along with risk-averse and blaming organisational cultures (Gillingham 2016; Lonne et al. 2013). A further challenge cited is the lack of social justice, and humane practice based on worker-client relationships (Featherstone et al. 2014).

Growing child protection demands, staffing shortages, and high turnover (Altman and Cohen 2016) alongside poor perceptions of child protection systems and practice, contribute to pressures on the workforce. Across these systems there is continued concern about the high rates of staff turnover, recruitment difficulties, and resultant costs (Griffiths et al. 2017). Staff turnover contributes to high proportions of inexperienced staff with limited support, and many workers leaving within months of commencing (Healy and Oltedal 2010; Lonne et al. 2013). These workforce issues have implications for service quality, client-worker relationships, and client outcomes.

Additionally, child protection workers face adversity through work stress, burnout, trauma, and vicarious trauma, with high rates of psychological dysfunction noted in multiple studies (Kim and Kao 2014). This adversity, and the resultant impact on workers, contributes to turnover (Lonne et al. 2013; Russ et al. 2009). Given the complex, emotionally charged, and adversarial nature of child protection work, stress and burnout are cited as common experiences adversely impacting staff (Sprang et al. 2011). Similarly, multiple or chronic experiences of trauma (e.g., threats, assaults and client deaths), and vicarious trauma (through observations, client disclosures, or case material), also adversely affect workers (Sprang et al. 2011). Even so, most staff manage this adversity effectively with many experiencing high levels of job satisfaction (Barth et al. 2008) .

The adversity and complexity experienced by workers impact on workforce turnover and clients. As indicated by Griffiths et al. (2017, p. 110), "turnover within the child welfare system threatens the ability to respond effectively". This threat involves gaps in service provision, and changes in the direction of case plans as workers change. Also noted, is the importance of the worker-client relationship in achieving intended objectives for children and families, and implications for clients of poor relationships (Featherstone et al. 2014; Ruch 2005). Each worker change requires a revisiting of relationship building, with a likely reduction in client trust particularly where issues that the client understands to have been addressed are revisited, or case goals and expectations of the client change. Workforce turnover impacts on worker-client relationships, contribute to inconsistent decision making and intervention, reduced service quality, and poorer client outcomes (Kim and Kao 2014). The personal costs to staff and clients, and systemic issues, suggest a significant impost of adversity on the effectiveness of the child protection system.

As Altman and Cohen (2016, p. 524) argued, "effective child protection requires retention of knowledgeable, competent and experienced workers". The retention of experienced workers enables the effective worker-client relationships that is required to achieve improved outcomes for children and families (Featherstone et al. 2014). Longer-term worker-client relationships allow workers to identify the progress and positive outcomes of clients that are likely to support a sense of efficacy, job satisfaction and thereby contribute to better understanding of and relationships with clients, and increased worker resilience. The benefits to clients of relationally-based practice and longer-term interventions, which rely on effective and experienced staff, have also been argued (Turney 2012). Where turnover is high, the ability to provide effective intervention is reduced (Kim and Kao 2014).

While the impacts of turnover are noted, there has been less attention to retention, which increases worker experience and longevity (Kim and Kao 2014). An increased focus on worker resilience and retention of experienced staff, may improve the capacity of the child protection workforce, thereby improving client outcomes. Focusing on the strengths and resilience of workers provides an alternative perspective to the predominant negative discourse, and encourages different approaches to staff support and retention (Collins 2017). In a study of experienced child protection workers, relationship-based and reflective practice was identified as contributing to their resilience, even where they faced significant adversity through their work (Russ 2016). These resilient workers had a high level of client and practice knowledge, consistently identified maintaining empathy, the worker-client relationship and commitment to positive client outcomes as important elements of their practice. An increased focus on resilience may enhance worker longevity, capacity and effectiveness, in this complex and adverse system, thereby reducing turnover and benefiting clients (Adamson et al. 2012; Russ 2016). Resilient workers are likely to benefit clients through consistency of case planning, longer-term interventions and an increased ability to maintain a strong commitment to empathetic practice and worker-client relationships critical to relationship-based practice. Relationship-based practice is in turn likely to increase worker satisfaction further contributing to resilience.

While enhancing worker resilience and strengthening relationship-based practice may contribute to improved workforce retention and client outcomes, this may be difficult to achieve in current systems. Alternative approaches that utilise relationship-based practice approaches, and recognise and build on the capacities and strengths of families and communities in the care of children, are also needed (Lonne 2013). Public health models that are aligned with socially just, humane, and ethical practice approaches, may be one such alternative.

2.7 Conclusions

This chapter has outlined the key issues inherent in current approaches to keeping children safe. All stakeholders in the system often report negative and coercive approaches inherent in the existing approach. As can be seen from the research reported above the interactions between child protection, families, carers and children themselves are often experienced as unhelpful. Furthermore, the restrictions imposed by the current service delivery models in the Anglophone world interact systemically; pressure in the frontline child protection services in terms of referral rates and administrative requirements leaves workers little time to focus on the essential component of their work, which is the developing of helping alliances with service users. The impact of this is experienced by foster carers and children, who can feel abandoned at times of stress; strain in foster care placements inevitably rebounds on children's experiences in a setting where measures of quality are unable to capture the uncertainties and insecurities that they feel. The circle is then squared when it comes to practitioner experience, where a combination of stress, disillusionment and a lack of confidence in the benefits of their interventions leads to a high turnover, thus adding to the instability of the system as a whole.

As Scott (2009) argued, tertiary child protection systems have screened huge numbers of referrals for child abuse and neglect to identify relatively small numbers of cases. Using a public health analogy she likened this to hospitals adding to their core function of acute care, the screening of large sections of the population for an ever increasing range of disease risk factors. The ever increasing number of children in state care is evidence, not of a system that is focused on preventing problems before they emerge, or intervening early to provide families with help they need but, rather, the state accelerating its use of formal regulatory powers, indeed its most extreme sanction – the removal of children. A public health approach that is informed by evidence, therapeutic and ecological in its orientation is an essential and urgent reform to increase children's safety and well-being.

References

Adamson, C., Beddoe, L., & Davys, A. (2012). Building resilient practitioners: Definitions and practitioner understandings. *British Journal of Social Work, 44*(3), 522–541.

Aldgate, J., & McIntosh, M. (2006). *Looking after the family: A study of children looked after in kinship care in Scotland.* Edinburgh: Social Work Inspection Agency Edinburgh.

Altman, J. C., & Cohen, C. S. (2016). "I could not have made it without them": Examining Trainee Cohort Perspectives on MSW Education for Public Child Welfare. *Journal of Public Child Welfare, 10*(5), 524–541.

Anglin, J. P. (2014). *Pain, normality, and the struggle for congruence: Reinterpreting residential care for children and youth.* London: Routledge.

Barth, R. P., Lloyd, E. C., Christ, S. L., Chapman, M. V., & Dickinson, N. S. (2008). Child welfare worker characteristics and job satisfaction: A national study. *Social Work, 53*(3), 199–209.

Bijleveld, G. G., Dedding, C. W., & Bunders-Aelen, J. F. (2015). Children's and young people's participation within child welfare and child protection services: A state-of-the-art review. *Child & Family Social Work, 20*(2), 129–138.

Bromfield, L., Arney, F., & Higgins, D. (2014). Child protection: Legal grounds for intervening in family life to ensure child safety. In A. Hayes & D. Higgins (Eds.), *Families, policy and the law: Selected essays on contemporary issues for Australia* (pp. 121–129). Melbourne: Australian Institute of Family Studies.

Bronfenbrenner, U. (1979). *The ecology of human development: Experiments by nature and design*. Cambridge MA: Harvard University Press.

Brown, J. D., & Bednar, L. M. (2006). Foster parent perceptions of placement breakdown. *Children and Youth Services Review, 28*(12), 1497–1511.

Buckley, H. (2017). In M. Connolly (Ed.),. *Beyond the risk paradigm in child protection Service users as receivers of risk-dominated practice*. London: Palgrave.

Buckley, H., Carr, N., & Whelan, S. (2011a). 'Like walking on eggshells': Service user views and expectations of the child protection system. *Child & Family Social Work, 16*(1), 101–110.

Buckley, H., Whelan, S., & Carr, N. (2011b). 'Like waking up in a Franz Kafka novel': Service users' experiences of the child protection system when domestic violence and acrimonious separations are involved. *Children and Youth Services Review, 33*(1), 126–133.

Butler, S., & Charles, M. (1999). The past, the present, but never the future': Thematic representations of fostering disruption. *Child and Family Social Work, 4*, 9–20.

Collins, S. (2017). Social workers and resilience revisited. *Practice, 29*(2), 85–105.

Connolly, M., & Masson, J. (2014). Private and public voices: Does family group conferencing privilege the voice of children and families in child welfare? *Journal of Social Welfare and Family Law, 36*(4), 403–414.

Cooley, M., Wojciak, A. S., Farineau, H., & Mullis, A. (2015). The association between perception of relationship with caregivers and behaviours of youth in foster care: A child and caregiver perspective. *Journal of Social Work Practice, 29*(2), 205–221.

Cossar, J., Brandon, M., & Jordan, P. (2016). 'You've got to trust her and she's got to trust you': Children's views on participation in the child protection system. *Child & Family Social Work, 21*(1), 103–112.

De Boer, C., & Coady, N. (2007). Good helping relationships in child welfare: Learning from stories of success. *Child & Family Social Work, 12*(1), 32–42.

Dillon, J., Greenop, D., & Hills, M. (2016). Participation in child protection: A small-scale qualitative study. *Qualitative Social Work, 15*(1), 70–85.

Doidge, J. C., Higgins, D. J., Delfabbro, P., Edwards, B., Vassallo, S., Toumbourou, J. W., & Segal, L. (2017). Economic predictors of child maltreatment in an Australian population-based birth cohort. *Children and Youth Services Review, 72*, 14–25.

Featherstone, B., & Evans, H. (2004). *Children experiencing maltreatment: Who do they turn to?* London: NSPCC.

Featherstone, B., White, S., & Wastell, D. (2012). Ireland's opportunity to learn from England's difficulties? Auditing uncertainty in child protection. *Irish Journal of Applied Social Studies, 12*(1), 5.

Featherstone, B., Morris, K., & White, S. (2014). *Re-imagining child protection: Towards humane social work with families*. Bristol: Policy Press.

Gibbons, J., Bell, C., & Conroy, S. (1995). *Operating the child protection system: A study of child protection practices in English local authorities*. London: HM Stationery Office.

Gilbertson, R., & Barber, J. (2003). Breakdown of foster care placement: Carer perspectives and system factors. *Australian Social Work, 56*(4), 329–339.

Gillingham, P. (2016). Social work and child protection in Australia: Whose job is it anyway? *Practice, 28*(2), 83–96.

Griffiths, A., Royse, D., Culver, K., Piescher, K., & Zhang, Y. (2017). Who stays, who goes, who knows? A state-wide survey of child welfare workers. *Children and Youth Services Review, 77*, 110–117.

Halsey, K., Murfield, J., Harland, J. L., & Lord, P. (2006). *The voice of young people: An engine for improvement? Scoping the evidence*. Reading: CfBT Education Trust.
Harker, R. M., Dobel-Ober, D., Lawrence, J., Berridge, D., & Sinclair, R. (2003). Who takes care of education? Looked after children's perceptions of support for educational progress. *Child & Family Social Work, 8*(2), 89–100.
Healy, K., & Oltedal, S. (2010). An institutional comparison of child protection systems in Australia and Norway focused on workforce retention. *Journal of Social Policy, 39*(2), 255–274.
Harris, P. L. (2012). Trusting what you're told: How children learn from others. Harvard University Press.
Healy, K., Harrison, G., Venables, J., & Bosly, F. (2016). Collaborating with families in differential responses: Practitioners' views. *Child & Family Social Work, 21*(3), 328–338.
Higgins, D., & Katz, I. (2008). Enhancing service systems for protecting children: Promoting child well-being and child protection reform in Australia. *Family Matters, 80*, 43–50.
Holtan, A. (2008). Family types and social integration in kinship foster care. *Children and Youth Services Review, 30*(9), 1022–1036.
Honey, K. L., Rees, P., & Griffey, S. (2011). Investigating self-perceptions and resilience in Looked After Children. *Educational Psychology in Practice, 27*(1), 37–52.
Hood, R., Goldacre, A., Grant, R., & Jones, R. (2016a). Exploring demand and provision in English child protection services. *The British Journal of Social Work, 46*(4), 923–941.
Hood, R., Grant, R., Jones, R., & Goldacre, A. (2016b). A study of performance indicators and Ofsted ratings in English child protection services. *Children and Youth Services Review, 67*, 50–56.
Hyde, A., Fullerton, D., Lohan, M., Dunne, L., & Macdonald, G. (2017). Young people's views on the impact of care experiences on their ability to form positive intimate relationships. *Adoption & Fostering, 41*(3), 242–253.
Jobe, A., & Gorin, S. (2013). 'If kids don't feel safe they don't do anything': Young people's views on seeking and receiving help from Children's Social Care Services in England. *Child & Family Social Work, 18*(4), 429–438.
Khoo, E., & Skoog, V. (2014). The road to placement breakdown: Foster parents' experiences of the events surrounding the unexpected ending of a child's placement in their care. *Qualitative Social Work, 13*(2), 255–269.
Kim, H., & Kao, D. (2014). A meta-analysis of turnover intention predictors among US child welfare workers. *Children and Youth Services Review, 47*, 214–223.
Kojan, B. H., & Lonne, B. (2012). A comparison of systems and outcomes for safeguarding children in Australia and Norway. *Child & Family Social Work, 17*(1), 96–107.
Leathers, S. J. (2006). Placement disruption and negative placement outcomes among adolescents in long-term foster care: The role of behavior problems. *Child Abuse & Neglect, 30*(3), 307–324.
Leeson, C. (2007). My life in care: Experiences of non-participation in decision-making processes. *Child & Family Social Work, 12*(3), 268–277.
Lonne, B. (2013). Reshaping our protective systems: Issues and options. *Communities, Children and Families Australia, 7*(1), 9–20.
Lonne, B., Parton, N., Thomson, J., & Harries, M. (2009). *Reforming child protection*. London: Routledge Taylor and Francis Group.
Lonne, B., Harries, M., & Lantz, S. (2013). Workforce development: A pathway to reforming child protection systems in Australia. *British Journal of Social Work, 43*(8), 1630–1648.
Magnussen, A.-M., & Skivenes, M. (2015). The child's opinion and position in care Order proceedings. *The International Journal of Children's Rights, 23*(4), 705–723.
Mannay, D., Evans, R., Staples, E., Hallett, S., Roberts, L., Rees, A., & Andrews, D. (2017). The consequences of being labelled 'looked-after': Exploring the educational experiences of looked-after children and young people in Wales. *British Educational Research Journal, 43*(4), 683–699.

Matthews, F. T. (2016). *What is important to looked-after young people during adolescence? A qualitatively driven photo-elicitation study*. Leeds: University of Leeds.
Melton, G. B. (2014). In J. Korbin & D. Krugman (Eds.),. Handbook of child maltreatment *Strong Communities for Children: A community-wide approach to prevention of child maltreatment* (pp. 329–339). New York: Springer.
Moore, T., McArthur, M., Death, J., Roche, S., & Tilbury, C. (2016). *Safe and sound: Exploring the safety of young people in residential care* (1925289990). Melbourne: Institute of Child Protection Studies, Australian Catholic University. Royal Commission into Institutional Responses to Child Sexual Abuse, Sydney. Retrieved from https://www.childabuseroyalcommission.gov.au/sites/default/files/file-list/Research%20Report%20-%20Safe%20and%20Sound%20Exploring%20the%20safety%20of%20young%20people%20in%20residential%20care%20-%20Causes.pdf
Moore, T., McArthur, M., Death, J., Tilbury, C., & Roche, S. (2017). Young people's views on safety and preventing abuse and harm in residential care:"It's got to be better than home". *Children and Youth Services Review, 81*, 212–219.
Morrison, R., & Shepherd, M. (2015). Exploring factors contributing to the outcomes of Looked After Children. *Communicare, 1*(2).
Moss, M. (2009). Broken circles to a different identity: An exploration of identity for children in out–of-home care in Queensland, Australia. *Child & Family Social Work, 14*(3), 311–321.
Munro, E. (2001). Empowering looked-after children. *Child and Family Social Work, 6*(2), 129–138.
Oke, N., Rostill-Brookes, H., & Larkin, M. (2013). Against the odds: Foster carers' perceptions of family, commitment and belonging in successful placements. *Clinical Child Psychology and Psychiatry, 18*(1), 7–24.
Pinto, C., & Woolgar, M. (2015). Looked-after children–a perspective into a more resilient future. *Child and Adolescent Mental Health, 20*(4), 181–181.
Richardson, J., & Joughin, C. (2000). *The mental health needs of looked after children*. London: RCPsych Publications.
Rostill-Brookes, H., Larkin, M., Toms, A., & Churchman, C. (2011). A shared experience of fragmentation: Making sense of foster placement breakdown. *Clinical Child Psychology and Psychiatry, 16*(1), 103–127.
Ruch, G. (2005). Relationship-based practice and reflective practice: Holistic approaches to contemporary child care social work. *Child & Family Social Work, 10*(2), 111–123.
Russ, E. (2016). *Witnessing resilience: Resilience of child protection workers in Queensland* (Unpublished doctoral dissertation). University of Queensland: Brisbane.
Russ, E., Lonne, B., & Darlington, Y. (2009). Using resilience to reconceptualise child protection workforce capacity. *Australian Social Work, 62*(3), 324–338.
Schofield, G., Biggart, L., Ward, E., & Larsson, B. (2015). Looked after children and offending: An exploration of risk, resilience and the role of social cognition. *Children and Youth Services Review, 51*, 125–133.
Scott, D. (2009). Regulatory principles and reforming possibilities in child protection: What might be in the best interests of children? *Communities. Children and Families Australia, 4*(1), 65.
Scott, D., Arney, F., & Vimpani, G. (2010). Think child, think family, think community. In F. Arney & D. Scott (Eds.), *Working with vulnerable families* (pp. 7–33). New York: Cambridge University Press.
Sinclair, I., & Wilson, K. (2003). Matches and mismatches: The contribution of carers and children to the success of foster placements. *British Journal of Social Work, 33*(7), 871–884.
Smithson, R., & Gibson, M. (2017). Less than human: A qualitative study into the experience of parents involved in the child protection system. *Child & Family Social Work, 22*(2), 565–574.
Sprang, G., Craig, C., & Clark, J. (2011). Secondary traumatic stress and burnout in child welfare workers: A comparative analysis of occupational distress across professional groups. *Child Welfare, 90*(6), 149–168.

Strijker, J., Zandberg, T., & van der Meulen, B. F. (2003). Kinship foster care and foster care in the Netherlands. *Children and Youth Services Review, 25*(11), 843–862. https://doi.org/10.1016/S0190-7409(03)00089-6.

Thomas, N. (2011). Care planning and review for looked after children: Fifteen years of slow progress? *The British Journal of Social Work, 41*(2), 387–398.

Thorpe, D. H. (1994). *Evaluating child protection*. Buckingham: Open University Press.

Turney, D. (2012). A relationship-based approach to engaging involuntary clients: The contribution of recognition theory. *Child & Family Social Work, 17*(2), 149–159.

Tusla Child and Family Agency [Ireland]. (2017). *The Prevention, Partnership and Family Support Programme: Collaborative leadership for better outcomes*. Retrieved from http://www.tusla.ie/uploads/content/PPFS_Low_Prevention_Services_Brochure.pdf

Winkworth, G., & McArthur, M. (2007). Developing communities of support for vulnerable children: Shifting the focus from risk. *Communities, Children and Families Australia, 3*(2), 44–54.

Withington, T., Burton, J., Lonne, B., & Eviers, A. (2016). Carer perspectives of factors affecting placement trajectories of children in out-of-home care. *Children and Youth Services Review, 65*, 42–50.

Withington, T., Duplock, R., Burton, J., Eivers, A., & Lonne, B. (2017). Exploring children's perspectives of engagement with their carers using factor analysis. *Child Abuse & Neglect, 63*, 41–50.

Wood, M., & Selwyn, J. (2017). Looked after children and young people's views on what matters to their subjective well-being. *Adoption & Fostering, 41*(1), 20–34.

Chapter 3
Assessing the Outcomes of Alternative Care and Treatment Responses

Amy Conley Wright and Melissa Kaltner

3.1 Introduction

Child protection as a function of the state is premised on a moral or ethical reason for government intervention (Kraft and Furlong 2012). Societal norms and legal protections give children's parent(s) the responsibilities and rights to care for them, and expect a minimum standard of parenting. This minimum standard is a line between acceptable parenting and abusive parenting, when parenting behaviours are considered as constituting or presenting a threat of child maltreatment (Wald 2014). If child maltreatment is suspected, a child protection intervention can be instigated, informally by extended family and community, or formally by government authorities. The outcomes sought through child protection interventions are essentially the same end values intrinsically valued by society for all children: safety, continuity, stability, permanency, and well-being (Testa 2010). However, the ability to achieve these outcomes through statutory interventions, particularly well-being, is highly dubious. Children in out-of-home care placements typically have poorer behavioural, educational and psychological functioning compared to other children, though it is not clear whether this is due to the maltreatment they may have experienced, the alternative placement intervention, or inadequacies of the child welfare system (Winokur et al. 2014).

Under the statutory intervention to child maltreatment characteristic of countries such as the USA, Australia, Canada, and the UK, removal to alternative care is the

A. C. Wright (✉)
Social Work and Institute of Open Adoption Studies, University of Sydney, Sydney, NSW, Australia
e-mail: amy.conleywright@sydney.edu.au

M. Kaltner
Department of Family and Community Services, Sydney, NSW, Australia
e-mail: Melissa.Kaltner@facs.nsw.gov.au

B. Lonne et al. (eds.), *Re-Visioning Public Health Approaches for Protecting Children*, Child Maltreatment 9, https://doi.org/10.1007/978-3-030-05858-6_3

primary treatment for children who are found by the court to be at unacceptable risk of maltreatment. Treatment responses are highly individualistic in nature, with significant resources expended in investigation of allegations to determine what happened with a specific child, and court action to determine alternative placement. Placement in alternative care is expected to address immediate safety concerns by putting a child in the care of a kinship or foster carer, or residential facility that has been assessed as capable of providing safe care. However, child removal as a form of treatment creates potential for iatrogenic harm to social and emotional well-being by disrupting the continuity of the parent-child relationship.

If a court deems that birth parents are unable to sufficiently mitigate risk conditions that predicated removal, their children will remain in long-term kinship or foster care, or in another permanency arrangement that confers parental responsibilities, such as guardianship or adoption. In making permanency decisions, continuity of relationships (with birth parents and kin) can be in tension with permanency and stability when considering alternative placements such as adoption. In short, child protection outcomes can be in competition with each other and child protection interventions can undermine the very goals they are meant to achieve. Moreover, there is unavoidable bias in the instigation of child protection investigation and allocation of interventions that makes it impossible to tease out the contributions of pre-existing factors versus interventions on child outcomes.

This chapter discusses research approaches used in child welfare and considers the particular challenges of assessing the causal impacts of alternative care. A public health approach to child maltreatment has promise for addressing some of the challenges facing statutory child protection systems. In particular, public health approaches coupled with technological advances in big data and political rhetoric favouring social investment suggest that the future is likely to hold more systematic efforts at monitoring population-level risk factors and outcomes associated with maltreatment as well as measuring the return on investment related to child welfare interventions.

3.2 Understanding Causal Impacts of Interventions on Outcomes in Child Welfare

Assessing the outcomes of alternative care and treatment in child welfare means asking the question 'What works best for whom in child welfare?' (Littell 2008, p. 66). What we want to know is the causal model, an estimate of the average effect of an intervention on outcomes (Testa 2010). The short answer is that given the current state of research, *we don't know the outcomes associated with alternative care and treatment in child welfare.* This section looks at research approaches to estimate causal impacts of interventions on outcomes and elaborates on why it is that we don't know the outcomes associated with statutory child protection interventions.

The accepted scientific approach to estimating causal effects of interventions on outcomes is a research review that synthesizes multiple studies. It is not enough to look at a single study, no matter how well designed, as any given study will have limitations in terms of utility and generalizability. To answer what works best for whom in broad terms requires careful synthesis of multiple studies to achieve the best possible estimates of program impacts and assessment of the conditions under which treatment effects may vary (Littell 2008). A research review can draw tentative conclusions about questions of *program efficacy* (e.g., Is there evidence for a genuine causal impact on outcomes?) and *program effectiveness* (e.g., Is there evidence of impact across different groups, different places, and different time periods?). It involves three general steps: (1) specifying the inclusion criteria of studies and searching for relevant studies, based on asking a well-specified research question; (2) assessing the validity of studies: for efficacy evaluation, internal validity regarding whether an observed statistical association between intervention and outcome is genuinely causal or influenced by spurious factors, and for effectiveness evaluations, external validity regarding whether causal relationships generalise across studies that look at different implementation contexts; and (3) critically synthesising research findings to estimate general overall conclusions about an intervention (Testa 2010).

Experimental research design is necessary to determine whether a treatment is effective on the measure of interest. Moreover, to make claims about efficacy of alternative care with any confidence would require multiple experimental studies synthesised in a research review, given limited generalisability arising from differences in service delivery among jurisdictions. The Cochrane Collaboration is a repository for research reviews that assess the evidence base of interventions. At present, there is only one registered review that assesses the outcomes of a form of alternative care: *Kinship care for the safety, permanency and well-being of children removed from the home for maltreatment*. The authors note that the findings of the review are "tempered by the pronounced methodological and design weaknesses of the included studies" and that "researchers and practitioners must do better to mitigate the biases that cloud the study of kinship care" (Winokur et al. 2014, p. 20). The same could be said for other forms of alternative care.

The PICO framework (or a variation) is commonly used to specify research questions to assess the evidence base of an intervention through a research review. PICO stands for *Population, Intervention, Comparison* and *Outcome*. See Box 3.1 for definitions and examples of each element. Assessing the impacts of alternative care on child outcomes requires a question that arranges these elements (in any order) into an answerable question. For example, does the statutory intervention of placement in out-of-home care (*I*) compared to no treatment (*C*) improve child safety in terms of experiencing child abuse or neglect (*O*) for children assessed as at risk of significant harm of child maltreatment (*P*)? There is an assumption of statistical independence, that the observed and unobserved *Population* characteristics are essentially the same in the *Intervention* and *Comparison* groups, so that the differences in *Outcome* between the two groups is a result of the intervention (Testa 2010).

Box 3.1 PICO Framework for Designing a Research Question on Child Welfare Outcomes. (Adapted from Testa 2010)

- *P*—The target **population** about which you wish to draw inferences, such as foster children aged 12 years or younger, abused and neglected children in intact families, or children in long-term foster care;
- *I*—The **intervention**, whose efficacy and effectiveness you are interested in evaluating, such as intensive family preservation, long-term foster care, kinship care, guardianship or adoption;
- *C*—The alternative course of action with which you want to draw a **comparison**, such as no intervention, regular services, or a different intervention; and
- *O*—The intended **outcome** you want to see achieved, such as child safety, family continuity, placement stability, adolescent well-being, or legal permanence.

Application of the PICO framework reveals the complications of assessing the outcomes of statutory child protection interventions. The statistical assumption of independence between intervention and comparison groups can only be met in a randomised control design studies, which are almost entirely lacking on the question of alternative placements. The research base on alternative care is therefore compromised by various forms of bias, particularly selection bias (Berger et al. 2009), where unobserved *Population* factors influence assignment to *Intervention* rather than *Comparison* group. These unobserved *Population* factors can have a direct impact on *Outcome*, so that instead of the true causal relationship between *I* and *O*, we get a mixture of $P + I$ (Testa 2010). There are also complications with specifying the *Intervention* and prioritising the desired *Outcomes*. The next section examines each of the PICO components with regards to how it influences interpretation of child welfare outcomes research.

3.2.1 Population

By its very nature, statutory child protection serves a population of children who are likely to have experienced adversity arising from parental substance abuse, mental health issues, and/or domestic violence (Barth et al. 2006). These prior experiences can independently be associated with outcomes of interest to child welfare, making it difficult to capture the effects of child protection interventions (Waldfogel 2000). Further, children removed from their homes and placed in out-of-home care are likely to differ from those who remain at home in a multiple of observable and unobservable factors (Berger et al. 2009). In statistical terms, the influence of other significant factors is known as confounding (Freedman 2005, cited in Testa 2010). For instance, if a research question is framed to consider the impact of out-of-home care on child well-being or functioning, there are *a priori* contributions of child maltreatment that may contribute to this outcome. Robust research suggests an association between early childhood adversity, including child maltreatment, and poorer health and mental health outcomes (Anda et al. 2006). It is difficult to tease out the contributions of prior experiences of child maltreatment from the contributions of alternative care placement as interventions on children's outcomes.

The complexity and lack of consistent definitions among child maltreatment types further complicates the issue. The commonly used categories of child maltreatment (physical abuse, sexual abuse, neglect, emotional abuse) are each umbrella terms for a broad range of parenting behaviours and child experiences. Neglect, for example, can be defined as in terms of parental omission of care, or child's experience of lacking in basic needs—there is not a clear and consistent definition used in the empirical literature. Research on neglect has tended to collapse different types of neglect into one category of general neglect, on the premise that different forms of neglect are manifestations of the same underlying issues; however, this may mask potentially significant differences among types. Further, research on neglect has generally treated it as a dichotomous variable (neglect or no neglect) rather than a continuous variable along a spectrum of meeting children's needs (Dubowitz et al. 2005). As this discussion illustrates, it is difficult to make a claim that an alternative placement has an impact on an outcome for a population of children when the parameters of what we mean by at risk of significant harm for a particular category of child maltreatment is not consistent across the literature.

It is also not possible to make a claim about the effectiveness of statutory child protection on a population basis because the underlying population of child maltreatment cases is poorly understood. Child maltreatment is acknowledgement to be an 'iceberg phenomenon': only a fraction of cases come to the attention of statutory authorities, with as many as half to 4/5 of child maltreatment cases going undetected (Trocmé 2008). There is the real demand and the recorded demand, and between those two figures is the latent demand (Mansell 2006). This volume makes the point that statutory child protection, with alternative placement as the primary intervention, cannot meet the true demand, which is perhaps misconstrued as a need for tertiary interventions for child protection rather than tiered public health investments for child well-being.

3.2.2 *Intervention*

Alternative care types as interventions are not well-specified, and each form of alternative care may vary significantly. While in general terms, foster care is defined as care provided by non-relatives for children in the statutory child protection system, it has different meanings in different jurisdictions. In the United States, foster care is considered under federal law to be a short-term intervention until a form of permanency through restoration to birth families, guardianship or adoption is achieved (though in practice many children will remain in long-term foster care). In other countries, such as Sweden, foster care is considered a preferable long-term option (Gilbert et al. 2011). Kinship care, understood in general terms as care provided by relatives or fictive 'kin' who may include family friends, is subject to varying levels of oversight, licensing and certification and varying level of financial support (Gibbs and Müller 2000). While adoption is recognised as creating a new legal relationship between the adoptive parents and the child and terminating the legal parenthood of birth parents, there may still be an expectation for a high level of court-mandated birth parent contact, as in New South Wales, Australia (del Pozo de Bolger et al. 2017) or limited and professionally mediated contact as is the norm in the United Kingdom (Neil 2002). In addition to the alternative placement types themselves, little is known and done to operationalise and measure impacts of routine agency practice on outcomes (McGhee et al. 2015).

Criteria for assignment to out-of-home care is not well delineated in the literature (Lawrence et al. 2006). Placement in alternate care may be associated with a single risk or incidence or multiple risks and/or accumulation of chronic maltreatment (Masten and Wright 1998). While there have been concerted attempts to standardise entry into alternative care through the use of actuarial risk assessment tools, in reality, there is still a large margin of subjectivity. Thresholds for intervention lack consistency even within jurisdictions: for example, professionals in the United Kingdom have reported political and financial pressure not to remove children (House of Commons Education Committee 2012). When assessing risk in child protection, it is inevitable that workers will sometimes get it wrong, due to partial information, bias and other factors (Munro 2008).

Moreover, there are ethical and practical constraints regarding assignment of a child to a form of alternative care. The type of alternative placement assigned to a child is typically based on the appropriateness and availability of kinship carers or foster carers (Barth et al. 2008). There are also preferences of potential carers. For example, likelihood of adoption is associated with (younger) child age and (lack of) diagnosis with an emotional or behavioural disorder (e.g., Connell et al. 2006).

3.2.3 Comparison

To know for certain the outcomes of alternative care and treatment in child protection would require a counterfactual: to observe the same child under conditions of the treatment or alternative care and under conditions where the treatment or alternative care were withheld. Because it is not possible to observe the same individual twice under different treatment conditions, approximations are needed. The best way that science has come up to infer causal effects is randomly assign intervention to comparison or treatment group (Rubin 1978). Yet in the field of child welfare, "there is not one single intervention that has generated a published peer-review article based on a study in which they accepted referrals from a child welfare agency, randomly assigned them to a treatment condition, and evaluated the outcome" (Wulczyn et al. 2005, p. 155). While arguments are made against controlled experiments in child protection on the basis of feasibility and ethics, the flipside argument can be made that current child protection approaches constitute uncontrolled experimentation that is no more ethical given the lack of evidence justifying current interventions (Testa 2010).

A major impediment to experimental research comes from "micro-macro tensions" around control (Testa and White 2014, p. 163). A randomised control trial takes control over assignment to the intervention condition out of the hands of the client or practitioner, in order to make causal claims about the average effect of an intervention on a macro scale. Micro practice in child welfare is predicated on the practitioner making a clinical assessment and causal assumptions about the need for a particular intervention. These tensions contribute to the difficultly in conducting experimental research, and generally result in the use of other research designs that leave some of the discretion regarding treatment in the hands of clients or practitioners, undermining the internal and externality validity of the resulting research (Testa and White 2014).

3.2.4 Outcome

One of the complications of assessing the outcomes of alternative care and treatment in child welfare is that there is not one intended outcome of child protection, but multiple, and often competing, outcomes (Gambrill 2008). If child safety was the only desired outcome, the question of whether the intervention of out-of-home care on safety would be sufficient. But as previously stated, there are a set of desired outcomes from child protection interventions: safety, continuity, stability, permanency, and well-being. These outcomes can be prioritised differently by different jurisdictions. For example, the Adoption and Safe Families federal legislation in the United States clearly prioritises child safety over continuity of care with the birth parents. However, in practice, child welfare practitioners are often juggling these competing priorities and there are multiple barriers to decision making (Gambrill 2008) that can influence what outcome they are seeking to prioritise and what intervention they therefore should put in place—for example, in-home family preservation services or out-of-home care.

Among the desired outcomes, child well-being or functioning has been the least well-operationalised and least measured. Child welfare research has tended to focus on measuring case status outcomes (e.g., reunification, re-entry or adoption), rather than child (client) outcomes (Altshuler and Gleeson 1999; Wells and Johnson 2001). Challenges associated with measuring child well-being are due to lack of conceptual clarity in the field of child welfare over what constitutes well-being (Webb 2010). If the true question is how to improve child well-being in terms of developmental trajectories (Wulczyn et al. 2005), then the limited interventions offered by statutory child protection are unlikely to yield desired outcomes. A new approach incorporating public health approaches, as this volume argues, would be needed to more holistically address the drivers of child well-being include contributions from schools, health services, and neighbourhoods (Harden 2004).

3.3 What Different Research Designs Can Tell Us

The proceeding discussion has stressed that the research base on alternative care needs to be approached with caution, given definitional issues, methodological limitations and potential bias. While randomised control trials provide the highest level of evidence about the causal relationship between an intervention and an outcome, in the case of alternative placement in child welfare, randomisation is not feasible or acceptable. At best, child welfare researchers can try to take advantage of natural experiments; for example, Doyle's (2008) study examining the impact of out-of-home care on children on the margin of entry to care, comparing those who remained in the home to those placed in foster care, using caseworker's propensity to remove as an instrumental variable to estimate causal effects (Berger et al. 2009). Yet given the rarity of these opportunities, child welfare must frequently rely upon other research designs.

Quasi-experimental research is a frequently used design in child welfare. It involves comparison of two groups, one which receives an intervention and one which does not, but the intervention is not randomly assigned (Baker and Charvat 2008). Statistical methods can be to adjust for selection bias when comparing children who have experienced alternative care to those who have not, commonly by controlling for known confounding variables or using propensity score matching to match a treatment to a comparison sample on observable background characteristics (Berger et al. 2009). However, when not all potentially relevant variables can be controlled, there is a risk of spurious findings, particularly in the context of complex interventions with heterogeneous groups (Weisburd 2010). Take for example research on family preservation. A meta-analysis of family preservation research found that with regards to the outcome of child removal, randomised control trials found a negative effect, whereas studies with an unmatched comparison group found a positive effect and studies with a matched comparison found no effect (Al et al. 2012).

Most of what we know about children who have experienced alternative placements or other treatments through the child welfare system comes from observational research. A causal model implies directionality – an intervention (independent variable) results in an outcome (dependent variable). By contrast, in an observational study, the independent variable and dependent variable (intervention and outcome) are naturally occurring in the sample without manipulation from the researcher. Observational research may detect correlation between two variables, but cannot prove directionality nor whether the association is due to an unmeasurable explanatory variable. While observational studies have been viewed as having less validity than experimental studies, meta-analyses in health suggest that observational studies do not systematically overestimate treatment effects when compared to randomised control trials on the same clinical topics (Concato et al. 2000), suggesting that well-designed observational research can be seriously considered for understanding outcomes of interventions (Landsverk et al. 2011).

Observational research may be cross-sectional, with data collection at a single point in time, or longitudinal, with data collection with the same individuals at two or more points in time (Baker and Charvat 2008). Cross-sectional research is limited to providing a snapshot of the child welfare population and their characteristics at a given point in time (Waldfogel 2000). Longitudinal research, on the other hand, allows for examination of how children's outcomes change over time, between individuals and within individuals (Altshuler and Gleeson 1999). Longitudinal research may be retrospective, looking to the past, or prospective, following a cohort into the future, which allows for examining events before and as they occur (Loeber and Farrington 1994).

Prospective longitudinal research studies which follow a cohort of children who have entered alternate care offers several advantages for studying children in alternative care. Examples of such study designs include Pathways of Care Longitudinal Study, in New South Wales, Australia, and the National Survey of Child and Adolescent Well-Being in the United States. Following a cohort of children over time can provide information on the outcome of well-being through repeated measurement that tracks deterioration or improvement in functioning (Altshuler and Gleeson 1999). Statistical methods can be used to control for the child's baseline functioning when measuring later levels of functioning, thereby adjusting for factors that are not directly observable but influence the outcome of interest at baseline and follow-up points (Berger et al. 2009). This research design also allows for studying protective factors that protect children from risk and promote resilience (Hunter et al. 2002).

The greatest need for data in child welfare, and where there is potential convergence with public health approaches, is for population-based research of children at risk of child welfare involvement—that is, children identified as needing secondary (targeted) services. As previously mentioned, there are studies that track cohorts of children who are involved with the statutory child protection system. There are also longitudinal studies that track a nationally representative sample of children; for example, the Longitudinal Study of Australian Children, the National Longitudinal Survey of Children and Youth in Canada and the Growing Up in Scotland study, to name a few. However, these studies tend not to collect information about child welfare involvement, or if they do, it is on a small sample of children. Population-based research on children identified as at-risk of child welfare involvement is needed to better understand not only the outcomes children experience once they become involved with statutory child protection but also the factors that bring them into the system (Waldfogel 2000).

3.4 The Promise of Public Health Approaches to Child Maltreatment

While not entirely overcoming the challenges highlighted in this chapter, there are ways that public health approaches could potentially improve upon service delivery for children identified as at-risk of serious harm and allow for more systematic research on the outcomes of such children. As discussed in this volume (*Cite editors' intro*), a public health approach to child maltreatment provides access to universal and targeted services to reduce the risk of harm to children. These primary and secondary levels of services can in turn reduce but not entirely eliminate the need for tertiary services such as alternative placement that constitute the focus of statutory child protection. The threshold for intervention would be more clearly specified and a stepped up or down response would be possible. This could enable better strategies for monitoring outcomes associated with interventions. Moreover, this approach could provide greater confidence that alternative placements are a last resort and only used for the children who absolutely need them.

Assessing the outcomes of a public health approach would have some major points of distinction to the current statutory approach. The focus of outcomes measurement in public health systems is at the population level. Moving from a statutory approach to a public health approach would necessitate a shift from research that attempts to measure individual-level outcomes to monitoring population-level outcomes (Peckover and Smith 2011). Another significant area of research under a public health approach is determining the true incidence of risk factors for child maltreatment in the population and ensuring routine data collection across the cohort of children identified as at-risk for child maltreatment.

The advent of 'big data' in the form of administrative data linkage holds significant promise for studying child maltreatment at a population-level. Administrative data are collected through the standard functioning of statutory child protection agencies, with commonly collected fields including the child maltreatment allegation, the investigation and service response if any, and background information about the child and parent or guardian. Data can be aggregated longitudinally to track contact with statutory child protection over time (Hurren et al. 2017). Critically, these data can be joined to other administrative data collected by systems such as health, education, and criminal justice to provide data on constructs of interest, such as measures of well-being over time, and enable calculations of incidence. For example, Putnam-Hornstein et al. (2011) joined birth records to administrative child welfare data in the state of California to determine the incidence of child maltreatment reports and related risk factors. Technological improvements in data storage and analysis have greatly increased the feasibility of conducting such research on a broad scale (Jonson-Reid and Drake 2008).

There are also political trends which may signal a shift favouring public health approaches to child maltreatment. Governments are increasingly adopting social investment thinking, with expectations that policy spending should result in return on investment (Midgley et al. 2017). Cost-benefit analysis can be used to compare investments in interventions, programs and organizational structures against child outcomes (Wulczyn et al. 2009). This approach can be used to measure cost savings and build the case for preventative interventions (Herrenkohl et al. 2015). More work is needed to develop priority-setting models that assess the performance and costs of alternative intervention approaches to allow for careful decisions on how best to allocate scarce financial resources in child welfare (Segal and Dalziel 2011).

These technological and political changes raise concerns about privacy and ethics. The surveillance focus of public health approaches are in tension with societal values of minimal interference with private family life (Peckover and Smith 2011). Big data raises ethical concerns that children and their families may be unaware that data on their child welfare experiences exists and can be shared with third parties for data linkage and analysis and additionally are not asked to consent (Berman and Albright 2017). There are also ethical concerns that expansion of child welfare toward a public health model would require significant additional resources for universal and indicated services at a time when jurisdictions are struggling to maintain investment in tertiary responses. There is a danger that instead of increasing resources, resources may be diverted away from the children who will need alternative care (Berrick 2008).

It is disturbing to reflect upon the fact that despite the millions of lives affected and billions of dollars spent on the statutory approach to child maltreatment, we do not know the true outcomes associated with alternative care. The promise of a public health approach to child maltreatment lies in a more systematic way of monitoring, identifying and intervening with children and families experiencing challenges to reduce the need for alternative placements in the first place.

References

Al, C. M., Stams, G. J. J., Bek, M. S., Damen, E. M., Asscher, J. J., & van der Laan, P. H. (2012). A meta-analysis of intensive family preservation programs: Placement prevention and improvement of family functioning. *Children and Youth Services Review, 34*(8), 1472–1479.

Altshuler, S. J., & Gleeson, J. P. (1999). Completing the evaluation triangle for the next century: Measuring child" Well-being" in family foster care. *Child Welfare, 78*(1), 125–147.

Anda, R. F., Felitti, V. J., Bremner, J. D., Walker, J. D., Whitfield, C. H., Perry, B. D., Dube, S. R., & Giles, W. H. (2006). The enduring effects of abuse and related adverse experiences in childhood. *European Archives of Psychiatry and Clinical Neuroscience, 256*(3), 174–186.

Baker, A. J., & Charvat, B. J. (2008). *Research methods in child welfare*. New York: Columbia University Press.

Barth, R. P., Wildfire, J., & Green, R. L. (2006). Placement into foster care and the interplay of urbanicity, child behavior problems, and poverty. *American Journal of Orthopsychiatry, 76*(3), 358–366.

Barth, R. P., Green, R., Webb, M. B., Wall, A., Gibbons, C., & Craig, C. (2008). Characteristics of out-of-home caregiving environments provided under child welfare services. *Child Welfare, 87*(3), 5–39.

Berger, L. M., Bruch, S. K., Johnson, E. I., James, S., & Rubin, D. (2009). Estimating the "impact" of out-of-home placement on child well-being: Approaching the problem of selection bias. *Child Development, 80*(6), 1856–1876.

Berman, G., & Albright, K. (2017). *Children and the data cycle: Rights and ethics in a big data world* (Innocenti Working Paper 2017–05). Florence: UNICEF Office of Research Florence.

Berrick, J. D. (2008). *Take me home: Protecting America's vulnerable children and families*. Oxford: Oxford University Press.

Concato, J., Shah, N., & Horwitz, R. I. (2000). Randomized, controlled trials, observational studies, and the hierarchy of research designs. *New England Journal of Medicine, 342*(25), 1887–1892.

Connell, C. M., Katz, K. H., Saunders, L., & Tebes, J. K. (2006). Leaving foster care—The influence of child and case characteristics on foster care exit rates. *Children and Youth Services Review, 28*(7), 780–798.

del Pozo de Bolger, A., Dunstan, D., & Kaltner, M. (2017). Descriptive analysis of foster care adoptions in New South Wales, Australia. *Australian Social Work*, 1–14.

Doyle, J. J., Jr. (2008). Child protection and adult crime: Using investigator assignment to estimate causal effects of foster care. *Journal of Political Economy, 116*(4), 746–770.

Dubowitz, H., Pitts, S. C., Litrownik, A. J., Cox, C. E., Runyan, D., & Black, M. M. (2005). Defining child neglect based on child protective services data. *Child Abuse & Neglect, 29*(5), 493–511.

Gambrill, E. (2008). Decision making in child welfare: Constraints and potential. In D. Lindsey & A. Shlonsky (Eds.), *Child welfare research: Advances for practice and policy* (pp. 175–193). Oxford: Oxford University Press.

Gibbs, P., & Müller, U. (2000). Kinship foster care moving to the mainstream: Controversy, policy, and outcomes. *Adoption Quarterly, 4*(2), 57–87.

Gilbert, N., Parton, N., & Skivenes, M. (Eds.). (2011). *Child protection systems: International trends and orientations*. Oxford: Oxford University Press.

Harden, B. (2004). Safety and stability for foster children: A developmental perspective. *The Future of Children, 14*(1), 31–47.

Herrenkohl, T. I., Higgins, D. J., Merrick, M. T., & Leeb, R. T. (2015). Positioning a public health framework at the intersection of child maltreatment and intimate partner violence: Primary prevention requires working outside existing systems. *Child Abuse and Neglect, 48*, 22–28.

House of Commons Education Committee. (2012). Children first: The child protection system in England. *Fourth Report of Session, 13*. Retrieved from https://publications.parliament.uk/pa/cm201213/cmselect/cmeduc/137/137.pdf.

Hunter, W. M., Cox, C. E., Teagle, S., Johnson, R. M., Mathew, R., Knight, E. D., Leeb, R. T., & Smith, J. B. (2002). *Measures for assessment of functioning and outcomes in longitudinal research on child abuse: Volume 2: Middle childhood*. Chapel Hill: LONGSCAN coordinating Centre, University of North Carolina.

Hurren, E., Stewart, A., & Dennison, S. (2017). New methods to address old challenges: The use of administrative data for longitudinal replication studies of child maltreatment. *International Journal of Environmental Research and Public Health, 14*(9), 1066.

Jonson-Reid, M., & Drake, B. (2008). Multisector longitudinal administrative databases: An indispensable tool for evidence-based policy for maltreated children and their families. *Child Maltreatment, 13*(4), 392–399.

Kraft, M. E., & Furlong, S. R. (2012). *Public policy: Politics, analysis, and alternatives*. Los Angeles: Sage.

Landsverk, J., Brown, C. H., Reutz, J. R., Palinkas, L., & Horwitz, S. M. (2011). Design elements in implementation research: A structured review of child welfare and child mental health studies. *Administration and Policy in Mental Health and Mental Health Services Research, 38*(1), 54–63.

Lawrence, C. R., Carlson, E. A., & Egeland, B. (2006). The impact of foster care on development. *Development and Psychopathology, 18*(1), 57–76.

Littell, J. H. (2008). How do we know what works? The quality of published reviews of evidence-based practices. In D. Lindsey & A. Shlonsky (Eds.), *Child welfare research: Advances for practice and policy* (pp. 66–94). Oxford: Oxford University Press.

Loeber, R., & Farrington, D. P. (1994). Problems and solutions in longitudinal and experimental treatment studies of child psychopathology and delinquency. *Journal of Consulting & Clinical Psychology, 62*, 887–900.

Mansell, J. (2006). The underlying instability in statutory child protection: Understanding the system dynamics driving risk assurance levels. *Social Policy Journal of New Zealand, 28*, 97.

Masten, A. S., & Wright, M. O. D. (1998). Cumulative risk and protection models of child maltreatment. *Journal of Aggression, Maltreatment & Trauma, 2*(1), 7–30.

McGhee, J., Mitchell, F., Daniel, B., & Taylor, J. (2015). Taking a long view in child welfare: How can we evaluate intervention and child well-being over time? *Child Abuse Review, 24*(2), 95–106.

Midgley, J., Dahl, E., & Wright, A. C. (Eds.). (2017). *Social investment and social welfare: International and critical perspectives*. Cheltenham: Edward Elgar Publishing.

Munro, E. (2008). Lessons from research on decision making. In D. Lindsey & A. Shlonsky (Eds.), *Child welfare research: Advances for practice and policy* (pp. 194–200). Oxford: Oxford University Press.

Neil, E. (2002). Contact after adoption: The role of agencies in making and supporting plans. *Adoption & Fostering, 26*(1), 25–38.

Peckover, S., & Smith, S. (2011). Guest editorial: Public health approaches to safeguarding children. *Child Abuse Review, 20*(4), 231–237.

Putnam-Hornstein, E., Webster, D., Needell, B., & Magruder, J. (2011). A public health approach to child maltreatment surveillance: Evidence from a data linkage project in the United States. *Child Abuse Review, 20*(4), 256–273.

Rubin, D. B. (1978). Bayesian inference for causal effects: The role of randomization. *The Annals of Statistics, 6*, 34–58.

Segal, L., & Dalziel, K. (2011). Investing to protect our children: Using economics to derive an evidence-based strategy. *Child Abuse Review, 20*(4), 274–289.

Testa, M. F. (2010). Evaluation of child welfare interventions. In M. F. Testa & J. Poertner (Eds.), *Fostering accountability: Using evidence to guide and improve child welfare policy* (pp. 195–230). Oxford: Oxford University Press.

Testa, M. F., & White, K. R. (2014). Insuring the integrity and validity of social work interventions: The case of the subsidized guardianship waiver experiments. *Journal of Evidence-Based Social Work, 11*(1–2), 157–172.

Trocmé, N. (2008). Epidemiology of child maltreatment. In D. Lindsey & A. Shlonsky (Eds.), *Child welfare research: Advances for practice and policy* (pp. 15–24). Oxford: Oxford University Press.

Wald, M. S. (2014). Beyond maltreatment: Developing support for children in multiproblem families. In J. Korbin & R. Krugman (Eds.), *Handbook of child maltreatment* (Contemporary issues in research and policy) (Vol. 2, pp. 251–280). Dordrecht: Springer.

Waldfogel, J. (2000). Child welfare research: How adequate are the data? *Children and Youth Services Review, 22*(9), 705–741.

Webb, M. B. (Ed.). (2010). *Child welfare and child well-being: New perspectives from the national survey of child and adolescent well-being*. Oxford: Oxford University Press.

Weisburd, D. (2010). Justifying the use of non-experimental methods and disqualifying the use of randomized controlled trials: Challenging folklore in evaluation research in crime and justice. *Journal of Experimental Criminology, 6*, 209–227.

Wells, S. J., & Johnson, M. A. (2001). Selecting outcome measures for child welfare settings: Lessons for use in performance management. *Children and Youth Services Review, 23*(2), 169–199.

Winokur, M., Holtan, A., & Batchelder K. E. (2014). Kinship care for the safety, permanency, and well-being of children removed from the home for maltreatment. *Cochrane Database of Systematic Reviews*, Issue 1. Art. No.: CD006546. https://doi.org/10.1002/14651858.CD006546.pub3.

Wulczyn, F., Barth, R. P., Yuan, Y. T., Harden, B. J., & Landsverk, J. (Eds.). (2005). *Beyond common sense: Child welfare, child well-being, and the evidence for policy reform*. Piscataway: Transaction Publishers.

Wulczyn, F. H., Orlebeke, B., & Haight, J. (2009). *Finding the return on investment: A framework for monitoring local child welfare agencies*. Chicago: Chapin Hall Center for Children.

Chapter 4
'Everybody's Responsibility': Exploring the Challenges of Community Engagement in Child Neglect

Nigel Parton and Sasha Williams

4.1 Introduction

There are two inter-connected themes that provide the focus for this chapter, both of which have central implications for the development of public healthapproaches to child protection. Firstly, it recognizes that the vast majority of work that comes into child protection agencies is framed in terms of child neglect indicating the importance of public health strategy focusing on this area of child maltreatment rather than simply child abuse. Secondly, it reflects the increased recognition that it is crucial to try and engage the wider community in day-to-day child protection policy and practice. Drawing on original research, the chapter explores how lay people understand the term child neglect and what they see as the best way of addressing the problem. The research suggests the importance for any public health model to identify and support clear roles for lay people and communities to respond to children considered to be at risk of maltreatment, rather than simply focus on service provision, and also forms a critique of current efforts to make child protection 'everyone's business' in England.

The last 30 years has witnessed an enormous growth in concern about child neglect such that it is now by far the biggest category of abuse being dealt with by child protection systems in 'western' jurisdictions. For example, in England the percentage of children who became the subject of a child protection plan categorized as child neglect increased from 30% (9,200 children) of the total in 1995 to 45% (28,360 children) in 2016. Similarly the percentage of children categorized as emotional abuse and subject to a child protection plan increased from 13% (3,800

N. Parton
Applied Childhood Studies, University of Huddersfield, Huddersfield, UK
e-mail: n.parton@hud.ac.uk

S. Williams (✉)
Children Team, Jones Myers Solicitors, Leeds, UK

B. Lonne et al. (eds.), *Re-Visioning Public Health Approaches for Protecting Children*, Child Maltreatment 9, https://doi.org/10.1007/978-3-030-05858-6_4

children) in 1995 up to 35% (22,420 children) in 2016. By 2016 the categories of child neglect and emotional abuse between them accounted for 80% of all child protection plans in England. In contrast the percentage of child protection plans categorized as physical or sexual abuse has gone down considerably. In 1995 physical abuse made up 40% (12,300 children) and sexual abuse 24% (7,200 children) of child protection plans while in 2016 physical abuse made up just 10% (6,200 children) and sexual abuse 5% (2,970 children) of child protection plans.[1] Similarly, in the US the most recent annual report of the National Child Abuse and Data System (NCANDS) has estimated that 75.3% of victims of child maltreatment in the US were neglected compared to 17.2% who were physically abused and 8.4% who were sexually abused (US Department of Health and Human Services 2017)

Concern has been prompted by the apparently "overwhelming academic and research evidence of the long-term damage of neglect" (Education Committee Stuart Report 2013, p. 23), which suggests that neglect is associated with deficits in children's neurological, cognitive, physical, behavioural, emotional and educational development (Gardner 2008; Meadows et al. 2011; Ward and Brown 2013) and impacts negatively on children throughout the age range (e.g., Brandon et al. 2013; Daniel et al. 2011; Rees et al. 2011). Research also seems to show that neglect is often found alongside other forms of serious maltreatment (Brandon et al. 2013) and can itself result in child death (e.g., Bridge Care Consultancy 1995; Ward 2008). Finally, research suggests that neglect may have significant financial implications for society as it appears to be associated with increased use of public services and resources throughout the lifespan (Burgess et al. 2012; Davies and Ward 2012; Meadows et al. 2011).

At the same time there has also been a growing focus on trying to engage the wider community in the effort to safeguard children. Not only can the community support neglected children and their families directly (thus avoiding the use of limited public resources) but it can also act as the eyes and ears of the child protection system (Burgess et al. 2012; Fisher and Gruescu 2011; Radford 2010). As Dhooper et al. (1991, p. 37) have pointed out: "only the operation of laymen - neighbours, friends, family, the general public - can bring the protection system to the service of the abused and neglected children early enough to be effective". In England numerous public inquiries and reviews have shown that lay people often hold key information about neglected children, and communication failures between lay people and professionals can have appalling consequences for children (Ofsted 2011; Ward 2008).

An explicit argument over recent years has been that 'child protection is everyone's business' (Macleod 1997; Council of Australian Governments 2009) or 'everyone's responsibility' (HM Treasury 2003; Laming 2009). Agencies have attempted to educate the public into their safeguarding role and about the importance of responding to child neglect. In the UK debates about neglect have been

[1] Figures for 1995 are based on the annual Department of Health *Children and Young People on Child Protection Registers Year Ending 31 March* and the figures for 2016 are based on the annual Department for Education *Characteristics of Children in Need.*

conducted in the popular media as well as the professional literature (Gardner 2008) and, the charity *Action for Children* championed a proposed amendment to the criminal law as a means to draw public, legal and political attention to neglect as an issue (Action for Children 2012). The importance of lay people playing a role in safeguarding all children was enshrined within the Children Act 2004 (as amended in 2009) with the requirement that Local Safeguarding Children Boards, who are the statutory bodies responsible for coordinating child protection work in local areas, must take reasonable steps to recruit two lay members. Lay members are there to facilitate contact between professionals and the community; their task is to "help to make links between the LSCB and community groups, support stronger public engagement in local child safety issues and an improved public understanding of the LSCB's child protection work" (HM Government 2015, p. 69).

Surveys for the *NSPCC* and *Action for Children* repeatedly suggest that the UK public is concerned about child neglect and about how best to respond to neglected children (e.g., Action for Children 2009; Burgess et al. 2012, 2013, 2014; Daniel et al. 2011; Gardner 2008; Hutchinson 2012), and, as we demonstrated earlier, there has been a considerable increase in the number of neglected children known to statutory agencies. However, despite these increases, prevalence studies suggest that a large number of children never reach the attention of the authorities despite experiencing levels of care or supervision that "could be regarded as problematic by the criteria applied in child protection and other professional contexts" (Cawson et al. 2000, p. 11). For example, the research by Radford et al. (2011) concluded that 5% of children under 11, 13.3% of 11–17 year olds and 16% of those aged 18–24 had experienced neglect at some point in their childhoods; and that under the broad category of emotional abuse 12% of children under 11, 17.5% of 11 to 17 year olds and 23.7% of 18 to 24 year olds had been exposed to domestic violence at some point in their childhoods. Finally, research in the US and UK suggests that only a small minority of children who experience neglect ever come to the attention of a child protection agency (e.g., Gilbert et al. 2009).

If neglect is indeed associated with the catastrophic effects outlined earlier, it is important to explore how lay people understand child neglect and what they perceive to be the most appropriate responses to it. Research in the UK suggests overwhelming public support for lay action of some kind: with 94% of respondents stating that people should become involved if they are concerned about a child (Burgess et al. 2012). There is evidence that some lay people may be meeting the needs of neglected children directly - a survey of parents found that 13% recounted having provided some level of care for a child they suspected was being neglected, e.g., providing a bed for the night, food and outings (Action for Children 2011). However, only just over 60% of those who had concerns about a child reported having told someone else, and those they approached initially tended to be partners, friends, neighbours and family members rather than professionals (Burgess et al. 2012, 2013, 2014). Lay people explained this reluctance as due to their feeling that the situation was none of their business, their fear intervention would cause trouble for the child and/or for themselves, their lack of certainty and/or proof about what was going on, and their lack of knowledge about where to go for help (Action for

Children 2009; Burgess et al. 2012, 2013, 2014). This lay reluctance to intervene is also reflected in studies carried out in the US (Korbin and Coulton 1996) and Bensley et al. (2004) and in Australia (NAPCAN 2010).

In order to make lay people partners in safeguarding children's welfare, we need to understand how they construct child neglect and the possible responses to it as a matter of practical, ethical and political importance.

4.2 Exploring Lay Constructions: Methodology

In 2013 one of us (Williams 2015) carried out qualitative research which aimed to explore how lay people construct child neglect and what they saw as the most appropriate responses to the problem. The data were collected from focus groups built around pre-existing groups of friends, neighbours and colleagues, hoping to capitalize on both the naturalistic data produced by focus groups (Smithson 2008; Stewart et al. 2007; Sussman et al. 1991; Wilkinson 2004) and the 'natural clusterings' (Kitzinger 1994, p. 106) in which lay conversations around child neglect might normally take place. In total the project recruited 46 people made up of 10 distinct natural clusters of friends, collegues and/or neighbours (the 'groups'). Each cluster formed a focus group of no fewer than three and no more than seven people and discussions within the groups were minimally moderated (Fern 2001; Parker and Tritter 2006).

Of the 46 participants, 34 described themselves as white British, English or Scottish, 38 as female, 8 as male, and 24 participants said they had been parents, guardians or carers. The participants were a heterogenous group ranging in age from 18 to 90, describing themselves as coming from a variety of socio-economic backgrounds, and currently living in rural and urban locations in the North, South East and South West of England. Rather than place a researcher-created definition of 'lay' to determine who should or should not participate in the research, participants were asked to exclude themselves if they had received professional training in child neglect. This process highlighted that the construction of 'lay' was complex and contingent. One group of participants were directly employed in education including both teachers and non-teachers yet did not consider themselves to be professionally trained in child protection, and stated that any concerns they had about children would be referred on to qualified safeguarding school staff. The construction of lay/professional boundaries in relation to child protection is worth exploring further.

Each of the 10 groups discussed the role of the media in constructing child neglect, the complexity of responding to children with unmet needs and to neglected children and the role of statutory children's services. Data were recorded and analysis followed Willig's (2008a, 2008b) framework for discourse analysis.

4.3 Constructing Child Neglect

The research indicated that participants constructed child neglect as occurring when children's physical, emotional, training and/or supervisory needs were not being met by a parental figure who was not behaving as a normal parent should (Williams 2015). Where these developmental needs (accepted by all participants) were unmet, children could be positioned as *Deprived, Unloved, Uncontrolled* or *Escaping* respectively. Deprived children were children whose physical needs were not being adequately met (for example for adequate food, shelter, clothing, etc.). Unloved children were those whose emotional needs were not being adequately met. Uncontrolled children were children whose training and socialization needs were not being adequately met (for example around laws, morals and social boundaries). Escaping children were children whose activities were not being properly supervised and regulated by adults. However, seeing a child as falling into one of these categories was not enough for a child to be positioned as neglected; for that, the unmet needs had to flow from a deficit in normal parenting. Normal parenting was seen as requiring both an appropriate parental disposition (in which the parent places the needs of the child ahead of their own needs), and appropriate skills and knowledge into how developing children need to be parented. Child neglect was seen to occur when parents lacked the appropriate parental disposition (*Underinvested Parents*), the appropriate parenting skills and knowledge (*Clueless Parents*) or both (*Unsuitable Parents*). Parents who possessed both the appropriate disposition and the required skills and knowledge but despite this were not meeting their children's needs were not constructed as neglectful but rather as *Overburdened.*

4.4 Constructing Child Neglect: The Role of the Media

The first question the research explored was where participants received the key messages about child neglect from, and what they made of these messages. For participants, information about child maltreatment was overwhelmingly distributed through the media. However, participants did not necessarily support the professional definitions of child neglect that they considered the media to be disseminating. Participants were extremely concerned by the long-term psychological effects of a failure to meet a child's emotional needs (*Unloved Child*) but felt that media stories ignored this aspect of neglect completely. There were stories about the *Uncontrolled Child* and *Escaping Child* in the media but the children concerned were not positioned as neglected. While several participants referred to *Escaping Child* stories (e.g., Madeleine McCann) as proper neglect stories (i.e., a failure to meet a child's needs due to deficits in normal parenting), they noted that in contrast the media tended to report such stories as tragedies (i.e., as not relating to a failure in parenting).

For participants, stories of child neglect in the media - whether emanating from charity campaigns or from case reporting - almost exclusively related to the *Unsuitable Parents/Deprived Child* combination. These stories were widely used and understood by participants: the story of Peter Connelly ('Baby P') and the NSPCC 'child in a cot' 'Make it Stop' campaign being most frequently alluded to and immediately recognized by others. The accounts and the campaigns were harrowing and memorable for participants (several repeated verbatim the words from the 'child in a cot' advert during the discussions). However, participants considered the stories to be extreme and the focus on them problematic. For some, these accounts had narrowed the neglect category to only the most extreme situations to the detriment of neglected children in less dire circumstances. This media focus distorted participants' ideas about the types of neglect cases professionals are interested and involved in. As Parton stated, the intense media focus on these 'heavy end cases' obscures the types of neglect cases that form the daily reality of children's social work (Parton 1995, p. 87).

As most serious cases involve both abuse and neglect (Brandon et al. 2013) there is little reason for the media to tease apart the two concepts for their audience. However, participants found it both difficult and important to separate out child neglect from child abuse. Child abuse and child neglect were positioned as two qualitatively different poles of child maltreatment, which meant that in some important way child neglect both was and was not child abuse. For several participants neglect was less serious than child abuse and cases that were clearly extremely serious or deliberately harmful were positioned as 'child abuse' and therefore not child neglect. Some participants constructed the binary in relation to adult intention. Finally, some participants constructed neglect in relation to omission and abuse to commission.

Participants struggled with the legal or expert splitting of child maltreatment into child abuse and child neglect, constructing divisions between the two, each of which served to minimize the importance of child neglect in relation to child abuse. Participants variously constructed child abuse as more intentional, harmful, serious and blameworthy than child neglect. This lay construction is similar to the way the criminal legal system tends to respond to child neglect (see Hoyano and Keenan 2010), despite a concerted and continuing effort spearheaded by children's charities to alert public, professionals and policy makers to the extreme seriousness and harmfulness of neglect as a form of child maltreatment (e.g., Action for Children 2014; Brandon et al. 2013; Burgess et al. 2012, 2013, 2014; Gardner 2008).

4.5 Responding to Child Neglect: Constructing the Lay Role

The research also explored what participants considered lay people should do if they were concerned that a child was being neglected. The participants were clear that lay people were responsible for doing something if they considered a child was clearly being harmed or maltreated. To refuse to get involved was in some important way to abrogate your duties as a member of society - to be guilty of child neglect.

This is in line with other research indicating that the public supports lay intervention to protect children from maltreatment (ComRes/Local Government Association 2009; Jütte et al. 2015; YouGov/NSPCC 2012). To this extent at least, for participants, child protection was indeed 'everybody's business/responsibility'.

Where participants saw the child as being in immediate physical danger, intervention was also seen to be required. Participants constructed scenarios where infants or young children were alone in unsafe conditions (infants in apartments/flats or trapped in hot cars) and in obvious distress as requiring assistance, and it being the responsibility of all adults to ensure that this was received. While the consensus within the groups was that child neglect was important and that it was everyone's business to try and stop it from happening, where there was no clear emergency to trigger a response, things were less clear.

The role adults could play in the lives of unrelated children was constructed as complicated. Participants who had not been parents were clearly aware of children within their communities and were able to produce many instances in which they had observed or heard children behaving in ways that could be constructed as *Deprived, Unloved, Uncontrolled or Escaping*. However, this awareness and concern did not translate into active relationships with children within local communities.

This lack of adult involvement in children's lives was attributed not only to social mobility and community fragmentation but also to fears of being positioned as a paedophile. Child protection surveillance appeared to inhibit the involvement of lay people, particularly men, in the lives of other people's children. Few were prepared to interact with children when to do so could cause them to be viewed with suspicion.

Participants who were parents spoke of providing an informal support network for friends and classmates of their own children, under the guise of 'one more won't hurt'. Importantly, this was constructed as support for *Overburdened* parents rather than tackling child neglect, participants did not report challenging other parents but rather saw themselves as helping out. This very much reflects the findings of the *Action for Children* (2011) poll in which parents reported informally helping to meet the needs of their children's peers and friends. Holland et al.'s (2011) research review also found that there was a great deal of informal childcare within communities. However, the ability of the wider public to meet children's needs informally in the way participants reported that they had done in the past, was constructed as very much reduced, to the detriment of children.

4.6 Intervening or Interfering: The Lay Dilemma

Where participants felt unable or unwilling to provide support for apparently struggling parents, they needed to decide whether or not to intervene in the situation in some other way. Participants positioned themselves as being forced to choose between 'do something' or 'do nothing'; 'doing something' was constructed as drawing the family to the attention of the authorities.

The default position for all participants was to ‘do nothing’. For participants to ‘do something’ they overwhelmingly positioned themselves as needing to be satisfied that what they were witnessing had crossed a line of some sort. Identifying this line or lines, was seen as complex, onerous, contested and dangerous. Even where participants spoke about being extremely concerned about children in situations that they identified as neglectful, they had felt unable to intervene.

This unwillingness to act was put down to a range of factors: participants spoke of the practical difficulties of identifying an unknown child to the authorities; of a lack of knowledge of the reporting process; evidential uncertainties; and of fears that in alerting the authorities to the situation they will make matters worse not only for the child but also for themselves (findings similar to those of Bensley et al. (2004) and Burgess et al. (2012, 2013, 2014)). Participants from all groups considered the family arena to be a private one in which outsiders should not interfere unless interference was absolutely justified. Intervention was constructed as something that would be contested and resisted by the parents concerned.

For some participants intervening would make them feel subjectively at fault and uncomfortable. The private family was seen as a vital mechanism in a liberal society, and parents should be allowed to rear their children free from state scrutiny and state regulation (Parton 1985, 1991, 2006). Participants constructed intervention as so serious an invasion of family privacy that there would need to be an overwhelmingly abnormal situation to justify it.

4.7 Not Working: Constructing Social Services

The final question that the research explored was how participants constructed the child protection professionals who were exhorting them to take action. Combined with the fear of interfering in private family life, participants expressed a lack of trust in authority to respond appropriately to the situation. For participants ‘doing something’ equated to ‘informing social services’ (the local authority statutory department of children’s services). The way in which participants constructed social services made it less likely that they would choose to do something about a child who they were concerned about. Social services were universally constructed as an investigatory body with draconian powers to separate children from abnormal parents. The involvement of social services was seen as provoking both fear and shame for families, and several participants spoke of the fear and shame associated with the potential of social service involvement in their own lives (usually arising from hospital visits after accidents). Social services were seen as inflexible, so that, for example, hospital staff were positioned as having no choice but to follow rigid child protection procedures even against their own medical judgement. As the local authority social services were not deemed to have any role to play in supporting ‘normal’ parenting, to refer someone to social services was to position them as abnormal, risking them feeling isolated and judged by neighbours.

Such views are not surprising as participants' knowledge and understanding of social work and social services was almost entirely informed by the media, and the dominant media discourse in relation to the social work profession and local authority social services in the UK is that they fail children (Franklin 2014; Franklin and Parton 2001). From the 1970s onwards, high profile public inquiries and reviews relating to abused and neglected children have exposed social workers to, at times, extraordinarily hostile critical scrutiny (Franklin 2014; Lonne and Parton 2014; Masson 2006; Parton 1985, 2006, 2014; Scourfield 2000). Social workers, particularly in England, have been depicted as either "ineffectual wimps incapable of protecting children … or alternatively as bullies whose unjustifiable interventions in the private affairs of families have resulted in their precocious break-up" (Franklin 2014, p. 27). Participants frequently drew on these media narratives to construct social services as overreacting or underreacting to concerns about children, so, therefore, either destroying 'normal' families or abandoning children to serious harm and death.

Time and again, social work practice was condemned in the media - social workers lacked training, experience and supervision, multi-disciplinary communication was ineffective, social workers wrongly prioritized the needs of adults over the needs of children (Parton 1995, 2014), and social workers were too tied up with meeting technological demands to do their jobs effectively (Jones 2014; Parton 2014; Shoesmith 2016). Participants drew on these concerns about the recruitment, training and support of social workers, the unmanageable size of social worker caseloads, and the lack of resources allocated to social work.

As a result, reporting a situation to social services was not to enlist the assistance of benevolent, professional and skilled workers, but rather to place oneself, the child and their family at the mercy of a dysfunctional institution. Participants constructed social services as also having a binary response to families: do nothing or remove the child. Neither option was seen as a desirable outcome - participants in all groups argued that the family should be preserved wherever possible. The removal of children by social services was seen as potentially transferring children from one unsuitable environment to another; removing children was seen to be fraught with difficulty and danger for the child.

4.8 Conclusions: Reconstructing Services for Children and Families

These findings suggest that professionals have a long way to go to persuade lay people to work together with them in order to safeguard children. Similar to other research findings (e.g., Burgess et al. 2014; Kendall-Taylor et al. 2014) the participants were aware of children's developmental needs and very concerned about children being neglected - perhaps more concerned than professionals might be (Williams 2017). However, the avenues for non-professionals to support children and their families informally within communities were seen as diminishing, and people felt that outside of those forums, becoming involved in the lives of children would appear 'abnormal', opening participants (particularly men) up to scrutiny and suspicion. This weakening of community is a concern, as informal community support for families can be a protective mechanism against child maltreatment (McLeigh 2013; Spilsbury and Korbin 2013) and enabling, supporting and investing in informal community networks must be an essential and invaluable addition to a public health approach (Melton 2013). Participants had a very negative and narrow view of social work and social services, constructing social work intervention almost exclusively in relation to child removal – an intervention which participants did not consider an appropriate response to the majority of children whose needs were unmet and/or who were being neglected.

This suggests that lay people would support a community-based strategy that seeks to support children and families largely through informal networks of care within non-stigmatizing, everyday settings. A similar strategy was proposed by The US Advisory Board on Child Abuse and Neglect in 1993. Entitled '*Strong Communities for Children*' and implemented initially in parts of South Carolina, it has demonstrated the potential for "a more effective child protection system grounded in neighbors care for one another" (McLeigh and Melton 2015, p. 2). Implementing a similar strategy in most jurisdictions would require a sea change for the way that professionals work, for they often "overlook resources for children and families that are not delivered by salaried professionals in agency settings" (Melton 2013, p. 1). Rather than focusing narrowly on children at risk, a public health approach must include those involved in universal and secondary services recognizing the important role they play in enabling, supporting, energizing and working with communities and the resources within them, building and reshaping them for the benefit of children and families.

Most importantly, professionals would need to engage with the lay community in determining how best to work together to safeguard children and what children can expect (Korbin et al. 2000). These are not questions for professionals to answer, but rather moral and political choices about what children are entitled to and how best to provide them with it (Parton 1995). There is a need to work together to reshape cultural norms to facilitate the engagement of everyone in ensuring children and families are cared for and nurtured within our communities. It is not enough to notice children whose needs are not being met, we also need to demonstrate care in the form of practical support (Kimbrough-Melton and Melton 2015). To be truly effective, child protection, rather than being everyone's business, needs to be reconstructed as part of everyday life (Melton 2013). In trying to develop public health approaches to child protection, the focus should not only be upon the way policies and practices might be rethought and restructured, but a recognition that the processes whereby change is brought about is key.

References

Action for Children. (2009). *Child neglect: Experiences from the frontline*. Retrieved from http://www.actionforchildren.org.uk/media/95084/child-neglect-experiences-from-the-frontline.pdf.

Action for Children. (2011). *Neglect in the summer holidays*. Retrieved from https://yougov.co.uk/news/2011/08/09/neglect-summer-holidays/.

Action for Children. (2012). *Keeping children safe: the case for reforming the law on child neglect*. Retrieved from https://resourcecentre.savethechildren.se/sites/default/files/documents/5896.pdf

Action for Children. (2014). *Why we should talk about child abuse, and not about Cinderella*. Retrieved from https://www.actionforchildren.org.uk/news-and-blogs/policy-updates/2014/april/why-we-should-talk-about-child-abuse-and-not-about-cinderella/

Bensley, L., Simmons, K. W., Ruggles, D., Putvin, T., Harris, C., Allen, M., & Williams, K. (2004). Community responses and perceived barriers to responding to child maltreatment. *Journal of Community Health, 29*(2), 141–153.

Brandon, M., Bailey, S., Belderson, P., & Larsson, B. (2013). *Neglect and Serious Case Reviews*. Retrieved from https://www.nspcc.org.uk/globalassets/documents/research-reports/neglect-serious-case-reviews-report.pdf

Bridge Care Consultancy (B.C.C.). (1995). *Paul: Death through neglect*. London: The Bridge Publishing House.

Burgess, C., Daniel, B., Scott, J., Mulley, K., Derbyshire, D., & Downie, M. (2012). *Child neglect in 2011: An annual review*. Retrieved from https://www.actionforchildren.org.uk/media/3361/childneglectin2011.pdf.

Burgess, C., Daniel, B., Scott, J., Mulley, K., & Dobbin, H. (2013). *The state of child neglect in the UK*. Retrieved from https://www.actionforchildren.org.uk/media/3270/2013_neglect_full-report_v12.pdf

Burgess, C., Daniel, B., Scott, J., Dobbin, H., Mulley, K., & Whitfield, E. (2014). *Preventing child neglect in the UK: What makes services accessible to children and families?* Retrieved from https://www.actionforchildren.org.uk/media/3214/preventing-child-neglect-in-the-uk_annual-review_march2014.pdf

Cawson, P., Wattam, C., Brooker, S., & Kelly, G. (2000). *Child maltreatment in the United Kingdom: A study of the prevalence of abuse and neglect*. London: NSPCC.

ComRes/Local Government Association (C.G.A.). (2009). *Social work and child protection survey for the Local Government Association*. Retrieved from http://webarchive.nationalarchives.gov.uk/20090809160520/http://www.lga.gov.uk/lga/aio/1738911

Council of Australian Governments. (2009). *Protecting children is everyone's business: National framework for protecting Australia's children 2009–2020*. Canberra: Commonwealth of Australia.

Daniel, B., Taylor, J., & Scott, J. (2011). *Recognizing and helping the neglected child: Evidence-based practice for assessment and intervention*. London/Philadelphia: Jessica Kingsley Publishers.

Davies, C., & Ward, H. (2012). *Safeguarding children across services: Messages from research*. Retrieved from https://www.gov.uk/government/uploads/system/uploads/attachment_data/file/183231/DFE-RR164.pdf

Dhooper, S. S., Royse, D. D., & Wolfe, L. C. (1991). A statewide study of the public attitudes toward child abuse. *Child Abuse and Neglect, 15*(1), 37–44.

Education Committee (Stuart Report). (2013). *Children first: The child protection system in England*. London: The Stationery Office Ltd.

Fern, E. (2001). *Advanced focus group research*. London: Sage.

Fisher, D., & Gruescu, S. (2011). *Children and the Big Society: Backing communities to keep the next generation safe and happy*. Retrieved from http://www.respublica.org.uk/wp-content/uploads/2015/01/Children-and-BS.pdf

Franklin, B. (2014). Citizen journalist or cyber bigots? Child abuse, the media and the possibilities for public conversation: The case of Baby P. In S. Wagg & J. Pilcher (Eds.), *Thatcher's grandchildren? Politics and childhood in the twenty-first century* (pp. 27–45). Basingstoke: Palgrave Macmillan.

Franklin, B., & Parton, N. (2001). Press-ganged! Media reporting of social work and child abuse. In E. Brunsdon, M. May, & R. Payne (Eds.), *Understanding social problems: Issues in social policy* (pp. 233–247). Oxford: Blackwell.

Gardner, R. (2008). *Developing an effective response to neglect and emotional harm to children*. Retrieved from http://www.nspcc.org.uk/Inform/research/nspccresearch/completedresearch/DevelopingAnEffectiveResponseToNeglectPDF_wdf56700.pdf

Gilbert, R., Widom, C. S., Browne, K., Fergusson, D., Webb, E., & Janson, S. (2009). Burden and consequences of child maltreatment in high-income countries. *The Lancet, 373*(9657), 68–81. https://doi.org/10.1016/S0140-6736(08)61706-7.

HM Government. (2015). Working together to safeguard children. *Journal of Interprofessional Care 14,* 363–373. Retrieved from https://doi.org/10.1080/13561820020003919

HM Treasury. (2003). *Every child matters*. Cm. 5860. London: The Stationery Office.

Holland, S., Tannock, S., & Collicott, H. (2011). Everybody's business? A research review of the informal safeguarding of other people's children in the UK. *Children and Society, 25*(5), 406–416.

Hoyano, L., & Keenan, C. (2010). *Child abuse: Law and policy across boundaries*. Oxford: Oxford University Press.

Hutchinson, D. (2012). *Helpline highlight: More people contacting the NSPCC with concerns about neglected children*. Retrieved from http://nspcc.org.uk/globalassets/documents/research-reports/neglect-serious-case-reviews-report.pdf

Jones, R. (2014). *The story of Baby P: Setting the record straight*. Bristol: Policy Press.

Jütte, S., Bentley, H., Tallis, D., Mayes, J., Jetha, N., O'Hagan, O., Brookes, H., & McConnell, N. (2015). *How safe are our children*. London: NSPCC.

Kendall-Taylor, N., Lindland, E., O'Neil, M., & Stanley, K. (2014). Beyond prevalence: An explanatory approach to reframing child maltreatment in the United Kingdom: The most prevalent form of maltreatment, child neglect, gets the least attention from the public and policymakers. *Child Abuse and Neglect, 38*(5), 810–821.

Kimbrough-Melton, R. J., & Melton, G. B. (2015). Someone will notice, and someone will care': How to build strong communities for children. *Child Abuse and Neglect, Elsevier Ltd, 41*(1), 67–78.

Kitzinger, J. (1994). The methodology of focus groups: The importance of interaction between research participants. *Sociology of Health & Illness, 16*(1), 103–121.

Korbin, J. E., & Coulton, C. J. (1996). The role of neighbors and the government in neighborhood-based child protection. *Journal of Social Issues, 52*(3), 163–176. https://doi.org/10.1111/j.1540-4560.1996.tb01584.x.

Korbin, J. E., Coulton, C. J., Lindstrom-Ufuti, H., & Spilsbury, J. (2000). Neighborhood views on the definition and etiology of child maltreatment. *Child Abuse and Neglect, 24*(12), 1509–1527.

Laming, L. (2009). *The protection of children in England: A progress report*.

Lonne, B., & Parton, N. (2014). Portrayals of child abuse scandals in the media in Australia and England: Impacts on practice, policy and systems. *Child Abuse and Neglect, 38*(5), 822–836.

MacLeod, M. (1997). *Child protection: Everybody's business*. Sutton: Community Care.

Masson, J. (2006). The Climbié Inquiry: Context and critique. *Journal of Law and Society, 33*(2), 221–243.

McLeigh, J. D. (2013). How to form alliances with families and communities: The provision of informal supports to families keeps kids safe. *Child Abuse and Neglect, 37*(5), 17–28.

McLeigh, J. D., & Melton, G. B. (2015). Children's safety in community context. *Child Abuse and Neglect, 41*(1), 1–2.

Meadows, P., Tunstill, J., George, A., Dhudwar, A., & Kurtz, Z. (2011). *The costs and consequences of child maltreatment*. Retrieved from https://www.nspcc.org.uk/globalassets/documents/research-reports/costs-and-consequences-child-maltreatment.pdf

Melton, G. B. (2013). Programs aren't enough: Child protection must become a part of everyday life. *Child Abuse and Neglect, 37*(5), 1–7.

NAPCAN. (2010). Help break down the wall community attitudes survey – Report to the Department of Families, Housing, Community Services and Indigenous Affairs. Retrieved from http://wcitlibrary.pbworks.com/f/NAPCAN_Survey_Report_FINAL_4_June_2010.pdf

Ofsted. (2011). The voice of the child: Learning lessons from serious case reviews: A thematic report of *Ofsted's evaluation of Serious Case Reviews from 1 April to 30 September 2010*. Retreived from https://www.gov.uk/government/publications/listening-to-children-in-serious-case-reviews

Parker, A., & Tritter, J. (2006). Focus group method and methodology: Current practice and recent debate. *International Journal of Research & Method in Education, 29*(1), 23–37.

Parton, N. (1985). *The politics of child abuse*. Basingstoke: Macmillan.

Parton, N. (1991). *Governing the family: Child care, child protection and the state*. London: Macmillan.

Parton, N. (1995). Neglect as child protection: The political context and the practical outcomes. *Children and Society, 9*(1), 67–89.

Parton, N. (2006). *Safeguarding childhood: Early intervention and surveillance in a late modern society*. Basingstoke: Palgrave/Macmillan.

Parton, N. (2014). *The politics of child protection : Contemporary developments and future directions*. Basingstoke: Palgrave/Macmillan.

Radford, J. (2010). *Serious Case Review in respect of the death of a child: Case No. 14 (Khyra Ishaq)*. Birmingham: Birmingham Safeguarding Children Board.

Radford, L., Corral, S., Bradley, C., Fisher, H., Bassett, C., Howat, N., & Collishaw, S. (2011). *Child abuse and neglect in the UK today*. Retrieved from http://doi.org/304.

Rees, G., Stein, M., Hicks, L., & Gorin, S. (2011). *Adolescent neglect: Research, policy and practice*. London: Jessica Kingsley.

Scourfield, J. (2000). The rediscovery of child neglect. *The Sociological Review, 48*(3), 365–382.

Shoesmith, S. (2016). *Learning from Baby P*. London: Jessica Kingsley.

Smithson, J. (2008). Focus groups. In P. Alasuutari, S. Bickman, & J. Brannan (Eds.), *The Sage handbook of social research methods* (pp. 177–198). London: Sage.

Spilsbury, J. C., & Korbin, J. E. (2013). Social networks and informal social support in protecting children from abuse and neglect: Community ties and supports promote children's safety. *Child Abuse and Neglect, 37*(S), 8–9.

Stewart, D. W., Shamdasani, P. N., & Rook, D. W. (2007). *Focus groups: Theory and practice*. London: Sage.

Sussman, S., Burton, D., Dent, C. W., Stacy, A. W., & Flay, B. R. (1991). Use of focus groups in developing an adolescent tobacco use cessation program: Collective norm effects. *Journal of Applied Social Psychology, 21*(21), 1772–1782.

US Department of Health and Human Services Administration for Children and Families, Administration on Children, Youth and Families, Children's Bureau. (2017). *Child maltreatment 2015*. Retrieved from http://www.acf.hhs.gov/programms/cb/research-data-technology/statistics-research/child-maltreatment

Ward, P. (2008). *Sheffield safeguarding children board serious case review: Child D: Executive summary*. Sheffield: Sheffield Safeguarding Children Board.

Ward, H., & Brown, R. (2013). Decision-making within a child's timeframe: A response. Family Law, February, 1181–1186.

Wilkinson, S. (2004). Focus group research. In D. Silverman (Ed.), *Qualitative research: Theory, method and practice* (pp. 177–198). London: Sage.

Williams, S. (2015). *Drawing the line: An exploration of how lay people construct child neglect.* PhD Thesis University of Huddersfield, Huddersfield. Retrieved from http://eprints.hud.ac.uk/25505 The research was was supported by the Economic and Social Research Council (ESRC) grant number ES/1024301/1.

Williams, S. (2017). Redrawing the line: An exploration of how lay people construct child neglect. *Child Abuse & Neglect, 68*, 11–24.

Willig, C. (2008a). Introducing qualitative research in psychology, (2nd ed.). Maidenhead: McGraw-Hill/Open University.

Willig, C. (2008b). Discourse analysis. In J. Smith (Eds.), Qualitative psychology: A practical guide to research methods (pp. 160–185). Los Angeles: Sage Publications.

YouGov/NSPCC. (2012). YouGov/NSPCC child abuse survey results. Retrieved from http://d25d2506sfb94s.cloudfront.net/cumulus_uploads/document/79o3owjw18/YG-NSPCC-Archive-results-141212-child-abuse-UK.pdf

Part II
Conceptualising Public Health Approaches

Chapter 5
Changing and Competing Conceptions of Risk and Their Implications for Public Health Approaches to Child Protection

Nigel Parton

5.1 Introduction

While risk to children has been the central focus for child protection systems and practices over the last 50 years, the way risk is understood has itself been subject to a number of competing and changing conceptions. Although initially the focus was almost exclusively concerned with protecting children from 'significant harm', this has broadened considerably over recent years to a much more positive approach which is concerned with supporting and promoting children's overall development and wellbeing. The latter is often central to approaches which aim to develop a public health approach. Public health approaches focus on reducing the *risk factors* that give rise to maltreatment and therefore prioritise preventive measures which can act on *risk factors* at all levels including the societal, the community, the family, the parents and the child. It emphasises the importance of primary prevention and thereby preventing the occurrence of the condition before it emerges and also secondary prevention, preventing the re-occurrence once the condition has occurred. In the process the objects of concern and the areas for possible intervention are considerably broadened and this has important implications for the role of a wide range of professionals and services.

While there is now clear evidence of public health approaches influencing thinking in a number of jurisdictions – including Australia's national framework for protecting children (Commonwealth of Australia 2009) and the Scottish Government's *Getting it Right for Every Child* (GIRFEC) policy (embedded in the Children and Young People (Scotland Act 2014) – this chapter will draw, primarily, on the example of England for critically analysing such developments. What will become evident is that public health approaches have important implications for the relationship

N. Parton (✉)
School of Human and Health Sciences, University of Huddersfield, Huddersfield, UK
e-mail: n.parton@hud.ac.uk

B. Lonne et al. (eds.), *Re-Visioning Public Health Approaches for Protecting Children*, Child Maltreatment 9, https://doi.org/10.1007/978-3-030-05858-6_5

between children, parents and the professionals with whom they come into contact. It opens up the likelihood of much greater surveillance and has a number of potential unintended as well as intended consequences, particularly in terms of the implications for the rights and civil liberties of children and adults. It will be argued that these constitute major challenges for public health approaches to child protection and that such developments need to be located in their political and social contexts. An analysis of the changing and competing ideas about risk are central for advancing our understanding of public health approaches to child protection and taking policy and practice forward.

5.2 From Dangerousness to Risk

A chapter written by Robert Castel, '*From Dangerousness to Risk*' (Castel 1991), published over 25 years ago, anticipated many of the themes which we will be discussing in this chapter. Castel argued that it was possible to identify an important shift in preventive strategies of 'mental medicine and social work' – from dangerousness to risk. Whereas dangerousness drew attention to the importance of trying to identify and contain individuals who were particularly prone to 'violent and unpredictable action', the contemporary focus on risk was rather different

> A risk does not arise from the presence of particular precise danger embedded in a concrete individual or group. It is the effect of a combination of abstract *factors* which render more or less probable the occurrence of undesirable modes of behaviour (Castel 1991, p. 287).

We can identify a similar shift in focus, from dangerousness to risk, taking place in relation to child protection in England from the mid-1990s until 2010.

The period from the early 1970s witnessed a considerable growth in concerns about child abuse and the failures of professionals to intervene appropriately to protect children. Following the high profile and very public criticisms of social workers and other health and welfare professionals in cases of child abuse in the 1970s and 1980s (Butler and Drakeford 2005; Parton 1985), the long-established state child welfare services in England were put under increasing pressure and came to be dominated by a reactive and forensically-orientated concern with child protection. Similar developments were evident in the other nations in the UK, as well as North America and Australia (Lonne et al. 2009; Waldfogel 1998).

By the early 1990s the child protection and child welfare systems could be characterised in terms of the need to identify 'high risk' cases so that these could be differentiated from the rest. Thereby children could be protected from abuse while ensuring that family privacy was not undermined and scarce resources could be directed to where, in theory, they were most needed (Parton 1991; Parton et al. 1997). 'High risk' was conceptualised in terms of 'dangerousness', for it was the small minority of 'dangerous families' (Dale et al. 1986; Parton and Parton 1989) subject to extreme family dysfunctions and violent personalities, who were seen as the primary cause of child abuse and which therefore needed to be identified so that children could be protected.

This was clear in the official government guidance for England and Wales at the time – *Working Together under the Children Act 1989: A Guide to Arrangements for Inter-Agency Cooperation for the Protection of Children from Abuse* (Home Office et al. 1991) – where the focus of attention was explicitly stated as 'the protection of children from abuse'. This was reinforced further in the only official guide on the purpose and content of professional assessments, *Protecting Children: A Guide for Social Workers Undertaking a Comprehensive Assessment* (Department of Health 1988). At the time Pithers commented that:

> The guide addressed the key issue of whether a family is considered safe for a child, or whether it can be made safe, or whether it is so potentially dangerous that alternatives have to be found (Pithers 1989, p. 18).

However, during the 1990s a major debate opened up about how policies and practices in relation to child protection integrated with and were supported by policies and practices concerned with family support and child welfare more generally (Audit Commission 1994; DH 1995). Rather than simply be concerned with a narrow, forensically-driven focus on child protection, it was argued there needed to be a 'rebalancing' or 'refocusing' of the work, such that policy and practice should be driven by an emphasis on partnership, participation, and prevention (Parton 1997). The priority should be on *helping* parents and children in the community in a supportive way and should keep notions of policing and coercive intervention to a minimum.

This change in thinking was evident in the official guidance published at the end of the decade, *Working Together to Safeguard Children: A Guide to Inter-agency Working to Safeguard and Promote the Welfare of Children* (DH et al. 1999). The words 'protection' and 'abuse' had been dropped from the title which was framed in terms of the general duty placed on local authorities by Section 17(1) of the Children Act 1989 'to safeguard and promote the welfare of children in their area who are in need'. The guidance underlined the fact that local authority social services had wider responsibilities than simply responding to concerns about 'significant harm' and identifying child abuse and was explicitly located in the much wider agenda for children's services being promulgated by the New Labour government (Parton 2006). The *Assessment Framework* (DH et al. 2000) published at the same time as the 1999 *Working Together*, attempted to move the focus from a narrow assessment of risk of 'significant harm' (DH 2001) to one which was concerned with the broader idea of risk of impairment to a child's overall development in the context of their family and community environment.

We can thus identify an important change in the nature of the risk which policy and practice was expected to respond to. The object of concern was no longer simply children at risk of abuse and 'significant harm'. Effective measures to safeguard children were seen as those which also promoted their welfare, and should not be seen in isolation from the wider range of support and services provided to meet the needs of all children and families. There was a broadening of concerns from 'child protection' to 'safeguarding', or, following Castel, from 'dangerousness to risk'.

5.3 Risk and Every Child Matters

The influence of public health thinking became more evident in the 2000s. In 2003/4 the government launched its *Every Child Matters: Change for Children* (ECM) programme (DfES 2004), following the consultative Green Paper *Every Child Matters* (Chief Secretary to the Treasury 2003) which had originally been launched as the government's response to a very high profile child abuse public inquiry into the death of Victoria Climbié (Laming 2003). However, the changes were much broader than simply being concerned with overcoming the problems with responding to cases of child abuse. The priority was to intervene at a much earlier stage in children's lives in order to prevent a range of problems both in childhood and in later life, including poor educational attainment, unemployment, crime and anti-social behaviour. The ambition was to improve the outcomes for all children and to narrow the gap in outcomes between those who did well and those who did not. The outcomes were defined in terms of: being healthy; staying safe; enjoying and achieving; making a positive contribution; and achieving economic well-being. Together these five outcomes were seen as key to improving 'well-being in childhood and later life'. It was a very ambitious programme and was to include *all children*, as it was felt that any child, at some point in their life, could be seen as vulnerable to some form of risk and therefore might require help. The idea was to identify problems before they became chronic. Two figures included in the Green Paper (Figs. 5.2 and 5.3) are particularly helpful in understanding how the reform of children's services was conceptualised.

All children in the population were included in the triangle in Fig. 5.1 and categorised according to their level of vulnerability; while in Fig. 5.2 services were organised according to whether they were specialist, targeted or universal. The idea was that problems would be identified as quickly as possible to ensure they did not escalate and that services were integrated to ensure that this took place.

The approach was heavily influenced by a public health model of prevention and was characterised as 'the paradigm of risk and protection-focused prevention' (France and Utting 2005) informed by risk factor analysis (RFA) (France et al. 2010), whereby the knowledge of risk factors derived from prospective longitudinal research was drawn upon to design particular programmes and re-orientate mainstream services. The work of David Farrington, Professor of Psychological Criminology at the University Cambridge, in relation to youth crime prevention was particularly influential (Farrington 1996, 2000, 2007). What was attractive to policy makers was that a range of overlapping personal and environmental 'risk factors' were identified, not only in relation to future criminal behaviour, violence and drug abuse, but also for educational failure, unsafe sexual behaviour and poor mental health (Dryfoos 1990; Goldblatt and Lewis 1998; Mrazek and Haggerty 1994). The Green Paper stated that:

> we have a good idea what factors shape children's life chances. Research tells us *that the risk of experiencing negative outcomes* is concentrated in children with certain characteristics (Chief Secretary to the Treasury 2003, p.17, emphasis added).

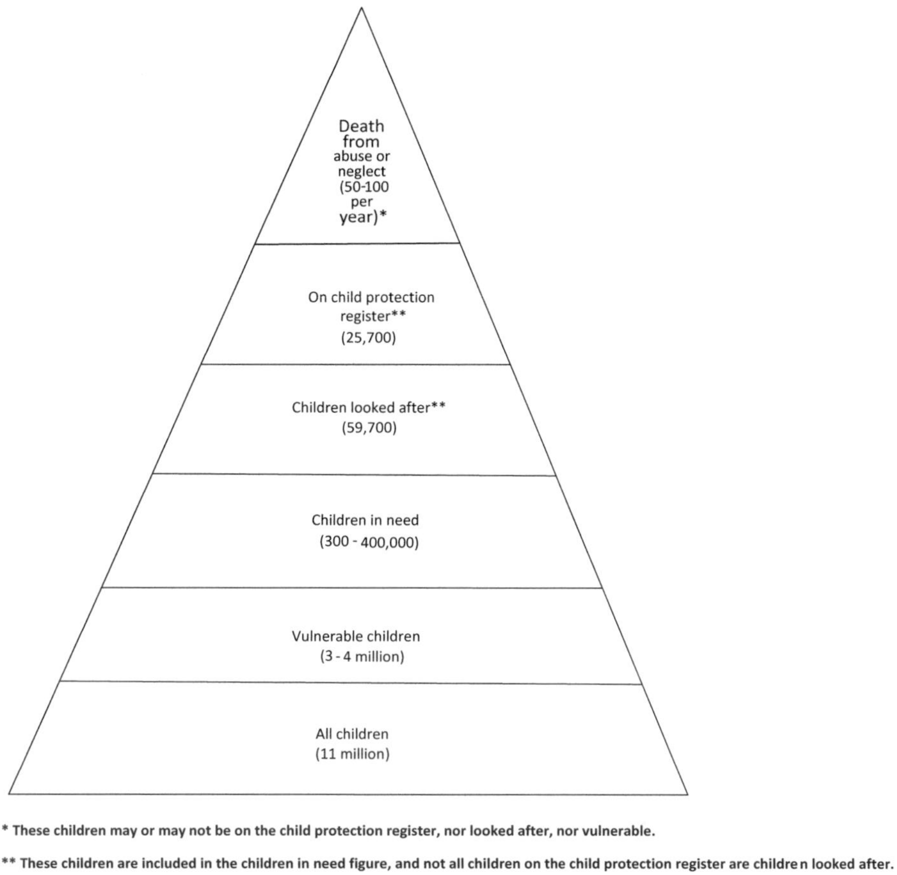

Fig. 5.1 'Every Child Matters': Categorising Children

and included:

- Low income and parental unemployment;
- Homelessness;
- Poor parenting;
- Postnatal depression amongst mothers;
- Low birth weight;
- Substance misuse;
- Individual characteristics, such as intelligence; and
- Community factors, such as living in a disadvantaged community.

The more risk factors a child had, the more likely it was that they would experience 'negative outcomes' and it was 'poor parenting' which was seen to play the key role.

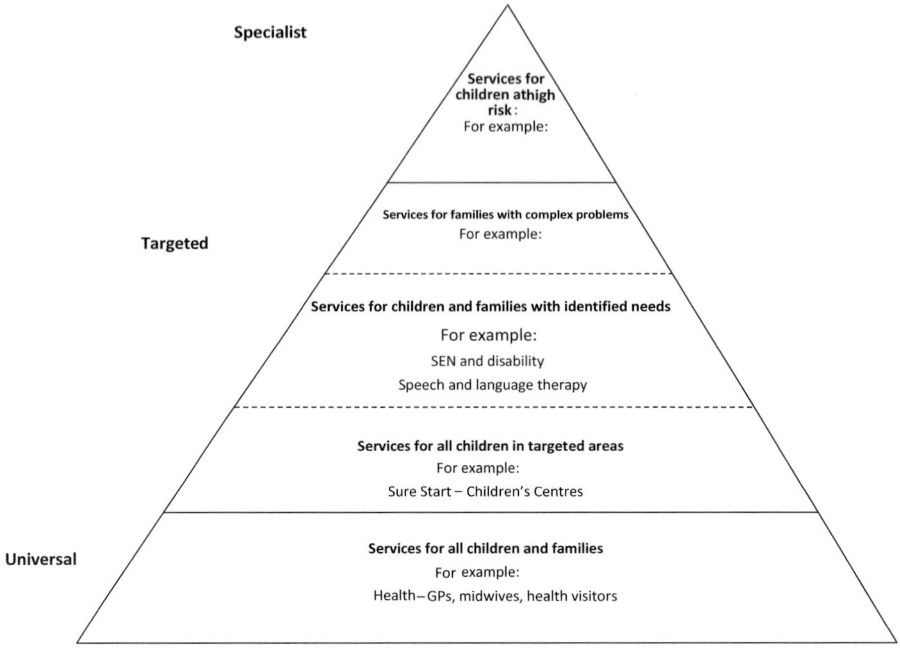

Fig. 5.2 'Every Child Matters': Targeted services within a universal context

However, the role of prevention was not only to combat the negatives involved but to enhance the positive opportunities for child development via maximising protective factors and processes. The approach was informed by the work of Michael Rutter (1990) who conceived of risk and protection as processes rather than fixed states and saw protectors as the basis for opening up opportunities. The timing of interventions was crucial, for – if they were to have the most impact – the 'early years' were key and success depended on recruiting parents – usually mothers – to the role of educators. The notion of protection was thus much wider than simply protection from harm or abuse. In trying to maximise childhood 'strengths' and 'resilience' the idea of risk was itself reframed in far more positive ways.

To achieve the outcomes, the ECM changes aimed to integrate health, social care, education, and criminal justice agencies and thereby overcome traditional organisational and professional 'silos'. Such a development required agencies and professionals to share information so that risks could be identified early and opportunities maximised. To take this forward a variety of new systems of information, communication and technology (ICT) were to be introduced – including the *Common Assessment Framework* (CAF) and *ContactPoint.*

The *Common Assessment Framework* (*CAF*) provides an important insight into the way 'risk' to children was rethought in the context of ECM and the way practice would be reconfigured as a result. The *CAF* was an electronic assessment form to be completed by any professional when they considered a child to have 'additional needs' that required the involvement of more than one service. It included a

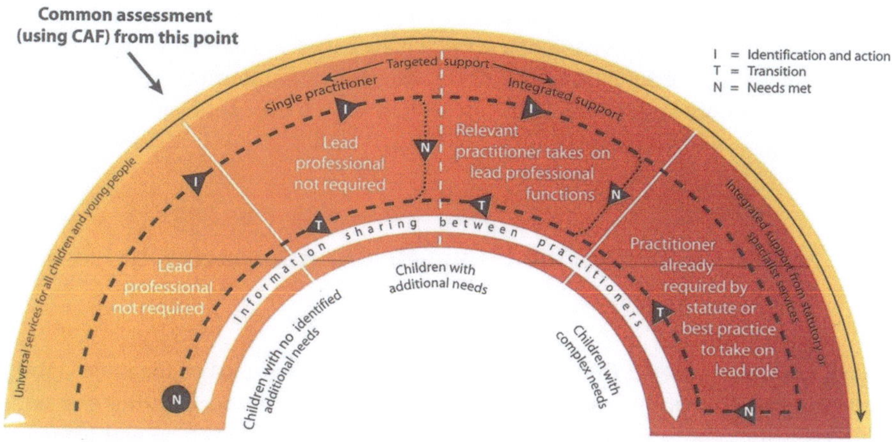

Fig. 5.3 Processes and tools to support children and families. (Source: The Common Assessment Framework for Children and Young People: Practitioners' Guide (CWDC 2009, p.8))

wide-ranging set of data covering most aspects of a child's health and development, including details about parents and siblings. The *CAF* was designed to identify those children who might not progress towards the five *ECM* outcomes without additional services.

The *CAF* was designed to identify 'children with additional needs' and therefore to operate at the level of secondary prevention (or targeted services). The diagram in Fig. 5.3, taken from the *CAF Practitioners' Guide* (CWDC 2009), provides a helpful picture of how the processes and tools designed to integrate children's services and support early intervention were conceived, particularly in the context of Figs. 5.1 and 5.2 earlier.

The *CAF* clearly demonstrates how the importance of early intervention and the growing use of ICT were seen as central for the transformation of children's services in England in the late 2000s. The focus of concern had broadened considerably from those children who might suffer 'significant harm' to include all children, particularly those who were at risk of poor outcomes and therefore who may not fulfil their potential. In the process, the systems designed to screen and identify those in need of attention had grown in size and complexity and the challenges and responsibilities placed upon a wide range of agencies and practitioners increased considerably.

In addition to the *CAF* local authorities were also expected to introduce a national computerised 'Information Sharing Index' which was eventually called *ContactPoint* covering all children. The electronic database would hold basic information on every child in the country, including: The child's name, address, gender and date of birth; a unique number identifying the child; the name and contact details of any person with parental responsibility or who had care of the child at any time; the name and contact details of any educational institution; primary medical services or any specialist or targeted services provided; the name of a nominated 'Lead

Professional' if there was one; and a recording of whether a *CAF* had been carried out. Finally, where the provision of a service had ceased and a decision was made to extend the periods of retention beyond the one year minimum this would indicate that the practitioner still had information to share which they believed to be relevant for others.

5.4 Major Challenges for Public Health Approaches to Child Protection

The *Every Child Matters Change for Children Programme* marked the most significant change in the philosophy and delivery of children's services in England since 1948 (Hudson, 2005) requiring a variety of organisational, practical and technical changes. However there were also major challenges arising directly from the rationales and assumptions which underpinned the changes. Four such challenges are discussed here related to (1) secondary prevention; (2) problem specificity; (3) screening and the identification of risk; and (4) surveillance, confidentiality and civil liberties – and each has implications for the way public health approaches to child protection might be developed.

5.4.1 Secondary Prevention

One of the problems for any attempt to apply a public health approach is that while the explanation of the risks to be addressed is often at the broader environmental level the actual preventive interventions introduced are usually at the secondary level (Freeman 1992; Hardiker et al. 1989). So the focus of ECM was not to bolster and invest in universal primary services as such, though clearly it was envisaged that universal services (particularly health and education) would play a key role in the identification of children with 'additional needs'; and, while investment did take place in relation to the introduction of some of the new organisational requirements and systems (such as the *CAF* and *ContactPoint)* investment in the provision of new services, apart from the funding of the new community based children's centres (Lewis 2011), was relatively minimal. However, as Fig. 5.1 earlier estimated there were between three and four million vulnerable children who may have 'additional needs', accounting for about a third of the population of children and young people. It is not clear that secondary prevention is able to take on such a large and strategic role in in the new landscape of children's services.

The assumption that money will be saved from the most expensive 'specialist' services (at the apex of the Fig. 5.2 triangle) which can be invested to expand secondary level services may be very difficult to deliver in practice. Attempts to reconfigure priorities are always in danger of being marginalised by the impact of high profile media and political criticisms arising from child abuse scandals (see for example Parton 2014 chapter 5; and Gainsborough 2010). However, beyond this there are two other related significant challenges.

First, to move resources and expertise from tertiary services in order to invest in secondary services until the secondary services have become established and their positive impact demonstrated is very difficult. This connects with the second issue, for it is not at all clear whether increased activity in the secondary level would have the effect of reducing demands on the tertiary level. Nor is it clear whether success should be measured by a reduction of referrals to the tertiary level for it can be argued that an important measure of the increased effectiveness of intervention at the secondary level would be that children and young people requiring 'specialist' tertiary level services were being identified who were previously ignored. It might therefore be that increased resources are required at both the secondary and tertiary levels. The success of such a development is likely to be dependent, in part, on the sensitivity of the screening processes which are put in place and the ability to identify different types and levels of risk, an issue I will address shortly.

5.4.2 Problem Specificity

A major attraction of public health approaches is their emphasis upon prevention. The idea of prevention rests on the view that ensuring that something does not happen is surely better than dealing with the consequences once it has. However, there is a danger that we miss the extent that prevention is not only a technical project but also a normative one so that while the general case for prevention may be unarguable the specific proposals may be seen as immoral, unjust or simply not worth it. For while prevention invites agreement and support at the general abstract level, specific proposals can invite disagreement and potential conflict.

As we have seen the period in England between the mid-1990s and the late 2000s, a considerable broadening of the objects of concern has occured – from significant harm to children and young people who might be at risk of not fulfilling their potential. In the process there was an elision of concerns about children and young people who might be 'at risk' from a whole range of different threats, including abuse, with concerns about children and young people who might pose a risk to others, particularly by falling into crime or anti-social behaviour (Munro 2010). The agendas around care and control of children, young people and their families and the relationship between different approaches which may be more welfare oriented and others which might have a more punitive focus became very blurred (James and James 2008; Sharland 2006).

Because the focus is upon identifying and intervening in the *risk factors* prior to the condition emerging the *risk factors* act as something of a proxy for the condition itself. In the process there can be much vagueness about the relationship between cause and effect and how outcomes can be predicted. The approach can fail to differentiate between quite different types of human problems, the moral and political differences involved and how far there is a social consensus on not only what the problem is but how it can best be addressed. This is associated with the related question of how far those identified as 'at risk' will be expected to participate fully in the help offered, or whether they will be *required* to receive the intervention. This is in a context where for many parents and children the problem is that the extra services and help they want and need, in the format and at the time they can use it, is simply not available. Who decides what the nature and priority of the risk is and what services are most appropriate can be highly contentious and subject to quite different views.

5.4.3 The Identification of Risk

Public health approaches heavily rely on epidemiological studies of the population in order to identify relevant *risk factors* (Aziz 2017). While this is important if the policies introduced are themselves located at the population level, invariably these *risk factors* are applied at the community, familial or individual levels. In predicting actual child maltreatment risk instruments have a high level of false positives (children inaccurately identified as high risk) as well as a small but significant number of false negatives (children who are at high risk but who are adjudged as safe) (Munro 2004; Parton 1989). David Farrington, whose research had been so influential in informing government policy in England has clearly stated that predictive accuracy is not sufficiently robust to support the screening of 'high risk' families when trying to predict future criminality (Farrington 2007). While research points to who might be 'at risk', this is a very inexact science. The major point is that *risk factors* are identified by research which is based on assessing a large number of aggregate data over time, which is very different to practitioners who are concerned with applying such *risk factors* to a *particular* child, family or community.

These challenges are well illustrated by the analyses that have been carried out over recent years in England of serious case reviews (SCRs). A SCR is a local enquiry carried out where a child has died or been seriously harmed and abuse or neglect are known or suspected, and there is cause for concern about professional practices. The most recent study (Sidebotham et al. 2016) was the fifth such study carried out by the same research team dating back to 2003–05. This particular study considered a total of 293 SCRs relating to incidents which occurred between 1 April 2011 and 31 March 2014. They were also analysed in the context of learning from SCRs since 2003, a total of 1,100 SCRs. One of the key findings was that only 12% of children at the centre of a SCR had a current child protection plan in place at the time of the death or serious harm, and this at a time when the number of child protection plans nationally had increased from 34,000 in 2007/8 to 63,310 in 2015/16. The report argues that while children are harmed within contexts of risk and vulnerability and that there are many opportunities to prevent abuse and protect children, it is clearly not possible to predict with any accuracy which particular children may be harmed, when or in what manner.

5.4.4 *Surveillance, Confidentiality and Civil Liberties*

A central feature of any public health approach is the need to increase the surveillance of the population and to gather and share information and thereby improve attempts at prevention. As we saw earlier the ECM reforms in England stressed the importance of professionals sharing information in order to identify risk and drew on newly created electronic systems to bring this about. This was seen to pose considerable challenges to maintaining confidentiality for the child, young person and the parents while also increasing the surveillance mechanisms by and over the professionals (Anderson et al. 2009; Broadhurst et al. 2010; Parton 2006; Wastell et al. 2010). In the process the boundaries between the public and the private, the state and the family become increasingly blurred and the rights of the child put at risk (Parton 2006; Roche 2008).

These are not simply legal issues of principal because issues of privacy and confidentiality have been identified as crucial as to whether clients engage with services and, even more significantly, whether clients, both children and adults, come forward in the first place. For example, research by Hallett and her colleagues (Hallett et al. 2003) clearly demonstrated that the most important factor which influences whether young people are prepared to discuss their problems is whether they feel they can trust the person they are telling to keep their problems confidential, particularly those working in statutory agencies. Other research exploring the views of young people found they would be reluctant to share information of a sensitive nature and some said they would prefer to forego vital services if their need for privacy was not respected (Children's Rights Alliance for England 2006; Hilton and Mills 2007). A major reason why confidential helplines have proved so popular with both adults and children is that they give the person making the call a large degree of control about what information they want to share (Wattam 1999).

In England concerns about state surveillance, the sharing of personal information and the potential undermining of civil liberties informed many of the high profile criticisms of the ECM changes. *ContactPoint* was subject to considerable debate and change (see for example Munro and Parton 2007), and when the Conservative/Liberal Democrat Coalition government came to power in 2010 one of its first actions was to withdraw *Every Child Matters*, cancel *ContactPoint,* and no longer made the use of the *CAF* compulsory.

5.5 Conclusions

This chapter has not focused on the advantages of public health approaches to child maltreatment; these will receive considerable attention elsewhere in this book. What it has done is try to identify some of the major challenges that such developments may face and has drawn particularly on the experiences of the ECM programme in England to illustrate. How we understand and respond to risk is seen as being of central importance. In doing so it suggests that there is a major tension between the much broader and more positive ideas about risk concerned with engaging the wider society in helping to maximise the well-being and development of all children when there is also a growing emphasis upon individualised notions of responsibility and accountability and which therefore has implications for the role and relationships between parents, professionals and the children and young people themselves. In particular it suggests that at a time when many of the long term universal health and welfare services are being cut back and withdrawn altogether we have to be very careful what we do in the name of public health and prevention.

References

Anderson, R., Brown, I., Dowty, T., Inglesant, P., Heath, W., & Sasse, A. (2009). *Database state*. York: Joseph Rowntree Reform Trust.

Audit Commission. (1994). *Seen but not heard: Coordinating community health and social services for children in need*. London: HMSO.

Aziz, H. A. (2017). A review of the role of public health informatics in healthcare. *Journal of Taibah University Medical Sciences, 12*(1), 78–81.

Broadhurst, K., Hall, C., Wastell, D., White, S., & Pithouse, A. (2010). Risk, instrumentalism and the humane project in social work: Identifying the *informal* logics of risk management in children's statutory services. *British Journal of Social Work, 40*(4), 1046–1065.

Butler, I., & Drakeford, M. (2005). *Scandal, social policy and social welfare*. Bristol: Policy Press.

Castel, R. (1991). From dangerousness to risk. In G. Burchell, C. Gordon, & P. Miller (Eds.), *The Foucault effect: Studies in governmentality*. Hemel Hempstead: Harvester-Wheatsheaf.

Chief Secretary to the Treasury. (2003). *Every child matters* (Cm. 5860). London: Stationery Office.

Children's Rights Alliance for England. (2006). *Children and young people talk about information sharing*. London: CRAE.

Children's Workforce Development Council. (2009). *Common assessment framework for children and young people: Practitioners' guide. Integrated working to improve outcomes for children and young people*. Leeds: CWDC.

Commonwealth of Australia. (2009). *Protecting children is everyone's business: National framework for protecting Australia's children 2009–2020*. Canberra: Australian Government.

Dale, P., Davies, M., Morrison, T., & Waters, J. (1986). *Dangerous families: Assessment and treatment of child abuse*. London: Tavistock.

Department for Education and Skills. (2004). *Every child matters: Change for children*. London: DfES.

Department of Health. (1995). *Child protection: Messages from research*. London: HMSO.

Department of Health. (1988). *Protecting children: A guide for social workers undertaking a comprehensive assessment*. London: HMSO.

Department of Health. (2001). *Studies informing the framework for the assessment of children in need and their families*. London: Stationery Office.

Department of Health (DH), Department of Education and Employment, Home Office. (2000). *Framework for the assessment of children and their families*. London: Stationery Office.

Department of Health, Home Office, and Department of Education and Employment. (1999). *Working together to safeguard children: A guide to inter-agency working to safeguard and promote the welfare of children*. London: Stationery Office.

Dryfoos, J. G. (1990). *Adolescents at risk: Prevalence and prevention*. Oxford: Oxford University Press.

Farrington, D. (1996). *Understanding and preventing youth crime*. York: Joseph Rowntree Foundation.
Farrington, D. (2000). Explaining and preventing crime: The globalisation of knowledge. *Criminology, 38*(1), 1–24.
Farrington, D. (2007). Childhood risk factors and risk-focused prevention. In M. Maguire, R. Morgan, & R. Reiner (Eds.), *The Oxford handbook of criminology* (4th ed.). Oxford: Oxford University Press.
France, A., Freiberg, K., & Homel, R. (2010). Beyond risk factors: Towards a holistic prevention paradigm for children and young people. *British Journal of Social Work, 40*(4), 1192–1210.
France, A., & Utting, D. (2005). The paradigm of "risk and protection-focussed prevention" and its impact on services for children and families. *Children & Society, 19*(2), 77–90.
Freeman, R. (1992). The idea of prevention: A critical review. In S. Scott, G. Williams, S. Platt, & H. Thomas (Eds.), *Private risks and public dangers*. Aldershot: Avebury.
Gainsborough, J. F. (2010). *Scandalous politics: Child welfare politics in the states*. Washington, DC: Georgetown University Press.
Goldblatt, P., & Lewis, C. (Eds.). (1998). *Reducing offending* (Home Office Research Study No.187). London: HMSO.
Hallett, C., Murray, C., & Punch, S. (2003). Young people and welfare: Negotiating pathways). In C. Hallett & A. Prout (Eds.), *Hearing the voices of children: Social policy for the new century*. London: Routledge Farmer.
Hardiker, P., Exton, K., & Barker, M. (1989). *Policies and practices in preventive child care, Report to the Department of Health, Supplement 11*. Leicester: University of Leicester School of Social Work.
Hilton, Z., & Mills, C. (2007). Ask the children. *Criminal Justice, 16*, 16–18.
Home Office, Department of Health, Department of Education and Science, and the Welsh Office. (1991). *Working together under the Children Act 1989: A guide to arrangements for inter-agency cooperation for the protection of children from abuse*. London: HMSO.
Hudson, B. (2005). Partnership working and the children's services agenda: Is it feasible? *Journal of Integrated Care, 13*(2), 7–17.
James, A., & James, A. (2008). Changing childhood in the UK: Reconstructing discourses of 'risk' and 'protection'. In A. James & A. James (Eds.), *European childhoods: Cultures, politics and childhoods in Europe*. Basingstoke: Palgrave/Macmillan.
Laming Report. (2003). *The Victoria Climbie inquiry: Report of the inquiry by Lord Laming* (Cm. 5730). London: Stationery Office.
Lewis, J. (2011). From Sure Start to children's centres: An analysis of policy change in English early years programmes. *Journal of Social Policy, 40*(1), 71–88.
Lonne, B., Parton, N., Thomson, J., & Harries, M. (2009). *Reforming child protection*. London: Routledge.
Lord Laming. (2003). *The Victoria Climbié Inquiry: Report of an inquiry by Lord Laming* (Cm. 5730). London: Stationery Office.
Mrazek, P. J., & Haggerty, K. J. (Eds.). (1994). *Reducing risks for mental disorders: Frontiers for preventive intervention research*. Washington, DC: Institute of Medicine/National Academy Press.
Munro, E. (2004). A simpler way to understand the results of risk assessment instruments. *Children and Youth Services Review, 26*(9), 877–887.
Munro, E. (2010). Conflating risks: Implications for accurate risk prediction in child welfare services. *Health, Risk and Society, 12*(2), 119–130.
Munro, E., & Parton, N. (2007). How far is England in the process of introducing a mandatory reporting system? *Child Abuse Review, 16*(1), 5–16.
Parton, C., & Parton, N. (1989). Child protection, the law and dangerousness. In O. Stevenson (Ed.), *Child abuse: Public policy and professional practice*. Hemel Hempstead: Harvester-Wheatsheaf.
Parton, N. (1985). *The politics of child abuse*. Basingstoke: Macmillan.

Parton, N. (1989). Child abuse. In B. Kahan (Ed.), *Child care: Research, policy and practice*. London: Hodder and Stoughton.
Parton, N. (1991). *Governing the family: Child care, child protection and the state*. Basingstoke: Macmillan.
Parton, N. (Ed.). (1997). *Child protection and family support: Tensions, contradictions and possibilities*. London: Routledge.
Parton, N. (2006). *Safeguarding childhood: Early intervention and surveillance in a late modern state*. Basingstoke: Palgrave/Macmillan.
Parton, N. (2014). *The politics of child protection: Contemporary developments and future directions*. Basingstoke: Palgrave/Macmillan.
Parton, N., Thorpe, D., & Wattam, C. (1997). *Child protection: Risk and the moral order*. Basingstoke: Macmillan.
Pithers, D. (1989). A guide through the maze of child protection. *Social Work Today, 20*(18), 18–19.
Roche, J. (2008). Children's rights, confidentiality and the policing of children. *International Journal of Children's Rights, 16*(4), 431–456.
Rutter, M. (1990). Psychosocial resilience and protective mechanisms. In J. Rolf, A. S. Masten, D. Cichetti, K. H. Nuechterlein, & S. Weintraub (Eds.), *Risk and protective factors in the development of psychopathology*. Cambridge: Cambridge University Press.
Sharland, E. (2006). Young people, risk taking and risk making: Some thoughts for social work. *British Journal of Social Work, 36*(2), 247–265.
Sidebotham, P., Brandon, M., Bailey, S., Belderson, P., Dodsworth, J., Garstang, J., Harrison, E., Retzer, A., & Sorensen, P. (2016). *Pathways to harm, pathways to protection: A triennia analysis of serious case reviews 2011–2014*. London: Department for Education.
Waldfogel, J. (1998). *The future of child protection: How to break the cycle of abuse and neglect*. Cambridge, MA: Harvard University Press.
Wastell, D., White, S., Broadhurst, K., Peckover, S., & Pithouse, A. (2010). Children's services in the iron cage of performance management: Streetlevel buruaucracy and the spectre of Svejkism. *International Journal of Social Welfare, 19*(3), 310–320.
Wattam, C. (1999). Confidentiality and the social organisation of telling. In N. Parton & C. Wattam (Eds.), *Child sexual abuse: Responding to the experiences of children*. Chichester: Wiley.

Chapter 6
Using an Injury Prevention Model to Inform a Public Health Approach to Child Protection

Carol W. Runyan and Desmond K. Runyan

6.1 Introduction

Although child abuse was first described in the French medical literature more than 150 years ago (Labbe 2005) a trio of American medical papers published between 1946 and 1962 are credited with creating national and international recognition and ushering in a new era of social service and law enforcement response with mandated professional reporting (Caffey 1946; Kempe et al. 1962; Woolley and Evans 1955). The problem has not abated. In 2000, the World Health Organization data estimated 57,000 child homicides globally (Krug et al. 2002). In the United States the rate of child maltreatment deaths was estimated at 2.25 per 1,000 children in 2015 (1,670 children).

Many more children are reported as abused or neglected; but even the large numbers of reported children appear to underestimate the size of the problem by a factor of 10 or more when surveys are conducted among parents and children (Gilbert et al. 2008; Theodore et al. 2005). Self-report data from parents and children estimate a global burden of child sexual abuse of 127 per 1,000 children and a burden for physical abuse of 226 per 1,000 children (Stoltenborgh et al. 2015). These rates yield global estimates of 241.3 million sexually abused and 429 million physically

C. W. Runyan (✉)
Colorado School of Public Health, Program for Injury Prevention, Education and Research, University of Colorado, Denver, CO, USA
e-mail: carol.runyan@ucdenver.edu

D. K. Runyan
Department of Pediatrics, University of Colorado, Denver, CO, USA

Department of Epidemiology, Colorado School of Public Health, Aurora, CO, USA

Kempe Center for the Prevention and Treatment of Child Abuse and Neglect, Denver, CO, USA
e-mail: Des.Runyan@ucdenver.edu

B. Lonne et al. (eds.), *Re-Visioning Public Health Approaches for Protecting Children*, Child Maltreatment 9, https://doi.org/10.1007/978-3-030-05858-6_6

abused children each year. More worrisome is that even these large numbers likely underestimate the scope as stigma and social desirability lead to under-reporting by parents or children. Clearly, even in countries with well-developed child protection systems, the scope of the problem is far greater than the availability of interventions and treatment. Prevention through public health solutions is not only critical to keep children safe; it is the only option to reduce this epidemic.

6.2 Public Health Perspective – Overview

Public health is a multidisciplinary field with a focus on preventing health problems in whole communities or societies. The key elements are a population perspective, a focus on primary prevention, and interventions that rely on evidence and attempt to solve the root causes of problems through large-scale social change. More detail on each of these points follows.

Last defined public health as 'the combination of sciences, skills, and beliefs that are directed at the maintenance and improvement of the health of all the people' (Last 1983). Beauchamp describes public health as being grounded in social justice in a classic paper that differentiates social justice from market justice (Beauchamp 1976). He argues that public health should strive to demonstrate principles of communitarian values (Beauchamp 1985) in which societies are engaged in promoting the welfare of the community rather than promoting individualism. Bernstein (2006) has contrasted these two approaches as the 'We're in this together' mindset (WITT) versus a 'You're on your own', or YOYO, mindset. These value differences are evident in the current discourse in contemporary culture; creating challenges for maintaining the approaches that public health has embraced for centuries.

6.2.1 Population Perspective

Public health is distinctive from medicine, which serves patients one at a time for identified health problems, in that the 'patient' for public health is the whole community, a 'population perspective' (McGavran 1958; Rose 1992). Adopting a population perspective requires a shift in mindset from a focus on individual responsibility to one that values communal action and communal goals. Examples in obesity prevention include making neighborhoods safe and walkable, as well as enhancing access to groceries with affordable healthy foods, which enable individuals to make healthy choices. Historically, much of the focus of population level change has involved interventions to improve physical environments (e.g., air, water, buildings, roadways, workplaces). However, changes in social environments also are important. Rather than relying on individuals or families to develop safer behaviors, the public health approach seeks to change how communities are organized and what structures are in place to assist families (e.g., affordable child care, quality schools, livable wages).

A 'population perspective' leads to conceptualizing health and disease differently with different questions than an individual perspective. The population approach examines whole communities, seeking to understand what the characteristics are of a community, nation, or culture that makes it healthier and safer, or alternatively, more dangerous than others. Gun violence is much higher in the United States than in Australia and is linked to differences in access, ownership, regulations about safe storage, and differences in socio-cultural beliefs about freedom and guns. Similarly, harsh corporal punishment patterns vary from one country or region to another (Runyan et al. 2010). By recognizing differences at this level, we can propose solutions that will impact the larger population (Rose 1992). This perspective may feel foreign for those oriented to working with individual level interventions or with individual clients, particularly realizing, as Rose points out, that any given individual may not benefit from the intervention – the 'prevention paradox'.

Rose argued that we can change the distribution of a health problem by reducing risk, even a little, for everyone rather than focusing only on the high-risk individuals. Lowering the median level of lipids in an entire population will have a salutary effect on risk of cardiac disease within the population and reduce the number of heart attacks. Following this logic, if we reduce the percentage of parents who hit their children, we will reduce the size of the tail-end of the distribution – those engaging in very harsh or abusive discipline. Reductions in the rates of corporal punishment in the United States mirror reductions in reported child abuse, serving as supportive evidence for the effectiveness of this population approach.

6.2.2 *Primary Prevention*

Preventing problems before they occur, rather than waiting to treat problems after they occur, is a touchstone of public health. This approach is referred to as 'moving upstream' – a metaphor derived from an 1895 poem by Joseph Malins, "The Ambulance in the Valley" as cited by Hemenway (2009). The poem describes ambulances waiting to rescue drowning people from a river in contrast with the alternative approach – going upstream to install a fence, preventing falls into the water.

Primary prevention, or preventing diseases or conditions before they occur, is the first of three levels of prevention. Primary prevention examples include: assuring proper nutrition, reducing workplace hazards, or supporting quality parenting. *Secondary prevention* involves identifying existing problems through screening and early intervention to reduce spread or exacerbation. Secondary prevention examples include screening for birth defects among newborns or for colon cancer in adults. In the realm of child abuse, secondary prevention includes telling children who have experienced unwanted sexual touching to tell someone. *Tertiary prevention* is treatment and rehabilitation to remediate harm. This describes the work of child protective services; employing medical, psychological, child welfare or legal services to stop the maltreatment and prevent further harm.

A somewhat different typology for categorizing prevention uses the labels *Universal*, *Selected*, and *Indicated*. These labels describe distinctions based upon the targets of the prevention activities rather than the timing of intervention. *Universal* approaches address all members of the community regardless of risk or disease status. *Selected* approaches are those directed at high-risk persons based on socio-demographic attributes or risky behaviors (e.g., teenage parents or those with a family history of domestic violence). *Indicated* approaches are directed at persons who have already demonstrated undesirable behaviors or outcomes; for example, parents who have already been reported for abuse.

6.3 Evidence-Based Practice

Public health interventions need to be derived from sound theory and/or empirical work. Just as automotive engineers rely on principles of physics and evaluation of different product designs, and physicians use the scientific method to develop new medications or procedures, public health draws upon research to formulate its approaches. Public health applies the principles of assessment (measurement), assurance of services, and policy development in an iterative cycle working to improve the health of the public (Institute of Medicine 1988). Assessing health problems in a population relies upon ongoing monitoring of the nature and magnitude of health problems – in public health parlance 'surveillance'. For example, child fatality review systems examine child deaths and look for patterns such as deaths associated with unsafe sleep practices, lack of use of child restraint devices, or events resulting in abusive head trauma (Christian and Sege 2010). By monitoring trends, public health professionals can observe patterns and direct interventions to change those patterns.

Sound evidence-based practice relies on strong conceptual and theoretical frameworks, rigorous evaluation of long- and short-term outcomes, and process evaluation of delivery or implementation. Once an intervention's effectiveness is established, widespread adoption of the intervention is needed for population level impact.

6.3.1 Conceptual Models Used in Public Health

The agent-host-environment model provides the basic conceptual foundation of the public health approach. Susser's and Andjelkovich (1973) book presented this simple ecological system, emphasizing the interaction among factors that contribute to health problems. In later papers, he compared his way of thinking to nested boxes to depict the notion of layers of influences (Susser and Susser 1996). This conceptualization closely parallels the social-ecologic theory articulated by Uri Bronfenbrenner in the context of child development (Bronfenbrenner 1979). The social-ecologic model, with slight variations in terminology, has been applied by others to injury and violence broadly (Runyan 2003) (Fig. 6.1) and child maltreatment specifically.

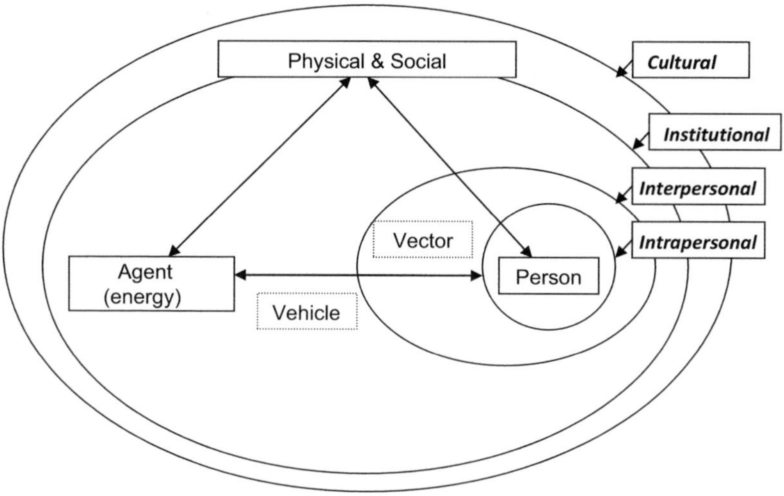

Fig. 6.1 Integration of Public Health Model with Bronfenbrenner's Social-Ecological Model. (Appeared in Runyan 2003)

These models address characteristics of the individual (i.e., the *intrapersonal*). For example, Barr et al. (2009) noted the pattern of inconsolable infant crying peaking at 3–4 months of age and suggested this is a risk factor for abusive head trauma. Similarly, other child characteristics such as activity level, gender, size, physical and intellectual capabilities, or disabilities may influence how the child is perceived by his or her caregivers and may alter engagement with the child or engender frustration.

The next conceptually encircling layer of the social-ecologic model is the *interpersonal level*. This layer refers to relationships among family members and peers. This may include, for example, the ways in which parents give or withhold emotional support to children and how they respond to challenges associated with the child's developmental characteristics or behaviors, or to intimate partner violence occurring between parents.

The *organizational or institutional level* considers the environment or communities in which people engage (e.g., schools, workplaces, religious organizations, or other community groups). Social networks may influence how parents engage with their children in that disciplinary practices observed by parents in childcare settings or demonstrated by other parents at the playground may serve as role models. Parenting education provided in high schools is intended to influence how teens learn future parenting. Employers may create more family-friendly businesses, either by design of the work or of the workplace, including flexible schedules, onsite childcare, supplements to support child care, paid parental leave, and health benefits--all of these factors may influence parenting.

At an even broader level are characteristics of the culture – referred to as the *socio-cultural level*. This level includes the cultural norms in a society such as disciplinary practices or norms about which parents perform which roles. The socio-political context influences issues such as corporal punishment in schools or social acceptability of spanking by parents, state-level policies for minimum wage or paid family leave, and how legal systems address child abuse and neglect (e.g., custody, foster care or prosecution of offenders).

Public health often employs multiple strategies together to address prevention. Recent documents from the US Centers for Disease Control and Prevention outline this approach to child maltreatment prevention with a variety of strategies to promote safe, stable, nurturing relationships and environments (Fortson et al. 2016).

6.4 Injury Prevention Models

6.4.1 Overview

Injury prevention draws on the public health host-agent-environment model, as well as the social-ecologic framework and employs multiple approaches to change risk. Education, regulation, legislation and litigation are all valid approaches, each of which can be employed in multiple ways. Education may be directed at individuals who are vulnerable and/or at those who make decisions. Examples include employers who make decisions related to employee welfare (e.g., family leave policy), the safety of their products (e.g., safety of cribs, toys, cars, prescription drugs, or marijuana), or their product packaging (e.g., marijuana or drug packaging to reduce ingestion by children). Education may also be directed at government policy makers to impact regulatory or legislative decisions. Changes in government regulations for institutions may include day care quality standards or corporal punishment policies in schools or professions (e.g., abuse reporting requirements). Legislation, a particular form of regulation, can shape safety for children (e.g., tax allocations for child care, legislating a minimum wage) and mandate rules for data collection or use of evidence in courts (e.g., mandated reporting of child abuse). Finally, litigation, or the threat of litigation, can be a powerful tool for change. For example, litigation has been used successfully to assure safer standards on multiple types of consumer products in the US as well as in encouraging better professional practices (e.g., medical malpractice) or addressing child protective worker caseloads or practices.

6.4.2 Haddon Matrix

Dr. William Haddon incorporated Susser's agent-host-environment public health model into a matrix that included timing of the intervention to address the prevention of injury (Haddon 1980). The agent in Susser's classic model is often an infectious organism, transferred to the host through either a vehicle or vectors. Vehicles are inanimate objects (e.g., unsanitary eating utensils, infected needle) whereas vectors are animate (e.g., mosquitoes carrying the malaria organism, plasmodium falciparum; or humans spreading colds directly from person to person).

In creating his matrix, Haddon drew on the work of Gibson (1961), a psychologist who defined the agent of injury as 'energy' that is transmitted to the human as analogous to how infectious diseases are transmitted by specific infectious agents. Just as there are bacteria and viruses, Haddon described energy of several types. One type is mechanical energy, such as in a car crash, a fall, or blunt trauma from being hit by a person or object where mechanical forces are transmitted in amounts that cause injury. Energy transfer may also take the forms of the transfer of chemical energy (e.g., poisoning by either ingestion or inhalation), thermal energy (e.g., touching a fire or hot stove); electrocution (e.g., lightning or contact with electrical outlets), and radiation energy (e.g., sunburn or X-rays).

Clearly, the transfer of energy may result in physical abuse (e.g., hitting a child transfers mechanical energy, cigarette burns result from thermal energy, pre-natal exposures to alcohol or other drugs are from chemical energy). Waller (1985) defined injury as processes resulting from the absence of an essential agent (e.g., oxygen in drowning or absence of heat in frostbite). Some forms of child neglect are more easily categorized in this way. Other forms of abuse (e.g., sexual assault or psychological abuse) are not easily classified as an energy transfer, although the concept of a vector (perpetrator) transmitting the abuse is still relevant and allows the problem to be considered within the context of the Haddon Matrix.

The Haddon matrix has been used in two ways – one to explain what the risk or protective factors might be for an injury problem; another to generate ideas about possible interventions. In the matrix, columns represent components of the host-agent-environment model as elements that can be changed, and the rows depict timing or phases in the prevention process. The rows are loosely derived from the principles of primary, secondary and tertiary prevention. While Haddon initially created the model to address motor vehicle safety, it can easily be applied to any public health problem, including child maltreatment, as shown in Fig. 6.2 (Runyan and Brandspigel 2016).

The first step in using the matrix is to delineate clearly what each row and column depicts. For example, in child maltreatment, one may define the host as children in the family, the vector as the abusing person(s), and the physical environment as where the child interacts with the vector (e.g., home, childcare facility, school, workplace, neighborhood). The social environment is the larger social and community environment in which this all takes place. The social environment may be conceptualized to include cultural norms and practices as well as laws and policies that may influence abusive or neglectful behaviors.

Second, the 'event' must be clearly defined. In the case of a motor vehicle crash it is easy – it is the crash itself, making it relatively simple to define what is pre-crash (the first row) and post-crash (the bottom row). For violence such as child maltreatment, where the events may be repetitive, it is helpful to think through whether the 'event' is the *first instance* or *any instance*. Often with violence,

Child Maltreatment Deaths				
Phases during which intervention has its effect ⬇	Factors to be changed			
	Person (child)	Vector (abuser) or Vehicle (implements used for abuse) as channels through which energy is transmitted	Physical and Social Environments (family/home, community/organizations, social/policy)	
			Physical Environments	Social Environments
Pre-event *(before maltreatment starts)*	• Address behavioral issues with children that may trigger negative parental reactions • Correct conditions that may make child more vulnerable to abuse (e.g., gastro-esophogeal reflux; chronic ear infections) • Early treatment of disabilities that create excess stress for caregivers	• Reduce parental use of substances • Help parents learn to identify proper caregivers • Encourage bonding between parents, caregivers, and their children • Parenting education, especially around early childhood development • Teach parents resilience, coping skills & help-seeking behaviors • Educate caregivers about handling difficult crying	• Ensure safe child care facilities are safe, stable and nurturing environments (safe toys, safe equipment, sturdy facilities) • Reduce crowded living arrangements that create stress • Design child care facilities to ensure supervision, child visibility and monitoring • Housing free of fall, burn, electrical, chemical, drowning, and other hazards (e.g., carbon monoxide and smoke detectors; locked medications & guns; pool fences, baby gates)	• Improve norms around positive parenting • Prohibit corporal punishment in schools • Accessible, affordable, and quality child care with well-trained staff • Accessible behavioral health services for parents, caregivers, and children & improved norms about help-seeking • Increase access to home visiting services & family resource centers • Prevent unintended pregnancies & increase high school completion • Create policies that are supportive of families (increase protective factors); increase positive support at the local level (government, schools, organizations, businesses) • Universal access to free kindergarten and preschool • Family friendly employment practices & policies (local government and local organizations/employers)
Event *(during a given maltreatment episode)*	• Teach children to de-escalate conflict with abusers • Teach older children how to get away from an abusing adult (self-defense skills) • Teach children to tell an adult about neglectful parenting practices or inappropriate discipline or sexual behavior	• Reduce access to lethal weapons in home • Teach parents to walk away when frustrated & need a break	• Cameras to allow early identification of abusive behavior by child care providers	• Change norms for bystanders' helping • Home visiting to assist abusive families • Public education about signs of child maltreatment and reporting laws & procedures
Post-event *(after specific incident of maltreatment takes place)*	• Teach children to tell adults about abuse that has occurred (e.g., Good touch/bad touch) • Mental health services for abused children • Teach everyone first aid skills and CPR	• Mental health services for abusive persons	• Easy access by EMS services to facilities where violence occurs (e.g., child care)	• Parents' Anonymous • Quality behavioral health treatment services for acute care & rehab • Access to social emotional health services and treatment • Increase health insurance coverage • Support child welfare

Fig. 6.2 Example of a Haddon Matrix applied to child maltreatment prevention

interventions after the event serve as pre-event strategies to prevent future events (e.g., removing the child from the home).

In filling in the matrix, the ideas listed in the first column are about changing the child in some way to prevent abuse from occurring or to minimize its effects. Often physical characteristics are hard to change (e.g., high pitched cry or disabilities), but there may be ways to alter behaviors, at least in older children (e.g., teaching children to avoid accepting rides from strangers or to avoid connecting with strangers met on the internet). The second column refers to the vehicles and vectors that transmit energy (the agent). In the case of motor vehicle safety this would be the car. In child abuse, the caregivers (e.g., parents) who interact with the child would be the focus of this column. Changes directed at the parent might include efforts to enhance parenting skills, change disciplinary practices, reduce substance use, or increase help-seeking behaviors when stressed. In the third column, one can identify ways to change the physical aspects of the environment the child encounters (e.g., greater visibility). Change here might be to reduce household crowding, ensure safe play areas without allowing sexual predators to interact with children unobserved, ensure safe child care facilities, or build neighborhoods where families easily interact and build social capital. The fourth column, the social environment, refers to factors such as policies, social norms, and values. For example, norms and laws around corporal punishment, policies that support economic security for families through living wages and parental leave, and abuse reporting policies.

The phases (or rows in the model) identify the time during which the intervention has its effect. If one defines the 'event' as the first occurrence of abuse or neglect, the first row (pre-event phase) refers to the time period before that incident. In the case of motor vehicle safety, for example, pre-event strategies include reducing speeds or reducing impaired or distracted driving. Pre-event strategies for child maltreatment prevention might include reducing teen pregnancy, pre-term delivery, or parental substance abuse, and providing quality health care to address health conditions that may make a child more vulnerable to abuse.

In Haddon's model, the event phase refers to efforts to arrest the process of an injury-producing event as an event is occurring. Making sure that passengers are properly restrained in cars is an event strategy because using a seatbelt or child restraint reduces the likelihood of injury in the event of a crash. Although restraint use is employed before the crash, its effect is during the crash. A similar example, for child maltreatment, is teaching children about 'good touch' or 'bad touch' so that a child who is being molested can recognize what is happening and take steps to get out of the situation and tell another adult. This method does not prevent the abuse from happening, but it may reduce the impact of the event and prevent future events.

The third row pertains to post-event strategies – those occurring after the event to address treatment and/or rehabilitation. In the case of a motor vehicle crash this might be first aid or emergency care. Similarly, child protective services intervention, foster care, or therapy for parents would fit in this row. An example of the matrix with examples relevant to child maltreatment appears in Fig. 6.2 (Runyan and Brandspigel 2016).

6.4.3 Making Decisions – Applying the Third Dimension

Haddon's Matrix is extremely useful in helping to identify an array of potential interventions and facilitate development of ideas that go beyond traditional approaches. Engaging professionals from different disciplines, with varying perspectives, can be helpful in developing the ideas using the matrix. Using the rules of brainstorming (not allowing critical comments in the idea-generation process) in completing the model allows the most creativity to emerge.

Once ideas are generated, there must be a method to sift or evaluate the ideas. This is where the third dimension for the matrix, shown in Fig. 6.3, comes in. The third dimension (Runyan 1992) helps organize decision-making in a more systematic way. This third dimension is derived from principles of policy analysis where analysts consider what value criteria are important and how to assess them, weighing different options in the context of those values underlying the decisions. To use the process, the first step involves identifying the important value criteria to use to choose among alternative strategies. This needs to be context-specific as what is appropriate in one setting, culture or point in time may not be suited to another setting or time. Each criterion needs to be carefully defined so the meaning is clear to all involved so that the options being considered can be evaluated in the context of that criterion. Decision makers considering interventions need to think carefully about the values underlying their value criteria in setting priorities. Too often decisions are made based on assumptions that everyone shares the same values or understanding of a particular criterion.

Some of the competing values are explained below for consideration by those thinking about using the third dimension as a tool to clarify what criteria are important in deciding among different options for preventive interventions.

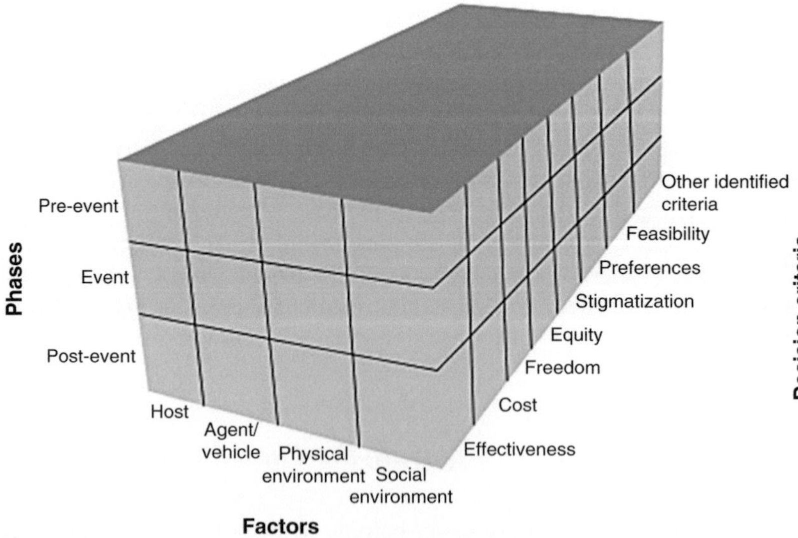

Fig. 6.3 Three–dimensional Haddon Matrix. (Runyan 1998)

6.4.4 Considering Values in the Third Dimension

Often, the first criterion considered is that of *effectiveness.* If the intervention under consideration is known to be effective based on sound evidence, it merits further consideration. Determining effectiveness relies on sound impact and outcome evaluations. Unfortunately, high quality evaluations employing randomized trials, quasi-experimental designs, or trend studies are frequently under-funded or not supported at all, requiring evaluators to rely on before and after studies without comparison groups, introducing multiple threats to validity. Even when studies are strong, there is often considerable room for uncertainty and questions about generalizability to the setting in which one is considering applying the intervention. If there is good evidence indicating an intervention is not effective, then alternative options should be considered. If the overall goal is one of primary prevention at a population level (as it typically is for public health interventions), making changes at the community and policy level is usually most appropriate; 'upstream' changes through social and organizational policy initiatives are more likely to get at the 'root causes' of the problem. This contrasts with a focus on individual behavior change or other individual approaches or strategies after the abuse has occurred which is much less likely to be successful.

Generally, the more effort required to provide safety, the less likely it is to be successful. A simple example is expecting that anyone bathing a baby will ensure that the temperature of the water is safe each and every time a bath is given. However, human behavior is highly fallible. A harried or distracted parent or babysitter may forget to check the temperature. In contrast, setting the temperature of the water at a safe level at the source (the water heater) is better protection because the temperature can never exceed a safe level and it doesn't require repetitive actions. Safety is assured even if the caregiver fails to check the temperature. Similar strategies are inherent in design of many products such as the use of airbags in cars. The airbag, a passive restraint device, enhances safety because it does not rely on human action.

Another value criterion often considered is that of *equity.* This can be *horizontal equity* where all persons are treated equally (e.g., with universal approaches like shaken baby education for all parents regardless of income or other social circumstances). Or, one may want to emphasize *vertical equity or fairness* in which unequally situated groups are treated unequally deliberately in order to equalize risk or opportunity. For example, a policy may provide lower income families access to subsidized childcare instead of providing subsidies to all, including affluent families. One might also differentiate on risk – targeting more prevention opportunities to those at higher risk – for example, assuring that families deemed high-risk for child maltreatment receive free home visiting services. In thinking about the balance of horizontal and vertical equity, consider the concepts discussed by Geoffrey Rose presented earlier in this chapter. To the extent the change is targeted at the whole population vs. high-risk groups, horizontal equity is more suitable. However, there are economic realities in using this approach (see the cost section below) and there may also be issues in addressing freedom of self-determination.

Freedom is a value factoring into many public health efforts. In most cultures, individual freedom is highly valued, presenting decision makers with difficult dilemmas when balancing limits on freedom with specific public health goals. For example, requiring child restraint devices in automobiles limits parental freedom to have passengers ride as they may wish or for children to sit wherever they desire. Nevertheless, most developed countries have decided that child restraints are a valuable means of preventing injury and that the freedom lost is worth the safety gains. Often, restrictions of freedom are more accepted when the safety of children is involved because of the rationale that children are unable to protect themselves. Examples of freedom restriction in the realm of child maltreatment prevention include requiring immunization, with failure to immunize viewed as a form of neglect, prohibiting child pornography possession, or banning corporal punishment in schools.

At times, different freedoms may be in conflict; for example, the freedom of parents to discipline a misbehaving child as they see fit may conflict with the freedom of the child to be protected from harm. Society must balance whose freedom is being restricted and whether that particular freedom is deemed highly important or relatively trivial. Many motor vehicle safety regulations are taken for granted and people do not feel limited by being unable to purchase a car without certain safety devices. Most people are not offended by giving up freedom to buy an unsafe product (e.g., an unsafe vs. safe barbeque grill) because of restrictions placed on manufacturers. However, suggesting restrictions on individual behaviors or personal choices over diet, smoking, use of motorcycle helmets, ownership of firearms, or childrearing practices (at least in the US) may trigger intense controversy because of perceived conflicts with personal choice.

It is useful to think about what elements of freedom are related to child maltreatment. For example, controversy arises over what constitutes neglect, such as at what age a child may be left at home alone or failing to accept cancer care for religious reasons when the form of cancer can be treated successfully. Who should get to make that determination? What protections should be in place when courts make decisions about removing children from the home?

Cost is another consideration in most intervention selections. As with freedom, cost can have multiple dimensions. Obviously, there are costs to implement a program or enforce a policy. But, there are also costs associated with not implementing the intervention (e.g., loss of life, medical care expenditures, or human suffering). This side of the equation is often not considered in cost considerations. Not all costs are the same; some are immediate, while others accrue over time. Interventions are often not equal in terms of who is responsible for paying and who benefits. Is it, for example, the parents themselves, taxpayers, manufacturers of a product, or organizations allowing flex time for employees that pays while other agencies or persons benefit from reduced foster care, fewer abuse or neglect investigations, fewer incarcerated persons, or reduced numbers of court cases? Intervention options may be evaluated differently depending upon who pays versus who benefits.

Stigmatization is another factor to consider when determining desirability of an intervention. Stigma may occur when an individual or a group is singled out as at risk or in need. Stigma can happen if it is not deliberately avoided. A school-based clinic requiring adolescents to acknowledge sexual activity before they access birth control services may stigmatize users. Programs identifying low-income children eligible for free school lunches may generate stigma. Public 'calling out' of negative behaviors, such as 'wife beating', drunk driving, or sex offending might be used to curb the behavior or allow neighbors to avoid the individual. In these circumstances, intentional stigmatization is used to achieve a goal. In considering a program or policy, one needs to think through the extent to which the effectiveness and cost of stigmatizing is balanced against both the potentially positive and negative social effects of the practice. For example, when the child maltreatment is neglect; public shaming of these families may result in further reductions in resources for the child and family. Similarly, singling out children or parents for post-event services based on their abusive history (vs. other care needs) may inadvertently stigmatize them in the care system.

Preferences of the affected group are also important to consider. This criterion relates directly to cultural norms and practices. Even if professionals favor banning certain parenting practices (e.g., spanking children under a certain age or removing guns from the homes of youth who are potentially suicidal) or favor providing other services (e.g., access, without parental consent, to long acting contraceptives to teenagers), these practices may be socially unacceptable in the community. Preferences of the community need to be factored into decision-making about whether and how to propose an intervention.

Although community preferences can change over time, it often takes a deliberative process within a community to change the culture to the point that a given intervention will be accepted or even promoted. General community acceptance of seatbelts, child restraint laws, and bans on smoking in public places did not happen overnight.

Planners need to carefully assess the preferences of the community in which an intervention is being proposed to determine both acceptability and what the competing values might be; for example, whether community concerns center on loss of a freedom, costs, fairness, or stigma associated with which persons will be affected. Engaging with community members through community meetings, surveys, key informant interviews, or focus groups will help to identify the acceptance potential or alternative approaches to addressing a problem. Incremental approaches may be a successful strategy; this worked for implementing limited smoking bans and then gradually expanding them to additional prohibited spaces. Similarly, mandated reporting of abuse and neglect was first proposed in the US for health and child care professionals and has been expanded in most states to include Emergency Medical Technician (EMT) personnel, police, and sports coaches.

After considering other criteria, the issue of *feasibility* should be addressed. This may include both technological feasibility and political feasibility. To be feasible, delivering a video-based shaken baby education program within hospitals requires time to interact with the new parents and whether there is access to video players. Short hospital stays and lack of resources may complicate delivering the education. While educating parents about shaken baby syndrome before birth through obstetrics offices may be more effective, the large numbers of provider offices and the resources needed in each may make this logistically infeasible. Often *technologic feasibility* gets in the way (e.g., relying on internet-based education may not be feasible in some populations). *Political feasibility* relates to community preferences and whether a community has the political will to endorse, implement, or enforce an intervention or policy (e.g., access to contraceptives by teenagers). It is important to not rule out otherwise good solutions too quickly on feasibility grounds; many feasibility issues can be overcome over time, with technology, or through education and/or advocacy to increase political will. Finally, depending on the setting or issue, other important value criteria may emerge and should be factored into the decision making process.

6.4.5 Using the Third Dimension to Make Decisions

Once criteria are defined, the decision-making group should examine interventions identified in the matrix and compare their relative merits in the context of the value criteria and how important they judge each criterion. The importance of any value criterion to the community might be labeled as high, medium or low or could be given a numeric score (e.g., from 1 to 10) to weigh its relative importance. Similarly, as intervention options are considered, the relative merits could be defined in degrees of positive or negative (e.g., +++, ++, +, –, ––, –––) or with numeric values. The point is to evaluate the merits of the intervention option in the context of its attributes relative to the value criteria identified and the importance of each criterion to the decision at that time and place. This process is described in more detail by Runyan (1998).

6.4.6 Dilemmas in Using the Third Dimension

Injury control has long demonstrated that changes to vehicles that confer energy transfer or physical environments are far more effective strategies for safety than changing individuals. This concept of active vs. passive intervention is critical to a public health and injury control approach (Runyan et al. 1993). This can be a useful companion to the Haddon Matrix in considering options for interventions.

To the extent possible, passive interventions are preferred as they rely less on individuals to engage in safe behaviors and afford protection automatically, often without individuals even being aware they have been protected. Water fluoridation is a passive intervention that provides dental protection without requiring individual action. Similarly, street lights and guard rails are unobtrusive means to provide safety. Other examples include altering the environment with the installation of nonflammable materials to protect against fires or structural features to prevent building collapse in an earthquake. These passive protections do not require human action or behavior change to afford protection. Advancing technology, such as development of both smart guns and smart cars, is making more of these types of interventions possible.

Mandating limitations on the level of fat in processed foods or sugar in beverages is an example of a *mandatory*, passive approach to obesity prevention. These approaches remove choices and limit freedom to select unhealthy options. Mandatory child-safe packaging of medications and recreational drugs, or mandatory lower temperatures on water heaters are examples of regulation that limits the harm that can occur to young children left unattended.

Voluntary, active interventions rely primarily on increasing the knowledge and/or intentions of individuals to engage in healthy or safe behaviors. These educational approaches are often the least effective. Human behavior change is difficult and even when people know the right thing to do, they make mistakes or do not act on their best intentions. Dr. C. Henry Kempe, a seminal clinician and writer in this field, observed "Abusive parents love their children very much, but not very well" (Krugman 2017). Creating environments that enable and foster positive parenting are likely to be more successful than individual remedial education.

An active mandatory approach is a frequent choice for preventing injury. Prohibiting corporal punishment, mandating video monitoring in day care settings, regulating water heater temperatures, and specifying that day care settings have few walls so that the children can be seen are examples of mandates to lower the risk of abuse or neglect.

6.5 Conclusions

Throughout this chapter we have explained key principles of public health and injury control approaches. We have focused on the population (vs. individual) and primary (vs. secondary or tertiary) prevention lens of public health. Through this lens, we explained how population approaches generate different questions about the health experiences of a whole population or achieving a goal of shifting 'the curve' for all, rather than focusing primarily on high-risk segments of the population. We stressed the importance of evidence-based planning and described the Haddon Matrix in detail, as a tool to identify multiple intervention approaches based upon the principles of both the public health and the social-ecologic frameworks. In presenting the third dimension to the Matrix, we introduced the notion of assessing which values are important to a given locale or culture in achieving health goals. Finally, we stressed the importance of passive approaches from policy and systems change, and consider examples from other public health issues as well as child maltreatment prevention.

Though discussion of implementation of these principles in actual community action is beyond the scope of this chapter, we recommend the book Prevention is Primary: Strategies for Community Well-being (Chehimi et al. 2007), the online Community Tool Box from the University of Kansas (http://ctb.ku.edu/en), and the technical package from CDC (Fortson et al. 2016) as useful tools that are consistent with the principles articulated in the chapter.

References

Barr, R. G., Rivara, F. R., Barr, M., Cummings, P., Taylor, J., Lengua, L. J., & Meredith-Benitz, E. (2009). Effectiveness of educational materials designed to change knowledge and behaviors regarding crying and Shaken-Baby Syndrome in mothers of newborns: A randomized, controlled trial. *Pediatrics, 123*, 972–980.

Beauchamp, D. E. (1976). Public Health as social justice. *Inquiry, XIII*, 3–14.

Beauchamp, D. E. (1985). Community: The neglected tradition of public health. *Hastings Center Report*, 28–36.

Bernstein, J. (2006). *All together now: Common sense for a fair economy*. San Francisco: Berrett-Koehler.

Bronfenbrenner, U. (1979). *The ecology of human development: Experiments by nature and design*. Cambridge, MA: Harvard University Press.

Caffey, J. (1946). Multiple fractures in the long bones of infants suffering from chronic subdural hematoma. *American Journal of Roentgenol, 56*, 163–173.

Chehimi, S., Chávez, V., & Cohen, L. (2007). *Prevention is primary: Strategies for community well-being*. Oakland: Copublished by American Public Health Association.

Christian, C. W., & Sege, R. D. (2010). The committee on child abuse and neglect: Child Fatality Review. *Pediatrics, 126*(3), 592–596.

Fortson, B. L., Klevens, J., Merrick, M. T., Gilbert, L. K., & Alexander, S. P. (2016). *Preventing Child Abuse and Neglect: A technical package for policy, norm, and programmatic activities*. Atlanta: National Center for Injury Prevention and Control, Centers for Disease Control and Prevention.

Gibson, J. J. (1961). *The contribution of experimental psychology to the formulation of the problem of safety – A brief for basic research. Behavioral approaches to accident research*. New York: Association for the Aid of Crippled Children.

Gilbert, R., Spatz Widom, C., Browne, K., Fergusson, D., Webb, E., & Janson, S. (2008). Burden and consequences of child maltreatment in high-income countries. *Lancet, 373*, 68–81.

Haddon, W. (1980). Advances in the epidemiology of injuries as a basis for public policy. *Public Health Reports, 95*(5), 411–421.

Hemenway, D. (2009). *While we were sleeping: Success stories in injury and violence prevention*. Berkeley: University of California Press.

Institute of Medicine. (1988). *The future of public health*. Washington, DC: The National Academies Press.

Kempe, C. H., Silverman, F. N., Steele, B. F., Droegemueller, W., & Silver, H. K. (1962). The battered-child syndrome. *Journal of the American Medical Association, 181*, 17–24.

Krug, E., Dahlberg, L., Mercy, J., Zwi, A., & Lozano, R. (Eds.). (2002). *World report on violence and health*. Geneva: World Health Organization.

Krugman, R. D. (2017). The more we learn, the less we know: A brief history of the field of child abuse and neglect. In J. B. Klika & J. R. Conte (Eds.), *The APSAC handbook on child maltreatment* (4th ed.). Thousand Oaks: Sage.

Labbe, J. (2005). Ambroise Tardieu: The man and his work on child maltreatment a century before Kempe. *Child Abuse & Neglect, 29*, 311–324.

Last, J. (1983). *A dictionary of epidemiology*. New York: Oxford University Press.

McGavran, E. (1958). The community as the patient of public health. *Texas State Medical Journal, 10*, 719–723.

Rose, G. (1992). *Strategies of preventive medicine*. New York: Oxford Press.

Runyan, C. W. (1998). Using the Haddon matrix: Introducing the third dimension. *Injury Prevention, 4*, 302–307.

Runyan, C. W. (2003). Back to the future: Revisiting Haddon's conceptualization of injury epidemiology and prevention. *Epidemiologic Reviews, 25*, 60–64.

Runyan, C. W., & Brandspigel, S. (2016). *Prevention toolkit for local child fatality prevention teams*. Distributed by the Colorado Department of Public Health and Environment.

Runyan, C. W., Fischer, P., Moore, J., Waller, P., & Hooten, E. (1993). Attempting to change local injury policy. *Family and Community Health, 15*(4), 66–74.

Runyan, D. K., Shankar, V., Hassan, F., Hunter, W., Jain, D., Paula, C., Bangdiwala, S., Ramiro, L., Muñoz, S., Vizcarra, B., & Bordin, I. (2010). International variations in harsh child discipline. *Pediatrics, 126*(3), 701–711.

Stoltenborgh, M., Bakermans-Kranenburg, M., Alink, L. R. A., & van Ijzendoorn, M. H. (2015). The prevalence of child maltreatment across the globe: Review of a series of meta-analyses. *Child Abuse Review, 24*, 37–50.

Susser, M., & Andjelkovich, D. (1973). *Causal thinking in the health sciences; concepts and strategies of epidemiology*. Oxford University Press.

Susser, M., & Susser, E. (1996). Choosing a future for epidemiology: II. From black box to Chinese boxes and eco-epidemiology. *American Journal of Public Health, 86*, 674–677.

Theodore, A., Chang, J. J., Runyan, D. K., Hunter, W. M., Bangdiwala, S. I., & Agans, R. (2005). The epidemiology of the physical and sexual maltreatment of children in the Carolinas. *Pediatrics, 115*(3), e331–e337.

Waller, J. (1985). Injury control – A guide to the causes and prevention of trauma. In*Lexongton*. Massachusetts: Lexington Books.

Woolley, P., & Evans, W. (1955). Significance of skeletal lesions in infants resembling those of traumatic origin. *Journal of the American Medical Association, 158*, 539–543.

Chapter 7
Intersecting Forms of Child Victimization and Public Health Prevention

Todd I. Herrenkohl and J. Bart Klika

7.1 Introduction

This chapter reviews existing literature on multi-type child maltreatment and poly-victimization, calling out some of the barriers to researching these issues. It also explores the public health model in relation to child maltreatment prevention, drawing on research about risk and protective factors that are documented in published studies and reports. The chapter concludes with a number of implications for future research that are intended to stimulate further work in this important area of child welfare scholarship.

7.2 Multi-type Child Maltreatment

A focus on multi-type maltreatment is a relatively recent development and few studies have addressed the issue comprehensively (Herrenkohl and Herrenkohl 2009). Most studies focus on a single type of maltreatment, or they include a general construct of child maltreatment that represents a combined average or sum of the frequency of abuse and neglect exposures in children of a particular age or developmental status (Higgins and McCabe 2001). As noted in our earlier publication on this topic, the study of child abuse and neglect has progressed in a 'stepwise' or piecemeal fashion in which attention has shifted from one type maltreatment to another, as

T. I. Herrenkohl (✉)
University of Michigan School of Social Work, Ann Arbor, MI, USA
e-mail: tih@umich.edu; tih@uw.edu

J. B. Klika
Prevent Child Abuse America, Chicago, IL, USA
e-mail: bklika@preventchildabuse.org

B. Lonne et al. (eds.), *Re-Visioning Public Health Approaches for Protecting Children*, Child Maltreatment 9, https://doi.org/10.1007/978-3-030-05858-6_7

awareness of the many ways children are harmed by adults responsible for their care has come into public view (Herrenkohl and Herrenkohl 2009).

According to Herrenkohl and Herrenkohl (2009), child physical abuse was first to receive attention from researchers in the 1960s. Child neglect, emotional abuse, and sexual abuse then followed, and each was taken up by researchers and child welfare professionals as it gained visibility in professional circles and in the news media. Children's exposure to domestic violence is, according to some state statutes, another type of child maltreatment (Herrenkohl et al. 2008), although there is still no consensus as to whether exposure to domestic violence should necessarily be considered abusive to children (Herrenkohl et al. 2008; Holden 2003). In fact, many practice and policy documents still do not list children's exposure to domestic violence as among the 'common types' of child maltreatment (see, for example Fortson et al. 2016), although children are routinely exposed to violence in the home and evidence suggest that even minor violence exposures can cause children lasting harm, particularly during sensitive periods of development (Herrenkohl et al. 2008). The reluctance to consider exposure to domestic violence as a form of child maltreatment stems partly from legal and definitional considerations, but also awareness that current welfare and service systems are not equipped to address the discrete needs of children and adults who have encountered violence.

The study of multi-type maltreatment emphasizes the point that the different types of child abuse (e.g., physical abuse, emotional abuse, sexual abuse) and neglect tend to cluster within families and that exposure to one type of maltreatment usually increases the likelihood of exposure to another (Dong et al. 2004; Herrenkohl and Herrenkohl 2009; Higgins and McCabe 2000, 2001). Evidence of this pattern is documented in both cross-sectional and longitudinal studies, which have used data from various sources, including child welfare case records, self-reports, and retrospective accounts of abuse victims themselves (Dong et al. 2004; Herrenkohl and Herrenkohl 2009; Higgins and McCabe 2001). Despite their many strengths and potential contributions, there have been relatively few longitudinal studies of multi-type maltreatment (Herrenkohl and Herrenkohl 2009). Cross-sectional studies are far more common, yet less robust and not at all positioned to investigate the developmental (causal) impacts of a child's risk exposure (Hardt and Rutter 2004; Widom and Shepard 1996). Still, much of what has been written on the topic comes from cross-sectional research, a limitation raised by Higgins and McCabe (2001) in their earlier review on the topic.

In their review, Higgins and McCabe (2001) explained that researchers who study the co-occurrence of maltreatment types do so in one of two ways: (1) by documenting the proportion of cases within a sample that experiences different combinations of abuse and neglect; or (2) by assessing the correlation between variables that represent different abuse and neglect subtypes. They found that a number of studies provide evidence of multi-type maltreatment, but results are difficult to compare because definitions and measures of abuse and neglect vary so widely. Moreover, their particular review was limited to 29 studies because so few studies included measures of all maltreatment types. Of the 29 studies, 13 had measures of two types of child maltreatment; 12 included measures of three types; and three included measures of four types of maltreatment. Only one study included measures of all five type together: sexual abuse, physical abuse, psychological maltreatment, neglect, witnessing family (domestic) violence. Further, the authors noted that researchers often failed to distinguish abuse and neglect that occurred in childhood and adolescence, which makes it unclear whether repeated exposures occur within a defined period, or over extended periods of development. They also noted a tendency for some researchers to rely on general constructs of abuse and neglect that do not actually identify which types of maltreatment have been recorded, thereby rendering results less meaningful. The use of general maltreatment constructs is understandable given its low base rate, but this approach is of little use to those who study co-occurrence and polyvictimzation.

In the review by Herrenkohl and Herrenkohl (2009), a similar set of conclusions were reached. The authors concluded that "maltreated children experience multi-type maltreatment relatively frequently…and that when assessed, the maltreatment types are often found to be correlated." Yet, they also noted evident inconsistencies in the operationalization and measurement of child maltreatment, as well as the analytic approaches used to investigate risk exposures in child victims. As did Higgins and McCabe, the authors recommended that the field adopt more uniform, consistent definitions and measurement strategies so that future research will advance what is known about the dynamics that underlie chronic victimization of vulnerable children.

7.2.1 Intersection of Child Abuse and Children's Exposure to Family Violence

As noted above, there has been a move in some settings to legally classify children's exposure to domestic violence as another type of child maltreatment (Holden 2003). Whether this will actually happen in unclear, but evidence even now suggests that the combined effects of child abuse and children's exposure to other forms of violence has a compounding, adverse effect on later development (Herrenkohl et al. 2008; Holden 2003; Wolfe et al. 2003). Knowing this to be true is important because it gives further weight to the argument for comprehensive policies and programs directed at the combined and overlapping risks encountered by those most vulnerable children and their families. More specifically, findings on the additive and cumulative effects of these and other forms of childhood adversity indicate that, to benefit children, prevention and intervention programs must focus not only increasing safety in the home, but also mitigating risks across the social ecology (Herrenkohl et al. 2015).

In their review of research, Herrenkohl et al. (2008) reported that there is a moderate to strong association (correlations around .50) between child abuse and children's exposure to other adverse experiences, which is generally similar to that of the different types of abuse and neglect mentioned earlier. However, it is hard to know for sure just how strongly correlated these experiences are because studies are so few and measures so inconsistent (Herrenkohl et al. 2008).

As important to documenting children's exposure to violence is learning 'why' and 'how' the violence occurred (Holden 2003). In one report, Holden (2003) developed a taxonomy of 10 different types of exposure. These include both direct (abuse) and indirect (witnessing abuse) exposures. Direct exposure occurs when a child witnesses a violent interaction or hears another family member being assaulted. Indirect exposure occurs when a child witnesses another's victimization, learns about violence from someone else in the family, or sees another person's injuries (Herrenkohl et al. 2008). While differing in proximity to the actual event, the consequences of indirect and direct exposure for children's development can be very similar (Herrenkohl et al. 2008). An added consideration in all such cases is whether a child has also been physically assaulted (Gewirtz and Edleson 2007; Holden 2003). In such cases, observing and being directly victimized by violence are part of the same overall experience (Gewirtz and Edleson 2007).

7.3 Polyvictimization

A closely related concept to multi-type maltreatment is that of 'polyvictimization', which refers to the clustering (within and over time) to differing forms of violence and assault (Finkelhor et al. 2011, 2013). The emphasis on repeated, compounding victimization experiences is important because it stresses the point that children can be traumatized many times over within a short period, or over their lifetimes. A report by Finkelhor et al. (2013) based on data from the National Survey of Children's Exposure to Violence (NatSCEV) II, a cross-sectional telephone survey of children 17 years of age and younger, found that nearly half (48.4%) of all children had been victimized at least once. Alarmingly, over 15% of youth participants reported six or more forms of victimization over their lifetimes. Data from a more recent iteration of the NatSCEV study showed that, in the past year, 37% of children experienced physical assault, 9% had an assault-related injury, 15% experienced maltreatment by a caregiver, and 6% witnessed assault between parents (Finkelhor et al. 2015). Children who are subject to repeated, of chronic forms of victimization represent a very high-risk and extremely vulnerable group that often lives in unsafe environments under constant threat of harm.

7.3.1 Adverse Childhood Experiences (ACEs)

In recent years, and with increasing interest in the biological embedding of stress, attention has focused on a related concept of adverse childhood experiences (ACEs) (Anda et al. 1999; Dong et al. 2004; Felitti et al. 1998). However, the method of studying ACEs using additive scales is akin to relying on general constructs of child maltreatment that do not differentiate among types of abuse and neglect, nor do they account for the developmental timing of risk exposure, frequency of exposure, or presence of other (protective) factors that can mitigate the effects of exposure. The fact that ACEs are typically retrospectively assessed is also problematic because few adults recall experiences of their past with much consistent accuracy. Yet, ACEs studies like the one by Felitti et al. (1998) are necessary because they reinforce the message that children are often victimized in many ways, often over extended periods.

7.3.2 *Child Maltreatment and Environmental Influences*

While the primary focus of this chapter is on child maltreatment and children's exposure to violence in the home, it is important to acknowledge that these experiences often occur in broader social ecology of risk (Aisenberg and Herrenkohl 2008; Block 2017; Herrenkohl 2011a). In fact, there is a relatively strong association between child maltreatment and neighborhood poverty and widespread unemployment, factors that impair the functioning of families (Coulton et al. 1999, 2007; Fortson et al. 2016; Freisthler and Merritt 2006). High residential turnover and social isolation among households are also neighborhood-level risk factors for child abuse and neglect, as well as predictors of psychopathology in children (Fortson et al. 2016).

In their review of the literature, Freisthler and Merritt (2006) documented other risk factors routinely encountered by children in poverty (see also Chap. 13 by Klevens and Metzler). These include poor supervision by adults, alcohol and drug availability in the community, and population density. They concluded that the most pressing question for the field at this moment is not whether neighborhood and environmental factors are related to child development (and psychopathology), but how they are related. They call on researchers to focus their efforts on studying mechanisms of risk transmission in order to determine 'causality' in the processes that underlie common problems in abused children.

Herrenkohl et al. (2018) proposed that "the effects of environmental risks on children's development are both direct and indirect. Indirectly, environmental risks can interfere or threaten children's development by negatively impacting how parents 'parent' and by reducing the functioning of families to a degree that children's needs go unmet" (p. 34).

7.4 Public Health Prevention

When children are maltreated and chronically victimized, as studies of multi-type maltreatment and polyvictimization show they are, consideration must be given to strategies that prevent and interrupt the 'cycle' of risk exposure that culminates in a child's being unable to function and contribute in meaningful ways to society. Yet, as is discussed throughout this book and in earlier publications, typical responses within the existing child welfare systems are reactive and generally ineffective

(Herrenkohl 2011a; Herrenkohl et al. 2015). They are ineffective because services follow an extended history of risk exposure in children and families are too poorly equipped to benefit from the relatively meager services they receive. While most children are inherently resilient (Herrenkohl 2011b), the emotional harm they endure from many years of victimization in highly toxic environments cannot be reversed (Herrenkohl et al. 2013a, b).

As noted by Higgins and colleagues in Chap. 1, a new model of engaging vulnerable families is desperately needed. Most practitioners and child maltreatment experts acknowledge that the most promising approach to prevent abuse use primary prevention strategies, which focus on eradicating abuse and neglect by addressing underlying risks (Herrenkohl et al. 2015). At a policy level, this requires a major shift in approach that allocates resources to programs focused on universal and early interventions rather than remediation and treatment (Herrenkohl et al. 2015). Yet, as noted by Herrenkohl et al. (2015) and Higgins et al. (this volume), changing child welfare to be more proactive and responsive to the needs of vulnerable children and families may not be sufficient to achieve major reductions in rates of child maltreatment. What is needed is a set of coordinated systems that emphasize primary prevention but also provide secondary and tertiary prevention for families at higher risk.

A public health approach provides a strong theoretical and empirical foundation for large-scale policy and systems reform to promote primary, secondary, and tertiary prevention. As described in a publication by the Centers for Disease Control and Prevention (CDC) (https://www.cdc.gov/violenceprevention/overview/publichealthapproach.html) (see Fig. 7.1), this model begins by defining the problem (e.g., child maltreatment); then identifying salient risk and protective factors related to the problem. It then moves to developing and testing interventions to address those risk and protective factors. A final stage supports widespread dissemination of research and adoption of empirically-supported preventive interventions consistent with a particular theory of change, such as improving family relationships and lessening environmental risks.

7.4.1 Risk and Protective Factors for Child Maltreatment

Over many years and across numerous studies, researchers have identified a host of risk and protective factors related to child maltreatment (Herrenkohl 2011a). Risk factors are variables that increase the likelihood of a negative outcome, such as child maltreatment, whereas protective factors do the opposite; they reduce the likelihood of that outcome (Herrenkohl 2011b; Heyman and Smith Slep 2001). Research shows that risk and protective factors interact, such that individual and family functioning depends on the balance of one to another (Leadbeater et al. 2004). When risk factors outnumber protective factors in the environment, functioning at the individual and family levels will generally decline; when protective factors outnumber risk factors, functioning will generally improve (Herrenkohl 2011b). This logic,

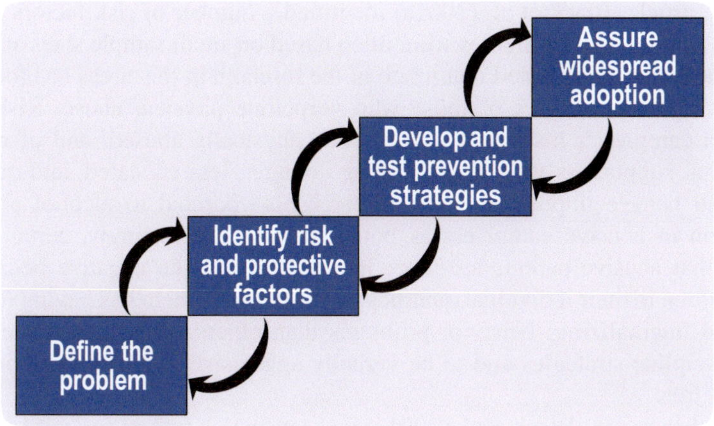

Fig. 7.1 Centers for Disease Control and Prevention (CDC): the public health approach to violence prevention

although somewhat more complicated than a simple ratio of risk to protective factors, is evident in the study of resilience in maltreated children, which shows a very high correspondence between a child's exposure to risk factors and her/his psychosocial adjustment (Herrenkohl 2011b).

According to a review by Herrenkohl and colleagues (2014), risk factors for child maltreatment are typically organized around domains of the social ecological framework first described by Bronfenbrenner (1979). This model emphasizes the layered environments and systems that shape the developing child, as well as transactions between and within systems that directly or indirectly influence a child's development. As explained by Belsky (1980), who adapted Bronfenbrenner's theory, risk factors for child maltreatment include those far removed from the day-to-day experiences and interactions of a child, such as norms and values that affect parenting and the use of harsh discipline, as well as those that are very proximal and directly related to a child's daily experiences, such as characteristics of the parent-child relationship, acute problems within the family, such as substance use and mental health problems of parent, and characteristics or qualities of the child him/herself, such as a difficult temperament or disabling condition.

In that child abuse and neglect experiences co-occur (cluster) within families, it is assumed they also share a common etiology; that is, they will be related to the same or similar set of risk and protective factors. However, few direct comparisons of risk and protective factors across maltreatment types have actually been conducted (Higgins and McCabe 2001). Authors of a special issue of Aggression and Violent Behavior in 2001 examined risk factors for child maltreatment subtypes in a series of literature reviews (see introduction by (Heyman and Smith Slep 2001)). The authors examined literature on physical abuse, psychological abuse, sexual abuse, and neglect. Their findings are briefly summarized to give readers some ideas of where risk and protective factors intersect.

In one article, Black et al. (2001a) identified a number of risk factors for child physical abuse, although studies were often based on small sample sizes and inconsistent measures. They noted that much of the research in this areas has focused on qualities or characteristics of those who perpetrate physical abuse. Risk factors include a caregiver's history of having been physically abused, and of receiving little social support, as well as their being younger, less educated, and quicker to anger and behave impulsively. The research also pointed to alcohol abuse and depression in abusive caregivers as potential risks. Interestingly, certain studies showed that abusive parents are more inclined to attribute negative behaviors of their children to their individual qualities and to perceive them has having (externalizing and internalizing) behavior problems than others. They also tended to use harsh discipline strategies and to be verbally aggressive in their interactions with their children.

In another review, Black et al. (2001c) focused on risk factors for child emotional or psychological abuse. Their review was somewhat less expansive because fewer studies on the topic were published at the time. However, they did find evidence of a link to hostility and aggression in abusive parents, as well as depression (dysthymic symptoms), and neuroticism. Their review also touched on an association between psychological abuse and a parent's own history of having had a less caring relationship with his or her parents, and of being yelled at more frequently as a child. Low family income was another risk factor they identified. Noting how few studies were included in their review, the authors cautioned against drawing any definitive conclusions or implications.

Although limited to only a few studies, Black et al. (2001b) reported on findings of yet another review focused on child sexual abuse. In this review, there appeared to be a connection to low family income, less education for parents, and parental unemployment. Mothers of those who were abused experienced more stress and were less socially connected and emotionally supported. They were also more angry and depressed. Sexual abuse victims were more likely than those not abused to come from single-parent families and stepfamilies. Findings also suggested that abusers were more likely to be from outside the family (acquaintances or strangers) rather from within. Research showed girls and older youth to be more often victims of sexual abuse than boys and younger children.

Finally, a review by Schumacher et al. (2001) focused on risk factors for neglect. Unfortunately, very little research had, at that time, examined neglect. In fact, the authors were able to identify only 10 relevant studies for their review. They concluded, "Although few factors have been examined in more than one study, when taken together, the findings suggest that parental behavioral and psychological characteristics may have the largest relations to neglect, and that limited socioeconomic resources are the most consistently documented risk factor for neglect" (p. 231).

A more recent meta-analysis by Stith et al. (2009) examined risk factors for both child physical abuse and child neglect. The authors found that factors such as parental anger/hyper-reactivity as well as conflict and cohesion in the family were associated with increased risk for child physical abuse. In addition to parental anger, child neglect was associated with a number of parental factors including stress, self-esteem, negative perceptions of the child, and the actual parent child relationship.

In summary, these articles, while not directly comparing risk factors for different subtypes of abuse and neglect, do provide evidence of possible etiological connections. Low family income, less education for parents, as well as mental health and substance use problems in the family, appear to place children at risk for several types of maltreatment. For the perpetration of physical abuse, parents' hostility and use of verbal aggression were also correlated risk factors. Knowing the factors that increase risk for child abuse perpetration and victimization help guide decisions on the timing, location, targets, and focus of prevention programs.

7.5 Protective and Mitigating Factors

Although fundamental to the study and amelioration of child maltreatment, there is far less research available on protective or mitigating factors—variables that lessen the risk of child maltreatment in vulnerable families (Herrenkohl 2011b; Herrenkohl et al. 2013a, b). Perhaps most well documented are the positive effects of social support, which consists of the presence of caring and supportive relationships from family members, as well as those outside the family (Black et al. 2001a; Herrenkohl et al. 2013a, b). Studies on social support suggest that families that well connected and adequately supported are generally at lower risk for maltreatment. In contrast, when parents are socially isolated—removed from a network of support—the risk of child abuse is much higher (Herrenkohl et al. 2014). Social support as well as positive coping strategies in parents and children are shown to be protective for vulnerable families (Munzer et al. 2017).

7.6 Consequences of Child Maltreatment

As with studies of risk and protective factors, those focused on the consequences of child maltreatment appear to show similarities across abuse types; if not uniformly the same in their expression at the individual level, then generally similar in what they represent about the emotional distress and sometimes physical impacts that abuse and neglect can have over the course of a lifetime. While there is variation in the outcomes that extend from child abuse and neglect, the effects for many children are generally quite serious (Herrenkohl 2011a). In fact, findings suggest that abuse, neglect, and children's exposure to family violence can individually and collectively increase the risk of attention problems and aggression in school-age children, as well as peer rejection, and low academic achievement. During adolescence, risks for mental health problems, including depression and anxiety, are notably higher for youth who were abused. The same is true of substance use problems and addiction. Problems of this sort are likely to continue and possibly escalate into early adulthood and beyond, if left unaddressed. For some, there is clear evidence of Post-Traumatic Stress Disorder (PTSD), which can include difficulties concentrating, sleeping and experiencing upsetting thoughts and memories (Herrenkohl et al. 2014).

The compounding effects of trauma in polyvictimized children is associated with ongoing problems in health and psychosocial functioning (Graham Bermann and Seng 2005; Higgins and McCabe 2001), and there is evidence that more victimization leads to worse outcomes. According to Graham-Bermann and Seng (2005), individuals who experience child abuse and other forms of violence can, and often do, develop chronic symptoms of PTSD. These symptoms, when carried forward from stressful experiences, can lead to symptoms of chronic health conditions and the early-onset of disease, such as coronary heart disease, diabetes, and autoimmune disorders (Shonkoff et al. 2009). Individuals who encounter violence and other traumatic events over many years and at different times in life are particularly vulnerable, in part because their minds and bodies experience constant stress and strain, what some have termed 'toxic stress,' thereby making them vulnerable to physical and mental health declines (Slopen et al. 2013).

7.7 Prevention of Child Maltreatment Using the Public Health Model

A question often asked by practitioners and policy makers is whether child maltreatment can be eradicated at a population level. As a general rule, one can expect that intervention programs targetingrisk factors that are shared across specified problems will have an effect on each and all of those problems if implemented with fidelity (Institute of Medicine 1994). In the case of child abuse and neglect, and, by extension, children's exposure to family violence, evidence from risk and protective factor studies suggests that common strategies are, in fact, viable, yet they remain understudied. Researchers have similarly discussed common approaches to the prevention of youth problems, such as substance abuse, violence, and teen pregnancy, which appear responsive to coordinated prevention systems (Hawkins 2006).

A common prevention strategy should be based on a strong theory and sound evidence. The Centers for Disease Control and Prevention developed a framework for public health child maltreatment and violence prevention that emphasizes the role of safe, stable and nurturing relationships and environments. The model, called Essentials for Childhood (EfC) (https://www.cdc.gov/violenceprevention/childmaltreatment/essentials.html), is a community-level prevention strategy that begins with a vision to end maltreatment and to ensure all children have access to relationships and environments that nurture and support their development. The vision is grounded in a set of complementary change strategies that involve collective impact, the use of valid and reliable data, effective programming, social norms change, and policies aligned to programs that support positive child development. The CDC views these areas as necessary components of a universal strategy to lessen child maltreatment.

Table 7.1 Technical Package Strategies and Approaches

Strategy	Approach
Strengthen economic supports for families	Strengthen household financial security
	Child support payments
	Tax credits
	State option for managing federal nutrition assistance programs
	Family friendly work policies
	Livable wages
	Paid leave
	Flexible and consistent schedules
Change social norms to support parents and positive parenting	Public engagement and education campaigns
	Legislative approaches to reduce corporal punishment
Provide quality care and education early in life	Preschool enrichment with family engagement
	Improved quality of child care through licensing and accreditation
Enhance parenting skills to promote healthy child development	Early childhood home visitation
	Parenting skill and family relationship approaches
Intervene to lessens harms and prevent future risk	Enhanced primary care
	Behavioral parent training programs
	Treatment for children and families to lessen the harms of abuse and neglect exposure
	Treatment for children and families to prevent problem behavior and later involvement in violence

Source: Fortson et al. (2016)

As noted by Herrenkohl et al. (2015), the EfC framework provide a strong conceptual foundation upon which large scale prevention efforts can be developed, tested, and scaled. While the field has not yet progressed to a point where common prevention approaches can be easily transported from one setting to another, findings support the use of certain approaches over others (Fortson et al. 2016). The CDC has outlined a set of core strategies and approaches to further goals of the EfC framework (see Table 7.1). These strategies include strengthening economic supports for families, changing social norms in support of positive parenting, providing quality child care and education, providing parents access to skills training to foster positive development in their children, and for intervening in cases of child abuse and neglect to lessen the consequences associated with the maltreatment. To accompany these broad-scale strategies are specific approaches which have demonstrated evidence of altering risk factors for child abuse and neglect. For example, one approach to strengthen economic supports for families is to provide families with paid leave following the birth of a new child. Research by Klevens et al. (2016) found that following implementation of paid family leave (PFL) in the state of California (compared to states without PFL) there were marked reductions in hospital admissions for pediatric abusive head trauma, an often fatal or life-altering form of child abuse. Building on this research, additional studies are needed to understand which strategies and approaches result in the greatest reductions in population-level rates of abuse and neglect and whether particular strategies are more or less successful in addressing particular forms and combinations of maltreatment and associated adversity.

One of the approaches noted in the CDC's technical package is the use of home visitation (Merritt et al. 2017). While home visitation models differ in the focus and goals of their approach (e.g., emphasis on health promotion versus early attachment), the credentials of the home visitor (e.g., nurse, paraprofessional), the timing of the services (e.g., prenatal, postnatal), and the target population of clients (e.g., first-time mothers, all families who give birth), these models generally agree that services should remain voluntary for families and that intervening early in a child's life is the best approach to ensure that maltreatment never occurs (Klika et al. 2017). Across models, home visitation demonstrates measurable impacts on maternal and child health, child injuries and maltreatment, school readiness and achievement, reductions in crime and domestic violence, improved economic self-sufficiency, and improved coordination and referrals for community supports (Sama-Miller et al. 2017). A major strength of home visiting is the simultaneous targeting of multiple risk factors and addressing multiple forms of trauma and adversity as outlined in this chapter.

Although home visitation remains a popular and theoretically complelling to child maltreatment prevention, findings on the effectiveness of home visitation remain mixed (Azzi-Lessing 2011; Casillas et al. 2016; Howard and Brooks-Gunn 2009; Sweet and Appelbaum 2004). For example, in a study by Green et al. (2017), those children who received a home visit had higher rates of unsubstantiated reports to child welfare than those children who did not receive a home visit. Interestingly, there were no differences noted between groups on rates of substantiated reports of child maltreatment. The authors explain these findings by suggesting a possible 'surveillance' effect of home visiting whereby questionable or concerning behaviors are reported to child welfare by the home visitor. In this way, it appears that home visiting increased, rather than decreased, child maltreatment. However, one could argue that home visitation in this instance accurately identified families who were 'at-risk' but not already engaging in abusive behavior, hence the unsubstantiated report. These findings raise important questions about how child maltreatment is defined and what qualifies as a reportable act of abuse or neglect. Assuming that unsubstantiated reports represent families at higher risk, they also raise questions about how to engage families proactively and whether current reporting procedures and practices lend themselves to activing on risks before they worsen and lead to substantiation.

Whether home visitation is more or less effective in preventing or addressing risk factors for different forms of maltreatment is not well understood. While many of the proxy measures used in home visiting studies examine issues related to physical abuse (e.g., child injuries) and neglect (e.g., accidental ingestions), less is know about whether sexual abuse is preventable through home visitation. In their review of the literature, Pecora et al. (2014) raise the possibility that different forms of maltreatment are more responsive to different prevention approaches. Interventions such as home visiting can be used to address many of the common risk factors associated with different forms of maltreatment, but targeted approaches may also be necessary.

Community-based prevention strategies, including those outlined in the CDC's technical package, begin to address risk and protection across multiple levels of the social ecology and hold great promise in reducing multiple forms of abuse and neglect. As Daro (2009) noted, no single strategy or intervention (e.g., home visiting) will succeed in eliminating abuse and neglect. Focus should be placed on creating integrated early childhood systems whereby children and families have access to resources such as home visitation, high quality childcare/education, and healthcare.

7.8 Conclusions and Future Directions for Research

As discussed earlier in this chapter, the study of multi-type child maltreatment and related concepts of polyvictimzation and cumulative risk provide important information for public health models of prevention. The public health model emphasizes proactive attempts to reduce risk factors and enhance protective factors in order to improve the functioning of families and to provide parents with tools to discipline nonviolently. At the same time, research has been slowed by a lack of consistency in definitions and analytic approaches used to examine the dynamic of multi-type maltreatment and its developmental impacts on children. The heavy reliance on cross-sectional data and tendency to limit investigations to a single subtype of child maltreatment have limited what we know and how we might develop targeted policies and programs. Often, studies of child maltreatment are focused on outcomes at later points in the life course, with a goal to establish how formative experiences shape later development. Absent corroborating longitudinal data, cross-sectional findings are extremely limiting and insufficient to draw causal inferences.

The study of risk and protective factors is fundamental to the publish health model. As reviewed in this chapter, there have been major developments in the field around these issues and evidence appears to suggest that the subtypes of child abuse and neglect share at least some common etiological factors. To the extent this is an accurate assessment, one can expect that prevention programs focused on those common factors have a relatively good chance of reducing child maltreatment of all types and forms. Of course, research has not advanced to the point where recommendations are necessarily based in strong and consistent evidence. Investigating common etiological factors and in the context of multifaceted preventive interventions is a key next step to advance the field.

Theories of social and environmental changes are important for intervention planning. Planning for large-scale prevention programs focused on child maltreatment is daunting but achievable. The Essentials for Childhood Framework developed by the Centers for Disease Control and Prevention in the USA is one example of a change model that is based on principles of public health practice. The framework can serve as a catalyst for policy and programmatic decisions in support of vulnerable children and their families.

Future research on the topics outlined in this chapter are desperately much needed, but research cannot simply reproduce knowledge the field already has. Developmental research focused on correlated subtypes of abuse and neglect will help establish the extent of co-occurrence that exists in families, as well as the impacts of these subtypes on child outcomes. Studies of developmental pathways will strengthen theories of child maltreatment consequences. And, tests of prevention models focused on common etiological factors will further establish whether assumptions about programs impacts are indeed warranted. There have been considerable advances in research on all fronts, yet much work left to be done in support of public health child maltreatment prevention.

References

Aisenberg, E., & Herrenkohl, T. I. (2008). Community violence in context: Risk and resilience in children and families. *Journal of Interpersonal Violence, 23*, 296–315.

Anda, R. F., Croft, J. B., Felitti, V. J., Nordenberg, D., Giles, W. H., Williamson, D. F., & Giovano, G. A. (1999). Adverse childhood experiences and smoking during adolescent and adulthood. *JAMA, 282*(17), 1652–1658.

Azzi-Lessing, L. (2011). Home visitation programs: Critical issues and future directions. *Early Childhood Research Quarterly, 26*, 387–398.

Belsky, J. (1980). Child maltreatment: An ecological integration. *American Psychologist, 35*, 320–335.

Block, R. W. (2017). No surprise: The rate of fatal child abuse and neglect fatalities is related to poverty. *Pediatrics, 139*, 357–358.

Black, D. A., Heyman, R. E., & Smith Slep, A. M. (2001a). Risk factors for child physical abuse. *Aggression and Violent Behavior, 6*, 121–188.

Bronfenbrenner, U. (1979). *The ecology of human development: Experiments by nature and design*. Cambridge, MA: Harvard University Press.

Black, D. A., Heyman, R. E., & Smith Slep, A. M. (2001b). Risk factors for child sexual abuse. *Aggression and Violent Behavior, 6*, 203–229.

Black, D. A., Smith Slep, A. M., & Heyman, R. E. (2001c). Risk factors for child psychological abuse. *Aggression and Violent Behavior, 6*, 189–201.

Casillas, K. L., Fauchier, A., Derkash, B. T., & Garrido, E. F. (2016). Implementation of evidence-based home visiting programs aimed at reducing child maltreatment: A meta-analytic review. *Child Abuse & Neglect, 53*, 64–80.

Coulton, C. J., Korbin, J. E., & Su, M. (1999). Neighborhoods and child maltreatment: A multi-level study. *Child Abuse & Neglect, 23*, 1019–1040.

Coulton, C. J., Crampton, D. S., Irwin, M., Spilsbury, J. C., & Korbin, J. E. (2007). How neighborhoods influence child maltreatment: A review of the literature and alternative pathways. *Child Abuse & Neglect, 31*, 1117–1142.

Daro, D. (2009). *Embedding home visitation programs within a system of early childhood services*. Chicago: Chapin Hall at the University of Chicago.

Dong, M., Anda, R. F., Felitti, V. J., Dube, S. R., Williamson, D. F., Thompson, T. J., et al. (2004). The interrelatedness of multiple forms of childhood abuse, neglect, and household dysfunction. *Child Abuse & Neglect, 28*, 771–784.

Felitti, V. J., Anda, R. F., Nordenberg, D., Williamson, D. F., Spitz, A. M., Edwards, V., et al. (1998). Relationship of childhood abuse and household dysfunction to many of the leading causes of death in adults: The Adverse Childhood Experiences (ACE) Study. *American Journal of Preventive Medicine, 14*(4), 245–258.

Finkelhor, D., Turner, H., Hamby, S., & Ormrod, R. (2011). *Polyvictimization: Children's exposure to multiple types of violence, crime, and abuse*. Retrieved from http://polyvictimization.org/wp-content/uploads/2015/07/235504.pdf

Finkelhor, D., Turner, H., Shattuck, A., & Hamby, S. (2013). Violence, crime, and abuse exposure in a national sample of children and youth: An update. *JAMA Pediatrics, 167*(7), 614–621.

Finkelhor, D., Turner, H., Shattuck, A., & Hamby, S. (2015). Prevalence of childhood exposure to violence, crime, and abuse: Results from the National Survey of Children's Exposure to Violence. *JAMA Peditriacs, 169*(8), 746–754.

Fortson, B. L., Klevens, J., Merrick, M. T., Gilbert, L. K., & Alexander, S. P. (2016). *Preventing child abuse and neglect: A technical package for policy, norm, and programmatic activities*. Atlanta: Division of Violence Prevention, National Center for Injury Prevention and Control, Centers for Disease Control and Prevention.

Freisthler, B., & Merritt, D. H. (2006). Understanding the ecology of child maltreatment: A review of the literature and directions for future research. *Child Maltreatment, 11*(3), 263–280.

Gewirtz, A. H., & Edleson, J. L. (2007). Young children's exposure to intimate partner violence: Towards a developmental risk and resilience framework for research and intervention. *Journal of Family Violence, 22*, 151–163.

Graham Bermann, S. A., & Seng, J. (2005). Violence exposure and traumatic stress symptoms as additional predictors of health problems in high-risk children. *Journal of Pediatrics, 146*(3), 349–354.

Green, B. L., Sanders, M. B., & Tarte, J. (2017). Using administrative data to evaluate the effectiveness of Healthy Families Oregon home visiting program: 2-year impacts on child maltreatment and service utilization. *Child & Youth Services Review, 75*, 77–86.

Hardt, J., & Rutter, M. (2004). Validity of adult retrospective reports of adverse childhood experiences: review of the evidence. *Journal of Child Psychology and Psychiatry, 45*(2), 260–273.

Hawkins, J. D. (2006). Science, social work, prevention: Finding the intersections. *Social Work Research, 30*(3), 137–152.

Herrenkohl, T. I. (2011a). Family violence and co-occurring risk factors for children exposed to violence. In T. I. Herrenkohl, E. Aisenberg, J. H. Williams, & J. M. Jenson (Eds.), *Violence in Context: Current evidence on risk, protection, and prevention* (pp. 73–91). New York: Oxford University Press.

Herrenkohl, T. I. (2011b). Resilience and protection from violence exposure in children: Implications for prevention and intervention programs with vulnerable populations. In T. I. Herrenkohl, E. Aisenberg, J. H. Williams, & J. M. Jenson (Eds.), *Violence in context: Current evidence on risk, protection, and prevention* (pp. 92–108). New York: Oxford University Press.

Herrenkohl, R. C., & Herrenkohl, T. I. (2009). Assessing a child's experience of multiple maltreatment types: Some unfinished business. *Journal of Family Violence, 24*, 485–496.

Herrenkohl, T. I., Sousa, C., Tajima, E. A., Herrenkohl, R. C., & Moylan, C. A. (2008). Intersection of child abuse and children's exposure to domestic violence. *Trauma, Violence, & Abuse, 9*(2), 84–99.

Herrenkohl, T. I., Hong, S., Klika, J. B., Herrenkohl, R. C., & Russo, M. J. (2013a). Developmental impacts of child abuse and neglect related to adult mental health, substance use, and physical health. *Journal of Family Violence, 28*, 191–199.

Herrenkohl, T. I., Klika, J. B., Brown, E. C., Herrenkohl, R. C., & Leeb, R. T. (2013b). Tests of the mitigating effects of caring and supportive relationships in the study of abusive disciplining over two generations. *Journal of Adolescent Health, 53*(Suppl. 4), S18–S24.

Herrenkohl, T. I., Hemphill, S. A., Florent, A., & Dee, T. (2014). Cultural, environmental, and psychosocial risk factors for child maltreatment. In J. Conte (Ed.), *Child abuse and neglect worldwide* (pp. 37–58). Santa Barbara: ABC-CLIO (Praeger).

Herrenkohl, T. I., Higgins, D., Merrick, M. T., & Leeb, R. T. (2015). Positioning and public health framework at the intersection of child maltreatment and intimate partner violence. *Child Abuse & Neglect, 48*, 22–28.

Herrenkohl, T. I., Kim, M., & Anderson, J. (2018). Child maltreatment in the context of poverty and other forms of adversity. In J. B. Klika & J. R. Conte (Eds.), *The APSAC handbook on child maltreatment* (4th ed., pp. 34–46). Thousand Oaks: Sage.

Heyman, R. E., & Smith Slep, A. M. (2001). Risk factors for family violence: Introduction to the special series. *Aggression and Violent Behavior, 6*, 115–119.
Higgins, D. J., & McCabe, M. P. (2000). Multi-type maltreatment and long-term adjustment of adults. *Child Abuse Review, 9*, 6–18.
Higgins, D. J., & McCabe, M. P. (2001). Multiple forms of child abuse and neglect: Adult retrospective reports. *Aggression and Violent Behavior, 6*(6), 547–578.
Holden, G. W. (2003). Children exposed to domestic violence and child abuse: Terminology and taxonomy. *Clinical Child and Family Psychology Review, 6*(3), 151–160.
Howard, K. S., & Brooks-Gunn, J. (2009). The role of home-visiting programs in preventing child abuse and neglect. *The Future of Children, 19*, 119–146.
Institute of Medicine. (1994). *Reducing risks for mental disorders: Frontiers for prevention intervention research*. Washington, DC: National Academy Press.
Klevens, J., Luo, F., Xu, L., & Latzman, N. E. (2016). Paid family leave's impact on hospital admissions for pediatric abusive head trauma. *Injury Prevention, 22*, 442–445.
Klika, J. B., Lee, S., & Lee, J. Y. (2017). Prevention of child maltreatment. In J. B. Klika & J. Conte (Eds.), *The American professional society on the abuse of children handbook on child maltreatment* (4th ed.). Thousand Oaks: Sage.
Leadbeater, B. J., Schellenbach, C. J., Maton, K. I., & Dodgen, D. W. (2004). Research and policy for building strengths: Processes and contexts of individual, family, and community development. In K. I. Maton, C. J. Schellenbach, B. J. Leadbeater, & A. L. Solarz (Eds.), *Investing in children, youth, families, and communities: Strengths-based research and policy* (pp. 13–30). Washington, DC: American Psychological Association.
Merritt, D., Maguire-Jack, K., & Negash, T. (2017). Effective program models for the prevention of child maltreatment. In J. B. Klika & J. Conte (Eds.), *The American professional society on the abuse of children handbook on child maltreatment* (4th ed.). Thousand Oaks: Sage.
Munzer, A., Ganser, H. G., & Goldbeck, L. (2017). Neglect social support, negative maltreatment-related cognitions and posttraumatic stress symptoms in children and adolescents. *Child Abuse & Neglect, 63*, 183–191.
Pecora, P. J., Sanders, D., Wilson, D., English, D., Puckett, A., & Rudlang-Perman, K. (2014). Addressing common forms of child maltreatment: Evidence-informed interventions and gaps in current knowledge. *Child and Family Social Work, 19*, 321–332.
Sama-Miller, E., Akers, L., Mraz-Esposito, A., Zukiewicz, M., Avellar, S., Paulsell, D., & Del Grosso, P. (2017). *Home visiting evidence of effectiveness review: Executive summary*. Retrieved from Washington, DC.
Schumacher, J. A., Smith Slep, A. M., & Heyman, R. E. (2001). Risk factors for child neglect. *Aggression and Violent Behavior, 6*, 231–254.
Shonkoff, J. P., Boyce, W. T., & McEwen, B. S. (2009). Neuroscience, molecular biology, and the childhood roots of health disparities. *JAMA, 301*(21), 2252–2260.
Slopen, N., McLaughlin, K. A., Dunn, E. C., & Koenen, K. C. (2013). Childhood adversity and cell-mediated immunity in young adulthood: Does type and timing matter? *Brain, Behavior, and Immunity, 28*, 63–71.
Stith, S. M., Liu, T., Davies, C., Boykin, E. L., Alder, M. C., Harries, J. M., et al. (2009). Risk factors in child maltreatment: A meta-analytic review of the literature. *Aggression and Violent Behavior, 14*, 13–29.
Sweet, M. A., & Appelbaum, M. I. (2004). Is home visiting an effective strategy? A meta-analytic review of home visiting programs for families with young children. *Child Development, 75*, 1435–1456.
Widom, C. S., & Shepard, R. L. (1996). Accuracy of adult recollections of childhood victimization: Part 1. Childhood physical abuse. *Psychological Assessment, 8*(4), 412–421.
Wolfe, D. A., Crooks, C. V., Lee, V., McIntyre-Smith, A., & Jaffe, P. G. (2003). The effects of children's exposure to domestic violence: A meta-analysis and critique. *Clinical Child and Family Psychology Review, 6*(3), 171–187.

Chapter 8
Universal Services: The Foundation for Effective Prevention

Deborah Daro and Cara Karter

8.1 Introduction

Prevention efforts have long been categorized using terms originally framed by clinical medicine – primary (preventing new cases of disease); secondary (reducing established cases of disease), and tertiary (decreasing the frequency and severity of a disease) (Commission on Chronic Illness 1957). More recently, Gordon (1983) developed a classification system based on population level risk – the notion of universal prevention strategies broadly available to everyone, selective prevention services focused on those demonstrating elevated risk for poor outcomes, and indicated interventions for those who have already experienced the negative effects of adversity (Doll et al. 2007). The interplay among these three strategies within a comprehensive public healthapproach has varied by topic as well as country. In some countries, universal access to health care, supportive services at the time a child is born, paid family leave, child care subsidies, and employment training programs are routinely offered at the population level as ways to reduce the rate and costs of chronic disease, enhance overall quality of life, share child rearing responsibilities, and improve productivity (OECD 2016). In other countries, such as the United States, primary emphasis is placed on offering universal access to educational opportunities as the most efficient way to improve literacy and promote economic mobility and long-term success (Mondale and Patton 2001).

More recently, the concept of universality has been extended in the United States as an alternative approach to preventing child maltreatment, improving parental capacity, and enhancing optimal child development (Daro and Dodge 2010). Historically,

D. Daro (✉)
Senior Research Fellow, Chapin Hall, University of Chicago, Chicago, IL, USA
e-mail: ddaro@chapinhall.org

C. Karter
Chapin Hall, University of Chicago, Chicago, IL, USA

B. Lonne et al. (eds.), *Re-Visioning Public Health Approaches for Protecting Children*, Child Maltreatment 9, https://doi.org/10.1007/978-3-030-05858-6_8

the US child welfare system has reflected a philosophy and public policy response that limits interventions into family life to families who have demonstrated an inability to care for their children or who face significant risk or limitations in meeting their child's basic needs (Myers 2006). In addition to protecting a zone of privacy around the family, targeted interventions are considered the most efficient and fair way to allocate scarce resources. These interventions limit public investments to those with demonstrated need. Unfortunately, evidence suggests that a singular reliance on targeted interventions has not reduced the prevalence of poor outcomes for children living in the most disadvantaged circumstances or who are served by a reactive child protection system (Waldfogel 2009). Health disparities based on gender, race, and socioeconomic status remain a major challenge. Indeed, concerns over variability in child health and well-being across subpopulations has propelled public health advocates to embrace notions of precision medicine, further targeting interventions to better address the unique needs of specific subpopulations (Xin 2017).

Refining targeted programs is one approach to addressing health disparities. However, another approach, advocated in this chapter, is to think of doing better with individual subgroups by first establishing a universal base of preventive services for all families. By recognizing the universal needs of all children and the universal challenges caretakers and communities face in addressing these needs, a more informed and effective policy can be developed, one which coordinates universal and targeted strategies in an intentional manner. Offering a new universal option is not about giving everyone a new entitlement; it is about raising awareness around a common need or shared concern and providing a mechanism to ensure families are provided access to the level of support they require.

This chapter begins with a theoretical overview of the challenges and benefits of adopting a universal response as a prerequisite for constructing an effective and efficient public health approach to preventing child maltreatment. The chapter then presents data on how universal strategies can work in partnership with more targeted efforts to maximize both participant outcomes and system efficiencies. The chapter concludes with recommendations on how to best use a universal foundation of support for all new parents to build more effective child protection policy.

8.2 The Targeted Versus Universal Dilemma

A preference for targeted prevention programs is often driven by the belief that the strategy offers the most appropriate and efficient way to allocate limited public resources, particularly in the areas of parent support and child maltreatment prevention (Guterman 2001). The need to avoid negative outcomes for children is best served, the argument goes, by limiting efforts to alter or control parental behaviors to those families who have already exhibited a given problem or who demonstrate known risk factors. Universal strategies are considered less optimal because they direct resources to those not needing assistance and exert unnecessary oversight of the "private" family. Under a scenario of fixed resource levels, serving everyone means having less to spend on those with the greatest need. Because the pool of available resources has been diluted across all families, those families at highest risk may not have access to the level of care required to alter their behaviors.

8.3 The Challenge in Predicting Risk

The efficiency argument regarding the benefits of limiting prevention services to those at highest risk is most appropriate in those circumstances when service access can be determined by a highly predictive and accurate risk assessment protocol or set of eligibility criteria. In the case of child maltreatment, this assumption is only partially met. Certain socioeconomic characteristics, such as income and young maternal age, have been repeatedly associated with an elevated risk for maltreatment, particularly child neglect (Chaffin et al. 1996; Parrish et al. 2011; Putnam-Hornstein and Needell 2011). Research also has demonstrated a link between parental functioning, in terms of a caretaker's mental health status, substance abuse issues, and exposure to domestic violence (Brown et al. 1998; Dubowitz et al. 2011; Kotch et al. 1999; Pears and Capaldi 2001; Renner and Slack 2006). There is little disagreement that an individual's past experiences and current realities influence their parental capacity and their ability to be responsive to their children's needs. Retrospective studies linking the frequency of various adverse conditions, including childhood maltreatment, to adult functioning and health outcomes support the hypothesis that those who have complex trauma histories face greater struggles in all domains of adult life than those without this history (Anda et al. 2006).

The complexity and plethora of causal pathways that contribute to maltreatment, however, suggest that limiting prevention efforts only to those with one or more risk factors is not a perfect solution to building an effective prevention system. In all of these areas, only a minority of those presenting with a given risk profile will, in the absence of intervention, mistreat their child. For example, research suggests only a third of those who experience maltreatment will go on to mistreat their own children (Kaufman and Zigler 1987; Jackson et al. 1999). A 30-year prospective longitudinal study conducted by Widom et al. (2015) and colleagues found the link between a history of reported maltreatment and abuse within subsequent generations to be uneven and related to other factors, such as the type of maltreatment being tracked and potential surveillance bias in administrative records. The predictive errors and stigmatization often associated with targeted prevention services is particularly problematic when risk is defined solely by easily observable socioeconomic characteristics such as race, marital status, young maternal age, and income (National Research Council 2014).

In other words, programs that limit their enrolment only to those who present with a predetermined list of concerns may not be as efficient as first thought. The individuals targeted for intensive, longer term prevention services include a mix of those truly in need of additional support and those who, while presenting with elevated risk, in fact have far more strengths and resources than their profile might suggest. When attempts are made to correct for this error by making eligibility criteria even more restrictive, sustaining a strength-based focus when enrolling and engaging potential participants is further compromised. Parents are offered assistance not based on the common needs they share with other parents, but rather on their documented deficiencies. Potential participants may begin to distance themselves from such interventions to avoid the stigma of enrolling in them, even if they believe they might benefit from support (Offord 2000).

Indeed, this tendency to avoid services viewed as being limited to "those with problems" may contribute to the struggles targeted prevention programs often face in enrolling and retaining those most challenged (McCurdy and Daro 2001; McCurdy et al. 2006). Because prevention programs are generally voluntary, participants are free to refuse offers of assistance or, once enrolled, to leave the program at any time. Research on targeted home visiting programs, for example, have found that although a very small percentage of those offered early assistance outright refuse such help, less than one-quarter receive the dosage many evidence-based models recommend (Daro et al. 2003, 2014). Some of those who leave do so because they no longer require services or are referred on to more intensive, clinical interventions better suited to their level of functioning. In the majority of cases, however, families are leaving programs early because of a disinterest in what the program is offering or because they are unable or unwilling to comply with the program expectations. The more prevention programs are viewed as being suitable for only the highest risk or most challenged families, the less interested families are in associating themselves with such assistance (Daro et al. 2015). Further, families facing the greatest challenges are often disconnected from social networks or formal service systems, limiting their access to voluntary preventive services. They typically do not utilize the public health clinics or nutrition programs that serve as primary referral sources for targeted prevention programs serving new parents. High-risk families can remain "invisible" to social services until they act in ways that result in a formal report to either law enforcement or child protective services.

8.4 Benefits of Universality

Creating a unified public health approach in which targeted services are provided as a second step in a combined universal-targeted system of care for new parents offers several advantages in addressing these problems (Daro 2000). First, formalizing a universal contact with all parents, ideally at the time a woman is pregnant or a child is born, reduces stigma. Politically, it reinforces the message that parenting is a tough job and that all parents, regardless of their status in life, can face difficulties in rearing their children. Offering an opportunity for all parents to reflect on these difficulties and providing parents a license to ask for help if needed creates a context in which seeking help is not a sign of weakness, but rather a preferred response when facing a complex challenge. Parenting is not something done in isolation, but rather a task best addressed by seeking out those formal and informal sources of support that best complement a parent's strengths and limitations. Within this framework, more intensive and targeted offers of assistance become one of many options available to all families following a careful assessment, not an option offered only to families with a demographic or behavioural risk profile sufficiently serious to merit public attention.

Second, a universal assessment of parental capacity can generate the types of data necessary to create an effective public health response. Determining an appropriate service mix within any community requires information on the population's full range of needs, the relative magnitude of these needs, and the perceived and real barriers to service access. Effective public health approaches require a robust database that can be used to determine the prevalence of certain conditions and the individual and environmental challenges that contribute to and mediate these conditions (Savel and Foldy 2012). At present, the determination of which targeted prevention programs to offer in a community, the capacity of these programs to meet current demand, and the appropriateness of a community's referral network are created based on what is perceived as the most critical need by agency managers or policy advocates. Some service needs are well known, such as access to medical services to resolve an illness, remedial services to address a developmental delay, or concrete supports to address basic needs such as housing or food. The appropriate resolution for other issues, such as maternal depression or lack of parenting skills, is more diffused, with the intensity or type of intervention a function of the problem's severity and a participant's capacity to engage in various forms of support. The appropriate mix and capacity of interventions or the best way to ensure full and fair access to service resources are often left to anecdotal comments gleaned from community providers or "thought leaders" based on their understanding of current research on program impacts, participant preferences, and service needs. A universal assessment of strengths and needs, coupled with offers of various options and levels of support that engages all new parents creates an opportunity to gather consistent, real-time data on parental needs and the community's capacity to address those needs. The process elevates the parent voice in these planning discussions and develops an empirical base for determining how public resources can most effectively be allocated.

Finally, a universal approach creates a context in which all children are assumed to be in need of collective attention—a concept at the heart of a public health approach to child well-being. Public health is the science of protecting and improving the health of people and their communities (Schneider 2014). Public health efforts are driven, in part, by the understanding that improving outcomes for all children requires a platform of support that addresses common needs and society's collective responsibility to address these needs. A public health perspective is grounded in the belief that collective goals are best realized when individuals act in ways supportive of their own health and the health of others (Wallack and Lawrence 2005).

Some threats to a child's well-being are best resolved through the development and dissemination of a single universal strategy. Universal interventions—such as immunizations, well-child care, and public education—have dramatically reduced child mortality and morbidity rates (Centers for Disease Control and Prevention (CDC) 1999). However, the prevention of child maltreatment and its corresponding mandate to strengthen parental capacity requires more than a single public intervention or service strategy or even a series of targeted prevention services designed to address individual risk factors. It requires a system of care that is built on the universal recognition that all parents face common challenges and that these challenges require both a collective and individual response. By beginning with a universal assessment to determine the capacity and needs of all parents, the public health response becomes more efficient at allocating limited resources and creating a social context more supportive to parents and more responsive to children.

8.5 Universal Strategies to Enhance Parenting

The utility of a universal approach in addressing social and health problems is far from consistent. Factors which determine when universal solutions may more easily be proposed and implemented include: high prevalence rates that cut across the total population, an evidence base that suggests a universal approach would be more cost-effective than screening for those at highest risk, and public support for the strategy's full implementation and acceptance (Offord 2000). In some instances, such as significant threats to public health, the adoption of a universal strategy, such as vaccinations, can be sufficient to make a significant and measureable improvement in the problem. One of the earliest compulsory vaccination success stories is the prevention of smallpox in the first half of the nineteenth century. Following the development of a smallpox vaccine by Dr. Edward Jenner in 1798, the vaccination became mandatory in many European countries. Because of these vaccination mandates, mortality rates due to smallpox declined over 88% by 1857 and eventually was eradicated from the population worldwide in 1977 (Hodge Jr and Gostin 2002). Throughout the next century, vaccines successfully reduced rates of many epidemic diseases. Indeed, the Centers for Disease Control and Prevention (1999) identified universal vaccinations as one of the ten greatest public health achievements in the United States during the twentieth century.

Broad acceptance and implementation of mandated vaccinations to prevent diseases has worked, in part, because the approach meets the criteria associated with adopting a universal intervention: the problem is widespread across the full population, the universal solution being proposed is well supported by research, and the public believes the strategy is required to protect their health. Vaccinations offer the added benefits of a low, per dosage cost and minimum patient inconvenience to implement.

Few of these conditions apply in the case of early family support services. While all parents benefit from support, evidence as to what exactly an individual parent needs and how best to meet those needs is limited and far from conclusive. And, in many cases, new parents may not understand the link between early supportive services and enhanced parental capacity. In response to the complexity of how best to strengthen parental capacity, many countries have elected to begin with a universal offer of assistance not as the solution to the problem but rather as an important first step in creating a network of family support that will vary by content and intensity. Supporting new parents through universal early home visiting in many parts of the developed world has long been a public policy component not of the child protection system but of comprehensive maternal and child healthcare (Kamerman and Kahn 1993). For example, universal offers of support to new parents through home visits are routinely offered in New Zealand (Royal New Zealand Plunket Society 2017); South Australia (Government of South Australia 2005) and the United Kingdom (National Institute for Health and Care Excellence 2014), among other locations. The purpose of these visits is to assess the health of the mother and child and facilitate the parent accessing additional support if needed. It has been argued that the provision of such assistance reduces the need for more costly interventions later and creates a collective appreciation for society's role in ensuring healthy child development (Kempe 1976). This base of universal support also has been associated with a reduced need for investing in intensive, multiyear home visiting programs that target recipients based on demographic risks, such as young maternal age and low income. A recent randomized trial in the US that compared outcomes for those at risk who received standard practice (a universal home visit shortly after birth and routine health care) and those also enrolled in intensive home visiting pre- and postnatally observed no differences in maternal smoking during pregnancy, low birthweight, emergency hospital use, hospital admissions, and timing of subsequent pregnancies (Robling et al. 2016).

In contrast, the United States does not ensure universal access to health care nor offer uniform follow-up contact with all new parents following a baby's birth. Although the majority of pregnant women do access prenatal care and infants are routinely connected to a medical home in some states, there is no systematic, universal attempt to assess the needs of all new parents or connect them to appropriate mental health, financial, or community services (Daro 2000; Daro and Benedetti 2014). Many new parents successfully navigate their community's service network and secure additional support such as voluntary home visiting programs, parent education services, child care, public assistance, and preventive medical care; others struggle to identify appropriate services or to manage complex intake procedures (Daro 1993). The end result is a mixed performance in terms of successfully linking families to appropriate services and reducing health disparities among children from different racial, ethnic, and socioeconomic backgrounds (Currie and Reichman 2015). Further, the absence of guaranteed health care for all individuals is often cited as a contributing factor to the high costs of health care in the US and the country's relatively poor health outcomes and prevalence of chronic diseases (Schneider et al. 2017).

Despite this lack of a national universal, public health response to supporting new parents in the United States, several local communities in the US have experimented with population-based early home visiting. Two such options – Durham Connects and Welcome Baby – offer an initial assessment at the time of birth for all new borns and their families within a specific geographic area and offer more targeted, on-going support as required. Research on both models suggests this approach can enhance child welfare outcomes and strengthen the community's capacity to offer a more supportive context for new parents.

8.6 Durham Connects/Family Connects

Durham Connects (being replicated across the United States as Family Connects) offers a home visit and additional support to all new parents within a specific geographic area. The initial contact occurs in the hospital following a baby's birth. Families are offered a nurse home visit, which consists of a physical assessment of the infant and mother, intervention and education on newborn care, assessment of family-specific needs, and, for families with significant nurse-identified risk, connections to relevant community resources to provide long-term support. If necessary, families receive up to two additional home visits to conduct further assessments or facilitate access to referrals. All families also receive a 1 month follow-up telephone contact from the staff to assess participant satisfaction and document referral outcomes (Dodge et al. 2014).

Critical program features include a universal service offer to all new parents and the use of a structure assessment tool, which rates family health and psychosocial risk through a high inference, family-friendly discussion. The assessment identifies problematic behavior or conditions in four primary domains commonly associated with elevated risk for maltreatment: healthcare, parenting and childcare, family violence and safety, and parent well-being. The home visit protocol also incorporates structured, validated screening instruments for psychosocial problems, including depression, substance abuse, and interpersonal/familial violence (Dodge et al. 2013a).

Repeated evaluations of the intervention, including two randomized clinical trials, have found the approach has significant and measurable impacts on parental capacity, utilization of community supports, and emergency care use. The initial randomized control trial conducted in Durham County, North Carolina offered the intervention to babies born on an even day of the week while babies born on odd days of the week served as the control group. Researchers, who were unaware of the family's study status, conducted interviews with a random sample of families when their infant was 6 months old. They found those in the treatment group reported a higher number of community service connections and more positive parenting behaviors. Based on observations of the parent-child interactions, researchers rated parenting quality higher in the intervention group (Dodge et al. 2014).

Administrative record review of all births in the county during the study period found the intervention group had 50% fewer emergency medical care contacts (including visits to the emergency room and overnight hospital stays) at 1 year of age than children in the control group (Dodge et al. 2013b). At 48 months post-enrolment, children in the intervention group had experienced 36% fewer reports to child protective services for suspected maltreatment than children in the control group (Dodge 2016). These findings underscore the potential long-term safety benefits for children that can be accrued when new parents are assessed early and directed toward a range of community-based resources that offer appropriate and continued support.

8.7 Welcome Baby

Public and non-profit organizations in Los Angeles County, California are collaborating on implementing a system of voluntary, evidence-based family strengthening home visiting services. The County Board of Supervisors and public agency directors, working in partnership with community-based agencies and First 5 LA, a publically funded entity focusing on improving early childhood outcomes, are developing a system for coordinating efforts across a range of universal and targeted home visiting programs serving new parents throughout the county (Ferrer 2017). The county's universal program, Welcome Baby, is funded by First 5 LA and offers early intervention services to all pregnant women and new parents living in one of 14 county communities, covering approximately one-third of the county's 150,000 annual births (Hill et al. 2014).

The program provides up to nine contacts with participants, including up to two prenatal visits and a follow-up phone contact; a visit in the hospital at the time of birth; a nurse home visit following the infant's birth; and additional visits by a parent coach when the infant is 1 month, 2 months, 4 months and 9 months of age. During the hospital visit, staff initiate a structured conversation covering several domains, including indicators of demographic risk (young maternal age, income, educational status); informal and formal support options and use; current maternal behaviour (smoking, substance abuse, pre-natal care, depression); and history of adversity (child maltreatment, domestic violence, mental health concerns) (Bridges for Newborns 2013). Following this assessment, participants in need of longer term, more intensive home visiting services are referred to these resources. Approximately 10% of all families assessed through Welcome Baby are referred on to intensive, multiyear home visiting services.

For those continuing in Welcome Baby, the first home visit is conducted by a nurse within 2 weeks of birth and involves an examination of the mother's and infant's health. While the nurse can be engaged in subsequent visits if necessary, the majority of the home visits and contacts are made by a parent coach, generally a professional with at least a bachelor's degree and experience in delivering home-based services. During the home visits, specific guidance is given around breastfeeding, home safety, and strengthening parent-child interactions and promoting child development. In addition, standardized assessments are conducted with the parent to identify potential concerns around the baby's development and maternal depression. The parent coach assists families in establishing a medical home, securing follow-up health visits, including well-baby care, and accessing other community resources (Hill et al. 2014).

Quasi-experimental evaluations of the program's initial implementation observed positive outcomes in studies conducted when the child was 12, 24, and 36 months of age. During the 12-month interviews, mothers receiving Welcome Baby services, in contrast to women without access to the program, were more likely to initiate breastfeeding and to have exclusively breastfed for at least 4 months. Standardized measures of the family's home environment at all three follow-up points found program participants maintained an environment more supportive of their child's development and engaged in more learning activities in and outside the home. The 36-month findings indicated program participants demonstrated more responsive, encouraging, and affectionate parenting than those in the comparison group. Standardized assessments of the children enrolled in the program found that Welcome Baby participants demonstrated stronger communication and problem-solving skills (Sandstrom et al. 2015).

8.8 Best Practice Standards

Both of these examples, while still evolving, highlight several important features to consider in crafting universal strategies capable of providing the infrastructure necessary for a robust public health response to preventing child maltreatment, enhancing parental capacity, and promoting optimal child development. First, effective universal systems have the capacity to achieve high penetration rates—they can attract and engage the vast majority of new parents within their target service area. They are well positioned to reach the full population (in this case, new parents) by offering services at a point of high receptivity. Offering such services in a hospital setting or prenatal clinics makes the concept of seeking out support when one has a new baby as commonplace and appropriate as asking questions about any other health concern, which avoids the stigmatization often associated with targeted services.

Second, these programs include a structured, uniform strategy for initiating user-friendly discussions about a parent's capacity to meet their child's most immediate needs. It is not a checklist of potential problems or adverse experiences. It is a conversation about behaviors and situations that invites new parents to reflect on what they require to help them facilitate their child's healthy development and how the absence of certain resources may impact their own emotional capacity to care for their child.

Third, these programs offer immediate solutions to immediate needs. They fill information gaps parents may have and they provide short-term 'teaching' on a range of basic skills required to meet the immediate needs of young infants—e.g., feeding, nurturing, monitoring, and safety. These interactions can boost new parents' confidence and reinforce the importance of asking questions and seeking help before problems surface. They give new parents license to ask for help and recognize that they need not face parenting challenges on their own.

Finally, these interventions facilitate linkages to other services based upon a family's unique needs and concerns. Both programs assist families in navigating the local service market by educating program participants about their service options and improving service access. Not all families will need referrals or additional assistance beyond these interventions. However, all families can benefit from an increased understanding that other resources do exist and that effective utilization requires some knowledge of the system and how to evaluate when and how to use available resources. These interventions improve a family's consumer skills and the system's overall efficiency by better matching program resources to individual participant need. Strengthening community service networks is a central function of both programs. Indeed, Family Connects requires their replication sites to spend as much time identifying and engaging a range of local service programs as they do implementing its home visiting component (Dodge et al. 2013a). Similarly, Welcome Baby is working to improve outreach and support to pregnant women and new parents, who face significant challenges by partnering with those county agencies serving the highest need families, such as the departments of public health, mental health, children and family services, and probation (Ferrer 2017).

8.9 Moving Forward

Adopting a more universal platform in building a robust public health response to addressing the disparities in child health and developmental outcomes will be challenging, particularly in countries that have adopted a residual model for justifying social service interventions. When a social service system begins from the premise that the efficient choice is to direct public investments solely to those with demonstrated risk, the system loses its potential to identify strategies that can galvanize and fully engage all citizens in resolving their problems and using the most appropriate array of preventive services. The acceptance of a universal strategy in addressing communicative diseases and threats to public safety is longstanding. Vaccinations to prevent disease, routine screening for genetic abnormalities that can led to serious health conditions, and safety regulations that prevent injury are well accepted by the public, as demonstrated by the passage and general acceptance of laws requiring individuals to comply with these public health directives. Similarly, parents accept their responsibility to enroll their children in primary and secondary education and to keep them in school or demonstrate that an adequate educational option is being provided in home school settings. While some percentage of the population challenges these regulations, the vast majority comply, in part because they understand the value of these recommendations in promoting healthy development.

In the social service domain, however, acceptance of a universal response is less consistent. Within this context, the primary response is that families will ask if they need help and that proactive offers of assistance are best limited to those who have demonstrated an inability to care for their children on their own. There is no universal infrastructure to explicitly weave the range of available targeted services into a coherent system of care for young children and support for all new parents. Due to this lack of infrastructure, prevention efforts are not as efficient and effective as they could be in achieving core outcomes and reducing the prevalence of key problems, including child maltreatment. Shifting the policy framework from an overemphasis on targeted prevention services to one including a strong universal platform for all parents will require aggressive implementation efforts in many domains, including the following:

- Progressive policies and strategies to reduce inequality in health outcomes will require a political environment in which families are encouraged and comfortable in both asking for help and providing help to other families, regardless of their economic circumstances;
- As a prerequisite, an efficient public health response requires robust, reliable, real-time data on family needs and local service capacity and a corresponding commitment to using these data to efficiently allocate resources commensurate with a community's collective needs;
- Methods should be developed to more effectively link this universal system to current programs that exist for families in poverty and parents facing difficult circumstances, such as mental illness, domestic violence, and substance abuse; and
- Meaningful system reform within the child protection system will be required to ensure that children in families unable or unwilling to avail themselves of preventive services receive timely and appropriate alternative care options.

References

Anda, R. F., Felitti, V. J., Bremner, J. D., Walker, J. D., Whitfield, C. H., Perry, B. D., et al. (2006). The enduring effects of abuse and related adverse experiences in childhood. *European Archives of Psychiatry and Clinical Neuroscience, 256*(3), 174–186.

Bridges for Newborns. (2013). *Welcome Baby Protocol.* Developed by LA Best Babies Network, Maternal Child Health Access and First5 LA. Retrieved from http://www.first5la.org/postfiles/files/AppendixG_ModifiedBridgesforNewbornsScreeningToolProtocol.pdf

Brown, J., Cohen, P., Johnson, J. G., & Salzinger, S. (1998). A longitudinal analysis of risk factors for child maltreatment: Findings of a 17-year prospective study of officially recorded and self-reported child abuse and neglect. *Child Abuse & Neglect, 22*(11), 1065–1078.

Centers for Disease Control and Prevention. (CDC). (1999). Impact of vaccines universally recommended for children–United States, 1990–1998. *MMWR. Morbidity and Mortality Weekly Report, 48*(12), 243.

Chaffin, M., Kelleher, K., & Hollenberg, J. (1996). Onset of physical abuse and neglect: Psychiatric, substance abuse, and social risk factors from prospective community data. *Child Abuse & Neglect, 20*(3), 191–203.

Commission on Chronic Illness. (1957). *Chronic illness in the United States* (Vol. 1). Cambridge, MA: Harvard University Press.

Currie, J., & Reichman, N. (2015). Policies to promote child health: Introducing the issue. *The Future of Children, 2*(1), 3–11.

Daro, D. (1993). Child maltreatment research: Implications for program design. In D. Cicchetti & S. Toth (Eds.), *Child abuse, child development and social policy* (pp. 331–367). Norwood: Ablex.

Daro, D. A. (2000). *Child abuse prevention: New directions and challenges.* In Nebraska symposium on motivation, 46, 161–220.

Daro, D., & Benedetti, G. (2014). Sustaining progress in preventing child maltreatment: A transformative challenge. In J. E. Korbin & R. D. Krugman (Eds.), *Handbook of child maltreatment* (pp. 281–300). New York: Springer.

Daro, D., & Dodge, K. (2010). Strengthening home-visiting intervention policy: Expanding reach, building knowledge. In R. Haskins & W. S. Barnett (Eds.), *New directions for America's preschool policies* (pp. 79–86). Washington, DC: NIEER and Brookings.

Daro, D., McCurdy, K., Falconnier, L., & Stojanovic, D. (2003). Sustaining new parents in home visitation services: Key participant and program factors. *Child Abuse & Neglect, 27*(10), 1101–1125.
Daro, D., Boller, K., & Hart, B. (2014). *Implementation fidelity in early childhood home visiting: Successes meeting staffing standards, challenges hitting dosage and duration targets.* Washington, DC: Children's Bureau, Administration for Children and Families, US Department of Health and Human Services. Contract No.: GS-10F-0050L/HHSP233200800065W. Retrieved from https://www.mathematica-mpr.com/our-publications-and-findings/publications/implementation-fidelity-in-early-childhood-home-visiting-successes-meeting-staffing-standards
Daro, D., Donnelly, A. C., Huang, L. A., & Powell, B. J. (2015). Common themes, questions and opportunities: Creating a context for continued improvement. In D. Daro, A. C. Donnelly, L. A. Huang, & B. Powell (Eds.), *Advances in child abuse prevention knowledge: The perspective of new leadership* (pp. 237–252). Dordrecht: Springer.
Dodge, K. (2016). *Universal postnatal home visiting: Evidence of impact and lessons learned.* In Invited plenary at national research conference on early childhood, Washington, DC.
Dodge, K. A., Goodman, W. B., Murphy, R. A., O'Donnell, K., & Sato, J. (2013a). Toward population impact from home visiting. *Zero to Three, 33*(3), 17–23.
Dodge, K. A., Goodman, W. B., Murphy, R. A., O'Donnell, K., & Sato, J. (2013b). Randomized controlled trial of universal postnatal nurse home visiting: Impact on emergency care. *Pediatrics, 132*(Supplement 2), S140–S146.
Dodge, K. A., Goodman, W. B., Murphy, R. A., O'Donnell, K., Sato, J., & Guptill, S. (2014). Implementation and randomized controlled trial evaluation of universal postnatal nurse home visiting. *American Journal of Public Health, 104*(S1), S136–S143.
Doll, L. S., Bonzo, S. E., Sleet, D. A., & Mercy, J. A. (Eds.). (2007). *Handbook of injury and violence prevention.* New York: Springer.
Dubowitz, H., Kim, J., Black, M. M., Weisbart, C., Semiatin, J., & Magder, L. S. (2011). Identifying children at high risk for a child maltreatment report. *Child Abuse & Neglect, 35*(2), 96–104.
Ferrer, B. (2017, June). *Maximizing and expanding home visiting services for families in Los Angeles County: Update.* Memorandum to the Los Angeles County Board of Supervisors.
Gordon, R. (1983). An operational classification of disease prevention. *Public Health Reports, 98*, 107–109.
Government of South Australia. (2005). *Family home visiting service outline.* Report prepared by the Children, Youth and Women's Health Services. North Adelaide.
Guterman, N. B. (2001). *Stopping child maltreatment before it starts: Emerging horizons in early home visitation services.* Thousand Oaks: Sage Publications.
Hill, I., Wilkinson, M., & Benatar, S. (2014, August). *First 5 LA Welcome Baby Expansion: Early Implementation Experiences.* Washington, DC: The Urban Institute.
Hodge, J. G., Jr., & Gostin, L. O. (2002). School vaccination requirements: Historical, social, and legal perspectives. *Kentucky Law Journal, 90*, 831. Retrieved from https://pdfs.semanticscholar.org/9289/8f3f9028fde3f0a8482dd126562b8e759cae.pdf.
Jackson, R. W., Triber, F. A., Turner, J. R., Davis, H., & Strong, W. B. (1999). Effects of race, sex, and socioeconomic status upon cardiovascular stress responsivity and recovery in youth. *International Journal of Psychophysiology, 31*(2), 111–119.
Kamerman, S. B., & Kahn, A. J. (1993). Home health visiting in Europe. *Future of Children, 3*(3), 39–52.
Kaufman, J., & Zigler, E. (1987). Do abused children become abusive parents? *American Journal of Orthopsychiatry, 57*(2), 186–192.
Kempe, C. H. (1976). Approaches to preventing child abuse: The health visitors concept. *American Journal of Diseases of Children, 130*(9), 941–947.
Kotch, J. B., Browne, D., Dufort, V., Winsor, J., & Catellier, D. (1999). Predicting child maltreatment in the first 4 years of life from characteristics assessed in the neonatal period. *Child Abuse & Neglect, 23*(4), 305–319.

McCurdy, K., & Daro, D. (2001). Parent involvement in family support programs: An integrated theory. *Family Relations, 50*(2), 113–121.
McCurdy, K., Daro, D., Anisfeld, E., Katzev, A., Keim, A., LeCroy, C., et al. (2006). Understanding maternal intentions to engage in home visitation programs. *Children and Youth Services Review, 28*(10), 1195–1212.
Mondale, S., & Patton, S. B. (Eds.). (2001). *School: The story of American public education*. New York: Beacon Press.
Myers, J. E. (2006). *Child protection in America: Past, present, and future*. New York: OUP.
National Institute for Health and Care Excellence. (2014, September). *Health visiting*. Local Government Briefing LGB 22.
National Research Council. (2014). *New directions in child abuse and neglect research*. Washington, DC: National Academies Press.
OECD. (2016). *Society at a Glance 2016: OECD social indicators*. Paris: OECD. https://doi.org/10.1787/9789264261488-en.
Offord, D. R. (2000). Selection of levels of prevention. *Addictive Behaviors, 25*(6), 833–842.
Parrish, J. W., Young, M. B., Perham-Hester, K. A., & Gessner, B. D. (2011). Identifying risk factors for child maltreatment in Alaska: A population-based approach. *American Journal of Preventive Medicine, 40*(6), 666–673.
Pears, K. C., & Capaldi, D. M. (2001). Intergenerational transmission of abuse: A two-generational prospective study of an at-risk sample. *Child Abuse & Neglect, 25*(11), 1439–1461.
Putnam-Hornstein, E., & Needell, B. (2011). Predictors of child protective service contact between birth and age five: An examination of California's 2002 birth cohort. *Children and Youth Services Review, 33*(8), 1337–1344.
Renner, L. M., & Slack, K. S. (2006). Intimate partner violence and child maltreatment: Understanding intra-and intergenerational connections. *Child Abuse & Neglect, 30*(6), 599–617.
Robling, M., Bekkers, M. J., Bell, K., Butler, C. C., Cannings-John, R., Channon, S., et al. (2016). Effectiveness of a nurse-led intensive home-visitation programme for first-time teenage mothers (Building Blocks): A pragmatic randomised controlled trial. *The Lancet, 387*(10014), 146–155.
Royal New Zealand Plunket Society, Inc. (2017). *Annual Report, 2017*. Wellington.
Sandstrom, H., Benatar, S., Greenberg, E., Hill, I., Howell, E., Triplett, T., et al. (2015). *Welcome baby home visiting: Findings from the 36-month child & family survey and 3-year longitudinal results*. Los Angeles: Urban Institute/University of California.
Savel, T. G., & Foldy, S. (2012). The role of public health informatics in enhancing public health surveillance. *MMWR Surveillance Summaries, 61*(Suppl), 20–24.
Schneider, M. (2014). *Introduction to public health* (4th ed.). Burlington: Jones and Bartlett Learning.
Schneider, E. C., Sarnak, D. O., Squires, D., Shah, A., & Doty, M. M. (2017). *Mirror, mirror 2017: International comparison reflects flaws and opportunities for better US health care*. Commonwealth Fund, US.
Waldfogel, J. (2009). Prevention and the child protection system. *The Future of Children, 19*(2), 195–210.
Wallack, L., & Lawrence, R. (2005). Talking about public health: Developing America's "second language". *American Journal of Public Health, 95*(4), 567–570.
Widom, C. S., Czaja, S. J., & DuMont, K. A. (2015). Intergenerational transmission of child abuse and neglect: Real or detection bias? *Science, 347*(6229), 1480–1485.
Xin, H. (2017). Editorial: Health disparities – An important public health concern. *Frontiers in Public Health, 5*(99). https://doi.org/10.3389/fpubh.2017.00099.

Chapter 9
Families – Private and Sacred: How to Raise the Curtain and Implement Family Support from a Public Health Perspective

Daryl Higgins, Matthew Sanders, Bob Lonne, and Dominic Richardson

9.1 Introduction

A cursory internet search quickly reveals the close intersection in public discourse between the concept of family, and notions of 'privacy' and sanctity/sacredness, and the tension with the role of the state. The UN Convention on the Rights of the Child (UNCRC) positions families are held up as the bedrock of society and pivotal to the socialization of children. Politicians, religious institutions, the judiciary and other social institutions are enjoined in the media to preserve 'the family'. To read that would make you think that family support services and strategies would be a high priority of governments globally. But that rhetoric of the priority of the family is confusingly juxtaposed with the notion of privacy. Families are the most important foundational element of society, but they must (largely) undertake the task of being a family (and in particular, caring for children) on their own – and while families are the most important thing, telling people *how* to be a family is frowned upon. Advising parents how to parent their children is presented in much of the public

D. Higgins (✉)
Institute of Child Protection Studies, Australian Catholic University, Melbourne, VIC, Australia
e-mail: daryl.higgins@acu.edu.au

M. Sanders
Parenting and Family Support Centre, University of Queensland, Brisbane, QLD, Australia
e-mail: m.sanders@psy.uq.edu.au

B. Lonne
School of Health, University of New England, Armidale, NSW, Australia
e-mail: blonne@une.edu.au

D. Richardson
UNICEF Office of Research-Innocenti, Florence, Italy
e-mail: drichardson@unicef.org

B. Lonne et al. (eds.), *Re-Visioning Public Health Approaches for Protecting Children*, Child Maltreatment 9, https://doi.org/10.1007/978-3-030-05858-6_9

discourse as unnecessary or unwanted state interference. To try and influence the choices families make about how they operate, and the quality of the interactions that go on within the family home are seen as 'beyond the pale'.

And yet, there is growing concern about the 'epidemic' of family violence, and escalating rates of notifications and substantiations of child abuse and neglect. Analysis of the 'drivers' or causal factors that contribute this this rise reveal a common set of family problems that typically lead to engagement with statutory service systems—that is, family violence, parental mental illness and addictions to alcohol, other drugs and gambling (Higgins 2015). The mechanism by which such problems affect children's development, and become abusive or neglectful, is due to the impact they have on parenting capacity. Although most aspire to be good parents, their knowledge about positive parenting behaviors and their confidence and skill to enact these is mixed at best. But there is rarely a focus on targeting these behaviors and enhancing these skills across society. In this chapter, we want to explore why, and how this can be changed.

A disconnect occurs in that a curtain has descended over the site where, from a public health perspective, prevention initiatives could—and rightly should—be implemented to address child maltreatment (and for that matter, family violence): the family home, and the behaviors that are enacted behind closed doors. To prevent harm to children, the major protagonists are parents, and their parenting skills and the way the 'do' family. But thankfully, the interventions don't need to happen behind closed doors. In his case for a public health approach to child safety and well-being, Higgins (2015) used examples of how other public health problems that are driven largely by personal, even *private* behaviors – such as smoking, drink-driving, unsafe sex – can effectively be shaped by *public* health strategies to prevent lung cancer, road fatalities and sexually transmissible infections (including HIV/AIDS). Just as these behaviors take place at a public bar (or the kitchen), in the car, in the bedroom, or in other personal or private spaces can be influenced by widely disseminated messages, attitude-change strategies, and avenues for seeking advice, help and support – so too can parenting behaviors.

Adopting a public health approach to preventing maltreatment inherently involves initiatives that seek to interfere with the 'private and sacred' notion of families, and make visible and influence the parenting practices, and safety conditions for children in the family home. In this chapter, we build on the arguments outlined in Chap. 1 and explain how statutory child protection responses to families in need of support, through diversion of reports or 'differential response' (i.e., funneling back supports to families after they've come to the attention of statutory authorities) is not necessarily the best and most efficient way of reaching those who would benefit from advice, help, and even more intensive support. Structural barriers to help-seeking also exist among families experiencing poverty, social dislocation or exclusion, which need to be taken into account when enacting the public health model through broad-based provision of parenting/family supports.

9.2 Population Health Approaches to Evidence-Based Parenting and Family Support

The goal of a population-approach to child maltreatment prevention is to reduce the *prevalence* of maltreatment and associated indicators across the entire population (not just within suspected 'high risk' groups or locations). To achieve that, prevention efforts are designed and implemented for *community-wide impact*. Such an approach relies on providing supports to enhance parenting capacity that are non-stigmatizing, drawing on specialized services where necessary, and emphasizing local networks and existing sources of support accessible by the majority of families (CFCA 2014; Herrenkohl et al. 2015).

9.2.1 Prevalence Reduction as the Ultimate Goal

A hallmark of population-health strategies is an emphasis on addressing community-wide prevalence. This type of metric is highly relevant to child maltreatment prevention, where the shared goal is reduction in the proportion of children experiencing adverse parenting and family environments. Child maltreatment prevention strategies need to be considered and evaluated in terms of the potential to reduce the prevalence of adverse outcomes (e.g., injuries, foster care placements, childhood mental health disorders) as well as to increase the prevalence of well-being outcomes (e.g., reaching developmental milestones, school achievement, behavioral self-regulation).

9.2.2 Broader Prevention to Overcome Low-Frequency Outcomes

Cases of child maltreatment in statutory systems, though troubling, nonetheless occur at relatively low rates in the population. Trying to prevent a relatively low-frequency outcome like child maltreatment that comes to the attention and meets the threshold of statutory services is further compounded by difficulties in predicting which parents will engage in abusive or neglectful behaviors and show up in a statutory child protection system. A population approach has the potential to address this challenge. Interventions that are designed for broad population reach increase the likelihood of engaging more parents who might mistreat their children. A related advantage is that population-based prevention can address a wider range of adverse parenting practices than can be achieved by targeting highest-risk families. Official cases of maltreatment represent only a small percentage of the children who are exposed to deleterious parenting. For example, in an anonymous telephone survey, Theodore and colleagues (2005) found that parents in the US self-reported physically abusive behaviors at a rate 40 times higher than the official substantiated rate of child abuse. Similarly, in a random household survey in the US, 10% of parents reported spanking their children with an object on a "frequent" or "very frequent" basis (Prinz 2016). In a similar Australian household survey of 4010 primary caregivers in the state of Queensland, 43.4% reported smacking with their hand and 7.7% smacking more than once or with an object (Sanders et al. 2007).

9.2.3 *Increased Normalization and Lowered Stigma of Seeking Help for Parents*

Singling out families for intervention on the basis of a risk profile may seem attractive to funders, but parents labelled as 'high risk' might have a different opinion. Common practices like participation in birth-preparation classes, use of car seats, and incorporation of physical exercise into schools have become normalized and thus benefit the whole population without stigmatizing individuals. Seeking out evidence-based parenting support (especially if such programs or services respect self-determination and a wide variety of acceptable parenting practices), needs to be normalized as a parent's pathway to happier, healthier children, rather than something that is punitive or that inadvertently marks the parent as deficient, incompetent, or misguided.

9.2.4 *Blending of Universal and Targeted Strategies in Prevention*

One of the concerns about adopting a strictly universal approach to child maltreatment prevention is that families in the population who might need more intensive services will be adequately addressed. A hybrid approach, called 'blended prevention' (or progressive universalism, or cascaded services), combines universal and targeted elements into an integrated strategy (Prinz 2015). Blended prevention can be found in other universal public policy areas, such as the use of car seats for infants and toddlers: car seats are legally mandated passage for all (i.e., universal), but it can be complemented by providing car seats at low-cost or free to parents who cannot afford them but are at high need, such as teen parents or care leavers (i.e., offering a higher intensity intervention to targeted groups with higher risk). The same concept can be applied to parenting support. Drawing on blended prevention, a well-integrated system of evidence-based parenting support would include broad-reach strategies such as large-group, low-intensity and media-based strategies, plus multiple levels of more intensive and extensive services and supports. In a well-crafted system, parents who do participate in the more targeted elements would also benefit from exposure to the universal facets of a public health strategy and reduces the likelihood of engagement being stigmatizing.

9.2.5 *Impact Multiple Outcomes with Same Intervention*

Evidence-based parenting support deployed in a blended prevention model can reduce child maltreatment – but concurrently can also reduce or prevent children's social, emotional and behavioral problems (which are more prevalent than child maltreatment but share many of the same contextual factors and prevention strategies). They can also improve children's readiness at school entry and reduce trajectories for adverse outcomes in adolescence such as substance abuse, delinquency, school dropout, and teen pregnancy.

9.2.6 *Application of Key Population Health Principles*

To be effective, key principles of a population approach need to be incorporated into child maltreatment prevention (Sanders et al. 2017). For example, interventions need to have:

- 'Minimal sufficiency' – incorporating low-intensity programs that have wide reach in terms of parental participation at an affordable cost;
- Universal elements such as a media and communication strategies that destigmatise parental involvement and that help to create "pull" demand from parents (legitimising the concept that all parents can benefit from help at some stage); and
- Cultural relevance – to the whole population, and adaptable to sub-population groups.

9.2.7 *Capitalizing on Multiple Settings, Delivery Formats, and Intensity of Interventions*

A population approach seeks to employ multiple different service delivery contexts as an opportunity to promote safe, nurturing relationships and effective parenting skills across the entire population. This involves using widely accessed, normative care contexts such as primary health care services, early childhood education and schools, drawing on various government and non-government sector organizations delivering parenting and family support services and programs and the media. Existing evidence relating to service access emphasizes the importance of non-stigmatizing entry points for services (Robinson et al. 2012; Stewart et al. 2011).

9.2.8 Evidence for Population Effects

Addressing child maltreatment through a population-based approach rests on two complementary lines of evidence. First, a large, growing evidence base over 40 years (including randomized controlled trials), shows that group and individual positive parenting programs (based on social learning and cognitive behavioral principles) produce sustained positive changes in both children and parents. There is also growing evidence that low-intensity interventions designed to have wide population reach and low-cost self-directed technology-assisted interventions (such as the Positive Parenting Program (Triple P) Online: <https://www.triplep-parenting.net.au/au-uken/find-help/triple-p-online/>) can be effective in changing parenting practices. Online platforms now provide greater flexibility in delivery of evidence-based programs and supports. Such technology-based suites can be delivered on a tiered continuum of interventions of increasing intensity and narrowing population reach. Such online platforms can provide an excellent foundation for the development and testing of a system of parenting support.

The second strand of evidence for a population-based approach is the small number of studies that document the outcomes of trials that have adopted a true population approach to deliver multiple levels of intervention to a defined geographical catchment area *and tracked outcomes at a population level*. For example, Prinz and colleagues demonstrated that community-wide implementation of evidence-based parenting support as a blended prevention strategy could reduce population prevalence of child maltreatment. "Place" in this study was a county with a population between 50,000 and 175,000 people. Randomizing 18 counties in South Carolina to either intervention or usual services, the US study implemented the full Triple P system, which is a tiered, multi-level approach to parenting support, through the existing workforce across several service sectors in the nine intervention counties. Controlling for the 5-year baseline period prior to intervention, the study found significant reductions in rates of confirmed child maltreatment cases in the statutory child protection service, out-of-home care placements (i.e., foster care), and hospital-treated child maltreatment injuries compared with the comparison counties (Prinz 2017; Prinz et al. 2009, 2016). Similarly, a quasi-experimental study conducted in Ireland, similarly showed that the implementation of a multi-level system that comprised social marketing, low-intensity seminars (mainly delivered through schools – a valuable hub for non-stigmatising population-based service delivery), topic-specific workshops on common developmental problems (e.g., shopping trips), and an 8-session Group Triple P intervention reduced the level of serious behavioural and emotional problems by 37% over a 2.5-year period, as reported by parents in an epidemiological household survey (Fives et al. 2014).

9.2.9 Challenges to Adopting a Population Approach

Marmot et al.'s (2010) principle of proportionate universalism is relevant to child maltreatment prevention as it implies all parents can benefit from support in parenting at various points in their parenting careers, but others need much more support. Having interventions based on the same core principles that vary in intensity can be very useful. Evidence-based strategies or programs range from low-intensity seminars and discussion groups about specific child rearing topics (e.g., bedtime problems), more moderately intensive multi-session active skills training programs for parents with more serious child behavior problems (e.g., children with oppositional behavior problems, conduct problems, developmental disorders), to more intensive programs where parenting problems are complicated by domestic violence and/or additional parental relationship, mental health or substance abuse problems (for examples of programs well-supported by evidence, see California Evidence-Based Clearinghouse for Child Welfare: http://www.cebc4cw.org).

Others might contend that screening, and then targeting services where children are at greatest risk is more likely to reap benefits. However, screening and targeted delivery is still very *expensive* to implement at a population level and runs the risk of introducing *stigma* in being identified as a parent who needs extra help with parenting. An alternative approach is to promote the idea that all parents experience difficulties and challenges in raising their children from time to time and that confronting and dealing with these challenges that come with everyday parenting is normal, and it is desirable to get involved in learning the skills and strategies that promote healthy development of children and families. However, not everyone needs the same level of support. By only targeting the most vulnerable families, the vast majority of parents experiencing difficulties with parenting will be ignored and it will be very difficult to impact on the prevalence of child maltreatment. Public health approaches that utilize universal services—or take a 'blended approach' as outlined earlier—will benefit a much larger proportion of the population who would benefit from parenting or other family supports.

9.2.10 Importance of Engaging Parents as Consumers

Practitioners and parents are the 'consumers' of parenting programs and support strategies. Actively involving target groups in planning an intervention can lead to more tailored or customized delivery of the program (Metzler et al. 2012). The aim of this approach is to enhance the ecological fit of the intervention to the intended audience.

9.2.11 Addressing Cultural Diversity

In culturally diverse settings, when parents and practitioners are asked to comment on Triple P, parents' ratings of the program's cultural relevance and acceptability tend to be higher than practitioners' ratings of these characteristics (Morawska et al. 2011). This may reflect the 'gateholder' phenomenon, whereby practitioners can be overprotective of communities they serve and may have opinions that differ from the parents involved. However, practitioners working with Indigenous groups have had to adjust the content and mode of delivery of the program (Turner et al. 2007). For example, in Australia, practitioners working with Aboriginal parents have focused on sensitivity to differences and cultural diversity, including strategies such as instituted longer sessions, relied less on workbook materials, and produced an Indigenous video to help engage parents (see Chap. 20).

9.2.12 Need for Effective Partnerships

Fives et al. (2014) identified the advantages and challenges in maintaining partnerships with partner organizations that supported the implementation of a public-health oriented parent-support strategy (i.e., the multi-level Triple P initiative). Organizations contributed in an unequal way, but were considered necessary to ensure that goals were reached. When establishing partnerships, different partners may make different contributions to a rollout of a strategy or intervention, and reviews should be conducted throughout the implementation process. Initial partnership goals may not go as expected, as they may be overambitious or under ambitious, and can be affected by factors such as funding cuts or how staff members were selected initially for training.

9.2.13 Training and Supporting a Workforce

Population effects are unlikely to be observed when programs are implemented with low fidelity. Traditionally, parenting programs were disseminated using a "train and hope" model in which staff would be trained in the program and then left to deliver the intervention without support from the training organization. Many of the steps to ensure the success of an intervention occur prior to—and after—training (Brown and McWilliam 2012). Implementation guidelines are needed, which can then be tested empirically. Each rollout of an intervention benefits from an implementation consultant, who follows an implementation framework and works directly with an organization to troubleshoot implementation challenges (e.g., reaching participation targets, managing crises). More empirical research is necessary to test the effectiveness of such implementation frameworks to determine if they improve population-level effects.

9.3 Alternatives to Statutory Child Protection Responses

There are tensions between population approaches to prevention of child maltreatment and tertiary level ones such as statutory child protection, particularly concerning notions of risk and safety, and the targeting of particular at-risk groups. Although the development of our protective systems over the past 50 years has been impressive regarding addressing physical and sexual abuse, it is less accomplished with the multi-facetted forms of child neglect, which is generally the largest type of maltreatment (Child Trends 2016; Stoltenborgh et al. 2013). However, in many jurisdictions there has also been growing awareness of the significant shortcomings with statutory and court-based responses, including judgmental and stigmatizing state interventions, and poor life outcomes for service users including children in care (see Chaps. 1, 2 and 3). Public inquiries into scandals and tragedies have often exposed systemic failures including slow and inadequate protective responses, under- and over-intervention into families and groups, slavish adherence to policy and procedure, and inability to provide necessary support and assistance to struggling families (Featherstone et al. 2014; Loman and Siegel 2015; Lonne and Parton 2014; Lonne et al. 2009).

Differential response pathways started to emerge during the 1990s. The aim of such pathways (or 'dual track' approaches) was both to decrease demand upon statutory child protection services and to provide alternatives to investigatory responses by channeling low-to-medium risk cases through a more supportive process (i.e., an alternative to the traditional 'investigatory' response) that could assist families by linking them to available community resources (see Chap. 12). A broad range of differential response systems exist, including services within or alongside child protection agencies, and those that are primarily operated by community-based systems, such as Victoria's Child FIRST (Cameron and Freymond 2014; Lonne et al. 2015; Winokur et al. 2014). And there is now substantial evidence to demonstrate efficacy of these responses concerning safety and enhanced family buy-in to intervention (see Chap. 12 in this volume and Cameron and Freymond 2014; Merkel-Holguin et al. 2014; Winokur et al. 2014).

But in all differential response systems, statutory child protection approaches remain the dominant service response, with its associated discourses of risk, safety, mandatory reporting, and accountability enforced through state intervention into the family on behalf of children. This backdrop of state authority and compulsion remains a critical issue with regard to willingness by many families to take up opportunities to access services. For example, marginalized groups such as Australian Indigenous people are understandably distrustful and wary of involvement with statutory authorities, fearing removal of their children (Bailey et al. 2017).

This contrasts with family support service approaches such as are found in Scandinavia and parts of Europe which restrict statutory involvement in favor of providing a broad range of voluntary measures to assist families to care for their children (Gilbert et al. 2011; Kojan and Lonne 2012). In our view, these approaches fit comfortably within public health models for early intervention and prevention of child maltreatment and population approaches to support parents.

Essentially, given the established efficacy of population-based parenting support programs, they need to be embedded within our protective systems, whether these have a child protection and safety emphasis or a family support one. Within such contexts there needs to be an overarching policy framework emphasizing accessible and helpful resources to support parents to meet their responsibilities for ensuring their children's health and well-being. This requires political will and institutional vision to:

- Recognize the limitations of 'protection-oriented' approaches;
- Embrace alternative discourses to dominant risk and safety ones and instead focus upon children's socialisation within healthy family and community environments, which is a foundational tenet in the UNCRC;
- Understand the importance of established efficacious population approaches to support families in the challenging tasks of parenting;
- Fund and equip universal support services adequately to enable all families and communities, but particularly those who have high needs, to easily access the non-stigmatizing assistance they require in a timely fashion;
- Establish the legal, organizational and policy frameworks to ensure that service delivery mechanisms are coordinated, integrated and operated; and
- Embed shared responsibility for family support, intervention and training across the institutions of government and community so that they all have a function in assisting families in need to utilize the available help.

Supporting parents at a whole-of-population level will ensure that the opportunities are optimized for families to seek and receive the help they need from compassionate health and welfare service providers, and that they can do so without fear of being stigmatized or marginalized. As outlined earlier, this requires collecting robust research and evaluation of processes and outcomes at both the population and the program level, ensuring program fidelity, and fostering a culture of service innovation.

9.4 Family Policies at the Government Level to Support Achievement of the UN 2030 Sustainable Development Goals

Since 2015, the global community has been working towards the achievement of 17 internationally agreed Sustainable Development Goals (SDGs), containing 169 social progress targets. Many of these goals relate to human development, such as reducing poverty, income inequality, and violence, and improving nutrition, health, education, and gender equality amongst other things. These goals follow-on from where the Millennium Development Goals left off, and for the first time include all countries of the world, not just the poorest ones. Relevant to the public health approach, the SDGs have the specific ambition of leaving no-one behind and improving population-wide outcomes.

Although the word 'family' is rarely mentioned in the goals and targets themselves, the family is a fundamental social unit, and is a key vehicle for public social intervention, in all countries of the world. In the most advanced welfare systems, family policies (including parenting programs, and child protection policies) constitute one of the largest public expenditures and, when including health interventions and education, housing and employment supports, human services and social protection make up over 60% of total public spending, on average, in high income countries (OECD 2015). In developing setting, developments in family policies, as well as investments in education and health interventions, continue to grow.

It is inevitable therefore that family policies, particularly those with a public health approach, will be key to achieving the SDGs. The question is, however, which ones should be prioritized in which contexts, for which goals, to hasten progress across the SDGs as whole? Focusing specifically on SDG 16, the goal for achieving Peace, Justice and Strong institutions, and on the target 16.2 that seeks to 'End abuse, exploitation, trafficking and all forms of violence against and torture of children' – how might national family polices support achievement of target 16.2?

Implementing family support to engage with the challenge of child maltreatment and address target 16.2 can be viewed from the perspectives of both prevention and treatment. Today, where stressors such as experiences of poverty, substance abuse, low education (including parenting skills) remain widespread, and can all influence the extent to which children are put at risk in the family home in the first instance, policies for prevention are have an important role to play. That said, present levels of violence against children are too high, and so a two-streamed approach to family policies is needed.

In terms of prevention, policies for identification of risk can be integrated into mainstream family policies early in the life course, such as the nurse family partnership and home visiting, and as children are, through the employment of school counsellors, counsellors in primary health care services, or family services centers. These policies, and with the addition of social workers and law officials such as the police, or the family courts, could effectively support the identification of both risk and experience of violence with appropriate resources (time finance, human capital) could represents effective means by which long-term risks and consequences of violence against children, for both the children and the communities in which they live can be addressed most effectively.

Prevention is also facilitated by improving family access family policies that reduce stressors, related to poverty, addiction and ill health. A recent study on synthesizing reviews of family policy effects on poverty, health, education, gender equity, youth employment and violence against children (Higgins forthcoming, cited in Richardson 2018) links family home-visiting policies, designed to end violence against children, to positive spill-overs in terms of access to health care, as well as educational and gender equity outcomes (as well as reducing violent discipline, and incidence of violence against children in developed and developing settings). The same study reviewed family policy designed to influence poverty, educational outcome and gender equity and showed these are important tools for reducing stressors and risk factors related to violence, such as to family stability, parental stress, mental health, material deprivation and income poverty, and externalizing behaviors in childhood (Richardson 2018).

Policies for treatment are inevitably dependent on the type and extent of violence experiences by the child. Out-of-home care for children, and medical and mental health treatment, of individual and family counselling policies (again dependent on the relationship of perpetrator to victim), may all be appropriate. A number of family policies, including foster care policies, parenting interventions, family counselling, are used in these instances, and can contribute to achieving the goals of the SDGs by breaking the cycle of violence experienced by these children.

When such a large part of public social expenditure is channeled through families, and societies choose to address healthy family functioning as a prerequisite to broader social progress, the public good attributes of effective family policies and programmes is underlined. And it is in acknowledging the public good nature of healthy families that the contention between private (and sacred) rights and public responsibilities for national policymakers lie. Nonetheless, given the weight of public policy behind family and human services, a balance here needs between to be struck, otherwise the efforts to achieve the SDGs while leaving no-one behind, may be in vain.

9.5 Meeting the Needs of Difference and Diversity

Public health approaches are founded upon the notions of prevention of harm and addressing the social determinants of health through targeted services to those with greater needs, particularly individuals and groups who are socially and economically marginalized. In doing so, there is an ideological and political stance taken to the presenting issues and their resolution. Yet, nations, communities and cultures embrace a variety of ideological viewpoints and political/institutional expressions. For example, Esping-Andersen's (1990) typology of 'ideal' types of welfare regimes (neo-liberal, social-democratic or conservative/corporatist) although limited in some respects, nonetheless alerts to the ideological differences and institutional diversity that societies use to operationalize the role of the state regarding citizen well-being. Nonetheless, in a rapidly changing world, the past few decades have witnessed increased neo-liberal practices utilized within government agencies, including an emphasis upon privatization, social impact investment, and increasing managerialism and interventions to lessen risk, rather than meet need.

The social constructions of children, childhood and families are highly contested and changing, with the role of the state in family life altering but general shift has seen an increased role for government intervention as well as the advent of the preventative surveillance state (Fox Harding 1996; Parton 2006, 2014). Fox Harding (1997) identified four historical value perspectives driving policy frameworks over time, each reflecting different emphases for the rights of parents and children, but with the increasing emergence on the rights of the child evident. This is illustrated by the UNCRC and its focus upon children's development being understood within a context of family, culture and community and the centrality of relationship (Melton 2010). However, despite the overall trends, tensions and how they have played out in different jurisdictions, Gilbert et al. (2011) identified in their study of child social policies and professional practices in ten Western nations a transnational child-focused orientation; the child is seen to have rights and an independent relationship with the state, which takes on a growing role regarding earlier intervention and prevention wider than just in regard to safety and risk, but also the child's overall development and well-being. Emerging knowledge from neuroscience and early childhood development are fostering these trends by providing insights into the importance of nurturing parent-child attachments in the developmental lifespan.

Yet, within these contested and evolving ideological and policy contexts, the state role has inherent tensions and conflicts concerning the primary, secondary and tertiary levels for intervening, particularly with respect to meeting the diversity of needs found amongst different groups, cultures and communities. Child protection illustrates well these public stresses concerning citizen privacy and the role of the state, but so too do public health approaches to family support and child well-being. For example, how should population interventions respond to the diversity of needs found amongst groups with respect to gender, race, ethnicity, culture, class, religion, sexual orientation, intellectual dis/ability and for those who live in, rural/remote communities? How ought difference be handled within universal programs, and what are the merits of using risk analysis to target secondary interventions? Might need be a better determinant of increased service provision? But, if so, how well would need fit within contemporary ideological and policy frameworks?

It remains the case that child maltreatment, particularly neglect, is highly associated with inequality and that over-representation of marginalized groups in child protection interventions is widespread (AIHW 2017; Featherstone et al. 2017; Gilbert et al. 2009). In our view, impoverished communities and marginalized groups experience the sorts of high and unmet needs that warrant greater support, intervention and training, but they need this to be delivered in accessible and non-stigmatizing ways. They also need to be involved as full participants in the process of devising, planning and delivering programs and services (see Chap. 20). This is imperative if the impacts of longstanding prejudice and discrimination are to be addressed in culturally safe ways. Without this, the familial and community distrust of social institutions and state interventions that we outlined earlier will continue to be a serious impediment to the take up of needed services and resources.

At present, many programs and services do not adequately address the needs of various groups, and the robust evaluation of these is lacking. Program fidelity is important. So too is ensuring that the delivery processes and interactions between service users and staff are undertaken in ways that are ethical, humane, inclusive and respectful of the differences found in values, cultural norms and practices, beliefs and significant life issues that services users confront. For example, trauma-informed practice with Indigenous peoples is contextually appropriate as a practice framework (see Chap. 20). Further research and development of evidence-based interventions is required to ensure that programs meet the needs of all service users, but particularly those who are from over-represented groups in protective systems.

9.6 Balancing the Need for Evidence-Based Programs with Evidence-Informed Models of Services/Supports

In trying to overcome the issue of how the view of family life and parenting skills as 'private and sacred' is the notion that it should only be if parents identify that they have a need, should they seek a service, and participate in a program. However, the reality is that many people who would benefit most are not necessarily the ones who enroll in, and/or complete such programs.

A particular benefit of the population-based approach, outlined earlier in this chapter, is that it provides the opportunity for 'intervention by stealth'. Recipients of the 'intervention' may not realize that they are actually receiving the intervention. Or it may be beneficial to frame it differently: not as an *intervention*, but an investment in the well-being of a population, applying the concepts of health promotion, asset-building. If tiered or multi-level models of support are implemented, then at the lower level of intensity, all parents can be benefitting from messages about the value of positive parenting, and what that entails. As well as the communications exercise (media campaigns, signage, flyers, etc.), good practice means equipping the existing workforce to operate consistent with the overall strategy and support parents in whatever way they can. For example, the early childhood educator could share with a parent during pick-up or drop-off how they are managing some early signs of a child's challenging behavior and invite the parent to join with them in creating a 'team approach' to this, asking questions like: "What do you do at home that works in that situation?". Similarly, a doctor or a school counsellor may see some positive interactions between a parent and child that they can comment on (positive reinforcement), and then suggest ways in which it could be expanded, or modified, to address different issues that the parent identifies.

Through such incidental interactions with services that the family is already engaging with, family support and parenting skill training embedded in these existing service platforms help bridge the divide between families as private and sacred, and families in need of support, intervention, and training. This is the backbone of a truly public health approach to maltreatment prevention – having a consistent strategy for supporting and equipping parents, with multiple points at which the intensity of support can be ramped up to meet the emerging needs. Such 'progressive universalism' or 'blended prevention' as we described earlier, is predicated on good interlinkages between existing universal service models and specific/targeted programs. To achieve this, it might mean opening up the premises of universal services—schools, child care centres, GP clinics, or maternal/child health centres—to be the venue for accessing some of the higher-intensity services. Accessible service hubs, or 'soft entry points' help overcome the stigma attached to reaching out to a separate service for parenting guidance (Robinson et al. 2012).

9.7 Implications and Conclusions

Public health messaging about the importance of family life, family supportive public policies, and strategies to support parenting knowledge and capacity can help 'raise the curtain' on what is otherwise seen as the taboo topic of *how* families do the business of being a family and raising children in a safe and supportive environment (Higgins 2015). Opening up discussion of parenting and the needs of families, particularly those at risk of venerability or in need of support, is critical. By focusing on the evidence about the risks, and importantly, the growing evidence about the efficacy of parenting strategies, and in particular, of population-level supports, accessed through non-stigmatising channels, can help overcome the 'privacy of families' mantra within many societies. Rather than only target strategies to the most vulnerable families, we are more likely to reduce the prevalence of child maltreatment if we give the vast majority of parents experiencing difficulties with parenting better supports.

One of the ways forward may be to frame the needs of families in terms of positive parenting skills being learnable, and the role of broader cultural drivers in supporting shifts in personal behavior – as we have seen with other population health initiatives related to smoking, or risky driving behaviors (e.g., no seat belts, drink driving). What we now need is research evidence to examine whether wholistic frameworks for parenting and childhood development based on a public health approach—such as Scotland's Getting it Right for Every Child – National Plan of Action for Child well-being (http://www.gov.scot/Topics/People/Young-People/gettingitright/what-is-girfec); or the Healthy Child Manitoba (2002) initiative—can improve well-being and prevent harm to children.

References

Australian Institute of Health and Welfare. (2017). *Child Protection Australia 2015–16, Child Welfare series no. 66. Cat. no. CWS 60*. Canberra: AIHW.

Bailey, C., Powell, M., & Brubacher, S. (2017). Reporting rates of child sexual abuse in Indigenous communities in two Australian jurisdictions. *Child Abuse & Neglect, 68*, 74–80.

Brown, J., & McWilliam, J. (2012, October). *An implementation framework for the Triple P—Positive Parenting Program*. Paper presented at the biennial Australian Implementation Conference, Melbourne, Australia.

Cameron, G., & Freymond, N. (2014). Accessible service delivery of child welfare services and differential response models. *Child Abuse & Neglect, 39*, 32–40.

CFCA. (2014). *Defining the public health model for the child welfare services context*. (CFCA Resource Sheet). Melbourne: Child Family Community Australia, Australian Institute of Family Studies. Retrieved from https://aifs.gov.au/cfca/publications/defining-public-health-model-child-welfare-services-context

Child Trends. (2016). *Child maltreatment: Indicators of child and youth well-being*. Retrieved from https://www.childtrends.org/wp-content/uploads/2016/09/40_Child_Maltreatment.pdf

Esping-Andersen, G. (1990). *The three worlds of welfare capitalism*. Princeton: Princeton University Press.

Featherstone, B., White, S., & Morris, K. (2014). *Reimagining child protection: Towards humane social work with families*. Bristol: Policy Press.

Featherstone, B., Morris. K., Daniel, B., Bywaters, P., Brady, G., Bunting, L., Mason, W., & Mirza, N. (2017). Poverty, inequality, child abuse and neglect: Changing the conversation. *Children and Youth Services Review*. Advanced access: https://doi.org/10.1016/j.childyouth.2017.06.009

Fives, A., Purcell, L., Heary, C., Gabhainn, N., & Canavan, J. (2014). *Parenting support for every parent: A population-level evaluation of Triple P in Longforth Westmeath. Final report*. Athlone: Longforth Westmeath Parenting Partnership.

Fox Harding, L. (1996). *Family, state and social policy*. Basingstoke: Macmillan Press Ltd.

Fox Harding, L. (1997). *Perspectives in child care policy* (2nd ed.). Essex: Longman.

Gilbert, N., Parton, N., & Skivenes, M. (Eds.). (2011). *Child protection systems: International trends and orientations*. Oxford: Oxford University Press.

Gilbert, R., Kemp, A., Thoburn, J., Sidebotham, P., Radford, L., Glaser, D., & Macmillan, H. L. (2009). Recognising and responding to child maltreatment. *The Lancet, 373*(9658), 167–180.

Healthy Child Manitoba. (2002). *Investing in early childhood development: 2002 progress report to Manitobans*. Healthy Child Manitoba. Retrieved from https://www.gov.mb.ca/healthychild/ecd/ecd_reports.html

Herrenkohl, T. I., Higgins, D. J., Merrick, M. T., & Leeb, R. T. (2015). Positioning a public health framework at the intersection of child maltreatment and intimate partner violence. *Child Abuse & Neglect, 48*, 22–28. https://doi.org/10.1016/j.chiabu.2015.04.013.

Higgins, D. J. (2015). A public health approach to enhancing safe and supportive family environments for children. *Family Matters, 96*, 39–52. Retrieved from: https://aifs.gov.au/publications/family-matters/issue-96/public-health-approach-enhancing-safe-and-supportive-family-environments-children.

Kojan, B., & Lonne, B. (2012). A comparison of systems and outcomes for safeguarding children in Australia and Norway. *Child and Family Social Work, 17*(1), 96–107.

Loman, L. A., & Siegel, G. (2015). Effects of approach and services under differential response on long term child safety and welfare. *Child Abuse & Neglect, 39*, 86–97.

Lonne, B., Brown, G., Wagner, I., & Gillespie, K. (2015). Victoria's Child FIRST differential response system: Progress and issues. *Child Abuse & Neglect, 39*, 41–49. https://doi.org/10.1016/j.chiabu.2014.08.003.

Lonne, B., & Parton, N. (2014). Portrayals of child abuse scandals in the media in Australia and England: Impacts on practice, policy and systems. *Child Abuse & Neglect, 38*(5), 822–836. https://doi.org/10.1016/j.chiabu.2014.04.020.

Lonne, B., Parton, N., Thomson, J., & Harries, M. (2009). *Reforming child protection*. London: Routledge.

Marmot, M. G., Allen, J., Goldblatt, P., Boyce, T., McNeish, D., Grady, M., & Geddes, I. (2010). *Fair society, healthy lives: The Marmot review. Strategic review of health inequalities I: England post 2010*. London: Marmot Review.

Melton, G. B. (2010). It's all about relationships! The psychology of human rights. *American Journal of Orthopsychiatry, 80*(2), 161–169.

Merkel-Holguin, L., Hollinshead, D., Hahn, A., Casillas, K., & Fluke, J. (2014). The influence of differential response and other factors on parent perceptions of child protection involvement. *Child Abuse & Neglect, 39*, 18–31.

Metzler, C. W., Sanders, M. R., Rusby, J. C., & Crowley, R. N. (2012). Using consumer preference information to increase the reach and impact of media-based parenting interventions in a public health approach to parenting support. *Behaviour Therapy, 43*(2), 257–270. https://doi.org/10.1016/j.beth.2011.05.004.

Morawska, A., Sanders, M., Goadby, E., Headley, C., Hodge, L., McAuliffe, C., & Anderson, E. (2011). Is the Triple P-Positive Parenting Program acceptable to parents from culturally diverse backgrounds? *Journal of Child and Family Studies, 20*(5), 614–622.

OECD. (2015). *Social Impact Investment: Building the evidence base*. Paris: OECD Publishing.

Parton, N. (2006). *Safeguarding childhood: Early intervention and surveillance in a late modern society*. Basingstoke: Palgrave Macmillan.
Parton, N. (2014). *The politics of child protection: Contemporary developments and future directions*. Basingstoke: Palgrave.
Prinz, R. J. (2015). Public health approach to parenting and family support: A blended prevention strategy to reduce child abuse and neglect. In A. Bentovim & J. Gray (Eds.), *Eradicating child maltreatment: Evidence-based approaches to prevention and intervention across services* (pp. 106–121). London: Jessica Kingsley.
Prinz, R. J. (2016). Parenting and family support within a broad child abuse prevention strategy. *Child Abuse & Neglect, 51*, 400–406.
Prinz, R. J. (2017). Assessing child maltreatment via administrative data systems: A case example of reproducibility. *Child Abuse & Neglect, 64*, 13–18.
Prinz, R. J., Sanders, M. R., Shapiro, C. J., Whitaker, D. J., & Lutzker, J. R. (2009). Population-based prevention of child maltreatment: The US Triple P system population trial. *Prevention Science, 10*(1), 1–12.
Prinz, R. J., Sanders, M. R., Shapiro, C. J., Whitaker, D. J., & Lutzker, J. R. (2016). Addendum to "Population based prevention of child maltreatment: The US triple P system population trial". *Prevention Science, 17*, 410–416.
Richardson, D. (2018). *Key findings on families, family policy and the Sustainable Development Goals*. Florence: UNICEF Office of Research, Innocenti. Retrieved from https://www.unicef-irc.org/publications/948-key-findings-on-families-family-policy-and-the-sustainable-development-goals-synthesis.html.
Robinson, E., Scott, D., Meredith, V., Nair, L., & Higgins, D. (2012). *Good and innovative practice in service delivery to vulnerable and disadvantaged families and children.* (CFCA Paper No 9). Melbourne: Australian Institute of Family Studies. Retrieved from https://aifs.gov.au/cfca/publications/good-and-innovative-practice-service-delivery-vulnerable-and-disadvantaged
Sanders, M. R., Markie-Dadds, C., Rinaldis, M., Firman, D., & Baig, N. (2007). Using household survey data to inform policy decisions regarding the delivery of evidence-based parenting interventions. *Child: Care, Health and Development, 33*(6), 768–783.
Sanders, M. R., Burke, K., Prinz, R. J., & Morawska, A. (2017). Achieving population-level change through a system-contextual approach to supporting competent parenting. *Clinical Child and Family Psychology Review, 20*(1), 36–44.
Stewart, J., Lohoar, S., & Higgins, D. J. (2011). *Effective practices for service delivery coordination in Indigenous communities*. (Closing the Gap Clearinghouse Resource Sheet No. 8). Canberra: Closing the Gap Clearinghouse, Australian Institute of Health and Welfare/Australian Institute of Family Studies. Retrieved from http://www.aihw.gov.au/uploadedFiles/ClosingTheGap/Content/Publications/2011/ctgc-rs-08.pdf
Stoltenborgh, M., Bakermans-Kranenburg, M., & van IJzendoorn, M. (2013). The neglect of child neglect: A meta-analytic review of the prevalence of neglect. *Social Psychiatry and Psychiatric Epidemiology, 48*, 345–355. https://doi.org/10.1007/s00127-012-0549-y.
Theodore, A. D., Chang, J. J., Runyan, D. K., Hunter, W. M., Bangdiwala, S. I., & Agans, R. (2005). Epidemiologic features of the physical and sexual maltreatment of children in the Carolinas. *Pediatrics, 115*, 331–337.
Turner, K. M. T., Richards, M., & Sanders, M. R. (2007). Randomised clinical trial of a group parent education programme for Australian indigenous families. *Journal of Paediatrics and Child Health, 43*, 429–437. https://doi.org/10.1111/j.1440-1754.2007.01053.x.
Winokur, M., Ellis, R., Drury, I., & Rogers, J. (2014). Answering the big questions about differential response in Colorado: Safety and cost outcomes from a randomized controlled trial. *Child Abuse & Neglect, 39*, 98–108.

Chapter 10
Child Sexual Abuse Prevention Strategies for Population-Level Change: Challenges and Future Directions

Antonia Quadara

10.1 Introduction

Despite a decade of concerted effort and policy investment, preventing child sexual abuse *before* it occurs – i.e. primary prevention – remains a fraught endeavour. This is not because child sexual abuse continues to occur, or that there have not been calls for a public healthapproach to child abuse and neglect (there have), but because a comprehensive, integrated and shared framework for the primary prevention of child sexual abuse does not yet exist. This can be contrasted with developments in the primary prevention of violence against women. Over the same decade, in line with a public health approach, research, policy and practice communities have worked together to:

- Determine the economic and health costs of domestic violence (Access Economics 2004; VicHealth 2004) and violence against women more broadly (KPMG 2009, 2016);
- Synthesise the extant empirical evidence on factors associated with victimisation and perpetration and map these across the social ecology (VicHealth 2007; Webster and Flood 2015);
- Integrate the evidence to develop an explanatory model of violence against women (OurWatch 2016);
- Develop primary prevention fameworks to guide programming across key settings such as schools, universities, local community settings, local government, workplaces and corporations, and recreation and sporting clubs (Our Watch 2016; VicHealth 2007);
- Evaluate initiatives and scale up promising or effective programs;

A. Quadara (✉)
Sexual Violence Research, Australian Institute of Family Studies, Southbank, VIC, Australia
e-mail: Antonia.Quadara@aifs.gov.au

B. Lonne et al. (eds.), *Re-Visioning Public Health Approaches for Protecting Children*, Child Maltreatment 9, https://doi.org/10.1007/978-3-030-05858-6_10

- Develop good practice standards for designing and delivering primary prevention programs (Carmody 2009; Carmody et al. 2009; Flood et al. 2009); and
- Develop tools, resources and communities of practice to support primary prevention action across key settings such as schools, local community settings, workplaces and sporting clubs.[1]

The aim in making this comparison is not to be needlessly critical about efforts to prevent child abuse and neglect. As with preventing violence against women, there has been a long-standing drive in countries like Australia to see child abuse and neglect as a public health issue and to use a public health framework to prevent child abuse and neglect occurring in the first place (e.g., ARACY 2008; Bromfield and Holzer 2008; O'Donnell et al. 2008), culminating in the development in Australia of the National Framework for Protecting Australia's Children 2009–2020 (COAG 2009). This is a 12-year blueprint to address child abuse and neglect to which all state and territory governments have committed. Further, primary prevention initiatives for child sexual abuse *are* being implemented, such as prevention education in schools to increase knowledge of sexual abuse and increase self-protective skills (see Walsh et al. 2013), as well as strategies to create child-safe organizations and ensure children's online safety. However, it is not clear to me that there is a shared understanding across key actors of the concept of primary prevention itself, how different prevention initiatives are – or should be – articulating together, or how to achieve sustainable, whole of population and societal change.

The purpose in this chapter is to examine why a shared and integrated approach to preventing child sexual abuse has been difficult to engender. Here, three key dimensions are examined: empirical issues, that is, the complex forms and dynamics of sexual abuse; theoretical and social policy issues in terms of where child sexual abuse "sits" as a social problem; and finally, practical issues relating to the translation of a public health approach to prevention into practice. From there, I outline what, in keeping with a public health approach, are the ways forward to address these issues. However, before examining the empirical complexity of what constitutes child sexual abuse, it is necessary to first describe the current challenge in the prevention of child sexual abuse.

10.2 Current Challenges

The lack of shared agreement about, and framework for, the primary prevention of child sexual abuse is not limited to the Australian context. Public health researchers at John Hopkins University recently described the US situation thus:

[1] See for example evaluations and resources available through OurWatch: https://www.ourwatch.org.au/Media-Resources; VicHealth: https://www.vichealth.vic.gov.au/our-work/preventing-violence-against-women, and Partners in Prevention Community Practice Network for prevention workers: http://www.partnersinprevention.org.au.

> The benefits of effective and widely adopted prevention programs for child sexual abuse are…sizeable, and it is not surprising that numerous efforts have been made to encourage the development of primary prevention programs during the past 30 years. What is surprising are the outright failures and significant limitations of these efforts. While some advances have been made, many existing primary prevention programs still suffer from a lack of rigorous evaluation, limited implementation settings, ineffective program content and inefficient skills practice. (Letourneau et al. 2014, p. 222)

Letourneau et al. (2014) noted that parents and adults protecting children are rarely the target of primary prevention programs, nor are potential offenders or bystanders. Moreover, efforts to extend etiological analyses beyond individual and familial risk factors to community or societal level-risk factors have been limited. The context in Australia arguably shares much with the above characterisation, namely:

- 'Sluggish' development of best-practice principles and approaches;
- Poor program and initiative design (e.g., lack of a theory of change; not evidence-informed; inappropriate 'dosage');
- Disconnected or ad hoc prevention activities;
- Disconnected 'communities of practice';
- Weak or inappropriate evaluation methodologies;
- Non-comparable evaluation and research findings; and
- Diverse or inconsistent criteria informing the funding of programs.

In combination, these issues mean that despite significant efforts at the program and practice levels, it has been difficult to develop a coherent understanding about "what works" or what is promising (i.e., programs based on theoretically sound, evidence-informed principles but yet to be examined empirically). Given the fervent commitment to preventing child sexual abuse, what are the challenges and obstacles? The following sections consider these issues.

10.3 Understanding the Dynamics of Child Sexual Abuse: Complexities and Challenges

10.3.1 Empirical Complexities

Child sexual abuse captures a broad range of behaviors (contact and non-contact, within a wide variety of victim/perpetration dyads (relationships, ages, genders) that are themselves located within diverse settings and contexts (familial, community, organizational, virtual). To date, there has been limited empirical and conceptual work to bring these diverse forms of sexual abuse together to consider what, if anything, these dynamics have in common and whether there are shared risk factors across them. This lack of "problem definition" or surveillance is presents a significant challenge to preventing child sexual abuse as it is the first step in a public health approach: the "systematic collection of information about the magnitude, scope, characteristics and consequences of violence" (WHO 2017), helps to define the territory for the next crucial step of identifying causes and risks factors. The following section endeavours to map out the diverse relationships and settings in which sexual abuse occurs.

10.3.2 Relationships

The available prevalence data in Australia indicate that significant numbers of the population have experienced some form of child sexual abuse, with 5.7–15.9% of males and 13.9–36% of females reporting non-penetrative sexual abuse and up to 7.5% of males and 12% of females reporting penetrative sexual abuse (Child Family Community Australia 2017).

As a category of child maltreatment, sexual abuse is comparatively more common than other single categories such as physical abuse, neglect or emotional maltreatment. However, compared to these forms of abuse and neglect, sexual abuse occurs across a wider range of relationships and settings. Child sexual abuse can thus take a range of forms, such as:

- Intra-familial abuse perpetrated by adult male family members in the immediate and extended family;
- Adolescents (or even children) who engage in harmful sexual behavior, again within and beyond the family;
- Abuse perpetrated by teachers, guardians and other non-familial carers;
- Adult men establishing exploitative sexual relationships with adolescents (typically female);
- Online grooming and sexual exploitation; and
- The production and circulation of child sexual exploitation material.

There are some key differences in perpetration dynamics when the perpetrator is an adult family member compared to non-family. Whether they are blended or biological, familial relationships are often characterised by privacy, complex attachments, frequent and intimate contact, and gender role expectations (e.g., paternal authority). Characteristics of sexual abuse that occurs within families include:

- Gender of victim: females are far more likely to be victimised where sexual abuse is perpetrated by a family member, while males are more likely to be sexually abused by non-familial perpetrators (see Australian Bureau of Statistics [ABS] 2006, 2013; Rosengard et al. 2007);
- Age of victim: age of first abuse is younger when the abuse is perpetrated by family members compared to non-family members;
- Demographics of perpetrator: parental perpetrators are older than extra-familial perpetrators, are often in marital or de facto relationships, or have participated in long-term intimate relationships with adults, which are typically regarded as protective factors (Goodman-Delahunty 2014); and

- Number of victims/frequency or duration of abuse: perpetrators of familial sexual abuse have fewer victims compared to non-familial perpetrators, but their offending is more likely to be frequent or occur against that victim for a longer period time. Although non-familial perpetrators may have a greater number of victims, they may only offend against that individual once or twice.

There is a tendency to view extra-familial sexual abuse as another way of saying 'stranger-perpetrated abuse'. However, many cases of extra-familial sexual abuse are also characterised by interpersonal relationships between perpetrators and victims. However, they are often characterised by somewhat looser or more formal social connections, such as schools, sports organizations or neighbourhood ties and take a variety of forms: (a) relationships based on care, supervision or authority; (b) interpersonal relationships, such as family friends, youth workers, or neighbours; and (c) peer relationships between young people (e.g., young students in school).

Impersonal relationships, where there is little to no initial relationship between the victim and perpetrator, such as 'stranger' child sex offenders who may approach children in public settings such as playgrounds, shopping malls or sporting events have been the archetype form of sexual abuse for several decades. Based on the available research, online settings appear to be a key way for adults to manufacture and cultivate a new relationship with a child or young person (in addition to enabling access to child exploitation material) (Bluett-Boyd et al. 2013; Quayle and Ribisl 2012). The speed of technology innovation makes detection, investigation, and prosecution difficult. Perpetrators may cross over from making connections with children/young people online to offline contact; or they may move from downloading of child exploitation material to virtual forms of child sexual abuse facilitated through instant messaging services or voice-over-Internet Protocol platforms. Further, as Bluett-Boyd et al. (2013) noted, online social networking platforms or other social media enable 'weak connections' between potential victims and perpetrators in the offline world to become more intimate, thus facilitating either contact abuse or the production of child exploitation material.

10.3.3 Contexts and Settings

Relationship dynamics are not sufficient to explain the occurrence of child sexual abuse. It is necessary to also look at the context or setting in which that relationship is located. Contexts (i.e., the situational environment in which the abuse occurs) influence the nature of the relationship between perpetrators and victims, providing a range of routine activities and interactions with children (Smallbone et al. 2008) and thus shaping how the opportunity to offend against a child presents itself (see Chap. 11). Quadara et al. (2015) identified two relevant contexts:

1. *Kinship and community contexts*: This extends the notion of the 'family' beyond the common western notion of the nuclear family. It refers to environments that are particularly relevant for Indigenous Australians. First, familial relationships

in Indigenous communities are broader than those in Anglo-European cultures, as well as having a complex arrangement of social interactions and roles (Dudgeon et al. 2002, 2010). This means that individuals who may not be biologically related are nevertheless considered to be family members within the particular kinship arrangements of an Aboriginal or Torres Strait Islander community. Second, a history of colonisation, disenfranchisement and child removal, and the subsequent secondary effects of these traumas means that the community context for many Indigenous children includes a range of risk factors associated with child sexual abuse.

2. *Organizational and institutional contexts*: This refers to settings such as schools, sporting or youth organizations, religious institutions, out-of-home care, child care, and so on where a relationship between children and adults is a feature of the organization or institution, and where, generally, there is a hierarchical relationship between children and adults.

10.3.4 Vulnerabilities and Grooming

Two further issues overlay relationships and contexts/settings: these are victim vulnerabilities, which are exploited by perpetrators and specific 'grooming strategies', which are more likely to be used by adult perpetrators. In line with Smallbone et al.'s (2008) theory that the opportunity for child sexual abuse requires both a motivated offender and a likely victim, victim vulnerabilities are likely to be consistent across the types of child sexual abuse, although they are likely to be particularly salient in relationships based outside the parental family unit. Victim vulnerabilities include: social isolation, family dysfunction, physical and intellectual disabilities, lack of secure attachments, history of maternal child sexual abuse, family violence, and older age (i.e., risk of sexual abuse increases with a child's age). Following on from this, there is a range of grooming tactics that adult perpetrators use. To an extent literature suggests broadly similar tactics across different types of child sexual abuse (e.g., Craven et al. 2006). These include:

- Making the child feel special (e.g., older or more sophisticated than other children; providing gifts);
- Creating a sense of trust and intimacy (this sense of trust can extend to the child's family);
- Gradual introduction to sexual content or sexual touch; and
- Keeping secrets (which can have a range of functions, such as creating trust, isolation from others, sense of complicity or used to blackmail).

However, there are some strategies perpetrators use that are more or less suited to particular relationships or contexts. For example, threats of harm to others may be particularly suited to familial relationships, whereas pretending to be a child or young person is suited to online contexts.

These four dimensions – relationships, context/settings, vulnerabilities and grooming – can help to map the parameters of child sexual abuse in terms of: types of relationships and settings; the possible intersections and overlaps between contexts; and perpetrators' exploitation of victim vulnerabilities and the opportunities afforded by both the relationship (e.g., a care/supervision relationship) and the setting or context (i.e., the type of youth-serving organization or institution). This typology can be used to help focus questions issues such as:

- The different programmatic areas at the policy level that exist to address these different dimensions and whether/how they interrelate; and
- The range of prevention approaches targeting these diverse circumstances.

10.3.5 Situating Child Sexual Abuse as a Social Issue: Theoretical and Political Complexities

A second challenge relates to the theoretical framings of sexual abuse as a social issue. The acknowledgement of child sexual abuse has a jagged history of being variously named, denied, minimised, re-explained, or attributed back to the victim. At the cusp of the twentieth century and into its early years for instance, medical professionals, first-wave feminists and child protectionists were certainly aware of sexual abuse occurring, noting the existence of venereal diseases such as syphilis and gonorrhoea among children living children's homes and wards. Dominant explanations, however, would typically veer around sexual abuse as the cause to infection by towels, lavatories and bedsheets (Smart 1999, 2000). Although Freud had initially been explicit about the seduction of children and its implications for psychopathology, he later rescinded this position, recasting the narratives of his patients as unconscious phantasies (Olafson et al. 1993). Indeed medical, psychiatric and sociological literature for most of the 20th century found ways of theorising away the existence of child sexual abuse: victims of child sexual abuse colluded in or initiated their own seduction; mothers were to blame for being sexually unavailable to their husbands; its occurrence was negligible; sexual abuse did not in fact cause harm (Myers et al. 1999).

From the 1970s, child sexual abuse became increasingly visible through the political analysis and activism of second-wave feminists regarding women's experiences of male violence over the life course, particularly men's use of sexual violence.[2] This activism, theoretical analysis and scholarship drew a connecting line through women's experiences of sexual abuse, street-based and sexual harassment, and rape and sexual assault (Itzin 2000). Those working in child welfare also worked to increase public awareness. For instance, in the state of Victoria (Australia), the

[2] The following paragraph draws from a conceptual mapping of the social, legal, cultural and institutional trends that influenced responses to child sexual abuse in institutions 1950–2014 (see Quadara 2017).

Children's Protection Society presented data on child sexual abuse for the first time in 1975 (see: http://www.cps.org.au/). From the 1980s, knowledge about child sexual abuse continued to expand in the form of empirical research studies that determined prevalence of child sexual abuse and started to theorise the traumatic impacts of these experiences. This scholarship demonstrated that sexual abuse was common and that the harm associated with it was significant. From this decade onward there has also been significant interest in child sex offenders – their motivations, criminogenic risk factors, treatment and surveillance and monitoring approaches.

This history means that as a social and policy issue, child sexual abuse crosses at least four domains—violence against women, family wellbeing and support, child protection, and criminal offending. There are subsequently "different, but independently legitimate, perspectives" (ISPCAN 2011, pp. 13–14) on the causes and appropriate responses to child sexual abuse. While this diversity of perspectives can bring a depth of expertise, knowledge, data, tools and strategies, when it is not integrated it can mean fragmentation, and, at the policy and program levels, it can mean that child sexual abuse falls between policy frameworks. Although there is agreement that primary prevention is the "change goal", the complex and multi-sectoral nature of child sexual abuse noted above influences understandings about what an effective prevention agenda should look like. For example, in statutory child protection services, the orientation is towards the rights of the child as well as the rights—and needs—of the parents. Where safety is an issue, the primary focus is the child's right to safety. By comparison, family services start from the idea that children are best cared for in the family. These different emphases can result in different issues triggering a service response. Further, when comparing sexual violence prevention (of which child sexual abuse is one example) to child protection, the target of intervention (i.e., those receiving a prevention initiative) differs. In sexual violence prevention, targets can be individuals, communities and organizations, or the broader social environment (e.g., media representations). In the child protection literature on prevention, the target is primarily seen as the family (ARACY 2008).

Further diverse activities and targets are identified as being "primary prevention". For example, some services consider the prevention of further offending by a perpetrator as being a form of primary prevention, or approaches being called primary prevention when they could more accurately be classified as secondary or tertiary prevention. In some cases, the long-term aims of primary prevention (such as "changing social norms" or population-level change) may be too abstract or difficult to apply to children, which may suggest that underlying determinants for child sexual abuse are not well identified. This can make it difficult to see how 'upstream' prevention efforts connect with a reduction in victimisation.[3]

[3]Acknowledging the challenge of drawing a line from addressing key determinants of violence against women to interim measures, to outcome measures, the national organization leading developments in preventing violence against women developed a guide for policy-makers, researchers, and other stakeholders on measuring population-level progress. This guide can be found at: https://www.ourwatch.org.au/What-We-Do/Counting-on-change-A-guide-to-prevention-monitorin

The following sections circle back to the current challenges of primary prevention for child sexual abuse and outlines future directions for prevention at the whole-of-population level.

10.4 The Trajectory of Prevention: Getting to Whole-of-Population Change

10.4.1 The Current Situation

There is a number of prevention activities specifically aimed at preventing the sexual abuse of children. These efforts are predominantly located within the following domains:

- *Protective behavior education for children*—increasingly referred to as "child abuse prevention education", which may also involve parents, and broader school personnel or systems;
- *Situational crime prevention*—applied to risky settings, organizations and institutions (see Chap. 11);
- *Therapeutic interventions for problematic sexual behaviors and sexually abusive behaviors*—targeting children and young people who are at risk of sexually offending, prior to their involvement with the criminal justice system;
- *Therapeutic work with offenders*— to prevent re-offending by targeting (a) young people who have come to the attention of the criminal justice system for sexually abusive behaviors and (b) detected and convicted adult sex offenders;
- *Criminal justice and other statutory responses*—to identify and monitor sex offenders and their engagement with children and young people; and
- *Therapeutic work with children and adolescents who have experienced sexual abuse*—to reduce their vulnerability to re-victimisation.

These efforts tend to lie at either end of the spectrum of prevention. On the one hand there is significant activity in educating children about child sexual abuse and increasing their capacity to deter potential perpetrators—what, from a public health perspective, could be considered *primary prevention.* On the other hand, there is significant focus on engaging with perpetrators, whether therapeutically or punitively: *tertiary prevention.* This situation is not unique to Australia. Finkelhor (2009) characterised the situation in the United States in similar terms. He concluded that criminal justice approaches to prevention (e.g., sex offender registration and monitoring) have not been effective, while the evidence on the effectiveness of educational programs in reaching "certain of their goals" has been promising, but decidedly unclear as to whether they result in a reduction in victimisation. Across prevention efforts specifically addressing child sexual abuse and child maltreatment more generally, similar issues have been raised about the right balance of prevention: a tendency to focus on individual-level risk factors rather than factors that occur, or are better addressed at the community or social level, such as partner violence and social norms (whether about the sexual nature of children, gender norms or the acceptability of violence towards children) (Klevens and Whitaker 2007; O'Donnell et al. 2008; Tomison and Wise 1999). The following section outlines what the evidence suggests about risk factors for child sexual abuse.

10.4.2 Understanding the Risk Factors and Correlates of Child Sexual Abuse

After problem definitions, the second key element on a public health approach is to determine the causes and correlates of the violence or harm being addressed, including the factors that increase or decrease the risk for violence, factors that could be changed through interventions. This requires looking at the factors that give rise to both victimization and perpetration. However, as noted by the International Society for the Prevention of Child Abuse and Neglect (ISPCAN 2013), the child protection field has historically paid more attention to "the management of the victim or the potential victim of child abuse than to the potential or actual perpetrator of violence" (p. 4). From a primary prevention point of view, it is essential that all factors and correlates associated with sexual abuse are identified and, importantly synthesised.

This section considers the risk factors for perpetration across the identified relationships and contexts. Before doing so, it is useful to consider the risk factors associated generally with child abuse and neglect. Work done by the US Centres for Disease Control and Prevention (CDC 2004) synthesised the evidence to describe risk factors across the social ecology. At the individual level, these risk factors include:

- Parents' lack of understanding of children's needs, child development and parenting skills;
- Parents' history of child maltreatment in family of origin;
- Substance abuse and/or mental health issues, including depression in the family;
- Parental characteristics, such as young age, low education, single parenthood, large number of dependent children, and low income;
- Non-biological, transient caregivers in the home (e.g., a mother's male partner); and
- Parental thoughts and emotions that tend to support or justify maltreatment behaviors.

At the familial level, relevant risk factors include social isolation; family disorganization, dissolution, and violence, including intimate partner violence; and parenting stress, poor parent–child relationships, and negative interactions. Community-level risk factors include community violence; and concentrated neighbourhood disadvantage (e.g., high poverty and residential instability, high unemployment rates, and high density of alcohol outlets), and poor social connections (adapted from Centers for Disease Control and Prevention 2004).

Although there is cross-over with child maltreatment risk factors, the literature on adult perpetrators of child sexual abuse also emphasises factors such as:

- Violence and delinquency;
- Maladaptive sexual behaviors, such as deviant sexual fantasies;
- Social deficits, such as lack of empathy and social skills deficits; and
- Attitudinal and cognitive variables, such as attitudes towards rape, the "sexual precociousness of children" and cognitive rationalisations (Whitaker et al. 2008).

In their meta-analysis of 89 studies of sex offender risk factors, Whitaker et al. (2008) found that sex offenders who target children (child sex offenders) were more likely than non-offenders to have poorer family functioning, more harsh discipline, poor attachment and generally worse functioning in their family of origin. Child sex offenders also demonstrated:

- Poorer social connectedness to others (e.g., loneliness, poor social skills);
- Significantly higher sexual externalising problems;
- Higher sex drive and preoccupation with sex;
- More deviant sexual interests;
- Greater sexualised coping;
- Attitudes that are more tolerant of adult–child sex; and
- Cognition that minimises perpetrator culpability.

Whitaker et al. (2008) concluded that while child sex offenders are different from non-offenders, they are *not* different from sex offenders who target adults. In other words, while both child and adult sex offenders share a number of risk factors with general (non-sexual) offenders, the point of difference relates to the sexual component of their behavior. This is echoed in other research on the attitudes of child sex offenders, which finds that their beliefs and attitudes in relation to children as sexual objects, general preoccupation with sex, and beliefs about entitlement, authority or control distinguish them from a range of other offenders (Helmus et al. 2013; Marziano et al. 2006; Ward and Keenan 1999).

Across the various contexts and settings of child sexual abuse, there are similarities in the risk factors to perpetration, as well as similarities in the behaviors engaged in by perpetrators. The research literature suggests that there are certain factors that are associated with the perpetration of multiple types of sexual abuse. These include:

- Biologically unrelated male;
- Highly sexualised environment;
- Neglect;
- Domestic violence in family;
- Poor family cohesion;
- Age (being young); and
- Violent behavior.

These common risk factors to perpetration can be outside the perpetrator's control: for example, being young, having a history of neglect or being a victim of domestic violence. However, there are also numerous ambiguous findings from the research regarding other risk factors. There is disagreement between researchers about the following:

- Substance misuse;
- Low socio-economic status;
- History of physical abuse;
- History of sexual abuse;
- Prior, non-sexual, criminal behavior; and
- Violent behavior.

This disparity may be due to differences in the research populations being approached for study.[4] Other individual-level factors include:

- Sexual interest: While neuropathology in concert with sexual interest may provide the environment for desire for sex with children to arise in a potential offender, numerous studies suggest that it is possible to screen for sexual interest in children, even if not consciously known to a person (Abel et al. 2012).

Neuropathology: Biological brain chemistry abnormalities have been raised in the literature as a cause (or even neuroplastic symptom) of child sexually abusive behaviors.

10.4.3 Moving Upstream: From "Risk Factors" to "Key Determinants"

In sum, there is a long list of risk factors associated with perpetration of child sexual abuse:

- Traditional or rigid gender values;
- Attitudes related to male sexual entitlement and sexual dominance;
- Biologically unrelated male;
- Highly sexualised environments (both within the family, online and more broadly);
- History of neglect;
- History of witnessing or experiencing domestic violence;
- Poor family cohesion during family of origin;
- Substance misuse;
- Low socio-economic status;

[4] For example, incarcerated males comprise only the known and currently apprehended child sexual abusers and are more likely to be from a low socio-economic status, whereas unapprehended child sexual abuse perpetrators are perhaps more likely to be from a more solid financial background (Briere and Spinazzola 2009; Schaefer et al. 2010).

- Being socially isolated;
- Growing up in a large family;
- Experiencing parenthood early;
- Physical abuse history;
- Psychological deficits (including psychopathology);
- Engaging in other violent behavior;
- Low educational attainment; and
- Living or working in closed familial and institutional settings.

We can see that some of these factors are common across child maltreatment, but their relationship to child sexual abuse appears to be weaker and less predictive. This is to be expected given the diverse circumstances in which sexual abuse occurs.

The overall goal of primary prevention is to reduce the actual incidence of child sexual abuse within the population. Working backwards then, it targets the factors that give rise to, or create, the conditions for sexual abuse and influence behavior. Although it is possible to address each of these factors, it would be very costly in time and funds to do so. It is necessary to move beyond risk factors to consider common underlying causes or conditions.

In tandem with the continued development of a shared understanding of prevention (and particularly primary prevention), a key direction relates to focusing efforts further "upstream". This refers to tracing problems back to the source. This is different to saying something is causally related. Causality is generally measured by how *direct* the relationship between a variable and an outcome is. Upstream determinants are those that occur at the macro level and include structural forces such as poverty, government policies, popular and news media. Their demonstrable influence is often less direct but they significantly shape people's opportunities in life.

When considering the 'upstream determinants' or those factors that create or support conditions that allow for an influence the behavior of child sexual abuse, it is instructive to refer to the literature on the social determinants of health—also sometimes understood as the "new public health". The World Health Organization [WHO] (2014) defined social determinants as:

> the conditions in which people are born, grow, live, work and age. These circumstances are shaped by the distribution of money, power and resources at global, national and local levels (p. 1).

Social determinants can also be referred to as the "causes behind the causes" (i.e., upstream determinants). This means looking to the underlying conditions giving rise to issues such as family dysfunction and instability, poor social skills, substance misuse, poor parenting and so on, all of which have been identified as risk factors for sexual abuse perpetration.

Focusing on social determinants enables prevention efforts to address root causes in a more efficient manner. In their review on gaps and directions in the prevention of child abuse and neglect, Klevens and Whitaker (2007)[5] argued that "preventative interventions targeting risk factors that are highly prevalent in a population will

---

[5] Note that in their review, Klevens and Whitaker (2007) did not include the prevention specifically of child *sexual*abuse.

generate a greater impact on the problem at the population level than targeting factors that are less prevalent" (p. 364), even if the risk factors appear to be less directly related. They further note that the reach and mode of delivery of prevention strategies are important dimensions not only for achieving population level behavior change (which is the aim of primary prevention), but are attractive from a "cost-containment" perspective. That is, initiatives are likely to be more cost-effective where: the deliverer is more whole-of-community (e.g., public institutions compared to individual service providers) and where the recipient is more expansive (e.g., a whole community compared to groups or individuals).

10.4.4 Identifying Key Determinants for Child Sexual Abuse

How does this thinking work in light of the many specific risk factors described above? Stepping back, it seems clear that child sexual abuse and its perpetration coalesces around the following key issues. These conditions give rise to many of the risk factors listed in the previous section, such as domestic and family violence; experiences of violence and abuse; substance misuse; social isolation and weak social ties; and poor family cohesion and insecure attachments.

Children's Structural Vulnerability Relative to Adults Within Social Domains such as Families, Organizations, and Institutions Social institutions such as families, schools, and broader civil society engender unequal relationships between adults and children. In many cases this inequality is way of protecting children and young people to optimise their development. However there are aspects of this structural inequality that increase children's vulnerability to sexual abuse such as:

- Beliefs in adults' superiority and natural authority over children;
- Attitudes that diminish children's views and self-expression about events, feelings and relationships; and
- Beliefs that children should not challenge adults, or that challenge is deliberative provocative.

These beliefs and attitudes can mean: assumptions that adults' treatment of, and engagement with, children and young people is appropriate or in the child's best interest; adults can manipulate a range of situations and groom children with little intervention; beliefs that children lie or are confused when they disclose incidents of sexual abuse.

Forms of Masculinity and Rigid Gender Attitudes that Endorse Men's Social Dominance, Entitlement (Including Sexual Entitlement), Authority and Control in a Range of Settings Rigid gender attitudes and attitudes and beliefs about sexual and emotional entitlement are commonly associated with domestic and family violence, sexual violence and child sexual abuse. Engaging men and boys in the development of gender-equitable relationships in the home, at work, and among peers in a key prevention strategy. *There are many initiatives occurring that do this in terms of violence against women.*[6]*In relation to child sexual abuse, two broad approaches can be taken:*

(a) Integrate key risk factors for child sexual abuse such as: sexual entitlement, entitlement to having emotional needs met in non-reciprocal ways; and age power and vulnerability, into the initiatives to prevent violence against women; and
(b) Integrate gender equity into family services, and maternal and child health services regarding gendered expectations about child care and division of labour following the birth of a child. Strategies to do this could have an effect on:
    - Family dynamics;
    - Women's social isolation following the birth of child;
    - Prevalence of family and domestic violence;
    - Men modelling gender-equitable behaviors to boys; and
    - Challenging norms that excuse the use of power, control and dominance in relationships.

Socio-Economic Disadvantage and Income Inequality, Including Gendered Socio-Economic Disadvantage Although socio-economic disadvantage is not associated with child sexual abuse to the same extent as child maltreatment more generally, it does increase the likelihood of sexual abuse occurring. Addressing social disadvantage could improve:

- Mothers' social isolation and gendered inequality compared to men;
- Prevalence of family and domestic violence;
- Collective efficacy and capacity to appropriately intervene in circumstances related to child sexual abuse (e.g., controlling behaviors exhibited by male partners); and
- Early intervention with perpetrators and young people who sexually abuse.

Poor or Non-Existent Mechanisms for Supporting Psycho-Social Needs for Trauma Arising from Child Abuse and Neglect (Including Sexual Abuse and Witnessing Family Violence) A significant and diverse body of literature suggests that exposure to childhood trauma can result in subsequent forms of victimisation.

---

[6] Key examples include respectful relationships education with children and young people in K-12 settings to teach skills in recognising and challenging gender stereotypes and in building respectful relationships (Ollis and Dyson 2017; Flood et al. 2009); prevention education programs with male-oriented sports such as Respect and Responsibility with Australian Football League (AFL clubs) (Dyson and Flood 2008); workplace prevention programs and initiatives to improve media representation of violence against women. More information about the designed to address the key determinants of violence against women can be found on the Victorian Health Promotion Foundation website: https://www.vichealth.vic.gov.au/search?category=Preventing%20violence%20against%20women; and the OurWatch website: https://www.ourwatch.org.au/What-We-Do

In addition to specialist trauma services, human services that are trauma-informed can support child sexual abuse prevention efforts by addressing:

- Maternal histories of child sexual abuse, which can affect parenting and protective capacities, is a risk factor for future victimisation for themselves and their children, and leads to a range of other negative outcomes for mothers; and
- Early acknowledgment of developmental risk factors for perpetration.

This identification of key determinants is not intended to replace or contradict the existing thinking on risk factors. Rather this thinking is indended to assist thinking through the challenges enumerated here and internationally regarding the overemphasis on individual-level risk factors and limited efforts at targeting more collective social structures such communities and society in addition to individuals, families and institutions.

10.5 Conclusions

Child sexual abuse is a complex phenomenon, both empirically (i.e., the actual circumstances in which it occurs) and conceptually. Numerous policies (e.g., COAG 2009), research studies, and expert commentary have noted that statutory responses are not sufficient, sustainable and often unable to prevent future harm (e.g., O'Donnell et al. 2008), and there is agreement that a public health model should be a framework through which to situate prevention of child abuse, including child sexual abuse. Developing an integrated approach to the prevention of child sexual abuse is a significant undertaking. However, without consensus about the aims, strategies and conditions for effective prevention (particularly primary prevention), specific initiatives will remain ad hoc and disconnected. Such a framework needs to be based on research evidence, have the support of the relevant practice and practice communities, and be an accessible reference for all key players working to prevent child sexual abuse.

References

Abel, G. G., Wiegel, M., Jordan, A., Harlow, N., Hsu, Y. S., & Martinez, M. (2012). Development and validation of classification models to identify hidden child molesters applying to child service organizations. *Children and Youth Services Review, 34*(7), 1378–1389.

Access Economics. (2004). *The cost of domestic violence to the Australian economy*. Partnership Against Domestic Violence – An Australian Government Initiative.

Australian Bureau of Statistics. (2006). *Personal safety survey Australia, 2005*. Canberra: ABS.

Australian Bureau of Statistics. (2013). *Personal safety survey 2011*. Canberra: ABS.

Australian Research Alliance for Children and Youth. (2008). *Inverting the pyramid: Enhancing systems for protecting children*. Canberra: ARACY.

Bluett-Boyd, N., Fileborn, B., Quadara, A., & Moore, S. (2013). *The role of emerging communication technologies in experiences of sexual violence: A new legal frontier?* Melbourne: Australian Institute of Family Studies. Retrieved from: https://aifs.gov.au/publications/role-emerging-communication-technologies-experiences-sexual-violenc

Briere, J., & Spinazzola, J. (2009). Assessment of the sequelae of complex trauma: Evidence-based measures. In C. A. Courtois & J. D. Ford (Eds.), *Treating complex traumatic stress disorders: An evidence-based guide* (pp. 104–123). New York: Guilford Press.

Bromfield, L., & Holzer, P. J. (2008). *A national approach for child protection: Project report*. Melbourne: Australian Institute of Family Studies.

Carmody, M. (2009). *Conceptualising the prevention of sexual assault though prevention*. (ACSSA Issues Paper, Vol. 10). Melbourne: Australian Institute of Family Studies.

Carmody, M., Evans, S., Krogh, C., Flood, M., Heenan, M., & Ovenden, G. (2009). *Framing best practice: National Standards for the primary prevention of sexual assault through education*. Sydney: Australia.

Centers for Disease Control and Prevention. (2004). *The social-ecological model: A framework for prevention*. Washington, DC: CDC. Retrieved from www.cdc.gov/violenceprevention/overview/social-ecologicalmodel.html.

Centers for Disease Control and Prevention. (2014). Child maltreatment: Risk and protective factors. Washington, DC: CDC. Retrieved from www.cdc.gov/violenceprevention/childmaltreatment/riskprotectivefactors.html.

Child Family Community Australia. (2017). The prevalence of child abuse and neglect. *CFCA Resource Sheet*. Retrieved from https://aifs.gov.au/cfca/publications/prevalence-child-abuse-and-neglect

Cossins, A. (2010). *Alternative models for prosecuting child sex offences in Australia*. Sydney: National Child Sexual Assault Reform Committee, University of New South Wales.

Council of Australian Governments (COAG). (2009). *Protecting children is everyone's business: National Framework for Protecting Australia's Children 2009–2020*. Canberra: Australian Government Department of Social Services. Retrieved from www.dss.gov.au/our-responsibilities/families-and-children/publications-articles/protecting-children-is-everyones-business.

Craven, S., Brown, S., & Gilchrist, E. (2006). Sexual grooming of children: Review of literature and theoretical considerations. *Journal of Sexual Aggression, 12*(3), 287–299. https://doi.org/10.1080/13552600601069414.

Dudgeon, P., Mallard, J., Oxenham, D., & Fielder, J. (2002). Contemporary Aboriginal perceptions of community. In A. T. Fisher, C. C. Sonn, & B. J. Bishop (Eds.), *Psychological sense of community. Research applications, and implications* (pp. 247–267). Boston: Springer.

Dudgeon, P., Wright, M., Paradies, Y., Garvey, D., & Walker, I. (2010). The social, cultural and historical context of Aboriginal and Torres Strait Islander Australians. In N. Purdie, P. Dudgeon, & R. Walker (Eds.), *Working together: Aboriginal and Torres Strait Islander mental health and wellbeing principles and practice* (pp. 25–42). Canberra: Australian Council for Educational Research.

Dyson, S., & Flood, M. (2008). *Building cultures of respect and non-violence: A review of literature concerning adult learning and violence prevention programs with men*. Melbourne: Victorian Health Promotion Foundation. Retrieved from: https://www.vichealth.vic.gov.au/media-and-resources/publications/building-cultures-of-respect-and-non-violence

Finkelhor, D. (2009). The prevention of childhood sexual abuse. *The Future of Children, 19*(2), 169–194.

Flood, M., Fergus, L., & Heenan, M. (2009). *Respectful relationships education: Violence prevention and respectful relationships education in Victorian secondary schools*. Melbourne: Victorian Health Promotion Foundation.

Goodman-Delahunty, J. (2014). *Profiling parental child sex abuse* (Trends and Issues in Crime and Criminal Justice). Canberra: Australian Institute of Criminology.

Helmus, L., Hanson, R. K., Babchishin, K. M., & Mann, R. E. (2013). Attitudes supportive of sexual offending predict recidivism: A meta-analysis. *Trauma, Violence & Abuse, 14*(1), 34–53. https://doi.org/10.1177/1524838012462244.

International Society for the Prevention of Child Abuse and Neglect. (2011). *ISPCAN Denver Thinking Space 2011: Child sexual abuse. An international perspective on responding to child sexual abuse: Executive summary*. Retrieved from tinyurl.com/l6dpsm3

International Society for the Prevention of Child Abuse and Neglect. (2013). *ISPCAN Denver Thinking Space 2013: Working with men and boys. A child protection strategy: Report on survey findings*. Aurora: ISPCAN. Retrieved from tinyurl.com/kkxnky2

Itzin, C. (2000). *Child protection and child sexual abuse prevention: Influencing policy and practice. Home truths about child sexual abuse* (pp. 405–449). London: Routledge.

Klevens, J., & Whitaker, D. J. (2007). Primary prevention of child physical abuse and neglect: Gaps and promising directions. *Child Maltreatment, 12*(4), 364–377. https://doi.org/10.1177/1077559507305995.

KPMG. (2009). The cost of violence against women and their children, safety taskforce, Department of Families, Housing, Community Services and Indigenous Affairs, Australian Government.

KPMG. (2016). *The cost of violence against women and their children: Final report*. Canberra: Australian Government. Retrieved from https://www.dss.gov.au/women/publications-articles/reducing-violence/the-cost-of-violence-against-women-and-their-children-in-australia-may-2016

Letourneau, E. J., Eaton, W. W., Bass, J., Berlin, F. S., & Moore, S. G. (2014). The need for a comprehensive public health approach to preventing child sexual abuse. *Public Health Reports, 129*(3), 222–228. https://doi.org/10.1177/003335491412900303.

Marziano, V., Ward, T., Beech, A. R., & Pattison, P. (2006). Identification of five fundamental implicit theories underlying cognitive distortions in child abusers: A preliminary study. *Psychology, Crime & Law, 12*(1), 97–105. https://doi.org/10.1080/10683160500056887.

McCartan, K. (2008). Current understandings of paedophilia and the resulting crisis in modern society. In J. M. Caroll & M. K. Alena (Eds.), *Psychological sexual dysfunctions* (pp. 51–84). New York: Nova Biomedical.

Myers, J. E., Diedrich, S., Lee, D., McClanahan Fincher, K., & Stern, R. (1999). Professional writing on child sexual abuse from 1900 to 1975: Dominant themes and impact on prosecution. *Child Maltreatment, 4*(3), 201–216.

O'Donnell, M., Scott, D., & Stanley, F. (2008). Child abuse and neglect: Is it time for a public health approach? *Australian and New Zealand Journal of Public Health, 32*(4), 325–330.

Olafson, E., Corwin, D. L., & Summit, R. C. (1993). Modern history of child sexual abuse awareness: Cycles of discovery and suppression. *Child Abuse & Neglect, 17*(1), 7–24.

Ollis, D., & Dyson, S. (2017). Respectful relationships education: A case-study of working in schools. In A. Taket & B. R. Crisp (Eds.), *Eliminating gender-based violence* (pp. 25–42). New York: Routledge.

Our Watch. (2016). *Change the story: A shared framework for the primary prevention of violence against women and their children in Australia*. Melbourne: Our Watch. Retrieved from https://www.ourwatch.org.au/what-we-do/national-primary-prevention-framework.

Quayle, E., & Ribisl, K. (2012). *Understanding and preventing online sexual exploitation of children* (1st ed.). London: Routledge.

Quadara, A., Nagy, V., Higgins, D., & Siegel, N. (2015). *Conceptualising the prevention of child sexual abuse*. Melbourne: Australian Institute of Family Studies. Retrieved from https://aifs.gov.au/publications/conceptualising-prevention-child-sexual-abuse

Quadara, A. (2017). *Framework for historical influences on institutional child sexual abuse: 1950–2014*. Sydney: Royal Commission into Institutional Responses to Child Sexual Abuse. Retrieved from: https://www.childabuseroyalcommission.gov.au/sites/default/files/file-list/research_report_-_frameworks_for_historical_influences_on_institutional_child_sexual_abuse_-_causes.pdf

Rosengard, A., Laing, I., Ridley, J., & Hunter, S. (2007). *A literature review on multiple and complex needs*. Edinburgh: Scottish Executive Social Research.

Schaefer, G. A., Mundt, I. A., Feelgood, S., Hupp, E., Neutze, J., & Ahlers, C. J. (2010). Potential and Dunkelfeld offenders: Two neglected target groups for prevention of child sexual abuse. *International Journal of Law and Psychiatry, 33*, 154–163.

Smallbone, S., Marshall, W., & Wortley, M. (2008). *Preventing child sexual abuse: Evidence policy and practice*. Cullompton/Devon: Willan Publishing.

Smart, C. (1999). A history of ambivalence and conflict in the discursive construction of the 'child victim' of sexual abuse. *Social and Legal Studies, 8*(3), 391–409.

Smart, C. (2000). Reconsidering the recent history of child sexual abuse, 1910–1960. *Journal of Social Policy, 29*(1), 55–71.

Tomison, A. M., & Wise, S. (1999). *Community-based approaches in preventing child maltreatment* (NCPC Issues Paper No. 11). Melbourne: Australian Institute of Family Studies. Retrieved from https://aifs.gov.au/cfca/publications/community-based-approaches-preventing-child-maltreatment

VicHealth. (2004). *Measuring the health costs of violence: Measuring the burden of disease caused by intimate partner violence – A summary of findings*. Melbourne: VicHealth.

VicHealth. (2007). *Preventing violence before it occurs: A framework and background paper to guide the primary prevention of violence against women in Victoria*. Melbourne: VicHealth.

Ward, T., & Keenan, T. (1999). Child molesters' implicit theories. *Journal of Interpersonal Violence, 14*(8), 821–838. https://doi.org/10.1177/088626099014008003.

Walsh, K., Berthelsen, D., Nicholson, J. M., Brandon, L., Stevens, J., & Rachele, J. N. (2013). Child sexual abuse prevention education: A review of school policy and curriculum provision in Australia. *Oxford Review of Education, 39*(5), 649–680.

Webster, K., & Flood, M. (2015). *Framework foundations 1: A review of the evidence on correlates of violence against women and what works to prevent it*. Melbourne: Our Watch.

Whitaker, D. J., Le, B., Hanson, K. R., Baker, C. K., McMahon, P. M., & Ryan, G. (2008). Risk factors for the perpetration of child sexual abuse: A review and meta-analysis. *Child Abuse & Neglect, 32*(5), 529–548. https://doi.org/10.1016/j.chiabu.2007.08.005.

World Health Organization. (2014). *What are social determinants of health?* Retrieved from www.who.int/social_determinants/sdh_definition/en/

Chapter 11
Youth-Serving Organization Safety Risks and the Situational Prevention Approach

Keith Kaufman, Marcus Erooga, Daryl Higgins, and Judith Zatkin

11.1 Introduction

Children spend a significant portion of their time in the care of adults outside of their family (Kaufman et al. 2012). Their involvement extends across a broad range of institutions and organizations for myriad reasons, for example, nearly 8.6 million children attend primary and secondary schools in the UK (Department of Education 2016) and 50.7 million children attend US public elementary and secondary schools (National Center for Education Statistics 2017). A majority of children are involved with organizations providing leisure-based services at any given time. In England, approximately 86% of children (5–15 years of age) participated in sports during the 4 weeks prior to a survey (Statista 2018). In the US, more than 60% of all children are regularly involved with community youth sports (Johnson 2015; Noble and Vermillion 2014; US Census Bureau 2009) and in Australia, estimates suggest that 70% of children aged 5–15 are involved in youth sports (Australian Bureau of Statistics 2009). In some cases, institutional involvement is mandated or necessitated by health or family concerns, with children spending time being cared for in

K. Kaufman (✉) · J. Zatkin
Portland State University, Portland, OR, USA
e-mail: cbkk@pdx.edu; jzatkin@pdx.edu

M. Erooga (✉)
Independent Safeguarding Consultant, West Yorkshire, UK

D. Higgins
Institute of Child Protection Studies, Australian Catholic University, Melbourne, VIC, Australia
e-mail: daryl.higgins@acu.edu.au

B. Lonne et al. (eds.), *Re-Visioning Public Health Approaches for Protecting Children*, Child Maltreatment 9, https://doi.org/10.1007/978-3-030-05858-6_11

hospitals, or placed in out-of-home care. Of course, a host of other leisure-focused youth serving organizations (YSOs) also help promote a variety of children's skills from academia to music, computer programing to recreational-based after school services.

The direct benefits derived from contact with many YSOs (e.g., schools, hospitals, mental health clinics) are complemented by evidence suggesting that for many children involvement with sports and leisure YSOs benefits are related to social, emotional, and personal development (e.g., self-confidence, self-esteem, positive social behaviors), skills development, and even academic advances (Durlack and Weissberg 2007; Durlak et al. 2010; Herrera et al. 2011). Although participation in these activities are often positive for children, there are also risks involved. Such risks include accidental injury and neglect, as well as physical and sexual abuse. Though it is difficult to pinpoint how many children are victims of such adverse events while in the care of a YSO, risk factors for victimization in organizational settings have been studied at length, and media reports regarding this type of abuse are common (Kaufman et al. 2012). In a series of national surveys of children's exposure to violence in the US, 6.4% of respondents indicated they had experienced some form of sexual violence or assault while in the care of a YSO (Shattuck et al. 2016). About 52% of cases of extra-familial sexual abuse in the UK occur in an organizational setting (Gallagher 2000). These findings demonstrate the need for organizational strategies to prevent child maltreatment. In this chapter, we identify setting-specific risks, as well as strategies to address risks that exist in all youth-serving organizational settings.

11.2 Organizational Child Sexual Abuse Risk Factors

The public health model (CDC 2017) emphasizes the critical role of risk identification as a foundation for the development of effective prevention initiatives. Typically, risks are defined as factors that increase the probability of child sexual abuse being perpetrated in a particular **setting** or against a particular **child**. Recently, we completed a comprehensive review of more than 400 research articles identifying risk factors related to the perpetration of child sexual abuse in youth serving organizations for the Royal Commission into Institutional Responses to Child Sexual Abuse in Australia (Kaufman et al. 2016). The following discussion provides a synopsis of findings in this area guided by the Royal Commission report and within the context of an ecological model.

11.3 Risk Factors Common Across Youth-Serving Organizations

Many risks are particular to a specific YSO, however some are common across organizational settings. Common individual risk factors for CSA victimization include gender, age, and disability status. The vast majority of CSA victims are female, accounting for approximately three-fourths of all victims (Finkelhor and Baron 1986). Children in late childhood and early adolescence are at the highest risk of CSA across a large number of settings (Kaufman et al. 2016). Children experiencing a range of disabilities, including mental illness, developmental delays and cognitive disabilities have been found to be at a higher risk of victimization (Black et al. 2001a, b, c) while youth with multiple disabilities have an even higher risk of abuse (Higgins 2010).

Studies have also identified a number of family-based risk factors for CSA victimization. These risk factors include low socio-economic status, parental mental illness, parental substance abuse, and the absence of a father or father figure in the home (Fater and Mullaney 2000; Feldman et al. 2001; Peter 2009).

Situational risk factors for CSA include the amount of time a child spends at a particular organization, as well as how central that organization is to their sense of identity (Wolfe et al. 2003). Other situational risk factors include an absence of well-developed present safety procedures, the training of staff, the condition of a facility, as well as the culture of a particular organization or institution (Kaufman et al. 2016).

Institutional risk factors that facilitate perpetration include staff role confusion and ambiguity, and facility cultures that do not emphasize youth safety (Erooga et al. 2012). Uneven power dynamics and hierarchical organization structures have also been associated with increased maltreatment risk in YSO settings (Parent and Bannon 2012; Stirling and Kerr 2009). For example, organizational cultures where questioning authority is discouraged may make it easier for supervisors and administrators to flaunt safety policies and perpetrate abuse. Further, high-status staff, professionals, board members, and donors, working with YSOs that ascribe to "top-down" organizational cultures, may be less likely to be held to YSO safety rules and policies (Kaufman et al. 2018). These individuals—including sports coaches, priests or church officials, foster parents, teachers, doctors, and organizational donors—have used their position and power to manipulate YSOs to foster their CSA offending behavior. Prominent cases include those of Jimmy Savile, a UK media personality and charity fund raiser (Erooga 2018); Jerry Sandusky, a US coach and children's youth sports foundation director (Freeh 2012); William Vahey, a UK international school teacher (Wonnacott and Carmi 2016); Miles Bradbury, a UK pediatric haematologist (Scott-Moncrieff and Morris 2015); and Terence Banks, UK, Chichester Cathedral Head Steward (Carmi 2014).

These cases and others like them reveal that individuals in positions of authority can be seen as "above the rules," and when this power goes unquestioned, abuse is more likely to go undetected.

Finally, common individual risk factors for perpetration are more challenging to identify, as there is no singular profile for CSA offenders (Marshall 1996). However, studies have linked a personal history of sexual abuse, a diagnosis of paedophilia and being male with a greater likelihood of CSA perpetration. At the same time, it is important to remember that most victims of abuse do not go on to abuse, not all who sexually abuse children are paedophiles, and most importantly that the presence of risk factors does not necessarily lead to abuse (Goldman et al. 2003).

11.4 Specific Risk Factors for Different Youth-Serving Organization Sectors

11.4.1 Faith-Based Settings

Faith-based YSOs reflect a broad array of organizations that share a common goal of meeting children's spiritual, social, educational, cultural, and recreational needs. Faith-based organizations have been the focus of a large number of international CSA related scandals reaching back more than 50 years (Carmi 2014; John Jay College of Criminal Justice 2004; Office of the Minister for Children and Youth Affairs 2009). In part, the huge number of children and teens who are involved in faith-based activities (as congregants, volunteers and employees) makes this a particularly rich area for research, prevention, and intervention (Brierley 2009; Office of the Minister for Children and Youth Affairs 2009). Evidence suggests that children may be at risk of CSA when participating in related activities which include volunteering, Sunday school, educational classes, youth camps, and any other activity where they come into contact with adults (Parkinson 2000). In general, faith-based settings reflect organizations where a large number of adults frequently interact with youth (Smith 2004), which may facilitate high risk situations vulnerable to the perpetration of CSA.

Though they are not the only CSA perpetrators in faith-based organizations, clergy clearly have considerable authority, which can facilitate access to potential victims, increase compliance in abusive acts, and reduce the potential for reporting (Harper and Perkins 2017). Other, risk factors may include clergy's perceived authority, their vows of celibacy, and some specific religious doctrines (Higgins 2001). CSA risks increase in religious organizations based, in part, on the extent to which individuals are granted power and authority, either directly from the church itself, or through their connection with a "higher power" (Guido 2008; McLoone-Richards 2012). This power is often unquestioned, allows perpetrators to act with limited oversight, and perpetuates the belief that those with authority in the church will be protected by church leaders (Parkinson 2014). Some perpetrators take this further, and directly use their 'special relationship with God' to groom their victims (Fogler et al. 2008). Historically, clergy have been poorly trained in matters of safety and rarely screened for their suitability to work with children, which has made this setting appealing to individuals with malevolent intentions (Bennett 2004; Dale and Alpert 2007).

It has also been suggested that the celibacy required of priests interferes with their sexual development, leading to them to seek-out intimacy in inappropriate ways and with under-aged partners (Doyle et al. 2006). This may lead church members to perceive priests as 'safe' (Scheper-Hughes and Devine 2003), a false assumption, as indicated by the number of clergy found to have committed CSA (Terry and Ackerman 2008).

Finally, religious doctrine represents another important contextual risk factor for faith-based child CSA. A number of elements of religious doctrine have been associated with CSA perpetration as well as with discouraging victim disclosure. Examples include the absence of women in leadership positions and patriarchal beliefs about the family, both of which foster more authoritarian beliefs and behaviours with regard to gender and barriers to questioning the behaviour of powerful member of faith-based YSOs. An emphasis on 'personal sin' and repentance can lead to a culture of victim-blaming that may shift responsibility from the perpetrator. Finally, reverence for church leaders can make reporting more difficult for victims (Higgins 2001).

11.4.2 Early Childhood Education and Schools

Schools represent a frequent setting for organizational CSA. There are incidence reports ranging from 3.7% to 50.3% of school staff engaging in sexual misconduct, and 9.6% of students being victimized (Shakeshaft 2004). Abuse risk varies both by victim gender and age: Males are more likely to be victimized while under the age of 12, while females are abused more often after the age of 13 years old (Ratliff and Watson 2014). Female students of colour and students with disabilities are at a particularly high risk for abuse in educational settings (Shakeshaft 2004). This may be due to the large amount of time they spend in one-to-one tutoring with school staff (Caldas and Bensy 2014). Technology that facilitates private communication between students and teachers/staff makes it more difficult to prevent and/or recognize early warning signs of grooming that is leading up to abuse (Quayle 2012).

Cultural and situational factors can also contribute to the potential for CSA in educational settings. Four factors in particular may be especially risky: (1) ineffective safety policies; (2) high-risk locations and settings; (3) unclear boundaries; and (4) ineffective responses to allegations of abuse (Shakeshaft and Cohan 1995). Researchers have identified high-risk locations in schools, including toilets, bathrooms, classrooms, hallways, offices, buses, cars, the private homes of educators and isolated outdoor locations (Shakeshaft et al. 1994; Shakeshaft 2004). Although schools can reduce risks related to these violence "hot spots" by shifting staff to these troublesome locations (Taylor et al. 2016), it is unclear how commonly this occurs.

11.4.3 Healthcare Settings

Millions of children are seen each year in health-care settings around the world and evidence suggests that about 1.6% of these children experience some type of maltreatment, including sexual abuse (Spencer and Knudsen 1992). High levels of occupational and environmental stress in health-care settings may contribute to the perpetration of child maltreatment (Blatt and Brown 1986). The status and authority of physicians may also contribute to both the perpetration of CSA and provide barriers to children reporting CSA (Scott-Moncrieff and Morris 2015).

Policy gaps and situational factors present in health-care settings can also contribute to the risk of CSA (Kaufman 2015), including some routine hospital procedures that leave children unsupervised or with only one adult present. Safety policies may be inadequate, absent, or poorly communicated to all hospital staff and volunteers. For example, some health-care clinics or hospitals may not provide "chaperones" for patients during sexually invasive procedures which may be particularly problematic for children or teens whose parents are not available to support or advocate for their children (e.g., during a hospitalization).

Patient and family vulnerabilities should also be considered when reviewing safety risks in health-care settings. Often parents and their children feel as though they cannot question the authority of medical professionals, even when they are uncomfortable with staff providing intimate and one-on-one care or in instances when parents are asked to leave the room to "give their teenage children some privacy" (Kaufman 2015; Scott-Moncrieff and Morris 2015). Finally, other victim-specific risk factors in healthcare settings include the vulnerability of children with chronic illnesses, motor and cognitive disabilities, mental illness, and a history of abuse (Colton et al. 2010; Feldman et al. 2001; Staley et al. 1986).

11.4.4 Out-of-Home Care

Children placed in out-of-home care (or "alternate care") may be at particular risk for CSA, given that foster parents or residential staff are often asked to act as stand-ins for unavailable or incapable parents. As such, these individuals often have a great deal of power over children in their care. Although necessary to provide adequate support and appropriate consequences, in the wrong hands such an arrangement can enable abuse of authority, intimidation of children in their care, and manipulation of child welfare staff (Green 2001; Stein 2006; Timmerman and Schreuder 2014). This may be further complicated in situations where children or adolescents are placed in out-of-home care due to serious behaviour management issues, where there is then little hope of being believed if abuse does occur (Brannan et al. 1993).

Fear of encouraging sexual provocativeness means children rarely are given adequate education on health sexuality (Green 2001, 2005), which places them at even greater risk of CSA and poorly positions them to report inappropriate advances (Higgins 2010; Lev-Wiesel et al. 2014).

Out-of-home care is traditionally under-resourced, leading to households and facilities that may have foster parents/staff who are inadequately trained or facilities that insufficiently staffed to provide adequate supervision (Green, 2001). This can lead to structural neglect and contribute to a climate in both residential and foster care where sexual abuse is more likely to occur (Bolton et al. 1981; Euser et al. 2013; Lepper 2013).

Females are more likely to be victims, whereas males are more likely to perpetrate inappropriate or abusive sexual behaviours (Hunter et al. 2003). When males are victims of CSA, however, they are much less likely to report their abuse. The prevalence of the sexist "boys-will-be-boys" attitudes in many out-of-home care settings fosters peer-to-peer abuse, where older boys sometimes perpetrate abuse, and female victims are blamed for not defending themselves (Timmerman and Schreuder 2014).

11.4.5 Youth Sports

The majority of children and adolescents regularly participate in community-based youth sports (70% in Australia, 61% in the USA; Johnson 2015; Noble and Vermillion 2014). It is estimated that between 2% and 22% of these youth have been victims of CSA (i.e., 900,000 children/teens at the low end of this estimate in the US (Friedrich 2006). Risks for CSA include low self-esteem and being female (Kirby et al. 2002; Noble and Vermillion 2014); however, abuse of young men is likely underreported due to prevailing gender stereotypes and fears of being seen as 'gay' (i.e., for male perpetrated abuse; Rhind et al. 2015).

A 'culture of silence' surrounding abuse, in which youth athletes are encouraged to place the good of the team and winning 'at all costs' over their own individual needs, in some cases discouraging reports of maltreatment due primarily to fears of backlash by team members (Kirby et al. 2002; Love 2016). The presence of hegemonic masculinity in sports, further contributes to maltreatment and presents a barrier to reporting, as it normalizes power, aggression, and competition, which can also lead to a toxic team culture (Mountjoy et al. 2015).

Situational factors, such as travel, shared hotel rooms, locker rooms and showering facilities also represent common risks for child maltreatment in sports. Moreover, a lack of safety policies and active safety practices regarding situational risk factors increases the potential for maltreatment to occur and go unreported (Brackenridge 2002, 2004). In fact, perpetrators often seek to capitalize on situational vulnerabilities as well as the lack of clear safety policies in perpetrating youth sports-based CSA (Kaufman et al. 2016; Toftegaard Nielsen 2001).

11.5 Situational Prevention Theory

Successfully addressing CSA prevention in youth-serving organizations requires consideration of the risks at each of the various ecological levels (e.g., individual; relationships; organizations; community; society) (Rogers et al. 2010). However, a number of CSA prevention models have highlighted the importance of a focus on situational prevention factors as a critical component in the amelioration of organizational CSA (Kaufman et al. 2018; Parent and Demers 2011; Smallbone et al. 2008). The following discussion briefly describes the 'Situational Prevention Approach' (SPA) and the process of tailoring prevention responses to address critical risks of CSA in YSOs (Kaufman et al. 2010, 2018).

Situational prevention involves a focus on environmental factors, risky situations, routine activities that may heighten risk, and policies (i.e., ones that are absent, in need of updating, or poorly communicated) that all may contribute to the perpetration of a crime (Kaufman et al. 2018). Situational prevention has been utilized as the foundation for more than 60 years of successful safe housing initiatives, as well as more than 25 years of successful community crime prevention efforts (see Kaufman et al. 2012 for a brief review). Cornish and Clarke's "Situational Prevention Model" (Clarke 1995; Cornish and Clarke 2002) forms the basis for much of this early literature. The model represents a criminological approach which focuses on contextual and situational risks that increase the chances of a crime occurring in a particular setting (Clarke 1995; Clarke and Homel 1997). Incorporating a number of theories, the model helps predict the likelihood of a crime occurring in particular contexts (Clarke 1995; Cornish and Clarke 2002). For example, according to Routine Activity Theory (Cohen and Felson 1979), three elements are required for crime to occur: (1) a motivated perpetrator; (2) a suitable victim; and (3) a lack of adequate supervision.

11.6 The Situational Prevention Approach

Clarke's model is powerful in that it applies to general criminal behaviour and has also been adapted for use with more specific criminal contexts. The Situational Prevention Model was adapted and expanded upon by Kaufman and colleagues to address the prevention of child sexual abuse (Kaufman et al. 2006), later to respond to CSA in youth-serving organizations (Kaufman et al. 2010, 2012, 2018), and most recently for use on college campuses to address sexual assault and other student harms (Kaufman 2017). Kaufman refers to his adaptation as the "Situational Prevention Approach" (SPA).

The SPA was designed as a sustainable prevention approach, to meet the diverse needs of a wide range of YSOs. Its overarching goal is to provide YSOs with a systematic strategy for identifying and responding to critical safety risks in such a way as to help shift the organizational focus and culture toward a proactive prevention approach. More specifically, the SPA assists YSOs in identifying and ameliorating safety risks before they can cause a child or adolescent harm. The SPA is a 4-step process: (1) brainstorming to identify existing safety risks; (2) developing affordable, effective, and do-able solutions to address identified risks; (3) prioritizing risk-solution pairs based on the level of concern and the availability of resources; and (4) developing simple implementation plans to guide action (Kaufman et al. 2012).

11.6.1 Step 1

Step 1 involves convening multiple stakeholder groups to brainstorm YSO risks. The goal here is to identify as many risks present in the YSO environment and in the surrounding neighbourhood that may, in the future, cause harm to youth. Groups typically include YSO staff and administrators, parents, and older youth (i.e., 12–17 years of age). Brainstorming is guided by asking participants to generate risks related to eight prompts (see Fig. 1): (1) characteristics of at-risk youth (e.g., presence of a cognitive disability, a parent with a substance abuse problem, emotionally needy); (2) high-risk locations (e.g., unused classrooms, rarely used stairs, slippery entry way); (3) facilitators (e.g., staff who call in sick at the last minute that affects staff-child ratios, trusted staff who break rules without consequences); (4) lifestyle and routine activities of youth and staff (e.g., young children who walk home alone at night, staff who give youth a ride home despite rules against it, staff who take younger children to the bathroom); (5) organizational policies and climate (e.g., a lack of organizational emphasis on safety, absence of staff policy re: phone/online); (6) health, mental health, accident prevention, and physical safety (e.g., mould in the building's walls, poor supervision in the gym that leads to injuries); (7) the larger community environment (e.g., gang activity that makes it unsafe to walk home after dark, busy streets with no traffic lights); and (8) community policies and climate (e.g., the YSO's use of the community pool when adults are in the pool, community playgrounds where equipment is old and broken).

11.6.2 Step 2

Risks identified by multiple groups are combined for use in Step 2 of the SPA process, which is to develop solutions for each of them. This involves the SPA workgroup, composed of a YSO administrator and staff, meeting to identify solutions for each identified safety risks. In this step, preference is given to the use of prevention solutions, since such solutions permanently resolve the risk. When prevention is not possible, however, risk-reduction solutions are utilized. For example, preventing YSO youth from leaving the facility by doors other than the front door (which is always staffed) will reduce risks related to missing youth. In contrast, strangers entering the building during a public event cannot easily be prevented, but risks may be reduced by asking all visitors to check-in and wear a name badge. Proposed prevention and risk-reduction solutions should draw first from existing YSO strengths and protective factors, before looking to create new solutions.

11.6.3 Step 3

The third SPA step is designed to assist with prioritizing risk-solution pairs in preparation for intervening to resolve them. A member of the YSO leadership team is asked to sort risk-solution pairs into two groups: less vs. more challenging to resolve. Next, the risk-solution pairs within each of the two groups are prioritized, based on level of concern and resources required to resolve the risk.

11.6.4 Step 4

In Step 4, the YSO leadership team is asked to develop simple implementation plans, identifying: the risk, the solution, the steps involved in carrying out the solution; who is responsible for each step in the solution process; who is supervising the process; any costs involved with solution steps (and sources of funds to meet the costs); due dates for each solution step; dates for when these steps were actually completed; and any ways in which existing policies need to be modified to accommodate the solution. The YSO is asked to work on resolving five risks at a time (i.e., always composed of three from the "less challenging" to resolve, and two from the "more challenging" to resolve group). The YSO uses this approach to work through their list of identified safety risks. YSOs are encouraged to repeat this process annually to both identify new safety risks and to ensure that solutions have continued to prevent the re-emersion of previously identified risks.

The advantages of SPA are: First, it is simple to implement and sustainable (i.e., the only costs for the process are related to staff time). Second, it incorporates existing YSO expertise and is a "self-tailoring" approach (i.e., it focuses exclusively on the YSO's risks and needed solutions). Third, by incorporating staff and administrators into the process, it also impacts and enhances the YSO's safety culture, increasing staff capacity and better orienting the organization to an everyday safety focus. Finally, it puts the process of enhancing safety in the hands of the organization and fosters the proactive management of risk, by shifting attention to identifying risks when they are 'small' and preventing their escalation into child or adolescent harm. Recently, the SPA was tailored for use by Boys and Girls Clubs of America (BGCA) as part of a 3-year prevention project funded by the Pennsylvania Coalition Against Rape. While not designed as an outcome study, preliminary results from the project were very promising. Sixteen clubs across four US states reported high satisfaction with the SPA, with a mean rating of 3.2 on a 4-point scale.

Further, when clubs using the SPA were compared with clubs in the same city waiting to implement the approach, the clubs using SPA identified 7–10 times more risks. They were also able to identify solutions to address each risk and in a relatively short period of time, were able to resolve most, if not all of the identified risks (Kaufman 2015). In general, staff felt that the SPA allowed them to quickly and efficiently develop and implement solutions for identified risks (Kaufman 2015). Beyond the BGCA study, the SPA has been used successfully at two large metropolitan children's hospitals, after incidents with abusive staff members (Kaufman et al. 2012). Finally, the SPA is currently the "centrepiece" of a multiyear US Department of Justice project designed to address campus sexual assault and other student harms. After working with 18 campus "units" (e.g., Athletics, Housing, International Studies, Greek System, Campus Safety) across three colleges and universities over the past year, it is clear that the SPA is useful for identifying campus safety risks and fostering the development of prevention solutions to address these concerns.

11.7 Conclusions

The overwhelming majority of children benefit from their involvement with YSOs and the adults with whom they come into contact. However, no system, however well organized, can hope to eliminate the inevitable residual risk. Vetting and screening are undoubtedly a key part of any process to maximise organizational safety but in themselves cannot be sufficient (Erooga 2009), despite their attractiveness as a seemingly simple solution (Price et al. 2013). Rather what is required is a whole-of-organization approach that is more 'organic', involving the entire organizational community in identifying where risk might occur and developing appropriate responses. Our field is an evolving and developing one but, if properly implemented in conjunction with appropriate with screening and vetting processes, the structured Situational Prevention Approach currently represents the most effective approach to maximising organizational safeguarding of which we are aware.

References

Australian Bureau of Statistics. (2009). *Children's participation in cultural and leisure activities.* Catalogue no. 4901.0. Canberra: ABS.

Bennett, R. S. (2004). *Report on the crisis in the Catholic Church in the United States.* Available from https://www.ncjrs.gov/app/publications/abstract.aspx?id=207962

Black, D. A., Heyman, R. E., & Smith Slep, A. M. (2001a). Risk factors for child physical abuse. *Aggression and Violent Behaviour, 6*(2), 121–188.

Black, D. A., Heyman, R. E., & Smith Slep, A. M. (2001b). Risk factors for child sexual abuse. *Aggression and Violent Behaviour, 6*(2), 203–229.

Black, D. A., Smith Slep, A. M., & Heyman, R. E. (2001c). Risk factors for child psychological abuse. *Aggression and Violent Behaviour, 6*(2), 189–201.

Blatt, E., & Brown, S. (1986). Environmental influences on incidents of alleged child abuse and neglect in New York State psychiatric facilities: Toward an ecology of institutional child maltreatment. *Child Abuse & Neglect, 10*(2), 171–180.

Bolton, F. G., Laner, R. H., & Gai, D. S. (1981). For better or worse? Foster parents and foster children in an officially reported child maltreatment population. *Children and Youth Services Review, 3*(1), 37–53.

Brackenridge, C. (2004). *Burden or benefit? An evaluation of SportScotland's Child Protection Programme with governing bodies of sport*. Edinburgh: SportScotland.

Brackenridge, C. (2002). '… so what?' Attitudes of the voluntary sector towards child protection in sports clubs. *Managing Leisure, 7*(2), 103–123.

Brannan, C., Jones, J., & Murch, J. (1993). Lessons from a residential special school enquiry: reflections on the Castle Hill Report. *Child Abuse Review, 2*, 271–275.

Brierley, P. (2009). *Safeguarding the church's children: The results of the 2009 survey*. Swanley: The Churches' Child Protection Advisory Service, Birmingham: Birmingham Safeguarding Children Board, UK.

Caldas, S. J., & Bensy, M. L. (2014). The sexual maltreatment of students with disabilities in American school settings. *Journal of Child Sexual Abuse, 23*, 345–366.

Carmi, E. (2014). *Case: CO1: Case review*. Chichester: Diocese of Chichester (UK).

Centers for Disease Control. (2017). *The public health approach to violence prevention.* Atlanta: CDC. Retrieved from https://www.cdc.gov/violenceprevention/overview/publichealthapproach.html

Clarke, R. V. (1995). Situational crime prevention. In M. Tonry & D. Farrington (Eds.), *Building a safer society: Strategic approaches to crime prevention. Crime and justice: An annual review of research* (Vol. 19, pp. 91–150). Chicago: University of Chicago Press.

Clarke, R., & Homel, R. (1997). A revised classification of situational crime prevention techniques. In S. P. Lab (Ed.), *Crime prevention at a crossroads* (pp. 17–30). Cincinnati: Anderson Publishing Co. and Academy of Criminal Justice Sciences.

Cohen, L., & Felson, M. (1979). Social change and crime rate trends: A routine activity approach. *American Sociological Review, 44*(4), 588–608. Retrieved from http://www.jstor.org/stable/2094589

Colton, M., Roberts, S., & Vanstone, M. (2010). Sexual abuse by men who work with children. *Journal of Child Sexual Abuse, 19*(3), 345–364. https://doi.org/10.1080/10538711003775824.

Cornish, D. B., & Clarke, R. V. (2002). Analyzing organized crimes. In A. R. Piquero & S. G. Tibbetts (Eds.), *Rational choice and criminal behaviour: Recent research and future challenges* (pp. 41–63). New York: Routledge.

Dale, K., & Alpert, J. L. (2007). Hiding behind the cloth: Child sexual abuse and the Catholic Church. *Journal of Child Sexual Abuse, 16*(3), 59–73. https://doi.org/10.1300/J070v16n03.

Department of Education. (2016). *Schools, pupils, and their characteristics*: January 2016. Retrieved from https://www.gov.uk/government/uploads/system/uploads/attachment_data/file/552342/SFR20_2016_Main_Text.pdf

Doyle, T., Sipe, A. W., & Wall, P. (2006). *Sex, priests, and secret codes: The Catholic Church's 2000-year paper trail of sexual abuse*. Los Angeles: Volt Press.

Durlak, J. A., Weissbuerg, R. P., & Pachan, M. (2010). A meta-analysis of after-school programs that seek to promote personal and social skills in children and adolescents. *Community Psychology, 45*(3–4), 294–309.

Durlak, J. A., & Weissberg, R. P. (2007). *The impact of after-school programs that promote personal and social skills.* Chicago: Collaborative for Academic, Social, and Emotional Learning. Retrieved from https://casel.org/the-impact-of-after-school-programs-that-promote-personal-and-social-skills-2007/

Erooga, M. (2018). Savile's sexual offending – what do we know? In M. Erooga (Ed.), *Protecting children and adults from abuse after Savile: What institutions and organizations need to do*. London: Jessica Kingsley Publishers.

Erooga, M., Allnock, D., & Telford, P. (2012). *Towards safer organisations II: Using the perspectives of convicted sex offenders to inform organisational safeguarding of children*. London: National Society for the Prevention of Cruelty to Children.

Erooga, M. (2009). *Towards safer organisations: A study of the literature about staff and volunteers who may present a risk to children in the workplace and implications for recruitment and selection to organisations where children may be vulnerable*. London: National Society for the Prevention of Cruelty to Children.

Euser, S., Alink, L. R., Tharner, A., Van IJzendoorn, M. H., & Bakermans-Kranenburg, M. J. (2013). The prevalence of child sexual abuse in out-of-home care: A comparison between abuse in residential and in foster care. *Child Maltreatment*, 1–11. https://doi.org/10.1177/1077559513489848.

Fater, K., & Mullaney, J. A. (2000). The lived experience of adult male survivors who allege childhood sexual abuse by clergy. *Issues in Mental Health Nursing, 21*, 281–295.

Feldman, K. W., Mason, C., & Shugerman, R. P. (2001). Accusations that hospital staff have abused pediatric patients. *Child Abuse & Neglect, 25*, 1555–1569.

Finkelhor, D., & Baron, L. (1986). Risk factors for child sexual abuse. *Journal of Interpersonal Violence, 1*(1), 43–71. https://doi.org/10.1177/088626086001001004.

Fogler, J. M., Shipherd, J. C., Rowe, E., Jensen, J., & Clarke, S. (2008). A theoretical foundation for understanding clergy-perpetrated sexual abuse. *Journal of Child Sexual Abuse, 17*(3–4), 301–328.

Freeh, L. (2012). *Report of the Special Investigative Council regarding the actions of the Pennsylvania State University related to child sexual abuse committed by Gerald A. Sandusky*. Washington, DC: Freeh Sporkin & Sullivan, LLP. Retrieved from: https://www.nsvrc.org/publications/reports/freeh-report-penn-state-university

Friedrich, B. (2006). Correlates of sexual behavior in young children. In K. Kuehnle & L. Drozd (Eds.), *Child custody litigation: Allegations of child sexual abuse*. New York: Haworth Press.

Gallagher, B. (2000). The extent and nature of known cases of institutional child sexual abuse. *British Journal of Social Work, 30*(6), 795–817.

Goldman, J., Salus, M., Wolcott, D., & Kennedy, K. (2003). *What factors contribute to child abuse and neglect? A coordinated response to child abuse and neglect: The foundation for practice*. Washington, DC: Office on Child Abuse and Neglect.

Green, L. (2001). Analysing the sexual abuse of children by workers in residential care homes: Characteristics, dynamics and contributory factors. *Journal of Sexual Aggression, 7*(2), 5–24.

Green, L. (2005). Theorising sexuality, sexual abuse and residential children's homes: Adding gender to the equation. *The British Journal of Social Work, 35*(4), 453–481. https://doi.org/10.1093/bjsw/bch191.

Guido, J. J. (2008). A unique betrayal: Clergy sexual abuse in the context of the Catholic religious tradition. *Journal of Child Sexual Abuse, 17*(3–4), 255–269.

Harper, C., & Perkins, C. (2017). Reporting child sexual abuse within religious settings: Challenges and future directions. *Child Abuse Review*. https://doi.org/10.1002/car.2484.

Herrera, C., Baldwin Grossman, J., Kauh, T., & McMaken, J. (2011). Mentoring in schools: An impact study of Big Brothers Big Sisters school-based mentoring. *Child Development, 82*(1), 346–361.

Higgins, D. J. (2010). Sexuality, human rights and safety for people with disabilities: The challenge of intersecting identities. *Sexual and Relationship Therapy, 25*(3), 245–257. https://doi.org/10.1080/14681994.2010.489545.

Higgins, D. J. (2001). A case study of child sexual abuse within a church community. *Journal of Religion & Abuse, 3*(1–2), 5–19. https://doi.org/10.1300/J154v03n01_02.

Hunter, J. A., Figueredo, A. J., Malamuth, N. M., & Becker, J. V. (2003). Juvenile sex offenders: Toward the development of a typology. *Sexual Abuse: A Journal of Research and Treatment, 15*, 27–48.

John Jay College of Criminal Justice. (2004). *The nature and scope of the problem of sexual abuse of minors by Catholic priests and deacons in the United States 1950–2002*. Washington, DC: City University of New York.

Johnson, S. (2015). Executive director, National Council of Youth Sports, Stuart, Florida. Personal communication, 18 October 2015.

Kaufman, K., Sitney, M., Glace, A., Stewart, K., Zatkin, J., & McConnell, E. (2018). Applying a situational prevention lens to the Savile case: Enhancing understanding and providing a template for strengthening organisational prevention of child sexual abuse. In M. Erooga (Ed.), *Protecting children and adults from abuse after Savile: What institutions and organizations need to do*. London: Jessica Kingsley Publishers.

Kaufman, K. (2017). *Enhancing students' safety: The campus situational prevention approach*. 36th annual research and treatment conference. Association for the Treatment of Sexual Abusers. Kansas City, Missouri.

Kaufman K. (2015). *Applying the situational prevention approach*: Enhancing safety in youth serving organizations. Safer childhood symposium. October, Atlanta, GA.

Kaufman, K., Erooga, M., Stewart, K., Zatkin, J., McConnell, E., Tews, H., & Higgins, D. (2016). *Risk profiles for institutional child sexual abuse: A literature review, Royal Commission into Institutional Responses to Child Sexual Abuse [online]*. Retrieved from http://www.childabuseroyalcommission.gov.au/policy-and-research/our-research/published-research/risk-profiles-for-institutional-child-sexual-abuse

Kaufman, K., Hayes, A., & Knox, L. A. (2010). The situational prevention model: Creating safer environments for children and adolescents. In K. L. Kaufman (Ed.), *The prevention of sexual violence: A practitioner's sourcebook*. Holyoke: NEARI Press.

Kaufman, K., Mosher, H., Carter, M., & Estes, L. (2006). An empirically based situational prevention model for child sexual abuse. In R. Wortley & S. Smallbone (Eds.), *Situational prevention of child sexual abuse: Crime Prevention Studies* (Vol. 19, pp. 101–144). Monsey: Criminal Justice Press.

Kaufman, K., Tews, H., Schuett, J., & Kaufman, B. (2012). Prevention is better than cure: The value of situational prevention in organizations. In M. Erooga (Ed.), *Towards safer organisations – Practical steps to prevent the abuse of children by those working with them*. London: Wiley Press.

Kirby, S. L., Greaves, L., & Hankivsky, O. (2002). Women under the dome of silence: Sexual harassment and abuse of female athletes. *Canadian Woman Studies, 21*(3), 132.

Lepper, J. (2013). Safeguarding in residential care. *Children and Young People Now*. [Online] https://www.cypnow.co.uk

Lev-Wiesel, R., Gottfried, R., Eisikovits, Z., & First, M. (2014). Factors affecting disclosure among Israeli children in residential care due to domestic violence. *Child Abuse & Neglect, 38*(4), 618–626.

Love, M. J. (2016). *Sexual abuse of male children in sports: Factors impacting disclosure*. Doctoral dissertation. Retrieved from ProQuest Dissertations & Theses, 3682472.

Marshall, W. L. (1996). The sexual offender: Monster, victim, or everyman? *Sexual Abuse: A Journal of Research and Treatment, 8*, 317–335.

McLoone-Richards, C. (2012). Say nothing! How pathology within Catholicism created and sustained the institutional abuse of children in 20th century Ireland. *Child Abuse Review, 21*(6), 394–404.

Mountjoy, M., Rhind, D. J. A., Tiivas, A., & Leglise, M. (2015). Safeguarding the child athlete in sport: A review, a framework and recommendations for the IOC youth athlete development model. *British Journal of Sports Medicine, 49*(13), 883–886.

National Center for Education Statistics. (2017). *Back to school statistics*. Washington, DC: US Department of Education. Retrieved from https://nces.ed.gov/fastfacts/display.asp?id=372

Noble, J., & Vermillion, M. (2014). Youth sport administrators' perceptions and knowledge of organizational policies on child maltreatment. *Children and Youth Services Review, 38*, 52–57. https://doi.org/10.1016/j.childyouth.2014.01.011.

Office of the Minister for Children and Youth Affairs. (2009). *Report of the commission to inquire into child abuse in Ireland*. Dublin: Stationery Office.

Parent, S., & Bannon, J. (2012). Sexual abuse in sport: What about boys? *Children and Youth Services Review, 34*, 354–359.

Parent, S., & Demers, G. (2011). Sexual abuse in sport: A model to prevent and protect athletes. *Child Abuse Review, 20*, 120–133.

Parkinson, P. (2000). *The problem of child sexual abuse in church communities*. In Project Axis: Child sexual abuse in Queensland: Selected research papers. Brisbane, Queensland: Queensland Crime Commission and Queensland Police Service, 59–72. Available from http://www.cmc.qld.gov.au/data/portal/00000005/content/38414001131403346713.pdf.

Parkinson, P. (2014). Child sexual abuse and the churches: A story of moral failure. *Current Issues in Criminal Justice, 26*, 119–138.

Peter, T. (2009). Exploring taboos: Comparing male-and female-perpetrated child sexual abuse. *Journal of Interpersonal Violence, 24*, 1111–1128.

Price, S., Hanson, R. K., & Tagliani, L. (2013). Screening procedures in the United Kingdom for positions of trust with children. *Journal of Sexual Aggression, 19*(1), 17–31.

Quayle, E. (2012). Organisational issues and new technologies. In M. Erooga (Ed.), *Creating safer organisations: Practical steps to prevent the abuse of children by those working with them* (pp. 99–121). London: Wiley.

Ratliff, L., & Watson, J. (2014). A descriptive analysis of public school educators arrested for sex offenses. *Journal of Child Sexual Abuse, 23*, 217–228.

Rhind, D., McDermott, J., Lambert, E., & Koleva, I. (2015). A review of safeguarding cases in sport. *Child Abuse Review, 24*, 418–426. https://doi.org/10.1002/car.2306.

Rogers, D., Green, J., & Kaufman, K. (2010). Using theory to strengthen prevention practice. In K. Kaufman (Ed.), *The prevention of sexual violence: A practitioner's sourcebook* (pp. 55–84). Holyoke: NEARI Press Inc.

Scheper-Hughes, N., & Devine, J. (2003). Priestly celibacy and child sexual abuse. *Sexualities, 6*(1), 15–40. https://doi.org/10.1177/1363460703006001519.

Scott-Moncrieff, L., & Morris, B. (2015). *Independent investigation into governance arrangements in the paediatric haematology and oncology service at Cambridge University Hospitals NHS Foundation Trust following the Myles Bradbury case*. Cambridge: Cambridge University Hospitals NHS Foundation Trust.

Shakeshaft, C. (2004). *Educator sexual misconduct: A synthesis of existing literature. PPSS 2004–09*. Washington: US Department of Education.

Shakeshaft, C., & Cohan, A. (1995). Sexual abuse of students by school personnel. *Phi Delta Kappan, 76*(7), 513–520.

Shakeshaft, C., Barber, E., Hergenrother, M. A., Johnson, Y., Mandel, L., & Sawyer, J. (1994). *Conceptions of community: Peer harassment and the culture of caring in the schools*. Paper presented at the annual convention of the University Council of Educational Administration, Philadelphia, PA.

Shattuck, A., Finkelhor, D., Turner, H., & Hamby, S. (2016). Children exposed to abuse in youth-serving organizations: Results from national sample surveys. *JAMA Pediatrics, 170*(2), 1–4.

Smallbone, S., Marshall, W. L., & Wortley, R. (2008). *Preventing child sexual abuse: Evidence, policy and practice*. Devon: Willan Publishing.

Smith, M. K. (2004). The case for youth work: Presentation to the Prime Minister's Strategy Group – September 2004. Retrieved from http://www.infed.org/archives/jeffs_and_smith/the_case_for_youth_work.html

Spencer, J., & Knudsen, D. (1992). Out-of-home maltreatment: An analysis of risk in various settings for children. *Child Youth Services Review, 14*(6), 485–492.

Staley, C., Ranck, E. R., Perreault, J., & Newgebauer, R. (1986). Guidelines for effective staff selection. *Child Care Information Exchange, 47*, 22–26.

Statista. (2018). Share of children (aged 5–15) participating in any sport in the last 4 weeks in England from 2008/09 to 2017/18. Retrieved December 24, 2018 from https://www.statista.com/statistics/421116/childrenssports-involvment-england-uk/.

Stirling, A., & Kerr, G. (2009). Abused athletes' perceptions of the coach-athlete relationship. *Sport in Society, 12*(2), 227–239.

Stein, M. (2006). Missing years of abuse in children's homes. *Child & Family Social Work, 11*(1), 11–21.

Taylor, B., Mumford, E., Liu, W., & Stein, N. (2016). *Assessing different levels and dosages of the shifting boundaries intervention to prevent youth dating violence in New York City middle schools: A randomized control trial, 2011–2014*. ICPSR36355-v1. Ann Arbor, MI: Inter-university Consortium for Political and Social Research [distributor], 2016-05-31. https://doi.org/10.3886/ICPSR36355.v1

Terry, K., & Ackerman, A. (2008). Child sexual abuse in the Catholic Church: How situational crime prevention strategies can help create safe environments. *Criminal Justice & Behavior, 35*(5), 643–657.

Timmerman, M. C., & Schreuder, P. R. (2014). Sexual abuse of children and youth in residential care: An international review. *Aggression and Violent Behavior, 19*(6), 715–720.

Toftegaard Nielsen, J. (2001). The forbidden zone: Intimacy, sexual relations and misconduct in the relationship between coaches and athletes. *International Review for the Sociology of Sport, 36*(2), 165–182.

United States Census Bureau. (2009). *Participation in selected sports activities*. Washington, DC.

Wolfe, D., Jaffe, P., Jette, J., & Poisson, S. (2003). The impact of child abuse in community institutions and organizations: Advancing professional and scientific understanding. *Clinical Psychology-Science and Practice, 10*, 179–191.

Wonnacott, J., & Carmi, E. (2016). Southbank International School Serious Case Review. Hammersmith and Fulham, Kensington and Chelsea and Westminster Local Safeguarding Children Board. Accessed on 26 July 2017 at 222.rbke.gov.uk/pdf/Southbank%20SCR%20REPORT%2012%201%2016.pdf.

Chapter 12
How Can Differential Response Inform a Public Health Approach to Child Maltreatment Prevention?

Lisa Merkel-Holguin, Tamara Fuller, Marc Winokur, Ida Drury, and Bob Lonne

12.1 Introduction

Previous chapters in this book have described the successes and limitations of contemporary child protection approaches around the globe, and have described the need for the conceptualization and development of public health approaches for preventing child abuse and neglect. In the United States (US), growing concerns

L. Merkel-Holguin (✉)
University of Colorado School of Medicine, Department of Pediatrics, Kempe Center for the Prevention and Treatment of Child Abuse and Neglect, Aurora, CO, USA

National Center on Family Group Decision Making, Aurora, CO, USA
e-mail: lisa.merkel-holguin@ucdenver.edu

T. Fuller
Children and Family Research Center, School of Social work, University of Illinois, Urbana-Champaign, IL, USA
e-mail: t-fuller@illinois.edu

M. Winokur
Social Work Research Center, School of Social Work, Colorado State University, Fort Collins, CO, USA
e-mail: marc.winokur@colostate.edu

I. Drury
University of Colorado School of Medicine, Department of Pediatrics, Kempe Center for the Prevention and Treatment of Child Abuse and Neglect, Aurora, CO, USA

University of North Dakota, Grand Forks, ND, USA
e-mail: Ida.drury@und.edu

B. Lonne
School of Health, University of New England, Armidale, NSW, Australia
e-mail: blonne@une.edu.au

B. Lonne et al. (eds.), *Re-Visioning Public Health Approaches for Protecting Children*, Child Maltreatment 9, https://doi.org/10.1007/978-3-030-05858-6_12

with several aspects of the traditional forensic approach to child protective services (CPS) led to the development of Differential Response (DR), which allows public child welfare systems the option of responding to screened-in reports of child abuse and neglect in more than one way. DR systems recognize that while some maltreatment reports require court involvement and are best approached through a traditional CPS investigation, many would be better served through an alternative approach. Specifically, a traditional response is better suited to addressing child sexual and physical abuse than neglect (Lonne 2015).

Families with allegations of neglect, which constitute the vast majority of families reported to CPS in the US, are typically eligible for the assessment response (AR), while those with allegations of sexual abuse or severe physical abuse typically receive a traditional response (TR). AR is an approach that emphasizes family-involvement and needs-driven service provision. AR does not conclude with a substantiation decision or placement on a central registry, which can have significant long-lasting economic and psychological impacts on families. Families in both response tracks are assessed for safety and provided with services and referrals ranging from housing assistance and home aides to out-of-home care for children who are unsafe at home. Since its initial development in the 1990s, DR has been implemented in more than half of the US and has been the subject of numerous rigorous evaluations.

This chapter describes the CPS context that gave rise to DR, provides a brief description of international variations of DR, and reviews the major research findings to date. Consideration is then given to the criticisms against DR and how they might be reframed to advance the current discussion instead of impede it. The chapter concludes with a discussion of how DR might inform a broader public health approach to child maltreatment prevention, including options, issues, and challenges in making the transition to a public health approach.

12.2 Child Protection in the USA and the Emergence of Differential Response

The modern era of child protection in the USA began in the 1960s, sparked by the publication of *The Battered Child Syndrome* by C. Henry Kempe and colleagues. Traditional child protection services systems were designed to respond to child maltreatment through several key functions: (1) maintaining a hotline for referrals of alleged child maltreatment; (2) screening these referrals to determine CPS response; and (3) investigating screened-in reports to determine (a) whether child maltreatment has occurred or the risk of future maltreatment is high and (b) what actions, if any, are needed to achieve child safety (US Department of Health and Human Services [USDHHS] 2003).

Soon after inception, pressures began to mount in the US child protection system as the number of annual child maltreatment reports increased from fewer than

10,000 in 1967 to more than four million in Federal Fiscal Year (FFY) 2015 (USDHHS 2017). By 1990, a US Advisory Board on Child Abuse and Neglect concluded child maltreatment was a "national emergency" and "the system the nation has devised to respond to child abuse and neglect is failing. It is not a question of acute failure of a single element of the system; there is chronic and critical multiple organ failure" (US Advisory Board on Child Abuse and Neglect 1990, p. 2). Blue ribbon panels of child welfare experts were convened and tasked with pinpointing problems and developing solutions. One such task force, the Harvard Executive Session, identified five major concerns of the CPS system: Over-inclusion, system capacity, under-inclusion, service orientation, and service delivery (Waldfogel 1998). In many ways the US led the world in developing child protection responses and similar issues were being identified elsewhere around the globe (See Chaps. 1, 2 and 3).

12.2.1 Overrepresentation of Lower Risk Cases in Child Welfare

As a wider range of child welfare concerns were included in state definitions of child maltreatment, "reports concerning relatively low-risk families unnecessarily add to the volume of cases flooding the CPS system" (Waldfogel 1998, p. 107); these reports were problematic not only because many families were being investigated that did not need to be, but they also impeded the ability of the system to respond effectively to other, higher-risk cases. This type of over-inclusion remains true today. In 2015, the vast majority of CPS investigations involve allegations of neglect (75%) and less than 30% require court action (USDHHS 2017). The CPS system continues to be a trigger for the intergenerational trauma faced by many families of color (e.g., African American, Native American, Latinx; See Chap. 20). The same is true in other child welfare systems, such as Australia. For example, half of all children in care in Western Australia are Aboriginal (Australian Institute of Health and Welfare 2017).

12.2.2 Adversarial Nature of CPS Investigations

Receiving a visit from CPS usually elicits feelings of fear, anger, shame, or humiliation from parents (Buckley et al. 2011; Gallagher et al. 2011; Harris 2012; Schreiber et al. 2013). This is particularly true when arriving unannounced and interviewing children and collateral contacts to corroborate evidence about the facts of the case. Thus, many parents find the investigation process intrusive, and respond by overtly resisting the intervention, hiding important information or concerns, or feigning cooperation out of fear of being negatively perceived by the worker and agency (Forrester et al. 2012; Harris 2012; Thoburn et al. 1995). The adversarial nature of traditional CPS investigations inhibits engagement, and makes parents less likely to accept services and less motivated to change their behavior (Schene 2005).

12.3 Family Engagement in Services

Although many parents who are investigated by CPS report feeling coerced into accepting services, most are not offered services at all. The vast majority of reports made to CPS are unsubstantiated, and rates of service provision even among substantiated cases are very low in many states (USDHHS 2017). This does not mean that investigated families have no service needs; many have underlying problems such as unstable housing, severe poverty, chronic physical and mental health conditions, and issues with substance abuse (Ringeisen et al. 2011). However, contact with the traditional child protection system does little to alleviate these problems (Campbell et al. 2010). As a result, many families come into repeated contacts with the child protection system while their needs and problems go unresolved.

12.4 International Perspectives and Variations of DR

Ideological, social, and institutional variations among social welfare systems are shaped by the values, beliefs and cultural norms found within their populations (Esping-Andersen 1990). Social constructions of families, children and childhood affect the value positions underpinning approaches toward the protection of children and social support for families and, more particularly, the role assigned to the state to intervene into the privacy of the family (See Chap. 9 and Fox Harding 1997; Parton 2006). Cameron and Freymond (2006) undertook an early international comparison of the different protective system orientations and identified three key types:

1. *Statutory child protection* – emphasizes the importance of state-authorized interventions to enforce protection of children and de-emphasizes community-based approaches that aim to support families and children. Dominating in most Anglophone countries, it places concepts of child risk and safety as paramount.
2. *Family services* – promotes voluntary participation and support, particularly through community-based services, in preference to state-authorized interventions. Scandinavian and other European countries embrace this approach, using a collectivist social obligation that de-emphasizes risk and safety concepts in lieu of rights to access family support.
3. *Informal community care* – relies upon the social care and support rendered via familial, community and cultural networks to those in need. This approach occurs in countries where formal protective systems are limited, and within neighbourhoods, being founded on relational involvement to assist struggling families.

It is important to recognize that while the genesis of DR was primarily driven by attempts to reform child protection approaches in the US, there were nonetheless reforms occurring throughout the globe as the shortcomings in each approach became more apparent. For example, when Gilbert et al. (2011) undertook their study of ten Western nations they found there was a convergence amongst the different systems towards public health approaches to prevent child maltreatment. The researchers also described an overall embracing of children's rights, with the child seen as having a relation with the state independent of their family, promoted through broader social policy frameworks focusing upon overall well-being and development rather than just safety and risk.

Given the key role of the US in the development of CPS internationally, it is unsurprising that innovations in DR have largely stemmed there. Nonetheless, the configuration of DR is quite varied dependent upon the ideological, social and institutional arrangements found in varied jurisdictions. While some states approach DR system development differently, the vast majority reserve the non-investigatory response for accepted reports initially deemed low or moderate risk (this construct is determined locally). These systems emphasize comprehensive family assessments and matching services to family needs. Safety and risk are generally constructed in a similar fashion to traditional responses, often mandating the same assessment instruments. The relationship between worker and family is established without the imminent threat of a substantiation decision about the child maltreatment report.

In contrast, Australian DR systems are structured to respond at the notification stage where CPS or community-based workers refer low-medium risk cases of suspected maltreatment to other universal services such as health and a diverse array of secondary-level non-government agencies providing services such as domestic violence, mental health, family support and disability assistance. Interventions are voluntarily accepted by service users. A variety of mechanisms and forums are used to coordinate case-related decision making, with early intervention and prevention seen as a high priority, and the voluntary nature of service user participation emphasized notwithstanding imprecise thresholds for statutory involvement (Lonne et al. 2015; Valentine and Katz 2015).

Scandinavian countries, however, developed social welfare systems with an emphasis on collective societal obligation to provide all families with services. The central question of this approach toward a family support and early intervention system, with a de-emphasis of safety and risk, is where does an investigation approach fit? Nonetheless, there is an increasing international trend toward earlier intervention and prevention, including DR (SPERU 2016).

12.5 Differential Response – The Evidence Base

DR has been one of the most rigorously evaluated child welfare interventions, with numerous published randomized controlled trials (RCT) published and over a dozen studies which have shown positive outcomes in terms of sustained child safety (as measured by re-involvement with the child welfare system) and improved family engagement (Center for Child and Family Policy 2009; Huebner et al. 2009; Loman et al. 2010; Loman and Siegel 2004; Murphy et al. 2013; Siegel et al. 2010; Siegel and Loman 1997, 2006; Virginia Department of Social Services 2008; Weiden et al. 2005; Winokur et al. 2015). For example, Winokur et al. (2014) found that AR families were more likely to score their caseworkers high on demonstration of family-centered practice skills and more likely to call CPS in the future than were TR families. This speaks to the primary and secondary prevention promise of DR, in that families have to be engaged for the service array to make a difference.

As for costs, several studies showed that initial costs were either higher or the same with the non-investigative pathway, but that higher follow-up costs were incurred with the investigative pathway (Fuller et al. 2013; Loman et al. 2010; Loman and Siegel 2004; Winokur et al. 2015). As a result, DR is classified to have promising research evidence by the California Evidence-based Clearinghouse for Child Welfare (www.cebc4cw.org).

The research to date is less promising in understanding community involvement with and support of DR, and whether views of CPS as a 'helping agency' have emerged from the implementation of DR practice models. Additionally, the research is limited regarding increased caseworker satisfaction, as it pertains to the opportunity afforded by DR to "get back to social work," and if caseworkers are more likely to stay in the field because of it. It is also unclear whether service users see DR as a way for child welfare to redeem itself and meet the aspirations of participatory and transparent child welfare practice. In addition, the evidence base on DR has been limited by non-standardized instruments and non-generalizable findings (Winokur and Gabel 2013), and a lack of longitudinal research (Loman and Siegel 2015).

12.6 The Contested Environment of Differential Response

Despite the strong evidence for DR effectiveness, a vocal anti-DR movement has emerged in the US Rather than encouraging a process that promotes dialogue whereby common ground can be reached, anti-DR proponents, pro-DR advocates, and independent researchers have 'dialogued' past one another. The resultant controversy is eerily similar to the family preservation vs. family safety discourse from the 1990s and the child rescue vs. family support dichotomy that has enveloped the child welfare system since its formal inception. This discourse outlines a dichotomy of thought around DR and the child welfare system as a whole, including the focus of financial resources and human capital, and the interaction between liberal thought (i.e., communal) and conservative thought (i.e., self-reliance).

Like any new system, theory, intervention, or change strategy being implemented in the child welfare system, leaders and advocates alike have an obligation to critically review the science of implementation, foundational principles, evidence, and impact. Yet, the polarized nature of the current DR debate in the US has proven neither helpful nor progressive for the child welfare system. This section examines the tenets of the debate, including differences and dilemmas that are not just inherent in DR, but instead belong to the *entire* system for the prevention and treatment of child maltreatment. These critiques may also serve as mileposts for rethinking the current child welfare system in terms of public health approaches.

Hughes et al. (2013) critiqued the extant DR research after conducting qualitative interviews with an undisclosed sample of key informants from across the country in all states then operating or previously operating a DR system. They formulated five critiques of DR and its research: (1) DR programs do not adhere to a uniform, standardized practice model, nor are programs implemented consistently across sites; (2) Methodological problems in the DR research limit confidence in research findings and conclusions; (3) There are insufficient data to confirm the safety of children served in alternative tracks; (4) DR programs appear to prioritize allocating services and resources for families in alternative tracks; and (5) DR literature misrepresents the traditional CPS response.

The critique that DR programs do not adhere to a uniform, standardized practice model is contrary to public health approaches to prevention and outreach, which emphasize community-tailored approaches to effective service delivery (Rippke et al. 2001). Furthermore, differences in laws, policies, and practices across jurisdictions are endemic to the child welfare system as a whole. To expect practice consistencies across States implementing DR is unrealistic, given that the federal guidance to states implementing DR, like other aspects of the child welfare system, is very broad. However, the vast majority of states implementing DR meet the core components of the intervention as outlined in 2014 by the National Quality Improvement Center on Differential Response in Child Protective Services [QIC-DR].

The critique that there are insufficient data to confirm the safety of children served in alternative tracks, could also be made regarding the safety of children served through the investigative track. There exist multiple forms of safety assessment across the US, *all of which* have the basis of clinical judgement and intuition. Essentially, the construct of safety across the child welfare system is challenging, at best, even in systems that do not implement DR. Although the standard proxies for determining 'safety' (e.g., re-reports of child maltreatment, recurrence of maltreatment) may be crude, they are the accepted norms for the child welfare field and are independent of DR implementation.

The next critique is that DR constitutes a misallocation of resources. This emphasis on harnessing resources to meet family needs has spurred child welfare caseworkers to learn about community resources, eligibility requirements of government programs, and to support families in accessing them. This is timely given that the resources to serve families who come to the attention of the child welfare system are scant, and in most communities, insufficient to meet the complex, demanding needs of families and children. One point of common ground is that all families who come to the attention of child welfare have resource needs, whether they receive an assessment or an investigation.

The last critique asserts DR proponents misrepresent traditional CPS in order to advance DR. Ultimately, DR adopters argue that any formal child welfare response should better match the reasons a family is referred to the system. Furthermore, 'champions' of DR do as one might expect: support the change and advocate for sustainability. This can be misinterpreted as "if change is needed, it must mean the 'old way' was wrong or deficient." To call this relationship advocacy is a fundamental misreading of the partnership necessary for program evaluation and contextual understanding of research questions and subsequent findings.

There is an emerging role for DR in informing the international trend toward public health approaches to preventing child maltreatment (Gilbert et al. 2011; SPERU 2016). DR is not about a need for statutory interventions or stripping away statutory resources, but who best to provide the support and assistance for struggling families to prevent their movement into the child welfare system. The key questions to be addressed are as follows:

1. Why do we need a system built around DR as the frontline prevention program?
2. How might such a system be structured and deliver early intervention and prevention services?

12.6.1 Values and Principles that Underpin Differential Response

In answering these questions, we recognize society's collective responsibility to create an interconnected and relational system that helps all families to be healthy and nurturing by providing the necessary social care and supports, particularly when they are struggling (Melton 2010a, 2014). This is family promotion rather than preservation. In this sense, helping others simultaneously assists the community at large because we are effectively rearing children and building a society where their socialization is undertaken through a system of mutual obligation, cultural education and relational connection, which are foundational aspects of the UN Convention on the Rights of the Child (See Chap. 9; Melton 2010b).

Preventing maltreatment is critical to these aims. But so is providing support and social care without intruding on family privacy or stigmatizing service recipients (see Chap. 9). Re-organizing the provision of services to children and families by taking low and medium risk out of CPS is a critical first step. However, this needs to be accompanied by delivering earlier interventions with community members serving on the frontline of social care provision. DR is poised differently than traditional CPS to link families to community-based resources and address poverty-related issues, which provides a way forward to re-vision the prevention of maltreatment.

12.6.2 Positioning Differential Response within Public Health Approaches – Options

Positioning DR to become the frontline early intervention delivery system within a public health model requires a fundamental reconfiguration of its roles, functions, and principles. There are four key principles of effective early intervention that are embodied by DR.

- *Acceptance of every family* – everyone needs non-stigmatizing support from others at some time or other;
- *Accessibility of social support* – getting the right sorts of help when needed is imperative;
- *Assessment of family and children's needs* – parenting is challenging and diverse needs across different cultural and community contexts are evident; and
- *Assistance to enhance parent capability* – support and resources need to build parental and community capacity to rear hearty and healthy children.

Organizational roles for DR will depend upon the jurisdiction's ideological stance toward welfare and its associated institutions, and may include being:

- The key agency for configuring and managing the system-wide responses for child maltreatment, including being the major funder of community-based agencies and programs providing prevention services;
- The frontline agency responsible for coordinating service systems and providing services to support communities and families to address maltreatment and/or unmet needs without involving statutory agencies;
- The developer and disseminator of primary-level public education campaigns to inform community understandings of child maltreatment and family support, and influence perceptions of social interventions at the neighbourhood level;
- The system coordinator of case-related information sharing between universal and secondary-level services, and those which undertake tertiary level interventions, including CPS, police, and other statutory agencies;
- A major policy creator and implementer of programs that redress the social determinants of health and inequalities associated with child maltreatment; and
- The primary evaluator, and researcher system, for program and service efficacy.

The functions will also depend on the community's ideological world view, and the institutional arrangements and cultures. For example, is there an ethically and socially just response to the community's approach, in which the idea of care and control come together? Another question is what the role of the community should be in the implementation of DR? Specifically, an increased role for the broader community that goes beyond being reporters of concerns to being vital and accessible help for those who are struggling. Furthermore, a new system provides potential opportunities and in some respects entails unseen challenges for all, including the following:

- Operationalizing service eligibility criteria that enable factors other than risk and safety to be brought forward, such as well-being, need, poverty, disability, child behaviour management, harm minimization, and an emphasis upon voluntary status;
- Facilitating community-level social care responses that enable marginalized groups to access the sorts of community development resources they require to properly nurture and raise their children, particularly where intergenerational trauma is evident (See Chap. 20);
- Promoting integrated and coordinated system responses that incorporate preventive interventions and allow for access to services and supports by community members from existing universal programs; and
- Developing cohesive public education programs focused on prevention and the enhancement of community ownership of the provision of social care.

12.6.3 Positioning Differential Response within Public Health Approaches – Issues

There are a number of structural and organizational issues that need to be addressed when operationalizing public health systems, including legal frameworks that regulate institutional roles and responsibilities (See Chap. 18). Having the political and administrative will to develop the institutional arrangements is critical, including establishing the agency that will best fit the new purpose and roles. Some have argued for this organization to be within a government's health or education structures (Lonne et al. 2009), so that services are accessible and non-stigmatizing, and thereby avoid the problems occurring when DR is part of the programs delivered by CPS.

In our view, a public health approach to child maltreatment prevention requires a single purpose institution because of the aggregation of voluntary early intervention and prevention services. It is best to distinguish this from CPS, and to enable it to lead initiatives for system collaboration, cooperation and communication (Ross 2009; Valentine et al. 2007; Winkworth and White 2010). Including this responsibility within the legal framework of the resulting agency can facilitate the necessary communication exchanges that reduce the potential for poorly targeted resource allocation, ineffective interventions, and organizational rivalries resulting from the lack of follow-up and monitoring of family's progress.

One system integration issue is determining organizational boundaries and thresholds for intervention through decision making that involves the personal, professional and organizational domains (Horwath 2007; Valentine and Katz 2015). These determinations impact whether or not children and families enter CPS (Kahn et al. 2017; Lonne 2015; Stoltenborgh et al. 2013). In a public health approach, the CPS system should only deal with those situations where the risk and safety issues warrant the removal of children.

Differential response set within a public health system is better positioned to rebuild trust, establish relationships, provide timely assistance, and match services to family needs. CPS systems commonly use time-limited case management interventions that do not necessarily match with family needs, particularly when dealing with chronic neglect. Truly voluntary public health services need not be driven by such factors, particularly when their remit is prevention of harm, and they have the resources available to address high need family and community circumstances. What is essential is that effective community development methods be broadly used to build the community capacity to intervene and provide informal supports to struggling families (Holland 2014; McDonell and Melton 2008). Done well, this has been found to reduce the service demands upon CPS (Melton 2014). This could benefit workers and organizations in terms of recruitment, retention, and operational resilience.

One example from Ireland exists to assist in this re-imagination of a public health approach. When developing their new agency to prevent child maltreatment and improve the well-being outcomes for children, the Irish government utilised a new word *Tusla*, to capture "a shared desire for a new beginning, forging a new identity" (See Chap. 23; Tusla 2014, n.p.). Language is important, particularly in jurisdictions that are intending to develop a new vision and role for a government agency embracing public health approaches to protecting children and supporting families and communities. Given the over-representation of Indigenous children in protective systems (See Chap. 20; Blackstock et al. 2004), considering Indigenous names for agencies has merit because community members can feel more comfortable in seeking voluntary assistance. This also provides an opportunity for parent, child, and community advocate voices to be prioritized in the development of the ongoing reform.

12.6.4 Challenges in Transitioning Differential Response to a Public Health System

Transitioning from an alternative track in a CPS-dominated system to a public health one involves significant challenges (see Chap. 15), particularly in jurisdictions experiencing continual change. Here we examine those that affect the people involved in delivering or receiving services. Organizations and practitioners will be required to alter their frameworks for intervention from risk and safety-based to those centred on relationships, caring, and support values (Featherstone et al. 2014). This new entity and other universal services will need to buy into the public health reform system, and provide high quality services where staff understand and can work with risk situations, while balancing the need to turn to the statutory system when warranted. Moreover, those working in universal agencies and CPS also need to buy into a public health system discourse and practices, and show commitments to cross-institutional communication and collaboration. They also need to be able to work in uncertain circumstances and avoid the temptation to unthinkingly shift risk back to CPS. These changes will occur in a period of uncertainty concerning how new institutional arrangements, policies and approaches are rolled out. Without ownership of the change processes by politicians, executives, and management, reform change processes will be fraught in the face of tragedies and scandals, where media pressure highlights systemic failings (See Lonne and Parton 2014).

Determining broad agreement for definitional thresholds and interventions by respective agencies and service is critical for ensuring the system functions effectively and efficiently (Valentine and Katz 2015). Ongoing staff and community education will be required to cement changed practice into place. These strategies may assist in helping the community to fully understand the shift toward voluntary service delivery and accessible assistance for struggling families, but more is needed to shift the perspectives of service users who are fearful of CPS involvement and wary of what voluntary interventions might involve.

Highly vulnerable groups and communities, particularly Indigenous peoples and other oppressed groups will need to have full partnerships in the change processes and re-configuration of the system discourses (See Chap. 20). This is especially acute given issues of indigenizing agencies, and addressing the overrepresentation of western views. Convincing those wary of the spectre of ongoing removal of children, should they not agree to voluntary services, is a very difficult task, especially when they distrust sharing of their private information with CPS.

In an increasingly digitalized world, there is potential for a public health system to favour being 'joined up' and thereby uncritically adopting information sharing of private family information as part of inter-agency protocols (See Chap. 14 and Featherstone et al. 2013; Wrennall 2010). A public health approach that fully utilizes DR values relies upon public trust and confidence that the assistance needed by struggling families and communities will be accessible, based on assessed need, and delivered in ways that are non-stigmatizing and understanding of human frailty. Transitioning to this is a real challenge given the chequered career that CPS has regarding outcomes for service users (See Chaps. 1, 2 and 3 in this volume).

12.7 Conclusions

In this chapter we have argued for DR to have a central place in public health systems for preventing child maltreatment because it reshapes the involvement of the state from focusing only on safety and risk discourses to increasing access to non-stigmatizing help through enhanced family engagement. The principles of these interventions are acceptance, accessibility, assessment, and assistance, which provide a cornerstone for building stronger children, families and communities. There is also the thorny issue of system cooperation, collaboration, coordination, and communication, which is a perennial and perhaps intractable problem. As such DR should not be viewed as a panacea, but as a fundamental component of a responsive preventative and protective CPS system. It's a mistake to portray DR as antithetical to effective protective systems because there is enough evidence to demonstrate that it is an effective alternative to a one-pathway system. In a public health approach, DR is well positioned to be the foundational, early intervention/prevention cornerstone.

References

Australian Institute of Health and Welfare. (2017). *Child protection Australia 2015–16, Child welfare series no. 66. Cat. no. CWS 60.* Canberra: AIHW.

Blackstock, C., Trocmé, N., & Bennett, M. (2004). Child maltreatment investigations among Aboriginal and non-Aboriginal families in Canada: A comparative analysis. *Violence Against Women, 10*, 901–916.

Buckley, H., Carr, N., & Whelan, S. (2011). 'Like walking on eggshells'. Service user views and expectations of the child protection system. *Child & Family Social Work, 16*, 101–110.

Cameron, G., & Freymond, N. (2006). Understanding international comparisons of child protection, family service and community caring systems of child and family welfare. In N. Freymond & G. Cameron (Eds.), *Towards positive systems of child and family welfare: International comparisons of child protection, family service, and community caring systems* (pp. 3–27). Toronto: University of Toronto Press.

Campbell, K. A., Cook, L. J., LaFluer, B. J., & Keenan, H. T. (2010). Household, family, and child risk factors after an investigation for suspected child maltreatment. *Archives of Pediatric and Adolescent Medicine, 164*, 943–949.

Center for Child and Family Policy. (2009). *Multiple response system (MRS): Evaluation report to the North Carolina Division of Social Services (NCDSS).* Durham: Duke University. Retrieved from http://www.ncdhhs.gov/dss/mrs/docs/2009%20MRS%20Report.pdf

Esping-Andersen, G. (1990). *The three worlds of welfare capitalism.* Princeton: Princeton University Press.

Featherstone, B., Morris, K., & White, S. (2013). A marriage made in hell: Early intervention meets child protection. *British Journal of Social Work*, Advance Access. https://doi.org/10.1093/bjsw/bct052

Featherstone, B., White, S., & Morris, K. (2014). *Reimagining child protection: Towards humane social work with families.* Bristol: Policy Press.

Forrester, D., Westlake, D., & Glynn, G. (2012). Parental resistance and social worker skills: Towards a theory of motivational social work. *Child & Family Social Work, 17*, 118–129.

Fox Harding, L. (1997). *Perspectives in child care policy* (2nd ed.). Essex: Longman.

Fuller, T., Nieto, M., & Zhang, S. (2013). *Differential response in Illinois: Final evaluation report.* Urbana: Children and Family Research Center, School of Social Work, University of Illinois at Urbana-Champaign.

Gallagher, M., Smith, M., Wosu, H., Stewart, J., Hunter, S., & Cree, V. E. (2011). Engaging with families in child protection: Lessons from practitioner research in Scotland. *Child Welfare, 90*, 117–134.

Gilbert, N., Parton, N., & Skivenes, M. (Eds.). (2011). *Child protection systems: International trends and orientations.* Oxford: Oxford University Press.

Harris, N. (2012). Assessment: When does it help and when does it hinder? Parents' experiences of the assessment process. *Child & Family Social Work, 17*, 180–191.

Holland, S. (2014). Trust in the community: Understanding the relationships between formal, semi-formal and informal child safeguarding in a local neighbourhood. *British Journal of Social Work, 44*, 384–400.

Horwath, J. (2007). The missing assessment domain: Personal, professional and organisational factors influencing professional judgements when identifying and referring child neglect. *British Journal of Social Work, 37*, 1285–1303.

Huebner, R. A., Durbin, L., & Brock, A. (2009). *Program evaluation of the multiple response system*. Unpublished manuscript. Kentucky Department for Community Based Services.

Hughes, R. C., Rycus, J. S., Saunders-Adams, S. M., Hughes, L. K., & Hughes, N. K. (2013). Issues in differential response. *Research on Social Work Practice, 23*, 493–520.

Kahn, N., Gupta-Kagan, J., & Hansen, M. (2017). The standard of proof in the substantiation of child abuse and neglect. *Journal of Empirical Legal Studies, 14*, 333–369.

Loman, L. A., & Siegel, G. L. (2004, November). *Minnesota alternative response evaluation: Final report*. St. Louis: Institute of Applied Research. Retrieved from http://www.iarstl.org/papers/ARFinalEvaluationReport.pdf

Loman, L. A., & Siegel, G. L. (2015). Effects of approach and services under differential response on long term child safety and welfare. *Child Abuse & Neglect, 39*, 86–97. https://doi.org/10.1016/j.chiabu.2014.05.014.

Loman, L. A., Filonow, C. S., & Siegel, G. (2010). *Ohio alternative response evaluation: Final report*. St. Louis: Institute of Applied Research. Retrieved from http://www.americanhumane.org/assets/pdfs/children/differential-response/pc-dr-ohio-section2-final-evaluation-report-1.pdf

Lonne, B. (2015). Mandatory reporting and the difficulties in identifying and responding to risk of severe neglect: A response requiring a rethink. In B. Mathews & D. Bross (Eds.), *Mandatory reporting laws and the identification of severe child abuse and neglect* (pp. 245–273). New York: Springer.

Lonne, B., & Parton, N. (2014). Portrayals of child abuse scandals in the media in Australia and England: Impacts on practice, policy and systems. *Child Abuse & Neglect, 38*, 822–836. https://doi.org/10.1016/j.chiabu.2014.04.020.

Lonne, B., Parton, N., Thomson, J., & Harries, M. (2009). *Reforming child protection*. London: Routledge.

Lonne, B., Brown, G., Wagner, I., & Gillespie, K. (2015). Victoria's Child FIRST and IFS differential response system: Progress and issues. *Child Abuse & Neglect, 39*, 41–49. https://doi.org/10.1016/j.chiabu.2014.08.003.

McDonell, J., & Melton, G. (2008). Toward a science of community intervention. *Family and Community Health, 31*(2), 113–125.

Melton, G. B. (2010a). Angels watching over us: Child safety and family support in an age of alienation. *American Journal of Orthopsychiatry, 80*(1), 89–95.

Melton, G. B. (2010b). It's all about relationships! The psychology of human rights. *American Journal of Orthopsychiatry, 80*(2), 161–169.

Melton, G. B. (2014). Strong communities for children: A community-wide approach to prevention of child maltreatment. In J. Korbin & R. D. Krugman (Eds.), *Handbook of child maltreatment* (pp. 329–339). New York: Springer.

Murphy, J., Newton-Curtis, L., & Kimmich, M. (2013). *Ohio SOAR Project*: Final report. Retrieved from http://www.hsri.org/files/uploads/publications/OHIO_SOAR_Final_Report.pdf

National Quality Improvement Center on Differential Response in Child Protective Services. (2014). *Final report: QIC-DR cross-site evaluation*. Retrieved from: www.differentialresponseqic.org

Parton, N. (2006). *Safeguarding childhood: Early intervention and surveillance in a late modern society*. Basingstoke: Palgrave Macmillan.

Ringeisen, H., Casanueva, C., Smith, K., & Dolan, M. (2011). *NSCAW II baseline report: Caregiver health and services*. Washington, DC: Office of Planning, Research and Evaluation, Administration for Children and Families, US Department of Health and Human Services.

Rippke, M., Briske, L., Keller, L., & Strohschein, S. (2001). *Public health interventions: Applications for public health nursing practice*. Minnesota: St Paul.

Ross, T. (2009). *Child welfare: The challenges of collaboration*. Washington, DC: The Urban Institute Press.
Schene, P. (2005). The emergence of differential response. *Protecting Children, 20*, 4–7.
Schreiber, J. C., Fuller, T. L., & Paceley, M. (2013). Engagement in child protective services: Parent perceptions of worker skills. *Children and Youth Services Review, 35*, 707–715.
Siegel, G. L., & Loman, L. A. (1997, November). *Missouri family assessment and response demonstration: Final evaluation report*. St. Louis: Institute of Applied Research. Retrieved from http://www.iarstl.org/papers/MoFamAssess.pdf
Siegel, G. L., & Loman, T. (2006). *Extended follow-up study of Minnesota's family assessment response: Final report*. St. Louis: Institute of Applied Research. Retrieved from http://www.iarstl.org/papers/FinalMNFARReport.pdf
Siegel, G. L., Filonow, C. S., & Loman, L. A. (2010, December). *Differential response in Nevada: Final evaluation report*. St. Louis: Institute of Applied Research. Retrieved From http://www.iarstl.org/papers/NevadaDRFinalReport.pdf
SPERU (Social Policy Evaluation and Research Unit). (2016). *Modernising Child Protection in New Zealand: Learning from system reforms in other jurisdictions. Wellington: SPERU.*
Stoltenborgh, M., Bakermans-Kranenburg, M., & van IJzendoorn, M. (2013). The neglect of child neglect: A meta-analytic review of the prevalence of neglect. *Social Psychiatry and Psychiatric Epidemiology, 48*, 345–355.
Thoburn, J., Lewis, A., & Shemmings, D. (1995). Family participation in child protection. *Child Abuse Review, 4*, 161–171.
Tusla. (2014). *About us*. Dublin: Tusla. Retrieved from http://www.tusla.ie/about
US Advisory Board on Child Abuse and Neglect. (1990). *A nation's shame: Fatal child abuse and neglect in the United States*. Washington, DC: The National Clearinghouse on Child Abuse and Neglect.
US Department of Health and Human Services [USDHHS], Administration for Children and Families, Administration on Children, Youth and Families, Children's Bureau. (2017). *Child Maltreatment 2015*. Retrieved from http://www.acf.hhs.gov/programs/cb/research-data-technology/statistics-research/child-maltreatment
US Department of Health and Human Services [USDHHS], Administration for Children and Families/Children's Bureau and Office of the Assistant for Planning and Evaluation. (2003). *National study of child protective services systems and reform efforts: Review of state CPS policies*. Washington, DC: US Government Printing Office.
Valentine, K., & Katz, I. (2015). How early is early intervention and who should get it? Contested meanings in determining thresholds for intervention. *Child and Youth Services Review, 55*, 121–127.
Valentine, K., Katz, I., & Griffiths, M. (2007). *Early childhood services: Models of integration and collaboration*. Canberra: ARACY.
Virginia Department of Social Services. (2008). *Evaluation of the differential response system*. Richmond: Author. Retrieved from http://www.dss.virginia.gov/files/about/reports/children/cps/all_other/2007/differentialresponsesystem_evaluation_annualreport_2007_12-07.pdf
Waldfogel, J. (1998). *The future of child protection: How to break the cycle of abuse and neglect*. Cambridge, MA: Harvard University Press.
Weiden, T., Nutter, B., Wells, L., & Sieppert, J. (2005). *Alberta response model implementation evaluation phase 1: Baseline data*. Calgary: Centre for Social Work Research and Professional Development, University of Calgary.
Winkworth, G., & White, M. (2010). May do, should do, can do: Collaboration between commonwealth and state service systems for vulnerable children. *Communities, Children and Families Australia, 5*, 5–20.
Winokur, M. A., & Gabel, G. (2013). A critical appraisal of issues in differential response: Moving the field forward. *Research on Social Work Practice, 23*, 531–534. https://doi.org/10.1177/1049731513475878.

Winokur, M., Ellis, R., Orsi, R., Rogers, J., Gabel, G., Brenwald, S., et al. (2014). *Program evaluation of the Colorado consortium on differential response: Final report*. Fort Collins: Social Work Research Center, School of Social Work, Colorado State University.
Winokur, M., Ellis, R., Drury, I., & Rogers, J. (2015). Answering the big questions about differential response. Safety and cost outcomes from a randomized controlled trial. *Child Abuse & Neglect: The International Journal, 39*, 98–108.
Wrennall, L. (2010). Surveillance and child protection: De-mystifying the Trojan Horse. *Surveillance and Society, 7*, 304–324.

Chapter 13
Bringing a Health Equity Perspective to the Prevention of Child Abuse and Neglect

Joanne Klevens and Marilyn Metzler

13.1 Introduction

Preventing child abuse and neglect (CAN) is a critical goal for societies seeking to achieve their full health, social, and economic potential. Achieving this goal requires ongoing examination of the question: Why are some children at greater risk for abuse and neglect than others? Children living in poverty are more likely to experience abuse and neglect than are children not living in poverty; differences in risk have also been documented by race/ethnicity in the US (Sedlak et al. 2010). Responses to these differences have traditionally focused on modifying parental behaviors or their risk factors, such as social isolation (Mikton and Butchart 2009). However, these approaches ignore the larger, structural factors that shape or constrain parents and place some groups at higher risk for CAN. Addressing only parental risk factors limits the effectiveness and reach of CAN prevention efforts. There is an increased recognition that in order to prevent CAN, it is also necessary to address the structural factors that lead to inequities in risk for CAN.

Authors' note: The findings and conclusions in this chapter are those of the authors and do not necessarily represent the official position of the Centers for Disease Control and Prevention.

J. Klevens (✉)
Division of Violence Prevention, Centers for Disease Control and Prevention (CDC), Atlanta, GA, USA
e-mail: jklevens@cdc.gov

M. Metzler
Division of Violence Prevention, Centers for Disease Control and Prevention/Karna, Atlanta, GA, USA
e-mail: mom7@cdc.gov; mom7@cdc.gov

B. Lonne et al. (eds.), *Re-Visioning Public Health Approaches for Protecting Children*, Child Maltreatment 9, https://doi.org/10.1007/978-3-030-05858-6_13

13.1.1 Expanding Our Understanding of the Root Causes of Poor Health

Over the past two decades, there is growing emphasis on understanding the root causes of health outcomes that systematically align along markers of advantage and disadvantage, including income, race/ethnicity, and education (e.g., Shonkoff et al. 2009; UNICEF 2012). The fact that risk for CAN is distributed along markers of social and economic advantage/disadvantage raises important questions about how the conditions in which some parents and caregivers are raising children may contribute to greater risk for harm. It is well documented that low income, inadequate education, insecure housing, and other social conditions increase risk for abuse and neglect (e.g., Doidge et al. 2017; Stith et al. 2009; Yang 2015), and that these interact to exponentially increase risk for CAN (Brown et al. 1998; Lamela and Figuereido 2015). Understanding how these conditions cluster and interact is critical towards the goal of preventing CAN.

Addressing the social and economic conditions in which many health issues are embedded and maintained is within the purview of public health research and practice. Public health aims to assure the conditions in which people can be healthy (National Academy of Sciences 1988; World Health Organization2018). This focus on conditions is not exclusive of clinical and behavioral interventions but recognizes that population health is largely determined by social conditions.

Emphasis on addressing the social determinants of health and health inequities has grown across the globe (see, for example, http://www.who.int/social_determinants/en/). In 2008, The World Health Organization's Commission on Social Determinants of Health (CSDH) published the landmark, *Closing the Gap in a Generation: Health Equity Through Action on the Social Determinants of Health,* where it defined the social determinants of health as "the conditions in which people are born, grow, work, live, and age, and the wider set of forces and systems shaping the conditions of daily life" (World Health Organization2008). To support action leading to health equity—meaning that everyone has a fair and just opportunity to be as healthy as possible (Braveman 2014)—the CSDH developed a framework for understanding and addressing the pathways and mechanisms contributing to inequitable health outcomes (Solar and Irwin 2010).

In this chapter, we use the CSDH framework as a tool for exploring and addressing inequities in risk for CAN drawing on, as previously noted, the US experience to illustrate key concepts and challenges. We begin with an overview of the theoretical underpinnings and major domains of the framework and then apply the framework to the problem of CAN. We provide concrete examples of how this framework has been used to guide and monitor activities to address inequities in risk for CAN. This discussion is relevant for all countries seeking to prevent CAN and achieve health equity.

13.2 A Theory-Driven Framework for Action on the Social Determinants of Health

No single theory can fully explain the complex pathways and relationships that may give rise to persistent, systemic health inequities. Multiple theories are needed to explain how health behaviors contributing to poor outcomes are patterned by social and economic conditions. Theories are also need to determine how these conditions, which are more or less available to groups based on their locations on social and economic hierarchies, are themselves patterned by structural policies and processes. For example, the ability to live in a safe neighborhood with equitable opportunities may be limited by housing and economic development policies that locate sidewalks, streetlights, and high quality schools in neighborhoods with more expensive homes compared to neighborhoods with more affordable homes.

To provide a comprehensive understanding of how social determinants impact health, the CSDH developed its framework to synthesize relevant evidence, theories, and pathways in order to support the development of effective actions (Fig. 13.1). The CSDH conceptual framework encompasses multiple interacting theories seeking to explain health inequities in current populations, as well as, and perhaps more significantly, how to decrease or eliminate future health inequities. These include psychosocial theories that address people's perceptions and experiences of being in hierarchies and living in social settings of inequality (Wilkinson and Pickett 2006); economic and political theories that focus on the impact of structural inequalities on health and disease (Kaplan et al. 1996); and, eco-social theories that seek to integrate social, biological, historical, and ecological perspectives in

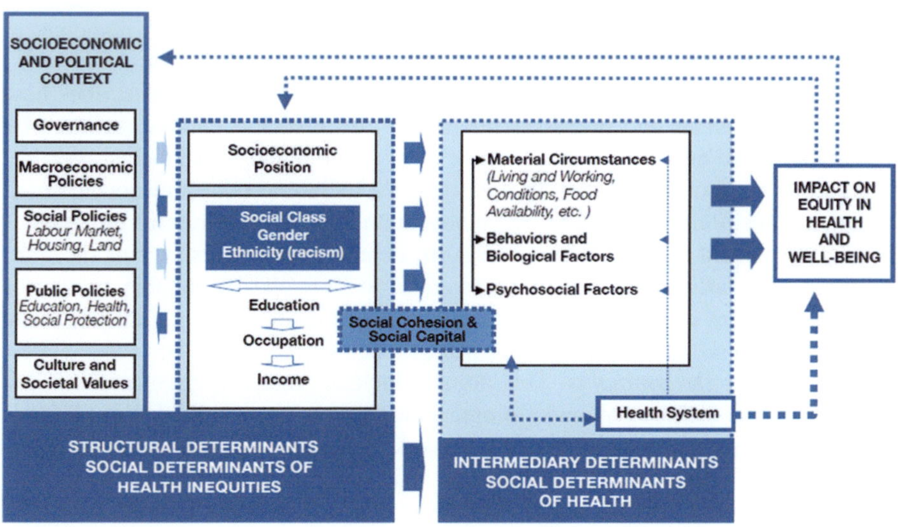

Fig. 13.1 Final form of the CSDH conceptual framework (used with permission). (World Health Organization, Commission on the Social Determinants of Health 2008)

order to develop new insights into determinants of population distribution of disease and social inequities in health (Krieger 2001). The CSDH framework draws on many models that preceded it and also provides needed specificity to inform in-depth explorations of the mechanisms and pathways through which structural policies and processes may contribute to differential exposure, differential vulnerability, and, consequently, differential and inequitable health outcomes.

13.2.1 Major Domains of the Framework

The CSDH framework suggests that the socioeconomic and political contexts determine who has more or less access to opportunities such as education and employment based on social characteristics that assign groups to their socioeconomic position. Both the context and the resulting hierarchies based on education, occupation, and income are considered 'structural determinants'. Structural determinants control who has better or worse access to healthy living conditions, mental health, and behaviors ('intermediary determinants'), which then lead to inequities in health outcomes.

Following is a brief overview of the major domains of the CSDH framework:

- *Structural Determinants: Socioeconomic and Political Context.* This domain includes the broad array of structural, cultural, and functional aspects of how societies are organized—governance structures, macroeconomic policies, social policies (including, for example, labor market and housing), public policies (including education, health and social protection), and cultural and societal values about children and the role of women. Policies at this level seek to maximize health and life opportunities through the fair distribution of society's resources to all members of a society.
- *Structural Determinants: Socioeconomic Position.* This domain describes how structural policies and processes interact to assign socioeconomic position, by groups, based on social characteristics (e.g., race/ethnicity, social class, gender) through more or less access to opportunities including education, occupation, and income. Policies that address socioeconomic position minimize the systematic assignment of this position based on social characteristics such as race/ethnicity (e.g., affirmative action), as well as to limit the inequitable burden of macro policies on members of society based on hierarchies (e.g., fair pay wage policies that seek to redress gender wage inequities).
- *Intermediary Determinants.* This domain includes material circumstances and psychosocial, behavioral, and biological characteristics of individuals and families. Broadly encompassing living and working conditions, such as the availability of food, this element also includes the health system, which has an independent and interacting effect on health. Policies at this level seek to limit the effects of excess vulnerability and exposure to existing conditions that disproportionately

impact groups disadvantaged by socioeconomic position (e.g., housing and food assistance, child care subsidies).
- *Cross-Cutting Determinants (including social capital and social cohesion).* This domain acknowledges the role of people in shaping policies and processes that effectively determine how societies are organized. The CSDH emphasized the need to include groups historically and currently excluded from decision-making processes that affect their health and life opportunities, and placed special emphasis on empowerment theory and models where collective action is informed by a human rights and social justice approach.
- *Health Equity.* This domain includes comparison of the health of populations based on hierarchies of social advantage and disadvantage (e.g., race/ethnicity, income, gender) in order to identify existing health inequities.

The goal of the CSDH framework is to explain how the differential impact of structural policies and processes influence socioeconomic position based on race, ethnicity, sex, and other social categories, and how this positioning creates vulnerability through more or less access to living and working conditions needed for health. This understanding of the contribution of structural determinants of health is needed in order to set reasonable expectations for health outcomes. For example, interventions addressing intermediary determinants may improve the situations of those currently living in unhealthy conditions, but addressing the structural determinants that give rise to these conditions in the first place is necessary to assure equitable, sustainable opportunities for health over the life course of current populations as well as for future generations. Finally, and importantly, the framework accounts for human agency in the generation of structures, policies, and processes that create and distribute life chances and opportunities for health by emphasizing the need to include groups historically and currently excluded from societal decision-making processes that effectively determine their health and life opportunities. This distinction between the determinants (e.g., macro-level policies) and the processes that give rise to their distribution (e.g., social and political power), is critical for the development of effective actions to eliminate health inequities.

The CSDH framework draws on many models that preceded it, including the socio-ecological model (SEM; Dahlberg and Krug 2002). The SEM also describes a series of nested relationships, acknowledging the complex interplay between the inner and outer spheres (i.e., individual, relational, community, societal) in conferring risk and protection. However, the CSDH framework provides greater specificity to inform more in-depth explorations of the mechanisms and pathways through which broader influences contribute to differential exposure, vulnerability, and inequitable health outcomes. In the CSDH framework, inequitable outcomes are explained by the differential impact of structural policies and processes leading to hierarchies in socioeconomic position based on income, race, ethnicity, gender, and other social categories, and how this positioning creates vulnerability through limited access to living and working conditions needed for health. This distinction between the structural and intermediate determinants is critical in reducing health inequities.

The CSDH has several limitations. Critiques include the absence of overarching determinants—including, for example, racism, sexism, classism—that not only inform how particular policies may be differentially implemented based on race, gender, and/or income, but also recognition that discrimination may be embedded in actual policies or social and political processes (Birn 2009; Krieger 2008). Despite its limitations, the CSDH has been a useful tool in applying an equity lens to efforts in reducing CAN. Given higher rates of CAN among lower income and Black families (Sedlak et al. 2010), throughout this chapter, we intentionally focus on the differential impacts of intermediary and structural determinants on families with low incomes and communities of color in order to address these observations.

13.3 Applying the WHO CSDH Framework to Address Inequities in Risk for Child Abuse and Neglect

The CSDH framework suggests what contexts might be empirically associated with CAN and the potential mechanisms through which these contexts create the conditions, leading to their differential distribution along racial and socioeconomic lines and increased risk of CAN for Black children and children in low socioeconomic families (Sedlak et al. 2010). Given the inequities in risk for CAN based on income and race/ethnicity, the CSDH framework can be used to look at more proximal/intermediary determinants to explore why some children are at greater risk than are others.

13.3.1 Intermediary Determinants: Living and Working Conditions

Poverty and low family income are associated with increased risk for CAN (Sedlak et al. 2010). While personal experiences are important, the choices parents make in caring for their children may also be shaped by the resources and opportunities available to them. These resources include more or less access to adequate income, stable jobs, secure housing, high quality affordable child care, high quality schools, and safe neighborhoods. Limited access to these resources can place undue stress on parents and contribute to increased rates of CAN. Living in poverty and low income conditions might contribute to CAN through multiple mechanisms. For example, insufficient income may determine limited or differential access to resources or supports that could directly prevent CAN (e.g., access to quality child care might prevent leaving children home alone; 'supervisory neglect'; Yang and Maguire-Jack 2016). Low income might also limit access to other important resources for childrearing such as family planning resources, health care, and mental health or substance abuse treatment. In addition, insufficient income may limit access to safe and stable housing and affordable and nutritious foods, impairing parents abilities to satisfy children's basic needs. Most states include the inability to provide adequate shelter or food in their definitions of child neglect (Child Welfare Information Gateway 2016). Therefore, child protective services may place children in foster care when families lack adequate housing or sufficient food (Fowler et al. 2013; also see: http://www.nccprblog.org/2017/12/two-giant-child-welfare-systems.html). Caregivers who have difficulty paying rent, double up, are evicted, or homelessness in the past 12 months are twice as likely to be investigated by child protective services (Yang 2015).

Insufficient income may also contribute to CAN given the psychological stress it can impose on families. Descriptions of the poor to those who are poor (Edin and Shaefer 2015) and 'near poor' (Newman and Chen 2007) show how parents struggle to balance work and family, experience long commutes, and end up with little time to positively interact with and monitor their children, both of which increased the risk for neglect and sexual abuse (Edin and Shaefer 2015; Newman and Chen 2007). Insufficient income may also lead to high cognitive load (Mullainathan and Shafir 2013). High cognitive load (i.e., the mental load imposed on an individual by a task such as figuring out how to pay the rent) drains mental resources from other tasks (Mani et al. 2013), such as the processing of information and cognitions related to social stimuli. As a result, high cognitive load can change how we perceive and react to stimuli, such as infant crying or non-compliance, which are common antecedents for physical abuse (Barr 2012; Klevens et al. 2000). High cognitive load interferes with inhibitory cues (e.g., empathy or foreseeing negative consequences) that could help people refrain from abusive behavior (Vasquez and Howard-Field 2016). High cognitive load also impedes impulse control (Hinson et al. 2003) and increases the likelihood of aggressing an innocent person (e.g., the child) as a result of being provoked in another setting (e.g., by an intimate partner or employer) and not being able or willing to respond to this provocation directly (Vasquez 2009). Inadequate financial resources may generate stress for additional reasons, including a mismatch between aspirations and opportunities, as a contributor to perceptions of being looked down on or devalued (Marmot 2004), or because of decreased control over life and work. Rising inequality may lead to longer working hours and increased debt because of status competition (the pressure to 'keep up with the Joneses') (Frank 2007). Families living in poverty or with low incomes also have fewer assets to serve as buffers during periods of unexpected financial hardship.

Access to a stable and predictable jobs that pay a living wage and allows workers some degree of control can be important for securing family income, reducing stress, and providing adults the opportunity to serve important societal roles. Unstable work schedules increases children's externalizing behaviors, making it more difficult to care for them (Evans and Wachs 2010). There is evidence that increased wages (Raissian and Bullinger 2017) and family-friendly work can prevent CAN (Klevens et al. 2016).

Unemployment is also a risk factor for child neglect (Connell-Carrick 2003), parental physical aggression towards a child (Black 2001), and physical abuse (Stith et al. 2009). Unemployment may contribute to CAN in many of the same ways as low income does (e.g., increased stress, greater material hardship).

In addition to family income level, one of the most consistent contextual factors associated with CAN is living in neighborhoods of concentrated disadvantage (Coulton et al. 2007; Freisthler et al. 2006). These include neighborhoods characterized by high poverty rates and high unemployment rates. Neighborhoods of concentrated disadvantage have fewer resources and services, leading to more stressors and less support for parents, both of which are risk factors for CAN (Stith et al. 2009). Residential instability is higher in neighborhoods of concentrated disadvantage and is consistently associated with CAN (Coulton et al. 1995; Deccio et al. 1994; Ernst 2001). Whether a direct result of low income or its correlate, residential instability makes it difficult for families to develop and maintain a local support network. Weak or lack of social support is a consistent risk factor for CAN (Stith et al. 2009).

In sum, multiple living and working conditions contribute to increased risk for CAN. Having established the connection between these conditions (or intermediary determinants) and increased risk for CAN, we turn to the question, "Which groups are more likely to experience poor living and working conditions?" Here, the CSDH framework points to the patterning of social hierarchies that effectively determine which groups have less, or more, access to conditions needed for health and safety. Examining these hierarchies can contribute to understanding that universal approaches alone may not be adequate to assuring all families have access to the conditions needed for health. Intervening with groups experiencing inequities may also be needed.

13.3.2 Structural Determinants and Socioeconomic Position

To understand how some families may have less access to opportunities for healthy living and working conditions, it is important to explore *how socioeconomic position is determined* in the United States. This includes understanding the underlying distribution of education that leads to occupational opportunities that determine income and effectively determines where groups land on social hierarchies that strongly correlate with race/ethnicity, class, gender, and other social characteristics. These social hierarchies are also systematically associated with multiple health inequities, including CAN. The CSDH framework examines how structural policies and processes interact to create these hierarchies.

A full exploration of all potential contributors to the distributions of socioeconomic status is beyond the scope of this chapter. But, even a brief look at a few policies related to education, employment, and income provides important insight into systemic and interacting policies and processes that may explain why some children and their families are less likely to have the conditions and resources needed for health, and how this may create differential risk for CAN. We provide a brief description of these policies and their effects below.

13.3.3 Policies Leading to Differential Access to Education

In the United States, all children are guaranteed the right to an education from kindergarten through high school. However, the research suggests the quality of this education is not an equal opportunity experience. Black and Latino students are more likely to attend racially segregated, high poverty schools (Orfield and Lee 2005). Nationally, the highest poverty school districts receive about 10 percent less per student (about $1200/student) in state and local funding than the lowest poverty districts; school districts serving the most students of color nationwide receive roughly 15 percent less per student (about $2000/student) in state and local funding than those serving the fewest (Ushomirsky and Williams 2015). Lower per-student spending is linked to lower achievement through exposure to poorer physical conditions, less qualified teachers, larger classroom sizes, and less consistency and order in school learning environments (Condron and Roscigno 2003).

For students who do complete high school and seek post-secondary education, the rising cost of college makes this aspiration costly: from 1987 to 2017, in-state college tuition at 4-year public schools increased 116 percent (College Board 2017) while median household incomes only increased 22 percent (Census Bureau 2017). Student borrowing has increased by more than 150 percent in the past decade (Experian 2017), making college a major cause of debt for low- and middle-income families with the situation likely to get worse as states cut funding for public colleges and universities and/or substantially increased college tuitions to balance their budgets (Mitchell et al. 2016).

In sum, children of color, and those who are poor, have fewer and lower quality educational opportunities. As a result, people who live below the poverty line are twice as likely to not complete high school as are those who live above the poverty line; Black non-Latino, American Indian/Alaska Native, and Latino students are at much greater risk of non-completion than are White, non-Latino and Asian/Pacific Islander students (Centers for Disease Control and Prevention 2011). Adults with just a high school diploma are half as likely to be employed as college graduates (Bureau of Labor Statistics 2017d); Latinos and Blacks are nearly twice as likely to be unemployed as are Whites (Bureau of Labor Statistics 2017e).

Furthermore, although education level can improve employment opportunities, it is not equally protective. At all levels of educational attainment, Black and Latinos earn less than Whites; Black and Latinos with Master's degrees have lifetime earnings lower than Whites with Bachelor's degrees (Carnevale et al. 2014). Level of parent or caregiver education may contribute to CAN through reduced income (mechanisms described in previous section) or because of less access to information that would enhance parental practices that contribute to optimal child development.

13.3.4 Policies and Practices Leading to Differential Access to Employment

While the cost of living rises every year, wages have stagnated for many. If the purchasing power of the minimum wage were equal to its peak in 1968, it would be $11.48, not $7.25 as it is today (Bureau of Labor Statistics 2017c). Far from the perception that minimum wage employees are teenagers, 94% are over 20 and 80% are over 25 years of age (Bureau of Labor Statistics 2017b). Low wages push many working families into poverty, with Blacks and Latinos twice as likely to be among the working poor, as compared to Whites (Bureau of Labor Statistics 2017a). This may be attributable, in part, to discriminatory hiring practices. Not much has changed over the past 25 years when the first rigorous field studies showed Whites applying for jobs received significantly more callbacks than Blacks, after controlling for potential confounders (Quillian et al. 2017). Even an advanced degree is not protective against employment-related discrimination. In an in-depth analysis of grant data from the US National Institutes of Health (NIH), Black Ph.D. scientists were less likely to receive NIH funding for a research idea than were White scientists from similar institutions with the same research records (Ginther et al. 2011). Discriminatory hiring practices may contribute to lower family income through reduced ability to secure employment. Both low income and unemployment are associated with increased risk for CAN.

13.3.5 Policies and Practices Leading to Differential Income

In addition to differential employment opportunities, other financial resources and opportunities affect household income. For example, access to banking services at a federally insured institution provides people with the opportunity to conduct basic financial transactions, save for emergencies and long-term security needs, and to access credit on affordable terms. However, many people in low-to-moderate income households do not have access to mainstream financial products such as bank accounts and low-cost loans, reducing opportunities to build credit histories and achieve financial security such as building wealth or investing in assets. In 2015, the Federal Deposit Insurance Corporation (2017) found that 27 percent of US households are currently unbanked (no one in household currently had a checking or savings account) or under-banked (those that have had a checking or savings account but also rely on alternative financial services); low-income and minority households were disproportionately represented in the findings. Most of these households used alternative financial services instead, including pawnshops, payday loans, and rent-to-own agreements. These services are not cheap—for example, a payday loan of $325 with a term of 2 weeks and an average interest rate of 16% costs the typical customer $52, translating to an Annual Percentage Rate of 400% (Parrish and King 2009). But these services are more geographically accessible in predominantly low income and minority neighborhoods, while traditional banks are more accessible in predominantly White neighborhoods (Cover et al. 2011).

The housing market also affects household income and wealth differentially. Home ownership is a key strategy for building wealth in the US. The 2007 subprime mortgage and foreclosure crisis affected people in the US (and elsewhere) across the socioeconomic spectrum, but those at the lower ends of social hierarchies experienced the greatest impacts. It is now well-documented that sub-prime mortgages were disproportionately marketed in communities of color; Blacks and Latinos were nearly twice as likely to have lost their homes to foreclosures compared to Whites (Gruenstein et al. 2010). An analysis of 2006 Home Mortgage Disclosure Act (HMDA) data for 100 metropolitan areas across the country documented striking racial disparities: in more than 70 percent of the communities, Black and Latino consumers were more likely to receive high risk, high cost loans than were White consumers *within their same income groups*. Similar patterns were observed between Latinos and Whites in 40 percent of the communities (National Community Reinvestment Coalition 2008). A companion study of 2007 HMDA data revealed similar mortgage lending inequities by gender, race, and class: in 84 percent of metropolitan areas examined, middle- to upper-income Black women were at least twice as likely to receive high-cost loans than were their White female counterparts. Latina women were at least twice as likely to receive high-cost loans as White females in nearly 62 percent of metro areas (National Council of Negro Women 2009).

High-cost loans translate into reduced buying power, making home ownership in neighborhoods of concentrated disadvantage the only option for many families. Given the magnitude of wealth lost due to mortgage lending disparities and increased rates of foreclosure, entire communities where families of color live and raise their children experience reductions in income and wealth.

Housing insecurity is not limited to those with mortgages. The US Department of Housing and Urban Development has established a 30 percent of net monthly income standard for housing affordability (Schwartz and Wilson 2006). Yet, low income families who rent often pay more than this. More than 5.6 million of the nation's lowest-income households pay more than 50 percent of their income in rent (Children's Health Watch 2011). As mentioned previously, caregivers who have difficulty paying rent or are evicted in the past 12 months are twice as likely to be investigated by child protective services (Yang 2015). Housing insecurity is directly associated with the risk for child neglect and increases risk for CAN directly and indirectly through maternal stress (Warren and Font 2015). Families who are behind on rent or mortgage must make trade-offs among household expenses, including whether to pay rent instead of paying for utilities, food, medical care or other life necessities. In some housing assistance programs, having utilities shut off is automatic grounds for eviction (Children's Health Watch 2011), leading to of the possibility of parents being charged with neglect for not meeting children's basic needs.

Another factor that adversely affects household income in communities of color is incarceration. Incarceration rates in the United States increased greatly over the past three decades in communities of color. Although Blacks and Whites have comparable rates of illicit drug use (Substance Abuse and Mental Health Services Administration 2014), the imprisonment rate of Blacks for drug charges is five times that of Whites (NAACP 2017). Time served in federal prison for drug offenses committed by Blacks is almost as long (58.7 months) as time served for violent offenses committed by Whites (61.7 months) (King and Mauer 2016), If current trends continue, 1 of every 3 Black males and 1 of every 6 Latino males born today can expect to go to prison in his lifetime, compared to 1 in 17 White males; the overall figures for women are lower, but the patterns are similar (Mauer and King 2007). Parental incarceration reduces parents' ability to provide economic support while incarcerated and reduces their ability to find employment when released undermining families' economic well-being (Travis et al. 2014). Male incarceration affects maternal mental health, also increasing the risk for CAN (Turney 2014).

In sum, expensive alternative financial services in communities of color, discriminatory mortgage lending practices, and differential incarceration rates affect household income. In addition, disproportionate housing costs can lead to housing insecurity. As noted in the section on living conditions, housing insecurity is independently associated with out-of-home placement of children and may lead to increased risk of child neglect directly and abuse and neglect through increased psychological stress on families.

13.3.5.1 Complex, Interacting Obstacles: Beyond the Ability of Families to Solve on Their Own

As previously explained, the literature shows associations between the intermediary determinants (living and working conditions) and increased risk for CAN. The CSDH framework is useful for exploring how the structural determinants may increase risk for CAN through their effect on the intermediary determinants. Using the framework, some paths to increased risk for abuse and neglect, such as low family income, are more readily apparent and clear-cut. Other paths can be explored from a theoretical perspective. For example, the relationship between differential incarceration rates and CAN might be mediated by lower household income. Complex, interacting policies and processes systematically and repeatedly create barriers for some groups over others in the ability to access life opportunities and essential resources needed for health. Understanding how these policies and processes effectively determine socioeconomic position and how they cluster based on, for example, race/ethnicity, is of critical importance in the quest to reduce the inequitable burden of CAN.

The excessive stress experienced by families and communities dealing with several or all of these compounding obstacles undoubtedly places children at greater risk for childhood adversity. However, families on their own cannot solve these societal obstacles. Addressing these structural determinants may seem to be beyond the scope of public health. However, assuring the conditions in which all people can be healthy and thrive is the mission and role of public health. As such, addressing the societal and sociopolitical factors that inhibit opportunities for health and wellness is critically important and inherent in the mission of public health research and practice.

13.4 A Public Health Approach to Addressing Inequities in Risk for Child Abuse and Neglect

Focusing on the conditions and contexts within which children are living, growing, playing, and learning is important in advancing public health's work to prevent childhood adversity. The Centers for Disease Control and Prevention (CDC) highlights societal-level factors that can lead to better health and wellbeing in their *Essentials for Childhood* vision, framework, and funding initiative (CDC 2014) for preventing CAN and other early adversities in our communities. While the CAN field has traditionally focused on reducing risk factors, the *Essentials for Childhood* vision focuses on what we want to promote: safe, stable, nurturing relationships and environments. Relationships are not limited to children and their parents, but also include children and other adults in their communities like teachers and mentors, and between parents and other adults in their communities. In fact, safe, stable, nurturing relationships among parents and other adults can break the intergenerational transmission of child maltreatment (Jaffee et al. 2013, 2014; Schofield et al. 2013). Safe, stable, nurturing environments at home, in child care, schools, and neighborhoods are also important factors in assuring children's health and wellbeing while the sociopolitical environment plays a role in creating the context within which children and families are able to achieve success and how easily they are able to do so.

13.4.1 Implementing Essentials for Childhood

The CDC Essentials for Childhood Framework suggests communities seeking to prevent CAN should: 1) raise awareness and commitment; 2) use data to inform actions; 3) create the context for healthy children and families through norms change and programs; and 4) create the context for healthy children and families through policies (CDC 2014). In 2013, five state public health departments (California, Colorado, Massachusetts, North Carolina, and Washington) received CDC funding to implement Essentials for Childhood (known as the Essentials Initiative) using a collective impact approach (Kania and Kramer 2011). CDC chose the collective impact approach because assuring safe, stable, nurturing relationships and environments for all children cannot be achieved by one agency or sector alone. Public health departments acted as the backbone agency along with a partner agency acting as a co-backbone (e.g., Children's Trust Fund, Prevent Child Abuse state chapter, Department of Human Services). Together, they identified and convened key stakeholders from both the public (e.g., early care and learning, education, justice) and private sectors (e.g., business, academia, philanthropy) and facilitated their reaching consensus around a common agenda (i.e., shared vision, goals, and strategies) to create safe, stable, nurturing relationships and environments for all children.

For the most part, the five states' common agendas converged on the four goals of Essentials for Childhood (numerated above). Workgroups were then created to implement the strategies chosen by the group of stakeholders which often led to reaching out to new stakeholders (e.g., community voices). The Workgroups identified what efforts needed to be aligned and coordinated so that they were mutually reinforcing; what efforts should be stopped; and what efforts needed to be developed or enhanced to fill gaps. Throughout this process, the backbones have facilitated progress and coordination through continuous communication (e.g., periodic meetings, newsletters, and websites).

To raise awareness and commitment (goal 1), CDC encouraged states to use *The Raising of America: Early Childhood and the Future of Our Nation,* a five-part documentary produced by California Newsreel (http:/www.newsreel.org). In conducting formative research for this documentary, the producers found that the dominant narrative around child development was individualistic—mostly a "blame the parents" frame if children were not faring well. However, as the research described previously shows, the producers realized that even the best intentioned parents may be handicapped by economic uncertainty; crowded, noisy and poor quality housing; food insecurity; segregation; unsafe neighborhoods, and lack of health care, child care and paid parental and sick leave. In order to help change the dominant "blame the parent" narrative, the documentary series reframes the conversation about early childhood health and development in America by tapping into the shared value of the nations' future prosperity. The documentary explains the importance of investing in early childhood to prevent adverse childhood experiences and suggests some policies that might protect children from adversity such as paid family leave to care for a newborn and high quality childcare and early education.

Use of this documentary was not limited to the five funded states. More than 730,000 people have screened *and* discussed one or more episodes of *The Raising of America* in structured settings since the series' 2015 release and its broadcast on public television (Saville et al. 2017). More than 3,200 organizations convened events in all 50 states as part of this public engagement initiative.

CDC's efforts to change the narrative precede the *Raising of America's* efforts. Since 2007, CDC has talked about 'safe, stable, nurturing relationships and environments' as its strategic direction instead of "prevent child abuse and neglect" to avoid triggering the 'blame the parent' frame. More recently, CDC and partners are learning how to talk about assuring stable and nurturing environments in ways that avoid triggering the 'blame the parent' frame or blame the child. CDC has shared messages with the states and states have developed message banks to share amongst their partners to consistently frame the problem of CAN and other adverse childhood experiences such as witnessing partner violence as a collective problem with shared responsibility for collective solutions. However, research is needed to establish the effectiveness of these frames and messages on changing the narrative and social norms around collective responsibility for children.

Changing the narrative around the problem of CAN may be key to building public commitment to strategies that are supportive of children and families and have been shown, through research, to prevent child maltreatment. CDC has compiled and disseminated the evidence around select policies that create safe, stable, and nurturing environments for families and children such as those that strengthen household economics, family-friendly work, and access to high quality childcare and early education (Fortson et al. 2016). States have used shared messaging and CDC's compiled evidence to educate their partners and decision-makers on policies and programs that can prevent CAN or lessen the harm for those children exposed. Data show that as awareness around the societal factors that lead to negative child outcomes increases, the public's commitment towards policies that support parents and children increases (Klevens et al. under review).

In order to evaluate the Essentials for Childhood framework, CDC is collecting data on state-level changes around high quality child care and early education, strengthening household economics, and family-friendly work. Since 2016, after the launching of *Raising of America*, we have observed one state passing one of the most equitable paid family leave policies in the nation (SB 5975); another state making their existing family leave policy more equitable (SB 63), and a third state working toward increasing awareness and commitment for paid family leave (https://ballotpedia.org/Massachusetts_Paid:Family_and_Medical_Leave_Initiative_(2018). Three states have also raised their minimum wage. As policies change and create a context supportive of families, we expect to see less children exposed to poverty, homelessness, and food insecurity (intermediary determinants). With improvements in the conditions in which children grow along with an increased reach of evidence-based programs, we can expect reductions in child maltreatment and other adverse childhood experiences to follow, and especially its inequitable burden for children living in low-income households.

13.4.2 Challenges to Implementing Essentials for Childhood

Despite their achievements, the CDC-funded states have encountered several challenges during the first 4 years of this initiative. The greatest challenge has been the complexity of this effort. The US is an individualistic culture (Oyserman et al. 2002). This can lead to solutions that address individual behaviors like programs that treat the symptoms of the problem only at the most proximate level (i.e., training individuals). In addition, individualistic narratives (e.g., 'pick yourself up by the bootstraps') are deeply ingrained in the American psyche (e.g., Bostrom 2004; Hunt 2007; Kluegel 1990; Tuch and Hughes 2011) and it will take many years of consistent and coordinated efforts to educate the public that a collective approach to supporting child development is also an effective approach.

Another challenge that the CDC-funded states have encountered has been maintaining the focus on primary prevention. As people learn more and more about adverse childhood experiences (ACEs), the reaction has been towards trauma-informed or trauma-responsive approaches for those who have already experienced CAN. While this is encouraging and benefits children (e.g., by banning suspensions and expulsions from school, keeping children in the juvenile justice system instead of treating them as adults), it is public health's role to prevent childhood adversity from occurring in the first place.

A key concern in this effort has been ensuring that efforts do not increase inequities. For example, family-friendly work policies like paid parental leave may be available only to employees of large companies (leaving out those self-employed like domestic workers or taxi drivers, for example) or cover a limited amount of employees' salary making those with lower incomes unable to take advantage of the benefit. Continuously including an equity lens in policy analysis and evaluation can help to make sure all benefit equitably. In addition to evaluating policies' impacts on child maltreatment, it is also important for researchers to examine the differential impact of policies among less advantaged groups compared to more advantaged groups.

Much more research is needed to inform what leads to norms and narrative change around supporting child development and preventing CAN. Although some formative research has increased our understanding of the kinds of messages that resonate with different audiences, more research is needed to test the effectiveness of messages to change the narrative and social norms related to CAN. Researchers might partner with community organizers to document the factors that differentiate successful efforts from unsuccessful ones.

13.4.3 Moving Forward

The Essentials for Childhood Framework and initiative is a work in progress with no evidence yet of its impact. Short- and long-term evaluation efforts are underway to determine if awareness and commitment increases (i.e., whether the narrative changes); whether increased awareness and commitment lead to adoption of programs and policies that research has shown prevent maltreatment; whether these changes lead to population-level improvements in children's living conditions; and whether improved living conditions lead to reductions in the inequitable burden of child maltreatment.

Although champions of child and family well-being have been involved in the Essentials Initiative, more might be accomplished by forging relationships with other community partners. For example, in 2011, Kansas City, Missouri Health Department (not a participant in the Essentials Initiative) partnered with Communities Creating Opportunity (CCO), a faith-based organization in the People Improving Communities through Organizing network (https://healthequityguide.org/case-studies/kansas-city-develops-mou-and-shares-space-with-community-organizers/).[1] Over the years, about one third of the Health Department staff had training in the classic community organizing technique of 'one-on-ones'. Since 2012, CCO offices are located inside the Kansas City Health Department. They participate in cross training of staff to build relationships and understanding between the fields of public health and community organizing. A community organizer is on the Health Department's Board and the Health Director is a member of CCO. Over several years, they developed a shared vision and a goal to promote family-friendly strategies in Kansas City. In 2016, CCO mobilized hundreds of people, including Kansas City's mayor, school superintendent and director of public health, to see a screening of the signature hour of *The Raising of America*. Following the screening, every viewer received a pledge card with suggested actions viewers could take. The bottom of the card listed dates of follow-up trainings. Nearly 18 months later city employees were granted 6 weeks of paid parental leave (Saville et al. 2017). This case study suggests that public health in partnership with community organizations can disseminate a compelling narrative that can lead to policy change, as long as their funding allows them to engage in such work (i.e., non-Federal sources). As one of the community organizers said, "The point of the story is not that we showed the film. …it was a moment in time that contributed to a much larger scope of work." (see https://youtu.be/zdEtAvlITRU).

The Essentials for Childhood Framework could extend its focus to other childhood adversity to take advantage of the growing movement around adverse childhood experiences (e.g., http://www.acesconnection.com/), which have been associated with more than 40 health outcomes as well as reduced access to life opportunities (Metzler et al., 2017). In addition to the 10 adverse childhood experiences examined in the original ACE study (Felitti et al. 1998), several researchers and practitioners have expanded childhood adversity to include poverty (e.g., https://developingchild.harvard.edu/), community violence, and peer victimization and rejection (Finkelhor et al. 2013). More research is needed to evaluate the effectiveness of safe, stable, nurturing environments achieved through policy change. For example, what interventions are most effective in improving housing stability and do they reduce child maltreatment and other adverse childhood experiences? We know mixed income and de-segregated neighborhoods improve children's school performance (Schwartz 2010) and educational attainment (Johnson 2011) but do they also reduce children's exposure to adversity? While we have some evidence on the effects of paid family leave (Klevens et al. 2016) and the Earned Income Tax Credit (Klevens et al. 2017), it is limited to abusive head trauma. Do these policies reduce other forms of CAN?

A key limitation to conducting policy research is the lack of sensitive uniform definitions of child maltreatment that do not change over time. CDC has proposed uniform definitions for child maltreatment which have been helpful to the field because they conceptually clarify what is meant by "child abuse and neglect" (Leeb et al. 2008). However, the specified International Classification of Diseases (ICD) codes proposed to identify cases of injuries and deaths miss too many cases of child maltreatment (Hooft et al. 2015; Raghavan et al. 2015), especially cases of neglect

[1] No federal funds were used for this effort.

(Klevens and Leeb 2010; Schnitzer et al. 2008). In addition, ICD codes were changed in 2015 (Centers for Medicaid and Medicare Services 2014). Reports to child protective services that are substantiated also miss too many cases (Theodore et al. 2005). Using rates of all children reported to Child Protective Services might be a better measure (Hussey et al. 2005; Kohl et al. 2009) but their reliability over time may be dependent on trust in the government, media coverage of high profile cases, the proportion of the population that comes into contact with mandated reporters, the number of calls that are abandoned (e.g., because of wait times) or deflected (e.g., because call volume is too heavy or staff is insufficient to take report); or racial or socioeconomic biases of mandated reporters. While the National Survey of Children's Health plans to collect information on adverse childhood experiences yearly, these exclude child maltreatment (https://mchb.hrsa.gov/data/national-surveys). For policy evaluation, a surveillance system based on self-reported perpetration of specific behaviors that qualify as child abuse or neglect such as those asked on the National Survey of Children's Exposure to Violence (Finkelhor et al. 2015) that would generate state-level estimates on a periodic basis might be the best data source. Self-reported perpetration of CAN identifies 16 times the number of maltreated children cases compared to substantiated cases and almost four times the number of cases reported to child protective services (Finkelhor et al. 2015; US Department of Health & Human Services 2016).

More research is needed around developing and testing interventions that increase safe, stable, nurturing environments at the community level and whether they achieve population-level reductions in CAN. A recent review of the evidence found just five interventions; three evaluated their effects on CAN using either a single group pre-post design, a pre-post design with non-randomly assigned control groups or a multiple time series post-test only with non-randomly assigned control groups with two showing positive effects (Van Dijken et al. 2016). One promising strategy that might help improve families' living conditions and reduce parental stress is removing barriers to needed economic supports. This includes automatically enrolling families into all programs for which they are eligible ("one stop shops"; Dorn 2008). Although an intervention like this showed positive improvements in parenting behaviors (Huston et al. 2003), the approach still needs to be evaluated for its impact on CAN.

13.5 Conclusions

Child abuse and neglect prevention requires a multi-level approach that includes strategies that move beyond programs focused on improving individual parenting behaviors. A public health approach with a health equity lens might encourage a multi-level approach by changing norms in ways that lead to community- and policy-level changes that improve the conditions in which parents are trying to raise their children. Essentials for Childhood is one example of such an effort. Short- and long-term evaluation will determine whether it is successful.

References

Barr, R. G. (2012). Preventing abusive head trauma resulting from a failure of normal interaction between infants and their caregivers. *Proceedings of the National Academy of Science, 109*(Suppl 2), 17294–17301.

Birn, A. E. (2009). Making it politic(al): Closing the gap in a generation: health equity through action on the social determinants of health. *Social Medicine, 4*(3), 166–182.

Black, D. A., Heyman, R. E., & Smith-Slep, A. M. (2001). Risk factors for child physical abuse. *Aggression and Violent Behavior, 6*, 121–188.

Bostrom, M. (2004). *Together for success*. Retrieved from http://www.topospartnership.com/wp-content/uploads/2013/03/TogetherforSuccess.pdf

Braveman, P. (2014). What are health disparities and health equity? We need to be clear. *Public Health Reports, 129*(2), 5–8.

Brown, J., Cohen, P., Johnson, J. G., & Salzinger, S. (1998). A longitudinal analysis of risk factors for child maltreatment: Findings of a 17-year prospective study of officially recorded and self-reported child abuse and neglect. *Child Abuse & Neglect, 22*(11), 1065–1078.

Bureau of Labor Statistics. (2017a). *A profile of the working poor, 2015*. Retrieved from https://www.bls.gov/opub/reports/working-poor/2015/home.htm

Bureau of Labor Statistics. (2017b). *Characteristics of minimum wage workers, 2016*. Retrieved from https://www.bls.gov/opub/reports/minimum-wage/2016/home.htm

Bureau of Labor Statistics. (2017c). *Consumer price index inflation calculator*. Retrieved from https://www.bls.gov/data/inflation_calculator.htm

Bureau of Labor Statistics. (2017d). *Unemployment rate 2.5 percent for college grads, 7.7 percent for high school dropouts, January 2017*. Retrieved from https://www.bls.gov/opub/ted/2017/unemployment-rate-2-point-5-percent-for-college-grads-7-point-7-percent-for-high-school-dropouts-january-2017.htm

Bureau of Labor Statistics. (2017e). *Unemployment rate and employment-population ratio vary by race and ethnicity*. Retrieved from https://www.bls.gov/opub/ted/2017/unemployment-rate-and-employment-population-ratio-vary-by-race-and-ethnicity.htm

Carnevale, A. P., Rose, S. J., & Cheah, B. (2014). *The college payoff: Education, occupations, lifetime earnings*. The Georgetown University Center on Education and the Workforce Web site. Retrieved from https://cew-7632.kxcdn.com/wp-content/uploads/2014/11/collegepayoff-complete.pdf

Census Bureau. (2017). *Income and poverty in the United States, Table A-2: Selected measures of household income dispersion 1967–2016*. Retrieved from https://www.census.gov/library/publications/2017/demo/p60-259.html

Centers for Disease Control and Prevention. (2011). CDC health disparities and inequalities report—United States, 2011. *Morbidity and Mortality Weekly Report, 60*(Suppl 1), 1–116. Retrieved from https://www.cdc.gov/mmwr/pdf/other/su6001.pdf.

Centers for Disease Control and Prevention, National Center for Injury Prevention and Control, Division of Violence Prevention. (2014). *Essentials for childhood framework: Steps to create safe, stable, nurturing relationships and environments for all children*. Retrieved from http://www.cdc.gov/violenceprevention/childmaltreatment/essentials.html

Centers for Medicaid and Medicare Services. (2014). *The ICD10 transition: An introduction*. Retrieved from https://www.cms.gov/Medicare/Coding/ICD10/Downloads/ICD10Introduction20140819.pdf

Child Welfare Information Gateway. (2016). *Definitions of child abuse and neglect*. Washington, DC: US Department of Health and Human Services, Children's Bureau.

Children's Health Watch. (2011). *Behind closed doors: The hidden health impacts of being behind on rent*. January, 2011. Available at https://childrenshealthwatch.org/behind-closed-doors-the-hidden-health-impact-of-being-behindon-Rent/.

College Board. (2017). *Annual survey of colleges*. Retrieved from https://trends.collegeboard.org/college-pricing/figures-tables/average-rates-growth-published-charges-decade

Condron, D. J., & Roscigno, V. J. (2003). Disparities within: Unequal spending and achievement in an urban school district. *Sociology of Education, 76*(1), 18–36.

Connell-Carrick, K. (2003). A critical review of the empirical literature identifying correlates of child neglect. *Child and Adolescent Social Work Journal, 20*, 389–425.

Coulton, C., Korbin, J. E., Su, M., & Chow, J. (1995). Community level factors and child maltreatment rates. *Child Development, 66*, 1262–1276.

Coulton, C. J., Crampton, D. S., Irwin, M., Spilsbury, J. C., & Korbin, J. E. (2007). How neighborhoods influence child maltreatment: A review of the literature and alternative pathways. *Child Abuse & Neglect, 31*(11–12), 1117–1142.

Cover, J., Fuhrman Spring, A., & Garshick Kleit, R. (2011). Minorities on the margins?: The spatial organization of fringe services. *Journal of Urban Affairs, 33*(3), 317–344.

Dahlberg, L. L., & Krug, E. G. (2002). Violence-a global public health problem. In E. Krug, L. L. Dahlberg, J. A. Mercy, A. B. Zwi, & R. Lozano (Eds.), *World report on violence and health* (pp. 1–56). Geneva: World Health Organization.

Deccio, G., Horner, W. C., & Wilson, D. (1994). High risk neighborhoods and high risk families: Replication research related to the human ecology of child maltreatment. *Journal of Social Service Research, 18*, 123–137.

Doidge, J. C., Higgins, D. J., Delfabbro, P., Edwards, B., Vassallo, S., Toumbourou, J. W., & Segal, L. (2017). Economic determinants of child maltreatment in an Australian population-based birth cohort. *Children and Youth Services Review, 72*, 14–25.

Dorn, S. (2008). How policy makers could use automation to help families and children. In *Big Ideas for children: Investing in our Nation's future*. Washington, DC: First Focus. Retrieved from https://firstfocus.org/wp-content/uploads/2014/06/Big-Ideas-2008.pdf.

Edin, K. J., & Shaefer, L. (2015). *$2.00 a day: Living on almost nothing in America*. New York: Houghton Mifflin Harcourt.

Ernst, J. S. (2001). Community level factors and child maltreatment in a suburban county. *Social Work Research, 25*, 133–142.

Evans, G. W., & Wachs, T. D. (Eds.). (2010). *Chaos and its influence on children's development*. Washington, DC: American Psychological Association.

Experian. (2017). *The state of student loan debt in 2017*. Retrieved from https://www.experian.com/innovation/thought-leadership/state-of-student-lending-in-2017.jsp

Federal Deposit Insurance Corporation. (2017). *2015 FDIC national survey of unbanked and underbanked households*. Retrieved from https://www.fdic.gov/householdsurvey/

Felitti, V. J., Anda, R. F., Nordenberg, D., Williamson, D. F., Spitz, A. F., Edwards, V., Koss, M. P., et al. (1998). Relationship of childhood abuse and household dysfunction to many of the leading causes of death in adults: The Adverse Childhood Experiences (ACE) Study. *American Journal of Preventive Medicine, 14*, 245–258.

Finkelhor, D., Shattuck, A., Turner, H., & Hamby, S. (2013). Improving the adverse childhood experiences study scale. *JAMA Pediatrics, 167*(1), 70–75.

Finkelhor, D., Turner, H. A., Shattuck, A., & Hamby, S. L. (2015). Prevalence of childhood exposure to violence, crime, and abuse: Results from the national survey of children's exposure to violence. *JAMA Pediatrics, 169*(8), 746–754.

Fortson, B. L., Klevens, J., Merrick, M. T., Gilbert, L. K., & Alexander, S. P. (2016). *Preventing child abuse and neglect: A technical package for policy, norm, and programmatic activities*. Atlanta, GA: National Center for Injury Prevention and Control, Centers for Disease Control and Prevention. https://www.cdc.gov/violenceprevention/pdf/CAN-Prevention-Technical-Package.pdf.

Fowler, P. J., Henry, D. B., Schoeny, M., Landsverk, J., Chavira, D., & Taylor, J. J. (2013). Inadequate housing among families under investigation for child abuse and neglect: Prevalence from a national probability sample. *American Journal of Community Psychology, 52*, 106–114.

Frank, R. (2007). *Falling behind: How rising inequality harms the middle class*. Berkeley: California University Press.

Freisthler, B., Merritt, D. H., & La Scala, E. A. (2006). Understanding the ecology of child maltreatment: A review of the literature and directions for future research. *Child Maltreatment, 11*, 263–280.
Ginther, D. K., Schaffer, W. T., Schnell, J., Masimore, B., Liu, F., Haak, L. L., et al. (2011). Race, ethnicity, and NIH research awards. *Science, 333*(6045), 1015–1019.
Gruenstein B. D., Li, W., & Ernst, K. S. (2010). *Foreclosures by race and ethnicity: the demographics of a crisis*. Retrieved from http://www.responsiblelending.org/mortgage-lending/research-analysis/foreclosures-by-race-and-ethnicity.pdf
Hinson, J. M., Jameson, T. L., & Whitney, P. (2003). Impulsive decision-making and working memory. *Journal of Experimental Psychology. Learning, Memory, and Cognition, 29*(2), 298–306.
Hooft, A. M., Asnes, A. G., Livingston, N., Deutsch, S., Cahill, L., Wood, J. N., et al. (2015). The accuracy of ICD Codes: Identifying physical abuse in 4 children's hospitals. *Academic Pediatrics, 15*, 444–450.
Hunt, M. O. (2007). African American, Hispanic, and White beliefs about black/white inequality, 1977–2004. *American Sociological Review, 72*, 390–415.
Hussey, J. M., Marshall, J. M., English, D. J., Knight, E. D., Lau, A. S., Dubowitz, H., et al. (2005). Defining maltreatment according to substantiation: Distinction without a difference? *Child Abuse & Neglect, 29*, 479–492.
Huston, A. C., Miller, C., Richburg-Hayes, L., Duncan, G. J., Eldred, C. A., Weisner, T. S., et al. (2003). *New Hope for families and children: Five year results of a program to reduce poverty and reform welfare*. New York: MDRC. Retrieved from https://www.mdrc.org/sites/default/files/full_457.pdf.
Jaffee, S. R., Bowes, L., Ouellet-Morin, I., Fisher, H. L., Moffitt, T. E., Merrick, M. T., et al. (2013). Safe, stable, nurturing relationships break the intergenerational cycle of abuse: A prospective nationally representative cohort of children in the United Kingdom. *Journal of Adolescent Health, 53*, S4e–S10e.
Jaffee, S. R., Takezawa, R., & Arsenault, L. (2014). Buffering effects of safe, supportive, and nurturing relationships among women with childhood histories of maltreatment. *Psychological Medicine, 47*(15), 2628–2639.
Johnson, R. C. (2011). *Long-run impacts of school desegregation & school quality on adult attainments*. NBER Working Paper No. 16664. Retrieved from http://www.nber.org/papers/w16664
Kania, J., & Kramer, M. (2011). Collective impact. *Stanford Social Innovation Review, 9*(Winter), 36–41.
Kaplan, G. A., Pamuk, E. R., Lynch, J. W., Cohen, R. D., & Balfour, J. L. (1996). Inequality in income and mortality in the United States: Analysis of mortality and potential pathways. *British Medical Journal, 312*(7037), 999–1003.
King, R. S., & Mauer, M. (2016). *Distorted priorities: Drug offenders in state prisons*. The Sentencing Project Web site. Retrieved from http://www.sentencingproject.org/wp-content/uploads/2016/01/Distorted-Priorities-Drug-Offenders-in-State-Prisons.pdf
Klevens, J., & Leeb, R. (2010). Child maltreatment fatalities in children under five: Findings from the National violent death reporting system. *Child Abuse and Neglect, 34*(4), 262–266.
Klevens, J., Bayon, M. C., & Sierra, M. (2000). Risk factors and context of men who physically abuse children in Bogotá, Colombia. *Child Abuse & Neglect, 24*(3), 323–332.
Klevens, J., Luo, F., Xu, L., Peterson, C., & Latzman, N. (2016). Paid family leave's effect on hospital admissions for pediatric abusive head trauma. *Injury Prevention, 22*, 442–445.
Klevens, J., Schmidt, B., Luo, F., Xu, L., Ports, K. A., & Lee, R. (2017). Earned Income Tax Credit's effect on hospital admissions for pediatric abusive head trauma. *Public Health Reports, 132*(4), 505–511.
Klevens, J., Ports, K., Metzler, M., Merrick, M. T., & Reidy, M. C. (under review). *Public explanations of why children struggle in America and support for family-friendly policies*.

Kluegel, J. R. (1990). Trends in Whites' explanations of the black-white gap in socioeconomic status, 1977–1989. *American Sociological Review, 55*(4), 512–525.
Kohl, P. L., Jonson-Reid, M., & Drake, B. (2009). Time to leave substantiation behind: Findings from a national probability study. *Child Maltreatment, 14*(1), 17–26.
Krieger, N. (2001). Theories for social epidemiology in the 21st century: An eco-social perspective. *International Journal of Epidemiology, 30*(4), 668–677.
Krieger, N. (2008). Ladders, pyramids and champagne: The iconography of health inequities. *Journal of Epidemiology and Community Health, 62*(12), 1098–1104.
Lamela, D., & Figuereido, B, (2015). A cumulative risk model of child physical maltreatment potential: Findings from a community-based study.*Journal of Interpersonal Violence* Published online 20 November 2015. https://doi.org/10.1177/0886260515615142
Leeb, R. T., Paulozzi, L., Melanson, C., Simon, T., & Arias, I. (2008). *Child Maltreatment surveillance: Uniform definitions for public health and recommended data elements*. Atlanta: Centers for Disease Control and Prevention/National Center for Injury Prevention and Control.
Mani, A., Mullainathan, S., Shafir, E., & Zhao, J. (2013). Poverty impedes cognitive function. *Science, 341*(6149), 976–980.
Marmot, M. (2004). *The status syndrome: How social standing affects our health and longevity*. New York: Henry Holt and Company.
Mauer, M., & King, R. S. (2007). *Uneven justice: state rates of incarceration by race and ethnicity*. Retrieved from http://www.sentencingproject.org/wp-content/uploads/2016/01/Uneven-Justice-State-Rates-of-Incarceration-by-Race-and-Ethnicity.pdf
Metzler, M., Merrick, M., Klevens, J., Ford, D., & Ports, K. (2017). Adverse child experiences and life opportunities: Shifting the narrative. Invited paper for special issue on the "Economic Causes and Consequences of Child Maltreatment". *Children and Youth Services Review, 72*, 141–149. https://doi.org/10.1016/j.childyouth.2016.10.021.
Mikton, C., & Butchart, A. (2009). Child maltreatment prevention: A systematic review of reviews. *Bulletin of the World Health Organization, 87*, 353–361.
Mitchell, M., Leachman, M., & Masterson, K. (2016). *Funding down, tuition up: State cuts to higher education threaten quality and affordability at public colleges*. Center on Budget and Policy Priorities. Retrieved from https://www.cbpp.org/research/state-budget-and-tax/funding-down-tuition-up
Mullainathan, S., & Shafir, E. (2013). *Scarcity: The new science of having less and how it defines our lives*. New York: Henry Holt and Co.
NAACP. (2017). *Criminal justice fact sheet*. Retrieved from http://www.naacp.org/criminal-justice-fact-sheet/
National Academy of Sciences. (1988). *The future of public health*. Washington, DC: National Academies Press.
National Community Reinvestment Coalition. (2008). *Income is no shield against racial differences in lending II: A comparison of high-cost lending in America's metropolitan and rural areas*. Housing Preservation Project Web site. Retrieved from http://www.hppinc.org/_uls/resources/Racial_Gap_Report.pdf
National Council of Negro Women. (2009*). Income is no shield, part III: assessing the double burden: Examining racial and gender disparities in mortgage lending*. Retrieved from http://www.ncnw.org/images/double_burden.pdf
Newman, K. S., & Chen, V. T. (2007). *The missing class: Portraits of the near poor in America*. Boston: Beacon Press.
Orfield, G., & Lee, C. (2005). *Why segregation matters: Poverty and educational inequality*. Cambridge, MA: The Civil Rights Project/Harvard University. Retrieved from https://cloudfront.escholarship.org/dist/prd/content/qt4xr8z4wb/qt4xr8z4wb.pdf.
Oyserman, D., Coon, H. M., & Kimmelmeier, M. (2002). Rethinking individualism and collectivism: Evaluation of theoretical assumptions and meta-analyses. *Psychological Bulletin, 128*(1), 3–72.

Parrish, L., & King, U. (2009). *Phantom demand: Short-term due date generates need for repeat payday loans, accounting for 76% of total volume*. Center for Responsible Lending. Retrieved from http://www.responsiblelending.org/payday-lending/research-analysis/phantom-demand-final.pdf

Quillian, L., Pager, D., Hexel, O., & Midbøen, A. H. (2017). Meta-analysis of field experiments shows no change in racial discrimination in hiring over time. *PNAS, 114*(41), 10870–10875.

Raghavan, R., Brown, D. S., Allaire, B. T., Garfield, L. D., Ross, R. E., & Hedeker, D. (2015). Challenges in using medicaid claims to ascertain child maltreatment. *Child Maltreatment, 20*(2), 83–91.

Raissian, K. M., & Bullinger, L. R. (2017). Money matters: Does the minimum wage affect child maltreatment rates? *Children and Youth Services Review, 72*, 60–70.

Saville, A. W., Adelman, L., & Poulain, R. (2017). *The Raising of America evaluation report*. Retrieved from http://www.raisingofamerica.org/take-action/evaluation-report

Schnitzer, P. G., Covington, T. M., Wirtz, S. J., Verhoek-Oftedahl, W., & Palusci, V. J. (2008). Public health surveillance of fatal child maltreatment: Analysis of 3 state programs. *American Journal of Public Health, 98*(2), 296–303.

Schofield, T. J., Lee, R. D., & Merrick, M. T. (2013). Safe, stable, nurturing relationships as a moderator of intergenerational continuity of child maltreatment: A meta-analysis. *Journal of Adolescent Health, 53*, S32–S38.

Schwartz, H. (2010). *Housing policy is school policy: Economically integrated housing improves school success in Montgomery Count, Maryland*. Retrieved from https://www.tcf.org/assets/downloads/tcf-Schwartz.pdf

Schwartz, M., & Wilson, E. (2006). *Who can afford to live in a home? A look at data from the 2006 American Community Survey*. Retrieved from http://www.census.gov/hhes/www/housing/special-topics/files/who-can-afford.pdf

Sedlak, A. J., Mettenburg, J., Basena, M., Petta, I., McPherson, K., Greene, A., et al. (2010). *Fourth National Incidence Study of Child Abuse and Neglect (NIS–4): Report to congress*. Washington, DC: US Department of Health and Human Services/Administration for Children and Families.

Shonkoff, J. P., Boyce, W., & McEwen, B. S. (2009). Neuroscience, molecular biology, and the childhood roots of health disparities: Building a new framework for health promotion and disease prevention. *JAMA, 301*(21), 2252–2259.

Solar, O., & Irwin, A. (2010). *A conceptual framework for action on the social determinants of health*. Social Determinants of Health Discussion. Paper 2 (Policy and Practice). Retrieved from http://apps.who.int/iris/bitstream/10665/44489/1/9789241500852_eng.pdf?ua=1&ua=1

Stith, S. M., Liu, T., Davies, L. C., Boykin, E. L., Alder, M. C., Harris, J. M., et al. (2009). Risk factors in child maltreatment. A meta-analytic review of the literature. *Aggression and Violent Behavior, 14*, 13–29.

Substance Abuse and Mental Health Services Administration. (2014). *Results from the 2013 National Survey on Drug Use and Health: Summary of National Findings*, NSDUH Series H-48, HHS Publication No. (SMA) 14–4863. Rockville, MD: Substance Abuse and Mental Health Services Administration. Retrieved from https://archive.samhsa.gov/data/NSDUH/2013SummNatFindDetTables/NationalFindings/NSDUHresults2013.htm#2.7

Theodore, A., Chang, J. J., Runyan, D. K., Hunter, W. M., Bangdiwala, S. I., & Agans, R. (2005). The epidemiology of the physical and sexual maltreatment of children in the Carolinas. *Pediatrics, 115*, e331–e337.

Travis, J., Western, B., & Redburn, S. (Eds.). (2014). *The growth of incarceration in the United States: Exploring causes and consequences*. Washington, DC: National Academies Press.

Tuch, S. A., & Hughes. (2011). Whites' racial policy attitudes in the twenty-first century: The continuing significance of racial resentment. *Annals of the American Academy of Political and Social Science, 634*, 134–152.

Turney, K. (2014). The consequences of paternal incarceration for maternal neglect and harsh parenting. *Social Forces, 92*(4), 1607–1636.

US Department of Health & Human Services, Administration for Children and Families, Administration on Children, Youth and Families, Children's Bureau. (2016). *Child maltreatment 2014*. Retrieved from http://www.acf.hhs.gov/programs/cb/research-data-technology/statistics-research/child-maltreatment

UNICEF. (2012). *The structural determinants of child well-being*. Florence: Author. Retrieved from https://www.unicef-irc.org/publications/678/.

Ushomirsky, N., & Williams, D. (2015). *Funding gaps 2015: Too many states still spend less on educating students who need the most*. The Education Trust. Retrieved from https://1k9gl1yevnfp2lpq1dhrqe17-wpengine.netdna-ssl.com/wp-content/uploads/2014/09/FundingGaps2015_TheEducationTrust1.pdf

Van Dijken, M. W., Stams, G. J., & de Winter, M. (2016). Can community-based interventions prevent child maltreatment? *Children and Youth Services Review, 61*, 149–158.

Vasquez, E. A. (2009). Cognitive load, trigger salience, and the facilitation of triggered displaced aggression. *European Journal of Social Psychology, 39*(5), 684–693.

Vasquez, E. A., & Howard-Field, J. (2016). Too (mentally) busy to chill: Cognitive load and inhibitory cues interact to moderate triggered displaced aggression. *Aggressive Behavior, 42*(4), 413–414.

Warren, E. J., & Font, S. A. (2015). Housing insecurity, maternal stress, and child maltreatment: An application of the family stress model. *Social Service Review, 89*(1), 9–39.

Wilkinson, R. G., & Pickett, K. E. (2006). Income inequality and population health: A review and explanation of the evidence. *Social Science & Medicine, 62*(7), 1768–1784. https://doi.org/10.1016/j.socscimed.2005.08.036.

World Health Organization, Commission on Social Determinants of Health. (2008). *Closing the gap in a generation: Health equity through action on the social determinants of health*. Retrieved from http://www.who.int/social_determinants/en

World Health Organization, Regional Office for Europe. (2018). *Public health services*. Retrieved from http://www.euro.who.int/en/health-topics/Health-systems/public-health-services

Yang, M. Y. (2015). The effect of material hardship on child protective service involvement. *Child Abuse & Neglect, 41*, 113–125.

Yang, M. Y., & Maguire-Jack, K. (2016). Predictors of basic needs and supervisory neglect: Evidence from the Illinois Families Study. *Children and Youth Services Review, 67*, 20–26.

Chapter 14
Critiques of a Public Health Model in Child Maltreatment

Mel Gray and Leanne Schubert

14.1 Introduction

Child protection systems are oriented toward the management of risk and control and placement of children outside the family. Scott et al. (2016) aptly summarized the current state of the art in child protection thus: Contemporary approaches to child protection are dominated by individualized forensically focused interventions that provide limited scope for more holistic preventative responses to children at risk and the provision of support to struggling families and communities. However, in many jurisdictions, it is frequently shown, often through public inquiries and program reviews, that investigatory and removal approaches are failing in critically important ways, particularly regarding reducing the inequities that underpin neglect and abuse (p. 408). Scott (2006) diagnosed the consequences of the resulting escalation in demand:

> Statutory child protection services have become demoralised, investigation-driven bureaucracies which trawl through large numbers of low income families to identify the small minority of cases which reach the criteria for statutory intervention (p. 9).

Practitioners in the medical field take a very different approach; rather than a violation of children's rights, health practitioners consider child maltreatment a public-health problem given it involves harm to individuals. As Reading et al. (2009) explained: Public-health approaches emphasise monitoring, prevention, cost-effectiveness, and population strategies; protective approaches concentrate on the legal and professional response to cases of maltreatment. Both approaches have

M. Gray (✉) · L. Schubert
School of Humanities and Social Science, University of Newcastle, Callaghan, NSW, Australia
e-mail: mel.gray@newcastle.edu.au; leanne.schubert@newcastle.edu.au

B. Lonne et al. (eds.), *Re-Visioning Public Health Approaches for Protecting Children*, Child Maltreatment 9, https://doi.org/10.1007/978-3-030-05858-6_14

been associated with improvement in outcomes for children, yet maltreatment remains a major global problem (p. 332).

The public health approach has emerged internationally as an alternative to statutory child protection. Many extol its value at a time of increased demand for child protective services in an environment of shrinking resources and quick-fix solutions (Barlow and Calam 2011; Cuccaro-Alamin et al. 2017; Dalziel and Segal 2012; Gelles 2017; Gilbert et al. 2009a, b; Higgins 2015; Moncrieff 2008; Putnam-Hornstein et al. 2011; Reading et al. 2009; Scott 2006; Shanahan et al. 2011; Vaithianathan et al. 2013). It seeks strategies based on health-promotion principles that maximise benefits for entire populations (Raphael and Bryant 2002; WHO 2018). In the case of child maltreatment, it aims to reduce and prevent the abuse and neglect of children at three levels:

- Primary – creating the underlying conditions for good-enough parenting for all parents to prevent the occurrence of child maltreatment;
- Secondary – targeted support for families at heightened risk and interventions where there is known risk of harm; and
- Tertiary – addressing the physical and psychological consequences of maltreatment.

For child protection, this entails:

1. Gaining a robust estimate of the extent of the problem in the population and the factors (at all levels or in all contexts) that drive the problem through large-scale epidemiological and aetiological data, and local routine health and social care data;
2. Public systems employing early intervention activities that promote secure and safe relationships, attachment, and positive parenting, including universal proportionate intervention models, where input is preventative and selective (a universal layer of intervention works in a preventive fashion to reduce the need for later more intensive treatment, based on appropriate data) (Lowe 2007). There have been few tests on universal proportionate models with child protection outcomes in mind, though one trial is examining the effectiveness of a universal proportionate parent-support model for reducing maternal depression and child social-emotional developmental difficulty (see Blower and Bywater 2018); and
3. Greater collaboration between, and integration of, services and professionals, working together to promote child welfare, locating the responsibility and activity for safeguarding children with all early years' education and health professionals working in multi-agency teams to deliver tiered early intervention programs. For example, health workers work with young mothers of newborn babies to develop relationships with families early on to educate them about child development before difficulties arise, while, simultaneously, social care and mental health professionals provide input to ensure the appropriate assessment of risks and avoidance of crises. At the same time, family support workers, health visitors, and other children's services professionals co-deliver evidence-based parent support and family resilience programs.

A public health approach targets *key risk factors* or social determinants for the whole population rather than focusing only on at-risk groups. Walden and Wall (2014) referred to it as 'an "upstream" approach to prevention' (p. 3). This element has attracted the attention of researchers and commentators in the child protection field, where the public suggests major changes in outlook and practice. Its proponents have noted several obstacles relating to child maltreatment, including difficulties in getting common understanding of the scope and nature of a public health approach, while reforms to include a public health approach have often not addressed the key social and structural dimensions of the problem (see Chap. 5). There are many concerns about the fit between the public health approach and child protection. Gelles (2017) argued that the focus of child protection should be on the child's welfare, while "engaging families and providing needed services" (Cuccaro-Alamin et al. 2017, p. 291). He viewed the child welfare system as deeply problematic. It has become a huge industry raising questions about who is benefiting from avoidable harm to children. While few would argue against the prevention of harm to children, doing so is intertwined with intractable, divisive political problems, including the lack of jobs that pay a living wage, rising housing costs, lack of healthcare, and poor-quality education. Despite the increased politicisation of child protection in response to child deaths, little is likely to change without concerted political action and the exposure of avoidable harms to children and families. Some advocates see a child rights perspective as preferable since it provides:

> … a framework for understanding child maltreatment as part of a range of violence, harm, and exploitation of children at the individual, institutional, and societal levels since it offers an inclusive approach to child (Reading et al. 2009, p. 332).

14.2 The Thin Line Between Prevention and Surveillance

The public health model couples prevention and intervention in the arena of child maltreatment. Working across these two arenas necessitates that practitioners work with the tension created by the diametrically opposed functions of prevention and surveillance, the new language of care and control. Verhallen et al. (2017) noted the tensions between preventive supportive care and controlling protective interventions, given their very different ideological and political underpinnings. They argued that there is a thin line between the two, hence, an understanding of the historical nature of this discourse is required for better understanding of these categories and how they influence practice. In their view, family support includes "services and interventions with poor or struggling families which aim to strengthen the care and capacities of their parents" (p. 2). In contrast, child protection comprises "interventions … directed at identifying and protecting children at risk of abuse or neglect" (p. 2). Notwithstanding their failure to recognise that the converse might be true—support can be controlling and protection caring—Verhallen et al. (2017) saw this dual approach as emerging in the responses to poverty in the late 1800s and early 1900s and the rise of the 'dangerous classes' arising from the forces of modernity.

This, coupled with the idealisation of the family, saw abuse accepted as a social problem. Initially the domain of voluntary and philanthropic groups, the state also became involved in intervention. Practice and related policies have always had elements of both approaches and at times fluctuated between the extremes of each (Baartman 2011, in Verhallen et al. 2017; Pelton 1997). Their work echoes the discussion of the basic functions of social work taken by Pincus and Minahan (1973) who suggested social workers engaged in a range of functions the most relevant to this discussion being:

- The helping function, where the worker assisted people to enhance and effectively use their capacity to cope and problem solve; and
- Their function as agents of social control.

This raises questions about what informs the basic framework of the public health model, an individualistic understanding of—or a structural approach to—the factors leading to, population health. Given research highlighting the relationship between poverty and child maltreatment, for example, would a public health model view poverty as a characteristic of individuals and under their control, or a function of inequitable economic and social systems that impact on individuals but for which the responsibility largely lies beyond them? There is a central debate regarding the public health perspective between advocates of an evidence-based approach, who see the need for improved predictive assessment and service funding and provision, and a critical public health approach that views child maltreatment as a reflection of power relations across society that occurs at all levels, not just among the poor. As Axford and Berry (2017) observed, "public health models involve protecting all children in the population from risks to their health and development, including those at high risk" (p. 14; see also: Barlow and Calam 2011; Berry 2008; Berry et al. 2013; Woodman and Gilbert 2013).

These views lead to divergent solutions. Advocates of "improving risk assessment and decision support" (Cuccaro-Alamin et al. 2017, p. 291) through predictive risk modeling believe policy makers should support and fund programs with tested success, such as universal home visiting (Donelan-McCall et al. 2009). This involves political decisions about who will pay, even though early intervention programs might decrease entry into the child welfare and juvenile justice system and the demand for welfare benefits. The prickly philosophical problem of distinguishing between acceptable and unacceptable behaviour in the context of child abuse and what policy makers should do about it is determined by the values and attitudes in society at any given time. This accounts for the myriad approaches to addressing child maltreatment. Perhaps the fiercest debates have centred on the relative merits of investment in social care or heavy-handed social control measures.

Contributing to this debate is the findings of research repeatedly highlighting the link between child maltreatment and low-income families. For example, Donelan-McCall et al. (2009), in their study of paediatric home visiting, found that low-income, unmarried women and their children (in their control group) were at much greater risk for problems of welfare dependence, substance abuse, and crime, and the home-visiting program:

> Was able to avert many of these untoward outcomes for this at-risk population. This pattern of results challenges the position that these intensive programs should be made available on a universal basis. Doing so is likely to be wasteful from an economic standpoint and may lead to a dilution of services for those families who need them most because of insufficient resources to serve everyone well. (p. 399)

Findings such as those of Donelan-McCall et al. (2009) challenge those who argue that automatically linking poverty and child maltreatment diverts attention away from its occurrence at all levels. It also challenges universal service provision and raises the thorny question of targeted care that critical commentators refer to as increased surveillance of low-income families (Wrennall 2010). What is the tipping point between early intervention care and disciplinary surveillance? All forms of treatment and intervention, including family support and home visiting, can be a means of social control, a disciplinary measure, or care, a helping measure. When does provision become intervention? This remains the thorny question for the child-focused public health approach of early intervention.

14.3 Public Health Approaches to Child Protection

Approaches advanced within the public health model range from whole-of-community interventions to a child-focused approach to intensive predictive risk modeling.

14.3.1 Strong Communities Approach

Typifying the former, Melton et al. (2008) described a 'strong comunities' approach that comprises four phases:

- Awareness-raising and identifying opportunities for enhanced family support;
- Mobilising the community to engage in developing and implementing plans to prevent child maltreatment;
- Increasing resources for families to access non-stigmatising help as and when they need it; and
- Institutionalising resource provision to sustain long-term family support.

The community-wide focus on child safety does not relate directly to child maltreatment and relies heavily on volunteerism (Melton et al. 2008). Melton et al. noted that "the penultimate goal is … to provide someone to watch over every family of a child younger than 6 years, if the family desires such help" (p. 85). Cynics might interpret this as a form of mass surveillance conducted by volunteers. It also highlights the difficulties in implementing whole-of-community public health approaches. As Melton et al. observed, the idea of a comprehensive, effective, and humane neighbourhood-based, child-centred, and family-focused system "may have changed the Zeitgeist in the field, but it appears to have had minimal effect on practice" (p. 85). Furthermore, multi-phased approaches, of the nature Melton et al. described, do not fit well within short-term policy and funding cycles. The whole-of-community approach requires fundamental attitudinal and behavioural changes across communities through long-term, sustainable primary level preventive intervention.

14.3.2 Child-Focused Approach of Early Intervention

The 'child-focused approach', which emerged in the 1990s, includes aspects of family support and child protection, while emphasising the child's independent relationship with the state (Gilbert et al. 2011, in Verhallen et al. 2017). It is seen in early-intervention policy service and practice, where 'parents' responsibilities as caregivers were both examined and supported to ensure they provide 'a good childhood' (Gilbert et al. 2011, p. 254, in Verhallen et al. 2017, p. 3). In the presence of concerns for a child, practitioners see family as inadequate and the state acts to provide support or intervention of a more authoritarian nature (Gilbert, in Verhallen et al. 2017). Verhallen et al. argued that this approach superficially combines family support and child protection and simultaneously provides substantial decision-making powers regarding the point at which one becomes the other. Their analysis highlights the very different outcomes emerging from a strengths or deficits-focused intervention process in assessing the risk to a child's development, given a child-centred focus requires not only prevention from harm but also making children resilient. As Panter-Brick (2002) noted, factors of risk and resilience "shape the long-term coping strategies of individual children, by developing their competence for negotiating high risk situations" (p. 163; see also Jenson and Fraser 2010; Richman and Fraser 2001; Rutter 1987, 2001). It leads to a focus on protective factors that help children cope with adversity, as well as

> the developmental and contextual processes by which some individuals manage to negotiate adversity (why and how they maintain self-esteem and self-efficacy; how they managed to have effective social networks). (Panter-Brick 2002, p. 163)

All too often, authorities presume that social support will suffice in reducing vulnerability and enhancing protection. However, resilience is defined by "in the active role taken by individuals under adversity … [that reflects] an individual's agency" (Panter-Brick 2002, p. 163). Panter-Brick argued there is too little knowledge about how interventions foster children's agency. Hence, Boyden and Mann (2000, cited in Panter-Brick 2002 p. 165) argued that:

> Public health concerns for children 'at risk' come with several important caveats. First, the risk discourse is helpful if one uses it less as a tool to categorize children and more as a tool to formulate questions of specific importance about children. For instance, one should ask not only what … put[s] children's health at risk, but also what processes enable children to cope with adversity. To turn the emphasis of risk on its head, how does one 'support the social and cultural expressions of resilience and coping in ways that effectively support children's wellbeing'?

Comparative and longitudinal studies on children's career outcomes would "appraise their different capabilities to face adversity. In this way, the concepts of risk and resilience would help to provide an overarching view of children whose rights are being jeopardized" (Panter-Brick 2002, p. 165) and focus on making children stronger by providing interventions that increase their coping capacities and resilience.

14.3.3 Predictive Risk Modelling

Predictive risk modeling to improve 'risk assessment and decision support' (Cuccaro-Alamin et al. 2017, p. 291) typifies the narrow focus. Its advocates see value in providing evidence on key risk factors to contribute to effective evidence-informed interventions (Axford and Berry 2017; Cuccaro-Alamin et al. 2017; Gambrill and Shlonsky 2000, 2001). Hence, it involves a system of monitoring through ongoing and systematic data collection, analysis, and interpretation for planning, implementing, evaluating, testing, and monitoring the effectiveness of public health interventions, including policy change (Axford and Berry 2017). Its critics see its focus on individualistic factors as compromising the essential structural or community approach to child protection. Nevertheless, balanced by a broader perspective, predictive risk modeling could be a useful accompaniment to the public health approach that leverages technology and uses available administrative data to improve assessment decisions (Cuccaro-Alamin et al. 2017).

In their review of the operational and statistical limitations of risk-assessment tools, Cuccaro-Alamin et al. (2017) presented evidence on predictive analytics – "data mining, modeling, and analytic techniques to existing data to discover patterns and make predictions" (p. 292) – to increase the accuracy of risk assessment. However, there are many ethical questions surrounding predictive assessment methods: Is it ethical to use predictive risk modeling if needed interventions do not exist? Is it unethical not to use risk modelling given that it is much more predictive than practitioner judgment alone? Gambrill and Shlonsky (2000) highlighted ethical issues surrounding the unnecessary involvement of, and disruptions to, families wrongly assessed of being at high risk, and parents who slip through the cracks of rigid assessments and go on to maltreat their children. Certainly, there is a huge focus on risk assessment and decision making to increase accuracy, despite the broader concerns about surveillance and targeting, already outlined (Cuccaro-Alamin et al. 2017; Dare 2013, 2015; Dare and Gambrill 2017; Gillingham 2016; Jenson and Fraser 2010; Vaithianathan et al. 2013). Regardless of the scale of the approach, its implementation rests on political decisions to support and fund programs with debates centring on who bears ultimate responsibility for child protection and who will pay.

14.4 Competing Knowledge Sources

Critical of the myopic focus on the shortcomings of the child protection system (e.g., reactive responses following child deaths, the tendency to rely on preconceptions rather than empirical data and evidence, and a lack of financial commitment to research and long-term treatment), Higgins (2015) and Garrison (2015) called for a knowledge-informed approach to address systemic weaknesses. However, there are many competing knowledge sources, as already shown, each of which has problems. For example, risk approaches tend to individualise, and surveillance approaches move the focus to 'troublesome' groups and communities. Broad approaches to address structural concerns are difficult to substantiate empirically and to implement. Individualistic approaches focused on electronic data collection and joined-up data systems can only be effective if married to research on high-risk factors for child maltreatment that tend to target such communities. In addition, there are legitimate ethical concerns surrounding privacy and the implications of electronic data collection for relationships between children, parents, the community, and the state (See Chap. 5). Of concern is the resultant increased surveillance and governance that has several unintended, and intended, consequences for the rights and civil liberties of children and adults within the normative child rights framework underpinning child protection. Many are critical of risk-based approaches because they infringe the civil liberties of targeted groups, typically poor families from impoverished communities, and lead to intrusive surveillance that further compounds issues for identified 'at-risk' groups and communities (Featherstone et al. 2014; Wrennall 2010). However, Holden et al. (1995) noted that, in the United States:

> … research on children in poverty has already shifted from comparisons between children in low-income and middle-income families to in-depth analyses of processes mediating poverty's influences on developmental and health outcomes (p. 176).

Axford and Berry (2017) made a similar observation, noting that:

> … the prevailing policy climate and organisational culture' fuelled by risk aversion is not a defining feature of early intervention, which aims to identify and build upon protective factors, while 'the process of addressing specified risk factors helps to meet need (p. 4).

This dominant focus on individualistic risk assessment and management is the main obstacle in moving toward a broader community focus, where child protection becomes 'everybody's business'. Evidence-based approaches, while useful and desirable, rest on quality evaluation studies of primary-level interventions that are all too often unavailable because they are extremely difficult to conduct. What is left is rhetoric that promises much but delivers little. Outweighed by individualised evidence, risk-based approaches gain precedence. Nevertheless, public health approaches, even the idea of them, has led to less stigmatising approaches to clients, especially with the social investment discourse adding to the emergence of universal and secondary early interventions (Gray 2014). However, the generational decline in social capital occurring in tandem with 'the ongoing crisis in the child protection system' (Melton et al.

2008, p. 84) compromises whole-of-community interventions that rest heavily on voluntary labour. For neoliberals, volunteering is desirable because it reduces costs and shifts responsibility from state to community (Gray 2010).

14.5 Critiques of the Public Health Approach

14.5.1 Failure to Address Structural Causes

While one view of a public health approach emphasises socioeconomic conditions as a health determinant without addressing the structural causes for differences in socioeconomic status or their consequences, others would argue that an emphasis on the structural causes underpinning socioeconomic conditions would support radically different policy and practice outcomes. Critics within the public health field note that:

> While models can be useful heuristic devices, there are risks involved in assuming that they provide a transparent means through which reality can be readily apprehended … many population health analysts seem to believe they are producing a neutral and universally acceptable research and policy paradigm, whereas they are actually bringing forward a specific, narrow, and … asocial combination of epidemiology and economics [that overlooks structural considerations] (Coburn et al. 2003, p. 393).

Because of its macro-level population focus and neglect of the broader socioeconomic context, it leads to a "political dead end" (Coburn et al. 2003, p. 393). Policy solutions, like public health population strategies within an evidence-based policy environment, "tend toward overly rationalist models in which greater knowledge is simply assumed to produce policies oriented to the enactment of this knowledge" (Coburn et al. 2003, p. 393). There is little "consideration of how such models can be connected to real people and groups in actual social contexts" (Coburn et al. 2003, p. 393). This amounts to 'context stripping' (Raphael and Bryant 2002). In general, "the field of population health has successfully marginalized … health promotion [approaches] … that placed greater emphasis on the active roles of individuals and communities" (Coburn et al. 2003, p. 393). Further, they don't address the question of

> why some capitalist countries with strong social democratic political parties and resilient welfare states, such as Sweden and Norway, have much lower health inequalities and better average population health than Canada or the United States (Coburn et al. 2003, p. 393).

Contrary to 'trickle-down theories of economic prosperity', there is "increasing awareness that national or regional wealth or economic growth cannot be equated with improved health or well-being" (Coburn et al. 2003, p. 393). Using social determinants of health diagnostically to identify risk in individuals must be balanced with interventions that attempt to address the inequalities of a class-based, capitalist system, that is, interventions must target social causes and not just blame disadvantaged individuals and groups for their problems.

14.5.2 Fit Between Public Health and Child Protection

The Australian Institute of Family Studies (AIFS 2014) highlighted the complexity of issues around child protection and consequent difficulties associated with categorising child protection responses as primary, secondary, or tertiary, noting the "need for some programs to be both primary and secondary, or secondary and tertiary". For the most part, applied to child protection, the public health approach has remained a tertiary response to investigation and removal options. The main approach remains investigative statutory child protection and programs targeted at high-risk, low-income families to prevent problems from escalating to child protection orders. Prevention targeting 'key risk factors or social determinants at a whole-of-population level through community-based and primary healthcare; universal early childhood support and education; universal nurse home-visiting programs; and home visits to help families develop solutions remains secondary (Axford and Berry 2017). Early intervention to detect and address early signs of child maltreatment, including family support and community engagement, and recording relevant, high-quality, 'real-time' data on implementation and outcomes takes a backseat to investigative work (Axford and Berry 2017).

14.5.3 Data Availability

The public health approach relies heavily on data collection and availability as a tool for predicting risk at various levels, but as Scott (2013) has highlighted, there is an absence of accurate prevalence data in Australia. Further, as already discussed, many question the ethics of collecting ever-more data on families and the conundrum surrounding what to do with it: What happens when at-risk family is identified (Gambrill and Shlonsky 2000)? Will service providers offer these families care and support? Are the services they need available? Do we know the quality of the services available and do the programs on offer work? It is the implications of the public health approach that needs addressing. For this reason, some believe that proponents of a public health approach underestimate the cost and difficulty of achieving meaningful change within an already constrained neoliberal environment of care provision.

14.6 Conclusion

This chapter has discussed the tensions within child protection. The public health approach aims to reduce and prevent the abuse and neglect of children across primary, secondary, and tertiary levels. However, contemporary approaches to child protection remain dominated by individualised forensically-focused interventions that occur predominantly at the tertiary level of intervention following the identification of maltreatment, particularly where state intervention is required. These interventions provide limited scope for more holistic preventative responses to children at risk and the provision of support to struggling families and communities. Child protection systems work diligently to focus only on remedial actions, while public health approaches aim at universal service provision to promote healthy families and communities. In this chapter, we highlighted the central debate underpinning the public health perspective, where advocates argue for evidence-based approaches and see the need for improved predictive assessment, service funding and provision, compared to those of a critical public health approach, which views child maltreatment as a reflection of power relations across society that occurs at all levels, not just among the poor. We showed the difficulties involved in reaching population-based public-health aspirations, in the face of these debates, which disagree on where the focus should lie: whether on targeted services for whole or 'troublesome' communities or better identification processes to identify 'at-risk' individuals, groups, and communities. We questioned the fit between public health and child protection and the complexity of the issues acknowledged with the route to resolution a mix of political action and further development of programs that work across primary, secondary, and tertiary levels to encompass these divergent views.

References

Australian Institute of Family Studies. (2014). Defining the public health model for the child welfare services context. *CFCA Resource Sheet*. Retrieved from https://aifs.gov.au/cfca/publications/defining-public-health-model-child-welfare-servi

Axford, N., & Berry, V. (2017). Perfect bedfellows: Why early intervention can play a critical role in protecting children – A response to Featherstone et al. (2014) 'A marriage made in hell: Child protection meets early intervention'. *The British Journal of Social Work, 48*, 254–273. https://doi.org/10.1093/bjsw/bcx003.

Baartman, H. (2011). Compassie en controle in de Jeugdzorg (Compassion and control in youth care). *Ouderschapskennis, 13*, 63–81.

Barlow, J., & Calam, R. (2011). A public health approach to safeguarding in the 21st century. *Child Abuse Review, 20*(4), 238–255.

Berry, V. L. (2008). *The relative contribution of family conflict to children's health and development*. Unpublished PhD thesis, University of Bath.

Berry, V., Blower, S., Axford, N., Little, M., & Kaoukji, D. (2013). The prevention of child maltreatment and neglect. In J. Conte (Ed.), *Child abuse and neglect worldwide*. Santa Barbara: Praeger.

Blower, S., & Bywater, T. (2018). *Enhancing social and emotional health in the early years*. ISRCTN Registry. https://doi.org/10.1186/ISRCTN11079129.

Boyden, J., & Mann, G. (2000, September 9–12). Children's risk, resilience and coping in extreme situations. *Background paper to the Consultation on Children in Adversity*. Oxford, UK.

Coburn, D., Denny, K., Mykhalovskiy, E., McDonough, P., Robertson, A., & Love, R. (2003). Population health in Canada: A brief critique. *American Journal of Public Health, 93*(3), 392–396.

Cuccaro-Alamin, S., Foust, R., Vaithianathan, R., & Putnam-Hornstein, E. (2017). Risk assessment and decision making in child protective services: Predictive risk modeling in context. *Children and Youth Services Review, 79*, 291–298. https://doi.org/10.1016/j.childyouth.2017.06.027.

Dalziel, K., & Segal, L. (2012). Home visiting programmes for the prevention of child maltreatment: Cost-effectiveness of 33 programmes. *Archives of Disease in Childhood, 97*(9), 787–798. https://doi.org/10.1136/archdischild-2011-300795.

Dare, T. (2013). *Predictive risk modelling and child maltreatment: An ethical review*. Auckland: The University of Auckland. Retrieved from http://www.msd.govt.nz/documents/about-msd-and-our-work/publications-resources/research/predictive-modelling/00-predicitve-risk-modellingand-child-maltreatment-an-ethical-review.pdf

Dare, T. (2015). The ethics of predictive risk modeling. In L. Waterhouse & J. McGhee (Eds.), *Challenging child protection: New directions in safeguarding children* (pp. 64–76). London: Jessica Kingsley.

Dare, T., & Gambrill, E. (2017). *Ethical analysis: Predictive risk models at call screening for Allegheny County*. Allengheny County Department of Human Services. Retrieved from: www.alleghenycounty.us/human-services/index.aspx

Donelan-McCall, N., Eckenrode, J., & Olds, D. L. (2009). Home visiting for the prevention of child maltreatment: Lessons learned during the past 20 years. *Pediatric Clinics of North America, 56*, 389–403. https://doi.org/10.1016/j.pcl.2009.01.002.

Featherstone, B., Morris, K., & White, S. (2014). A marriage made in hell: Early intervention meets child protection. *British Journal of Social Work, 44*(7), 1735–1749.

Gambrill, E., & Shlonsky, A. (2000). Risk assessment in context. *Children and Youth Services Review, 22*(11–12), 813–837. https://doi.org/10.1016/S0190-7409(00)00123-7.

Gambrill, E., & Shlonsky, A. (2001). The need for comprehensive risk management systems in child welfare. *Children and Youth Services Review, 23*(1), 79–107.

Garrison, M. (2015). Reforming child protection: A public health perspective. *Virginia Journal of Social Policy & the Law, 12*(3), 590–637.

Gelles, R. (2017). *Out of harm's way: Creating an effective child welfare system*. Oxford: Oxford University Press.

Gilbert, R., Kemp, A., Thoburn, J., Sidebotham, P., Radford, L., Glaser, D., & MacMillan, H. L. (2009a). Recognising and responding to child maltreatment. *Lancet, 373*, 167–180.

Gilbert, R., Spatz Widom, C., Browne, K., Fergusson, D., Webb, E., & Janson, S. (2009b). Burden and consequences of child maltreatment in high-income countries. *Lancet, 373*(9657), 68–81. https://doi.org/10.1016/S0140-6736(08)61706-7.

Gilbert, N., Parton, N., & Skivenes, M. (2011). *Child protection systems: International trends and orientations*. Oxford: Oxford University Press.

Gillingham, P. (2016). Predictive risk modelling to prevent child maltreatment and other adverse outcomes for service users: Inside the 'black box' of machine learning. *British Journal of Social Work, 46*, 1044–1058. https://doi.org/10.1093/bjsw/bcv031.

Gray, M. (2010). Social development and the status quo: Professionalisation and third way co-optation. *International Journal of Social Welfare, 19*(4), 463–470. https://doi.org/10.1111/j.1468-2397.2009.00714.x.

Gray, M. (2014). The swing to early intervention and prevention and its implications for social work. *British Journal of Social Work, 44*(7), 1750–1769. https://doi.org/10.1093/bjsw/bct037.

Higgins, D. (2015). A public health approach to enhancing safe and supportive family environments for children. *Family Matters, 96*, 39–52. Retrieved from https://aifs.gov.au/publications/family-matters/issue-96/public-health-approach-enhancing-safe-and-supportive-family-environments-children

Holden, E., Horton, L., & Danseco, E. (1995). The mental health of homeless children. *Clinical Psychology: Science and Practice, 2*(2), 165–178.

Jenson, J. M., & Fraser, M. W. (Eds.). (2010). *Social policy for children and families: A risk and resilience perspective* (2nd ed.). Thousand Oaks: Sage.

Lowe, R. (2007). *Facing the future: A review of the role of health visitors*. London: Queen's Nursing Institute.

Melton, G. B., Holaday, B. J., & Kimbrough-Melton, R. J. (2008). Community life, public health and children's safety. *Family & Community Health, 31*(2), 84–99.

Moncrieff, J. (2008). *The myth of a chemical cure: A critique of psychiatric drug treatment*. New York: Palgrave.

Panter-Brick, C. (2002). Street children, human rights, and public health: A critique and future directions. *Annual Review of Anthropology, 31*(1), 147–171. https://doi.org/10.1146/annurev.anthro.31.040402.085359.

Pelton, L. (1997). Child welfare policy and practice: The myth of family preservation. *American Journal of Orthopsychiatry, 67*(4), 545–552.

Pincus, A., & Minahan, A. (1973). *Social work practice: Model and method*. Itasca: F.E. Peacock Publishers Inc.

Putnam-Hornstein, E., Webster, D., Needell, B., & Magruder, J. (2011). A public health approach to clinical maltreatment surveillance: Evidence from a linkage project in the United States. *Child Abuse Review, 20*, 256–273. https://doi.org/10.1002/car.119.

Raphael, D., & Bryant, T. (2002). The limitations of population health as a model for a new public health. *Health Promotion International, 17*(2), 189–199.

Reading, R., Bissell, S., Goldhagen, J., Harwin, J., Masson, J., Moynihan, S., Parton, N., & Santos Pais, M. (2009). Promotion of children's right and prevention of child maltreatment. *Lancet, 373*(9660), 332–343. https://doi.org/10.1016/S0140-6736(08)61709-2.

Richman, J. M., & Fraser, M. W. (2001). Resilience in childhood: The role of risk and protection. In J. M. Richman & M. W. Fraser (Eds.), *The context of youth violence: Resilience, risk, and protection* (pp. 1–12). Westport: Praeger.

Rutter, M. (1987). Psychosocial resilience and protective mechanisms. *American Journal of Orthopsychiatry, 57*(3), 316–331.

Rutter, M. (2001). Psychosocial adversity: Risk, resilience and recovery. In J. M. Richman & M. W. Fraser (Eds.), *The context of youth violence: Resilience, risk, and protection* (pp. 13–41). Westport: Praeger.

Scott, D. (2006). Towards a public health model of child protection in Australia. *Communities, Children and Families Australia, 1*(1), 9–16.

Scott, D. (2013). *The prevalence of child abuse and neglect. CFCA fact sheet*. Melbourne: Australian Institute of Family Studies. https://aifs.gov.au/cfca/publications/prevalence-child-abuse-and-neglect

Scott, D., Lonne, B., & Higgins, D. (2016). Public health models for preventing child maltreatment. *Trauma, Violence, and Abuse, 17*(4), 408–419.

Shanahan, L., Copeland, W. E., Costello, E. J., & Angold, A. (2011). Child-, adolescent-, and young adult-onset depressions: Differential risk factors in development? *Psychological Medicine, 41*(11), 2265–2274. https://doi.org/10.1017/S0033291711000675.

Vaithianathan, R., Maloney, T., Putnam-Hornstein, E., & Jiang, N. (2013). Children in the public benefit system at risk of maltreatment: Identification via predictive modeling. *American Journal of Preventive Medicine, 45*(3), 354–359. https://doi.org/10.1016/j.amepre.2013.04.022.

Verhallen, T., Hall, C. J., & Slembrouck, S. (2017). Family support and child protection approaches: Historicising perspectives on contemporary discourses of social work. *Qualitative Social Work*, 1–16. https://doi.org/10.1177/1473325017712798.

Walden, I., & Wall, L. (2014). *Reflecting on primary prevention of violence against women: The public health approach* (ACSSA Issues No. 19). Melbourne: Australian Centre for the Study of Sexual Assault, Australian Institute of Family Studies. https://aifs.gov.au/publications/reflecting-primary-prevention-violence-against-women/public-health-approach

Woodman, J., & Gilbert, R. (2013). Child maltreatment: Moving towards a public health approach. In BMA Board of Science (Ed.), *Growing up in the UK: Ensuring a healthy future for our children* (pp. 84–105). London: British Medical Association.

World Health Organisation. (2018). The public health approach. *Violence Prevention Alliance: Global campaign for violence prevention.* Accessed 27 Aug 2018. http://www.who.int/violenceprevention/approach/public_health/en/

Wrennall, L. (2010). Surveillance and child protection: De-mystifying the Trojan Horse. *Surveillance & Society, 7*(3/4), 304–324. http://www.surveillance-and-socety.org.

Part III
Addressing Operational and Systemic Issues

Chapter 15 What Are the Risks and Obstacles in Implementing a Public Health Approach to the Well-Being and Protection of Children?

Maria Harries and Melissa O'Donnell

15.1 Introduction

Our research, policyimplementation and practice work have been informed by more than a decade of persuasive scholarship on the need to adopt a public health approach to the care and protection of children (Garrison 2005; Hammond 2003; Scott 2006). We have also been engaged with and excited by the attempts to adopt a public health approach as described in Chap. 1 and throughout this book, and also captured succinctly in the ground-breaking National Child Protection Framework (COAG 2009, p. 13):

> Conceptually, the National Framework claimed to be based on a public health model, under which: priority is placed on having universal supports available for all families (for example, health and education). More intensive (secondary) prevention interventions are provided to those families that need additional assistance with a focus on early intervention. Tertiary child protection services are a last resort, and the least desirable option for families and governments. Just as a health system is more than hospitals so a system for the protection of children is more than a statutory child protection service.

M. Harries (✉)
Senior Honorary Research Fellow, Social Policy and Practice Research Consortium (SPPRC), School of Population and Global Health, The University of Western Australia, Perth, WA, Australia

School of Occupational Therapy, Social Work and Speech Pathology, Curtin University, Perth, WA, Australia
e-mail: maria.harries@uwa.edu.au

M. O'Donnell
National Health and Medical Research Fellow, Telethon Kids Institute, University of Western Australia, Perth, WA, Australia
e-mail: Melissa.odonnell@telethonkids.org.au

B. Lonne et al. (eds.), *Re-Visioning Public Health Approaches for Protecting Children*, Child Maltreatment 9, https://doi.org/10.1007/978-3-030-05858-6_15

Importantly, our thoughts are underpinned by an appreciation of decades of earlier evidence about the systemic failures of approaches to protecting children (Lonne et al. 2009; Scott and Swain 2002) and particularly what has become known as the 'paradox of modernity' (Keating and Hertzman 1999). The latter is a concept recognising that despite rising prosperity, there are equivalent rises in contemporary disparities and rising inequalities in child health and well-being outcomes. Relating this paradox to child abuse and neglect, Li et al. (2008, p. 65) observed that:

> Factors precipitating child abuse and neglect are similar to those associated with other indicators of poor outcomes, including living in single-parent households, low income and financial stress, parental substance abuse, social isolation and lack of family support.

There are many international examples of projects aimed at addressing these identified systemic concerns. Dating from the late 1990s the innovative Australian research project '*Pathways to Prevention*' is one of them and is informed by the clear evidence as well as the common sense idea that "mobilising resources to support children, families and their communities before problems emerge is more effective than intervening when problems have become entrenched" (Homel et al. 2006, p. 36).

Based on the emerging knowledge from these projects and ongoing evidence of the failure of the contemporary Anglophone paradigm of child protection, there is also considerable international scholarship now dedicated to methods of deconstructing (Pelton 1998), re-strategising (Melton and Barry 1995), 'reforming' (Lonne et al. 2009), re-imagining (Featherstone et al. 2015), or re-thinking (Daniel 2010) our efforts at protecting children. Asher Ben-Arieh (2014) refers to the now compelling evidence of the need for a policy move from preventing risk factors and negative behaviour to promoting protective factors and positive behaviours.

Additional urgency about the need to think and act differently emerges from the disturbing evidence of scholars such as Bywaters et al. (2016). Commenting on the outcomes of the now considerable research on family and child poverty, they support the earlier and prescient observations of Pelton (1989), noting that a child and family have a far greater chance of being the object and target of child protection services if they are in any way disadvantaged by circumstances such as poverty.

15.2 The Challenging Arena for Change

Implementation of any reform process is difficult. In human service delivery of any sort, reforms are inevitably mediated within varying jurisdictional structures each with their own distinct legislation, public policy frameworks, organisational structures and arrangements and, political ideologies (Kennedy and Richards 2016). New ways of working require courage and a thorough appreciation of the perceived and actual risks in disturbing traditional ways of working. Unarguably, in order to implement changes, current arrangements need to be understood in order to appreciate the ties that potentially hold them in place and the perceived threats that will restrict opportunities for change.

In most contemporary Anglophone approaches to child protection, originating in the 1960s, most of them now guided by mandatory reporting requirements, it is a legislative requirement and professional obligation, to 'notify' or 'report' concerns about risks to children to the appropriate statutory authority. In nearly all jurisdictions that have adopted this forensic approach to the protection of children, the largest proportion of such reports are not substantiated, that is, they are assessed not to be ones that provide a risk to the child that warrants statutory intervention and the removal of the child to a place of safety (Bilson et al. 2017). The critical question about the point at which the grave and coercive act of removing a child from family and community is justified is predicated on the acceptance that significant harm has been done or is very likely to occur.

Given such actions of state coercion are highly intrusive in the lives of children, families and communities, a reasonable assumption must be that prior to such action, everything possible has been done to mitigate the chances of harm by ameliorating the adversities seen to be linked with them. The evidence is uncontroversial that that such amelioration is generally absent in large part due to the burden of overwhelming numbers of notifications and associated deluge of demands for risk assessments (Allen Consulting Group 2003; Munro 2011). Almost 20 years ago, Leroy Pelton warned us of the dangers in the developing child protection system and described it thus: "The fundamental structure of the public child welfare system is that of a coercive apparatus wrapped in a helping orientation" (1998, p. 126).

The need for earlier discernment prior to and alongside meeting the statutory requirements for reporting is critical in the implementation of a public health approach (Bromfield et al. 2014). Within a public health approach, a pivotal question is when the statutory authority needs to be engaged? For some children, this might need to be sooner than under current structural arrangements. However, the vast number of children and families may not need statutory intervention at all because preventative strategies addressing structural determinants of abuse will have a better chance of reducing adversity through earlier assistance before problems become entrenched.

Marsha Garrison, a US expert on law and policy relating to families and children observed "a quarter of a century ago, researchers and reformers reported that the results achieved by the CP system were far removed from its goals" (Garrison 2005, p. 590). She stated that incremental changes had proven unsuccessful to the point when – even then – the 'grave threat' of child abuse was out of control. She attributed the failure in 'halting the epidemic' of child maltreatment to the erroneous adoption of an acute medical care model by a statutory body that focused on an individualised 'cure' for a problem that was ill understood and highly linked to adverse environmental conditions. In outlining a new approach she identified the need to abolish the residual model and focus instead on prevention, research, evidence based work, support and "long-term, intensive and multifaceted intervention" (2004, p. 630).

Increasingly, scholars, professionals, researchers, and, importantly families themselves have promoted the value of the alternative public health approach. There are numerous descriptors for what defines such an approach and these are covered elsewhere in this book. Within such an approach, the care and protection of children is seen as 'everyone's business' and it is only when community and other services and systems prove unable to generate safety for children that the formal, statutory child protection system is utilised. Within this model, statutory child protection and allied health, alcohol and drug, education and correctional services – all involved in various ways with the well-being of children – along with universal services – need to work differently together and in partnership with community-based agencies to re-focus their service delivery.

However, the challenges that face executive leadership in all these arenas as they try to implement new ways of working, without de-stabilising already overloaded systems and workers, are immense. These leadership challenges are no less significant, although different, from those facing frontline workers. Everyone in both child and adult services is confronted with the need to accept new roles and negotiate and adapt to new role relationships across professional boundaries and agencies.

One of the many challenges facing leadership is how to introduce innovative practices using promising levers for change and develop replicable interventions and also build the evidence for successful new ways of working. Those responsible for moving to a model that seeks to protect children by acknowledging the need for comprehensive, universal services for them and their families to be provided in the first instance and intervening with their families and communities much earlier and differently have to manage a complex process of change that requires building new partner relationships (Anaf et al. 2014). Such changes require leaders and those with political will to acknowledge that changes to established organisational structures and relationships require the naming and addressing of structural impediments to child well-being. At the same time they need to continue to contain the anxiety about the injury or death of a child on their watch. What if it all goes wrong? Who will be blamed?

15.3 Obstacles to Change

In this section we highlight structural, funding and organisational challenges that can easily become barriers to the important system changes noted above. We do this by reflecting on our experiences of engagement with jurisdictional authorities that have attempted the process of implementing major change to their child safety arrangements by introducing a public health approach. In describing the steps agencies have taken, we obtained feedback from stakeholders involved. They were able to explain and highlight the complexity of the roadmap to change when problems encountered easily default to customary solutions.

15.3.1 Political Will and Courage

Generally, the demand for change occurs as a result of public outrage about a failure in the child protection system followed by an outcry for reform. Children are seen to be at risk because of the failure of workers to assess and intervene in a timely fashion. The first and immediate call is for an inquiry that ascertains the reasons for failure and identifies culpability. This is often followed by a demand for more child protection staff. Such solutions are often politically expedient and provide an immediate sense of relief as 'something is being done'. This, we argue is the first obstacle. Inquiries and more staff simply operate to shore up the system that is already unworkable. Political will and courage are required to think and act differently.

15.3.2 Conceptualisation of a Public Health Approach

The alternative to shoring up the failing system by instead conceptualising a public health approach to replace it, faces its second obstacle in the problems with the language of public health itself. The public health scholarship as applied to child protection to date has been preoccupied with describing the concept and promoting the essence of its relevance, central ideas and principles rather than how to implement it. A public health approach has indeed provided a metaphor for a change in orientation of services but scholarship to date has not yet adequately embraced the complexities of method of application. In particular there is the potentially problematic incorporation of the language of 'health' in a human service arena that has traditionally worked within a community paradigm rather than a medical one. Despite the fact that the formal acceptance of the notion of 'the battered child' which led to the current child protection rescue paradigm (Scott and Swain 2002) emerged from the work of paediatrician Henry Kempe et al. (1962), different mindsets have traditionally informed medical (health) and community services (child protection) arenas.

An important method of overcoming some elements of this ideational obstacle has been to utilise the work of scholars such as Baum (1998) who have long promoted the concept of the 'new public health' model which moves the concept from a medical framework to a socio-environmental one. In her ground-breaking work, Baum presented a social model of health and well-being and emphasises the importance of social, economic and environmental issues in growing the capacity of communities to support and sustain lasting change in conditions that affect the well-being of all. Her model resonates well with those who work within a community development paradigm (Lang and Rayner 2012).

15.3.3 Gaps in Evidence

Once the notion of a 'new public health approach' has been even cautiously held by those who are responsible for creating change in child protection systems, a range of questions immediately arise which separately or combined, provide a series of further potential obstacles. Where is the evidence of such a model working to protect children? Does early prevention actually reduce the incidence of abuse and neglect? What sorts of interventions assist what sorts of families? Broadley and Goddard (2015) captured the importance of what he saw as some of these fundamental evidential prerequisites for implementing a public health approach to the protection of children. He included the need for the following to be available: an understanding of the magnitude of child maltreatment; the ability to identify at-risk populations; evaluation of the effectiveness of prevention and intervention activities; and evidence to inform, evaluate and improve the response to at-risk children and families.

It would be ideal if all of these data were available and satisfied those wanting firm and convincing evidence prior to implementing necessary changes. Although it is important to implement as comprehensive as possible a public health model when re-orienting services, it is not possible nor reasonable to expect that we can only commence when all the evidence is in. While the lack of a full repertoire of evidence may reduce our understanding of the nuancing for the adoption of the public health approach and adds to the difficulties of informing its ongoing development and refinement it should not prevent a public health approach from being implemented. In Australia, the report of the Victorian Auditor-General into Early Intervention Services for Vulnerable Children and Families (2015) amongst others, provided encouraging evidence of promising interventions as well as identifying the need for more monitoring and reporting of outcomes. In terms of the evidence for the financial value of such interventions, the data from Masters et al.'s (2017) systematic review of cost savings from public health affirm that the return on investment in public health approaches are significant.

It is evident that many prevention and early intervention services have not been adequately measured for their effectiveness. The reasons for this are numerous but generally these often well intended and innovative services are funded and delivered by organisations that lack the capacity and resources to collect data on the effectiveness of services (Seivwright et al. 2016). There is clearly a need for this capacity to be developed and resourced in order to ensure that prevention and early intervention services are effective in delivering services for families including those families at greatest need. It also requires a more nuanced understanding of the capacity of the system to respond to the needs of select cohorts and groups whose outcomes may not be effected by agencies and who may require different or more tailored approaches.

15.3.4 Universal Service Provision

No public health model is possible without an appreciation of the need for universal services and population-wide strategies that prevent or limit the occurrence of childhood adversities in the first place. This argument has been clearly outlined in Chap. 8 by Daro and Karter. The essentials include adequate housing, home visiting supports, financial resources, and access to education, as well as adequate child care for all families. These and others are fundamental. Such services maximise opportunities for child health and well-being and limit the risks of harms occurring that then need to be mitigated.

Child protection services in Anglophone countries are costly and to add additional costs, even with the prediction this will limit tertiary-level costs, demands additional investment in the first instance. In 2008 the ARACY report 'Inverting the Pyramid' highlighted the fact that the child protection system is heavily resourced toward the top of the pyramid, focused on investigating families and removing children from families found to have maltreated their child or at high risk of doing so (The Allen Consulting Group 2008). In a public health approach it is necessary to invert the pyramid, focusing resources on the bottom of the pyramid to provide universal services to support all families which will therefore reduce the risk of maltreatment across the population including high risk families. Figure 15.1 is adapted from the work of Morrison (O'Donnell and Stanley 2007) and captures the important location of universal services:

Unarguably, there are ideological and political obstacles to supporting and funding universal services (See Chap. 8 in this volume). Funding such services may be controversial and particularly so for conservative governments that hold fast to promoting individual initiative and limiting the role of government in society (See Chap. 9 in this volume). Persuading such governments to increase the level and

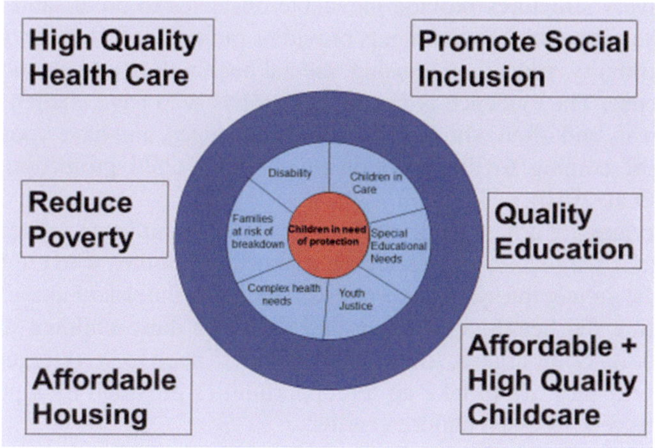

Fig. 15.1 Locating the importance of the universal services

adequacy of resourcing of universal services is, however, possible if there is sufficient evidence of the value of such an investment and the guardians of the government purse can be so assured.

15.3.5 Resourcing

Disagreement about the need for adequately resourcing of universal services at the bottom of the pyramid is only one obstacle that is put in the way of implementing a public health approach. Governments will also need to resource the middle of the pyramid including targeted services for vulnerable families, early intervention for families deemed at low-moderate risk as well as continue to fund the top of the pyramid, the statutory responses for high risk families (Bromfield et al. 2014). The current child protection system provides limited responses to those families who are deemed low to moderate levels of risk or who may require long term support. As described earlier, the contemporary forensic system is one in which low-moderate risk families with little support often re-present as higher risk families requiring resources in the form of statutory investigation and response with the potential for children to end up in out-of-home care. Investigating and intervening with high risk families often with complex problems is exceedingly resource intensive both in funds and in caseworker time. However failure to do this prevention and early intervention work will result in a larger number of families who reach the threshold for statutory responses resulting in a greater burden of resources on the system.

15.3.6 Service Delivery Structures

Service delivery structures provide inevitable obstacles in predictable and unpredictable ways. Generally, governments provide a range of targeted services in areas including disability, education, housing, mental health, drug and alcohol domestic/family violence. The evidence is clear that families who have challenges in these and other areas, and often who have multiple challenges, and have young children, are at risk of coming to the attention of statutory child protection authorities (Bromfield et al. 2010).

Adult services are not generally funded to support families to reduce the risk of maltreatment. Unarguably, the greater the support for families who are facing these challenges the greater the systems response in reducing the risk of abuse and neglect and supporting the health, well-being and safety of these children and families (Scott 2009). As Scott argues, these 'adult services' need to work together as well as differently if they are to take up the opportunities provided by a public health model to intervene to assist children earlier.

These adult services, of course, argue persuasively that if they are to expand their role to work closely together and facilitate interventions that include the prioritising of the needs of children of the adults currently accessing them, they will need increased funding (Darlington et al. 2005; Spath et al. 2008). Strong arguments and evidence are required to convince funders that investment is well spent on prevention and early intervention by all services in order to improve family circumstances and the well-being and safety of children.

Changing the ways that services are delivered within government is only one of a number of obstacles in the way of adopting a new way of working in child protection. Universal prevention services and secondary early intervention services are provided by services such as primary health services, as well as via different levels of government including federal and state/province. Non-government agencies are often the ones contracted to deliver family support services. This is not an obstacle per se because often local community agencies have the trust of their local communities and families, however the challenge lies in the type and focus of the funding models in place. Models of funding may be based on the numbers of families or individuals to whom a service is delivered. In this instance, the focus is not on outcomes but on the outputs of the agency. Often the families who most require support and services are those families who are the most challenging to engage in services or who have the most complex needs and issues. These families are resource intensive for non-government agencies and outcome goals hard to achieve. When agency resources are stretched, these families are often seen as too high a risk and so may well be the least well serviced – with the obvious consequence that the children are more likely to enter statutory care (Hamilton and Braithwaite 2014).

In the absence of adequate resourcing for family support services there are less options for child protection workers when they are faced with keeping a child in the home with support versus removing a child. The system therefore becomes much more focused on a punitive response to risk then a therapeutic approach to working with families. This was clearly outlined in the Child Protection Outcomes Project report (Allen Consulting Group 2003) which argued that a regulatory approach by the child protection system is very effective in identifying and responding to children who are at high risk with immediate safety concerns, such as sexual or severe physical abuse.

However, it is a less effective approach when working with families who experience chronic problems complicated by factors such as adverse living conditions as well mental health problems, substance misuse, parental disability, etc. The regulatory process of investigation, and court processes add a further burden on such families who often do not have the resources and capacity to effectively represent their issues and circumstances (Hamilton and Braithwaite 2014).

A further obstacle for agencies providing services to vulnerable families is that often under contractual obligations they are seen to become an extension of the child protection surveillance system. This can create a lack of trust by families with challenging issues who open the door to agencies for support, often disclosing risks which may then set off another investigation into the family by child protection. This also creates role confusion for agency staff working with families as they do require families to build a level of trust and rapport to engage them in services and they will be at their most effective when families can disclose the risks that need to be reduced and mitigated. However their dual role of supportive engagement and surveillance will mean that they will be under obligation to report families deemed at risk thereby creating distrust with families who require the support.

15.3.7 Workforce Matters

In most child protection inquiries the focus of concerns and the subsequent recommendation have been on training, recruitment and retention of frontline child protection workers employed in statutory authorities. In adopting a public health approach, a vital requirement is those engaging 'differently' with families with the complex needs so evident in such families, have the skill and training to make assessments and work in new ways – and to do so working within a variety of service locations. Tailored responses are required which may lie outside the expertise of any one agency. In these cases multi-agency responses are required. With siloed funding models this resource need is often not addressed. Agencies are competing with other agencies for contracts to maintain their funding and this may discourage multiagency strategies for families with complex needs. Unless this is specifically written into contractual agreements and the agencies are funded to do collaborative work with joint outcomes and reimbursed for the complex and resource intensive work with complex families this will remain a challenge (Institute of Public Care 2012).

It is axiomatic that without an able and strong workforce that can adapt to new ways of working, policies and plans made with the best of intentions will not result in the changes that are required when introducing a public health approach. A comprehensive workforce development plan incorporating recruitment, training and retention strategies' including supervision, and support and management structures is essential – across all sectors. What is required is an integrated cross-sectoral workforce development plan across the continuum of universal, secondary and targeted services between government and non-government. Often agencies provide a 'one size fits all' approach to service delivery however families with complex needs will require flexible service responses to deal with a constellation of challenges and issues (Mason and O'Rinn 2014; Munro 2011).

15.3.8 Community and Family Partnerships

Article 18 of UNCROC states that for the purpose of guaranteeing and promoting children's rights, governments should provide "appropriate assistance to parents and legal guardians in the performance of their child rearing responsibilities". These articles in the Convention are important in ensuring that we support families, particularly vulnerable families, to enable children the opportunity to grow up in their own family and maintain their relationships. By partnering with families and supporting them in their child rearing responsibilities we are effectively serving the best interests of the child through enabling parents to care and ensure the safety of their children.

In countries where there is a strong focus on a family services approach such as Sweden and Denmark, relationships with parents are about developing a partnerships with parents are less adversarial (Allen Consulting Group 2003). This approach highlights ensuring that services meet the needs of families and resources are available to more families at an earlier stage. An example is the role of the maternal-child health nurse who visit mums with newborn babies or young children and other associated home visiting programs. There is evidence that home visiting programs can reduce or prevent child maltreatment particularly for women engaged prenatally (Peacock et al. 2013). Home visiting is an effective strategy for reaching all families including high-risk families to provide information, emotional support, and access to other services which are factors associated with ameliorating the risk of maltreatment (Howard and Brooks-Gunn 2009).

Central to a community-wide concept of prevention and early intervention is the importance of family engagement in services: a politic focused on relationships and removing the power of the expert. Indeed, as Tobis (2013) observed, the engagement is not sufficient: community engagement and participation requires shared leadership with those who are the 'targets' of services. Many services engaged with attempts to move services for children to a public health model have emphasised the importance and difficulty of operationalising the rhetoric of engaging community and participation. The prevailing view with which they struggle is the contrasting one in which parents are seen to be perpetrators who deserve punishment through an adversarial system. Inevitably, there are situations in which families do perpetrate terrible abuse and adversarial approaches are essential and urgent. However the majority of situations facing child welfare workers are ones in which there are chronic problems in which families are struggling to meet their child rearing responsibilities and with support and assistance the well-being and safety needs of the child could be met (Price-Robertson and Bromfield 2011).

To meet the needs of families it is the families themselves who know best what their needs and challenges are (Hamilton and Braithwaite 2014). It is therefore essential that innovative models of service delivery and provision can be achieved. This includes government agencies and NGO's working collaboratively to co-design services as well as engaging the end users, individuals and families, in the design of the service to meet their needs. In Australia both New South Wales and Western Australian child protection systems are utilising a co-design approach to redesign services with NGO's and communities, particularly Aboriginal communities to provide culturally safe and supportive services (Department for Child Protection and Family Support 2016; Family and Children Services 2015). This is a move away from the child protection system viewing itself as the expert and knowing or dictating what families need to do and how they should do it. Within a public health approach, co-design which includes both NGOs and families who are the end users will hopefully result in more effective and useful services for families.

15.3.9 Organisational and Cultural Change

Many of the obstacles identified above coalesce around a much larger and perhaps more complex challenge and that is the need for a change in organisational culture individually and collectively. A change of the magnitude required to 'shift the juggernaut of child protection' (Humphreys et al. 2009) requires a new language for services as well as a re-orientation of human services. All services, not just those traditionally engaged with the task of protecting children, need to move to enable a culture of engagement rather than a culture of 'notification', surveillance, monitoring, and processing – one that does not alienate and create fear in families but instead provides and sustains emotional support alongside the shared protection of children. Families will be more likely to engage in services with such an approach and less likely to feel stigmatised and shamed (Featherstone et al. 2013). Such a cultural change, it is proposed, requires a comprehensive re-framing by all services.

Importantly, changes in culture are predicated on a more nuanced engagement with what is now known as the culture of risk in child protection services. Significantly, leaders of these reforms are implementing changes in what are already risk saturated practice environments. In the era of risk management, our child protection systems have been focused on managing risks to workers, agencies and governments as well as the more obvious issue of risks to children. Indeed, there has been criticism that risk management by the child protection system is less about effectively supporting families and protecting children and more about protecting child protection systems from blame when adverse outcomes occur (Price-Robertson and Bromfield 2011). Highly publicised child deaths influence the risk assessment of the system and the workers within it (Connolly and Doolan 2007). Risk assessment drives child protection practice, can be very subjective and will vary markedly between child protection workers. It can be influenced by a variety of factors including experience, practice knowledge, ambiguity of information (Dorsey et al. 2008). Understandably, in a public health model where the expectation is that concerns about any and every risk to a child are not simply 'posted' to a statutory authority but are to some extent, and unless they are significant, managed by other agencies, there is a need for other agencies to accept more risk.

15.4 Overcoming the Obstacles

The calls for reform have come from inquiries, families, care leavers, practitioners, and researchers. Central to doing things differently is acknowledging the complexity of shifting the juggernaut – a shift that requires political will, the incremental accumulation of evidence, the engagement of communities and families and the promotion of positive developmental opportunities for children. Changing the focus and culture of a system that primarily relies on an investigative and adversarial approach to engaging creatively and working with families who have complex needs and issues is probably the largest hurdle to jump. As outlined this requires changes in service delivery structures, a focus on universal service provision and a community development approach to the public health model. It requires the development of multiagency strategies for working with families as well as the development of skills and flexible approaches for engaging complex families. The aphorism 'child protection is everyone's business' has tended to mean that everyone is responsible for reporting their concerns about risks to children to a statutory child protection authority. A public health approach requires the adoption of a nuanced understanding of this – one in which the well-being and safety of children is accepted as the business of all services and the whole community.

The current system is focused on managing risk, risks for children, families, child protection workers and processes. The need to engage families in supportive systems at lower levels of risk is required to reduce the pressure on the tertiary end of the system. "Research studies support the common sense notion that when protective factors are established in a family, the likelihood of child abuse and neglect diminishes" (New York State Office of Children and Families 2013, p. 1). It also involves agencies across systems increasing their capacity to support families, managing moderate levels of risk and working collaboratively with families to strengthen their parenting and ability to deal with multiple adversities. Importantly the system, services and agencies need to understand that a tertiary child protection system only requires the investigation of families at the highest levels of risk and those families which do not reach this threshold will inevitably have to be supported and served by agencies across government and community based services. The World Health Organisation has advocated that 'broader government policy and a whole-of-society approach should focus on developing nurturing and safer environments for children in families, communities and societies', this requires 'a shift in societal responses from one of child protection, culpability and blame to one that promotes welfare support to help families and children develop healthily and realize their full potential' (World Health Organisation2013, p. 93).

References

Allen Consulting Group. (2003). *Protecting children: The child protection outcomes project.* Melbourne: The Allen Consulting Group.

Allen Consulting Group. (2008). *Inverting the pyramid: Enhancing systems to protect children.* Melbourne: The Allen Consulting Group.

Anaf, J., Baum, F., Freeman, T., Labonte, R., Javanparast, S., Jolley, G., Lawless, A., & Bentley, M. (2014). Factors shaping intersectoral action in primary health care services. *Australia and New Zealand Journal of Public Health, 38*(6), 553–559.

Baum, F. (1998). *The new public health: An Australian perspective.* Melbourne: Oxford University Press.

Ben-Arieh, A. (2014). Social policy and the changing concept of child well-being. The role of international studies and children as active participants. *Zeitschri Fur Padagogik, 60*(4), 569–581.

Bilson, A., Cant, R. L., Harries, M., & Thorpe, D. H. (2017). Accounting for the increase of children in care in Western Australia: What can a client information system tell us? *Child Abuse and Neglect, 72*, 291–300.
Broadley, K., & Goddard, C. (2015). A public health approach to child protection: Why data matter. *Children Australia, 40*(1), 69–77.
Bromfield, L., Lamont, A., Parker, R., & Horsfall, R. (2010). *Issues for the safety and well-being of children in families with multiple and complex problems*. Melbourne: Australian Institute of Family Studies.
Bromfield, L., Arney, F., & Higgins, D. (2014). Contemporary issues in child protection intake, referral and family support. In A. Hayes & D. Higgins (Eds.), *Families, policies and the law: Selected essays on contemporary issues for Australia*. Melbourne: Australian Institute of Family Studies.
Bywaters, P., Brady, G., Sparks, T., & Bos, E. (2016). Child welfare inequalities: New evidence, further questions. *Child & Family Social Work, 21*(3), 369–380.
Connolly, M., & Doolan, M. (2007). Responding to deaths of children known to child protection agencies. *Social Policy Journal of New Zealand, 30*, 1–11.
Council of Australian Governments. (2009). *Protecting children is everyone's business: National framework for protecting Australia's children 2009–2020*. Canberra: Author. Retrieved from https://www.dss.gov.au/sites/default/files/documents/06_2012/nfpac_ar_2010_11_may_0.pdf
Daniel, B. (2010). Concepts of adversity, risk, vulnerability and resilience: A discussion in the context of the 'child protection system'. *Social Policy and Society, 9*(2), 231–241.
Darlington, Y., Feeney, J. A., & Rixon, K. (2005). Practice challenges at the intersection of child protection and mental health. *Child and Family Social Work, 10*(3), 239–247.
Department for Child Protection and Family Support. (2016). *Building safe and strong families: Earlier intervention and family support strategy*. Perth: DCPFS.
Dorsey, S., Mustillo, S., Farmer, E., & Elbogen, E. (2008). Caseworker assessments of risk for recurrent maltreatment: Association with case-specific risk factors and re-reports. *Child Abuse and Neglect, 32*(3), 377–391.
Family and Children's Services. (2015). *Guiding principles for strengthening the participation of local aboriginal community in child protection decision making*. Sydney: Family and Children's Services.
Featherstone, B., Morris, K., & White, S. (2013). A marriage made in hell: Early intervention meets child protection. *British Journal of Social Work, 44*(7), 1735–1149.
Featherstone, B., White, S., & Morris, K. (2015). *Re-imagining child protection: Towards humane social work with families*. Bristol: Policy Press.
Garrison, M. (2005). Reforming child protection: A public health perspective. *Virginia Journal of Social Policy and the Law, 12*, 590–637.
Hamilton, S., & Braithwaite, V. (2014). *Complex lives, complex needs, complex service systems, RegNet Occasional Paper No 21*. Canberra: Regulatory Institutions Network, Australian National University.
Hammond, R. (2003). Public health and child maltreatment prevention: The role of the centers for disease control and prevention. *Child Maltreatment, 8*(2), 82–83.
Homel, R., Lamb, C., & Freiberg, K. (2006). Working with the indigenous community in the pathways to prevention project. *Family Matters, 75*, 18–23.
Howard, K., & Brooks-Gunn, J. (2009). The role of home-visiting programs in preventing child abuse and neglect. *The Future of Children, 19*(2), 119–146.
Humphreys, C., Harries, M., Healy, K., Lonne, B., Mendes, P., McHugh, M., & Sheehan, R. (2009). Commentary: Shifting the child protection juggernaut to earlier intervention. *Children Australia, 34*(3), 5–9.
Institute of Public Care. (2012). *Commissioning for families with complex needs*. Oxford: Oxford Brookes University.
Keating, D. P., & Hertzman, C. (Eds.). (1999). *Developmental health and the wealth of nations: Social, biological and educational dynamics*. New York: Guildford Press.

Kempe, C. H., Silverman, F. N., Steele, B. F., Droegemueller, W., & Silver, H. K. (1962). The battered-child syndrome. *The Journal of the American Medical Association, 181*(1), 17–24.

Kennedy, R. J., & Richards, J. (2016). *Integrating human service law and practice, South Melbourne* (4th ed.). Melbourne: Oxford University Press.

Lang, T., & Rayner, G. (2012). Ecological public health: the 21st century's big idea? An essay by Tim Lang and Geof Rayner. *British Medical Journal, 345*, e5466. https://doi.org/10.1136/bmj.e5466.

Li, J., McMurray, A., & Stanley, F. (2008). Modernity's paradox and the structural determinants of child health and well-being. *Health Sociology Review, 17*(1), 64–77.

Lonne, B., Parton, N., Thomson, J., & Harries, M. (2009). *Reforming child protection*. London: Routledge.

Mason, R., & O'Rinn, S. E. (2014). Co-occurring intimate partner violence, mental health, and substance use problems: A scoping review. Co-occurring intimate partner violence, mental health and substance abuse problems: A scoping review. *Global Health Action, 7*, 24815. https://doi.org/10.3402/gha.v7.24815.

Masters, R., Anwar, E., Collins, B., Cookson, R., & Capewell, S. (2017). Return of investment of public health interventions: A systematic review. *Journal of Epidemiology of a Community Health, 71*, 827–834.

Melton, G. B., & Barry, F. D. (Eds.). (1995). *Protecting children from abuse and neglect: Foundations for a new national strategy*. New York: Guilford Publications.

Munro, E. (2011). *The Munro review of child protection: Final report, a child-centred system CM, 8062*. London: The Stationery Office.

New York State Office of Children and Families. (2013). *Promoting the well-being of children, youth and families in child welfare*. Retrieved from http://ocfs.ny.gov/main/cfsr/Promoting%20Well-Being2013.pdf

O'Donnell, M., & Stanley, F. (2007). *Ministerial community roundtable on child protection presentation*. Perth, Western Australia.

Peacock, S., Konrad, S., Watson, E., Nickel, D., & Muhajarine, N. (2013). Effectiveness of home visiting programs on child outcomes: A systematic review. *BMC Public Health, 13*, 17.

Pelton, L. H. (1998). Four commentaries: How we can better protect children from abuse and neglect. *The Future of Children, 8*(1), 126–129.

Price-Robertson, R., & Bromfield, L. (2011). *Risk assessment in child protection*. Melbourne: Australian Institute of Family Studies.

Scott, D. (2006). Towards a public health model of child protection in Australia. *Communities, Children and Families Australia, 1*(1), 9–16.

Scott, D. (2009). 'Think child, think family': How adult specialist services can support children at risk of abuse and neglect. *Family Matters, 81*, 37–42.

Scott, D., & Swain, S. (2002). *Confronting cruelty: Historical perspectives on child protection in Australia*. Melbourne: Melbourne University Press.

Seivwright, A., Flatau, P., Adams, S., & Stokes, C. (2016). *The future of outcomes measurement in the community sector in Western Australia* (Social impact series: No 6). Perth, Western Australia.

Spath, R., Werrbach, G. B., & Pine, B. A. (2008). Sharing the baton, not passing it: Collaboration between public and private child welfare agencies to reunify families. *Journal of Community Practice, 16*(4), 481–507.

Tobis, D. (2013). *From pariahs to partners: How parents and their allies changed New York City's child welfare system*. New York: Oxford University Press.

Victoria. Auditor-General. (2015). *Report of the Auditor-General: Early intervention services for vulnerable children and families*. Melbourne: Victorian Auditor-General's Office.

World Health Organisation. (2013). *European report on preventing child maltreatment*. Denmark: World Health Organisation.

Chapter 16
The Role, Importance and Challenges of Data for a Public Health Model

Debbie Scott and Agatha Faulkner

16.1 Introduction

Public healthresponses are based on a 'feedback loop' that identifies risk, measures the health outcome and/or associated risk factors, intervenes, assesses the effect of the intervention by re-assessing, modifies the intervention accordingly and cycles through this process again. The public health framework also consists of a continuum of services delivered in accordance with the risk of the adverse health consequence occurring in a population. Universal services are directed at whole populations, secondary services target populations at increased risk of the occurrence of the health outcome (usually because of their exposure to risk factors associated with the condition), and tertiary services target those populations where the health outcome exists and serve to minimise the effects of that outcome. Data relating to risk factors, the health outcome in question and affected populations are therefore integral to the implementation of the public health model.

The measurement of known risk factors associated with a public health outcome can assist in understanding the related outcome and inform future public health planning and policy. For example, reductions in the smoking rate in a population could be a proxy indicator of lower levels of future lung cancer incidents and may impact health service prioritisation. Similarly, within a child protection context, levels of poverty, substance misuse, maternal education, teen pregnancy and unemployment have all been associated with child maltreatment (Walker and Shepherd 2008) and therefore changes in these risk factors may also affect rates of maltreatment, and may be points of intervention.

D. Scott (✉) · A. Faulkner
Monash University, Box Hill, VIC, Australia

Turning Point, Richmond, VIC, Australia
e-mail: debbie.scott@monash.edu; Agatha.Faulkner@justice.tas.gov.au

B. Lonne et al. (eds.), *Re-Visioning Public Health Approaches for Protecting Children*, Child Maltreatment 9, https://doi.org/10.1007/978-3-030-05858-6_16

Before attempting to use or interpret data in any field of public health, understanding the unique challenges and limitations associated with data measurement is essential. As a concept, child maltreatment is broadly understood, but not well defined. There is no universal definition of child abuse or maltreatment and, although this doesn't impede measurement of population rates at a jurisdictional or 'study' level, it does impact on the comparability of rates over time and across studies or jurisdictions.

An extremely important component of a public health model is the evaluation of outcomes associated with program or policy interventions. Where sufficient high-quality data exist, outcomes can be measured for populations associated with specific risk factors, geographic regions or population types (e.g., culturally diverse, gender, age groups). Measuring client satisfaction with a program is valuable but may not provide outcome measures. Few programs have been evaluated for child protection outcomes (MacMillan et al. 2009).

16.2 Definitional Issues

A fundamental issue in capturing data on child maltreatment is the lack of a universally accepted definition (CFCA 2015). Definitions of maltreatment vary by jurisdiction, agency/organisation, context and culture (Pinheiro 2006). Researchers, legislators, practitioners and policy makers use various definitions depending on the context in which the definition is used (e.g., to extract a research sample from an administrative dataset, to identify families requiring tertiary intervention, or to identify children at risk in families where a parent is receiving treatment for mental health issues) (Scott 2012). Definitions of maltreatment are further complicated when the developmental stage of the child is considered, for example, when considering supervisory neglect, supervision for a toddler is quite different than would be expected for an adolescent. There is an additional layer of complexity in defining maltreatment when it is broken into subcategories. Tertiary child protection systems usually include neglect, sexual abuse, physical abuse, emotional maltreatment, exposure to family violence, however it may be reasonably argued that bullying, sibling abuse, exposure to community violence, organised exploitation (child prostitution, child workforce), institutional abuse (within institutional structures such as foster care, religious institutions, volunteer organisations), and state sanctioned abuse (e.g., Residential schools in Canada or Stolen Generation in Australia, female genital mutilation in some parts of Africa) are also child maltreatment (CFCA 2015) and should be considered in any public health response to child maltreatment.

Without a universally accepted definition of child maltreatment, measuring the incidence and prevalence in any population is difficult. Using data to understand the impact of any public health intervention or comparisons between jurisdictions then also becomes fraught because the outcome will be dependent on the source of the data, the population where it is being measured and the definition within that dataset.

Although definitional issues are important for any research or policy evaluation, there are still numerous sources of data that can contribute to the understanding of the magnitude, risks associated with maltreatment and the impact of policy and practice on outcomes – provided the limitation of the datasets are clearly understood.

16.3 Measurement Issues

Various methods are utilised for the measurement of child maltreatment in research and statistics, some of which stem from the definitional differences described above while others may be project and/or context-based dependent:

- Forms of maltreatment: Various forms of maltreatment exist, however the failure to consider each form can lead to underestimates of maltreatment, and fails to provide insight into how various forms of maltreatment often co-occur and influence each other;
- Harm or risk of harm: Some studies consider only children who have experienced some form of measurable harm, while others consider 'substantial risk of harm' in their measures;
- Incidence or prevalence: Reporting based on incidence (e.g., how many cases of maltreatment are recorded in a given time period) or prevalence (e.g., lifetime maltreatment occurrence) will result in different measures and may not be comparable; and/or
- Family level or individual level: Measurement can occur at the family level, or individual child level.

These measurement variations are most problematic when methods of a given study are not clearly described in study outlines or in trying to generate interjurisdictional comparisons (Fallon et al. 2010).

16.3.1 Administrative Data

Administrative datasets can be a rich source of information, provided the limitations are understood and accounted for. Not all jurisdictions will have accessible or reliable administrative data and in some cases, there is no data collected at all, for example, developing economies or jurisdictions where policies and practices do not require the collection of information. Where data exist, the quality is likely to differ between and within jurisdictions. Factors such as how data is captured (e.g., measurement of maltreatment), the systems that capture data (e.g., electronically vs paper-based), and how those systems function (e.g., in-built accuracy checks), differing service needs and funding levels (e.g., agencies with limited funding but high workload may not have the resources for reliable, well maintained systems) and staff engagement in seeing the value of accurate and timely documentation, are all factors that can impact on data quality/reliability. Additionally, those who are visible in one 'system' or dataset are more likely to be visible in others. For example, those who receive disability support may be more likely to appear in other income support databases. Research has shown that children who are already known to the child protection system and/or children who live in families with low socio-economic status or unemployment predicts engagement and, often, re-entry to the child protection system. Other research has demonstrated an institutional bias in child protection systems that supports the over representation of cultural minorities (e.g., Black, Indigenous, Culturally and Linguistically Diverse (CALD)) in child protection datasets (Hill 2004; Tilbury and Thoburn 2009).

Administrative data collections are seldom designed for statistical understanding of risk factors or outcomes, but for case management, business and administrative reasons and some may not be suitable for other purposes, particularly where the information may be affected by accuracy of the information recorded. Collecting research data can be perceived as an unwanted and unwarranted burden by those who are not directly involved in the research, this can affect the data quality and completeness. The representative capture of those cases of interest in the research within the data must also be carefully considered as this can affect the representativeness of the results. Additionally, where a database is created for one purpose, it may not be suitable for use in other contexts. Therefore, the use of any dataset must be considered carefully and the limitations considered in the context of the research being conducted. Liaison with data custodians is critical to understand the subtleties of these data and should form part of the process of any analysis.

16.3.2 Child Protection

Tertiary child protection systems in most jurisdictions collect data on services they provide to children and families, often providing the best available indicator of the extent of the child maltreatment. However, such data is fraught with issues of underreporting and cannot be used as an accurate measure of how many children in a community are subject to maltreatment. A number of studies in Australia have highlighted the issue of underreporting and point to various contributing factors; including the difficult or traumatic experience of disclosing such experiences to researchers and requiring the evidence to back up their claims; posing a significant challenge in many circumstances. Similar to other administrative data, child protection data relies on the detection and reporting of maltreatment incidents and consequently provides an underestimation of actual figures. Generally speaking these datasets capture reported and substantiated incidents of maltreatment and the system response to those substantiations, for example, court orders and children placed in out-of-home care. Data on the type of reported and substantiated harm is also available, but depends on system capacity and so may only include the most serious form of maltreatment, rather than all forms.

Some systems capture details on associated risk factors for the child and/or the family (such as alcohol and other drug misuse (AOD), family violence or homelessness), although this may not appear in the coded data but in the textual data held in client notes. Systems may also vary in whether they capture incidents of maltreatment at the family level, or the individual child level. An individual child is likely to have various incidents recorded in administrative data, and how these multiple incidents are aggregated or disaggregated needs to be established when reporting figures. It is also important to recognise that aggregate figures of a maltreatment event, using child protection/welfare data, can be reported at either the child-level or family-level. Figures at a child-level may appear inflated when compared with a jurisdiction that reports at the family level. Jurisdiction comparisons should therefore be disaggregated in a consistent manner to allow comparisons (Fallon et al. 2010).

Child protection administrative data are reflective of system capacity and areas where activity is directed therefore numbers will increase until system capacity is reached – and then they will level off. If additional child protection workers are employed to respond to community concerns of maltreatment, there will be a corresponding increase – until those additional workers reach their capacity, then numbers will level off again. The legislative framework and policies that child protection authorities respond to maltreatment will affect the data as well. For example, in a jurisdiction where all reports of 'harm' were collected for a period of time and the threshold raised to 'serious harm' the numbers of reports will appear to fall, not because there is a change in community behaviour but due to policy and practice changes. In a jurisdiction where the child protection system captures exposure to family violence under emotional abuse, if legislation is changed to require police reporting of all family violence there may be a corresponding increase in reports of emotional abuse but the actual levels of emotional abuse in the community remain unchanged.

16.3.3 Health

Morbidity or health data is a reliable source of information on population health, both nationally and internationally (Scott et al. 2009), and these data can be a rich source of information on child maltreatment. This is particularly true for physical abuse, but other health conditions associated with maltreatment can also be captured in health data. There are numerous forms and sources of health data that can be used to identify maltreatment related morbidity. These include ambulance data, emergency department data, hospital admission data, and mental health treatment data.

Health data is derived from the patients' clinical notes and, therefore, it is dependent on the treating clinician recognising or asking if the presentation is related to child maltreatment and consequently documenting that response. Furthermore, it is reliant on a coding system with the ability to capture the information with sufficient detail, reliability and consistency to enable statistical analysis (Scott et al. 2009).

There are subsets of morbidity data that can also be used, for example injurysurveillance or trauma registry data, to provide an additional level of information that will enable more granular analysis and detail that is otherwise unavailable without a medical record review. When utilising administrative hospital and morbidity data it is critical to note that there may be variation in both reliability and consistency between jurisdictions, over time and even within departments. Concerns about documentation of maltreatment suspicions have been identified in research studies (Scott and Fraser 2015) and are known to affect the reliability of morbidity data (McKenzie and Scott 2011a, b; McKenzie et al. 2012; Scott et al. 2009).

16.3.4 Police

Some child protection issues are reported to police (most commonly family violence and sexual assault) and so police data may provide insight into these issues. Family violence is considered a police issue in many jurisdictions and police and child protection workers often work together to respond to families where there are reports of 'disturbances' and children are present (Osofsky 2003). One Canadian study found that police were the second most likely professional group to report child abuse (16% of reports) after school personnel (17%) but before social workers (10%) and health care professionals (8%) (Tonmyr et al. 2010). The accessibility of these data as coded variables in police databases will vary and may require text searches in some jurisdictions.

16.3.5 Other

Data sources are potentially only limited by the imagination of the researcher and the willingness of the data custodian to work with researchers to provide meaning and utility to those data. Some datasets will not have direct reference to child protection issues, for example, education, vaccination registers, adult AOD treatment, however linking multiple datasets can provide rich information about correlates, risk factors and outcomes. The limitations of a single dataset can be overcome by performing data linkage and 'gaps' in one dataset may be offset by combining with another (see for example Cadzow and Armstrong 2000; O'Donnell et al. 2010, 2011; Parrish et al. 2011; Putnam-Hornstein 2011; Putnam-Hornstein and Needell 2011; Schnitzer 2004).

16.4 Survey Data

As described above, data to describe the magnitude of the problem and to assess the impact of any intervention is critical to a public health approach. In any research, the utility of the results are reliant on the quality of the data and how they can be generalised to populations of interest. Survey data is an alternative where administrative or death data does not meet the study needs, particularly when aiming to provide estimates of prevalence or incidence of child maltreatment, attitudes and cultural understandings of maltreatment or specific details on program participant experiences of an intervention. For example, national estimates of incidence or prevalence of maltreatment will be underestimated if administrative data from health or child protection systems are used, however a well-designed community survey may provide better quality data if the response rate reflects a significant proportion of the community.

Administrative data is often seen as a preferable option to surveys because the routine nature of the data collection minimises potential bias and is less likely to cause additional distress to individuals. However, these are offset by recognition that survey data asks the question researchers want in a routine and systematised way minimising potential error.

16.4.1 Survey Modality

Face-to-face interviews and pencil and paper surveys were once the only survey tools available for researchers. Advances in technology and increased global access to the internet have increased the modes of surveying available and have had a significant impact on study costs, data management, data accuracy and access to a wider demographic of survey participants.

Survey samples were once overrepresented by easy-to-access groups such as university psychology students, but with increased phone use and access to the internet a wider demographic of study participants are now just as easily accessible. In the field of public health, where the aim is to draw conclusions at a population level, this is a critical progression.

With progression comes a set of additional complexities and considerations when interpreting data, such as sampling bias and comparability of data between various modes of surveying (e.g., issues of confounding). Sampling bias can occur when some populations are more likely than others to respond to one modality (such as mobile phone only surveys) compared to another modality (such as mobile and landline combined). Additionally, research is currently ongoing about the impact of survey modality on responses to questionnaire items (Bates and Cox 2008; Livingston et al. 2015). In particular, face-to-face or pencil and paper surveys are likely to yield different responses compared to online only surveys. There are several reasons for this, including anonymity and confidentiality of information which may be perceived differently across survey modalities. Some evidence suggests when asking participants sensitive questions, such as those relating to sexual behaviours, responses are most accurate (or internally valid) when surveying is conducted through an online setting compared with face-to-face surveying (Richman et al. 1999). Survey studies of child maltreatment may therefore require careful consideration when interpreting or comparing data from studies that utilise differing survey methodologies. Of note, however, when content is considered less sensitive or neutral, differences in survey modality appear to have minimal impact on internal validity (Bates and Cox 2008).

16.4.2 Questionnaire and Study Design

Definitional issues in the field of child maltreatment were discussed previously and of additional significance in survey research is the need for consistency in questionnaire design to allow cross-jurisdictional comparisons. This includes how questions are worded and the consistency of response options. This can be particularly difficult to attain across cultures and language but the iCAST tool and its implementation in the BECAN study and Dunne et al.'s 2009 work in Asia as described below are examples of how this can be done.

To measure and compare prevalence and incidence of child maltreatment requires similar forms of measurement. Due to the lack of consistency in recent approaches, the World Health Organization (WHO) and the International Society for the Prevention of Child Abuse and Neglect (ISPCAN) established a set of recommendations to enable internationally comparable and reliable data on measuring children's exposure to violence (Butchart et al. 2006).

In addition to an agreed international standard to allow comparability, other factors need to be considered in study design: Surveys need to be non-threatening, consider the balance between not enough vs too much detail in terms of likelihood of distress. Language skill should be considered and when considering technology-based surveys, how competent some groups may be in using such technology. This is particularly important across various cultural groups that may have varied experience with technology and differing literacy levels.

16.4.3 Working with Children

Surveying of children for the purposes of participants' experiences of child maltreatment can be controversial and the risk of conducting any such survey needs to be balanced by the importance of giving children and youth a voice. Concerns about involving children in survey research include the potential that children may not have the experience or ability to contextualise an event as maltreatment. Should a child disclose a situation where they are in an abusive situation, researchers must have a process in place to respond to that disclosure and provide for the safety of the child. The requirement that a research participant give an informed consent may make assessing the potential consequences in terms of risks and benefits of participation impossible for children, particularly young children, therefore parental consent may be required. Parents who fear that a child may disclose abuse are likely to refuse consent to participate – potentially forming a source of bias for the study.

The challenges associated with such studies are reflected by the limited number of internationally validated survey instruments involving children and young people's experiences of maltreatment. The Juvenile Victimization Questionnaire (Hamby et al. 2005) has been developed for youth and adults, covering a broad range of 'victimizations' including child maltreatment.

The ICAST tool, is a 38 item self-report measure for children developed by ISPCAN for prevalence studies across diverse contexts (Dunne et al. 2009; Nikolaidis et al. 2018). The tool was developed to provide internationally comparative survey data and has been implemented and tested across multiple countries.

Implementing such surveys among children has its challenges and may have implications on final outcomes. Recruiting a representative sample of children may be difficult and can involve recruitment through schools or other means. In some countries such as Australia, schools are increasingly difficult to access by researchers, as curriculums are becoming 'overloaded'. School samples are also prone to bias, for example children most at risk of maltreatment are likely to have low school attendance and may not be well represented in such samples (Fantuzzo et al. 2011). The content of the survey needs to be considered, and whether schools are an appropriate place to run surveys where distress is a possible outcome among peers. Other options include random selection procedures such as random-digit dial telephone surveys, as implemented in a US study. A short interview was conducted with a caregiver, before a child was interviewed (Finkelhor et al. 2005). However, the presence of a parent nearby may have significant impact on children's responses and it is noted that counsellors or support staff cannot be physically present in case of a serious disclosure and/or distressful outcome.

16.4.4 Adult-Related Surveys

Survey studies involving adults are somewhat more straightforward and can involve parents and other caregivers or those in specialist fields of practice such as child protection workers. Surveys can include questions relating to attitudes and/or beliefs related to child maltreatment or measures related to family risk and protective factors. Studies (Finkelhor et al. 2005); have demonstrated it is possible to survey parents and other caregivers (Finkelhor et al. 2011; Straus et al. 1998) regarding their own or other caregiver's behaviours of maltreatment even when acts have been committed against their own children. However, the authors noted the importance of creating a safe and confidential environment for caregivers as a means of improving the likelihood of participants responding openly and honestly; parents and caregivers may feel embarrassment, shame or even fear of potential consequences. However, Finkelhor et al. (2011) also noted that for some families (particularly for some cultures), violence and maltreatment that includes hitting, punching or yelling at children is not always considered unusual or wrong. It's important that researchers in the field keep 'in check' their own values and assumptions when designing surveys and communicating with participants. Adapting the survey to fit specific cultural settings and organisation needs is also a consideration, as is recommended by Mathews et al. (2016) in their recommendations to the Australian Royal Commission into Institutional Child Sexual Abuse.

There are various studies involving those from specialist fields. For example, the CIS (Canadian Incidence Study of Reported Child Abuse and Neglect)/NIS (National Incidence Study of Child Abuse and Neglect) – North America and Canada National surveys- conducted with child protection workers and asks about their experiences in their role, regarding their investigations of alleged child maltreatment (Fallon et al. 2010). The CIS uses a serial survey methodology, asking the same set of questions are various points in time (Fallon et al. 2010). A new sample of children are selected for each study round, limiting the conclusions that can be drawn longitudinally (e.g., causality).

16.4.5 Cultural Factors

Previously, we mentioned the need for international consistency as a means of accurately measuring prevalence and incidence of maltreatment. An overly Westernised approach may be fraught with issues, such as the conceptualisation of maltreatment. Child maltreatment in one society may not be so in another, as we have touched on previously. The nuances may be experienced within and across countries and should always be a consideration in interpreting administrative and survey data.

Cultural awareness is therefore critical and relevant to the content of a survey and mode of surveying. The mode of inquiry can have a significant impact on how well the participant engages with the study content and the researcher. In some cultures asking sensitive questions relating to maltreatment is not well understood because it is an unspoken topic or considered a deeply private family issue. For example, In Aboriginal cultures the content itself may be highly sensitive, and would require the input of from elders and others in the community. In such settings, a paper and pencil questionnaire may not be understood because some community members are not exposed to such forms of communication, or may have limited literacy, and therefore the only mode of inquiry would be face-to-face interviews. Cultural customs such as not looking someone in the eyes need to be acknowledged, and where possible, the researcher and the participant should be matched on gender and cultural background in a way that builds trust and openness to responses.

16.5 Death Data

Understanding the mortality statistics associated with a condition are an important component of a public health approach. There are significant challenges in obtaining timely, reliable death data, particularly for deaths associated with child abuse and neglect. WHO (2016) estimates 41,000 violence-related deaths globally every year in children under the age of 15.

Mortality statistics are reliant on the complete capture of deaths in a population. Statistical reporting of child death is possible using coded mortality data from WHO member states. A recent study found that high quality data was available for only 20 countries of 83 who capture death data at all and the statistics are likely to represent only 28% of the global population (Bhalla et al. 2010). In countries where birth and death registration is less well established there is little research to describe the reliability and completeness child maltreatment death data. These countries are likely to rely on either a community survey for cause of death information or perhaps, verbal autopsies where the cause of death is determined/assigned by a doctor (if present) or a tribal elder (CFCA 2017). Mortality statistics are reliant on the ICD coding of the death certificate and an additional impediment to these statistics relates to the coding rules for ICD10. Where there is any doubt as to the intent, coding rules require that the default code assigned is ‘accidental’ where no clear determination of ‘intentional’ is made, therefore the ICD codes for maltreatment are often not assigned (Scott et al. 2009). Research has supported this with a recent study finding that difficulties in determining intent between unintentional and inflicted injury may result in the misclassification of cause of death (Fraser et al. 2014).

Child death review teams (CDRT) are well established in the United Kingdom, Canada, USA and Australia. CDRT primarily take one of two forms (Scott 2017);

1. Review of a specified groups of deaths associated with a defined population. These may be related to children within a certain age range (e.g., under 5 years), those associated with a cause of death (e.g., perinatal or Sudden Unexplained Death in Infancy), or a certain risk factor (e.g., child maltreatment) with a view to identifying systemic issues for modification to reduce deaths. These reviews may be on a case-by-case basis or include a group of children within a specific jurisdiction and often the findings are not made public.
2. Review of all deaths. This type of review uses a public health approach and may consider systemic issues but include recommendations related to other risk factors as well. For example, a review of deaths associated with external causes will include those deaths that may be due to inflicted injury be self or others (physical abuse) or failure to supervise (supervisory neglect). These reviews are often reported publically and recommendations may include preventive messages (e.g., safe sleep practice, pool fencing) but may also include recommendations for systems or policy improvement (e.g., formation of a review panel for consumer product safety issues, changes to legislation relating to quadbike use).

CDRTs that examine only those deaths where the child was known to 'the system' may be missing a broader opportunity. Where a death is due to or has a significant contribution from risk factors associated with maltreatment it is important to consider why the child wasn't known to authorities who could have intervened to prevent the death. A public health response that considers all child deaths and risk factors in the social ecological model like that recommended by Bronfenbrenner allows for a broader understanding of child, familial, community and societal factors that can be modified to prevent these deaths (Krug et al. 2002).

Child death review teams are an important source of information on not only child maltreatment deaths, but all child deaths. However, the data are of limited use to contribute to the understanding of national rates of maltreatment death because of the different forms of review and definitions for inclusion in the reviews.

16.6 Ethical Considerations

There are important ethical considerations in the use of administrative data. In large, epidemiological studies it may not be feasible, or possible to obtain consent for the data to be used by third parties, and so it is critically important that confidentiality of the records is maintained with careful attention paid to presentation of the results to ensure no individual is compromised or potentially identified. It is also important to report research results sensitively so as not to stigmatise or 'blame'.

In survey research, all researchers must consider potential risks, benefits and harms of both the conduct of the survey itself and the use of the data resulting from the survey. Consideration must be given to:

- What distress is the survey likely to cause for participants and interviewers?
- How can distress be minimised?
- What balance can be provided between anonymity of study participants and disclosures of harm or wrong doing?
- What harms are likely to occur with the circulation of outcomes of the study and how will the results be reported and used? What are potential unintended consequences be (e.g., stigmatisation of a minority group)?
- Do the benefits outweigh the potential harm to individuals?

Research that involves children is increasingly being seen as an important component of a public health model for child protection, and child wellbeing more broadly (Graham et al. 2013). The right of children to be involved in research that affects them is upheld by the United Nations Convention on the Rights of the Child (UNCRoC) (United Nations 1989). It is important, however to balance the tension between respecting the right to be heard and the need to be protected from harm in research. The issue of informed consent is also critical when conducting research with children. Children should be able to understand the risks and benefits of participation, and parental consent may also be required. There is no 'one size fits all' approach to conducting research with children; it will require researchers to consider their practice beyond simple ethical approval processes and identify how their conduct influences, balances the need for information and the need to be kept safe, and responds to children participating in research. An important document that can guide and inform ethical research with children is 'Ethical Research Involving Children' available through UNICEF at https://childethics.com/.

16.7 Conclusions

A public health model is cyclical and relies on data that is accurate, valid, reliable, timely, relevant and complete. Data are used to understand the initial magnitude of child protection, the prevalence and association with risk factors and, after intervention, the impact of an intervention of outcomes. Any implementation of a public health model for child protection will require the use of data to provide an evidence base, support public health responses, and measure outcomes post intervention.

There are multiple potential sources of data that can inform the measurement of child maltreatment and associated risk factors; and of program and policy intervention outcomes, enabling public health practitioners to draw on a broader set of evidence to rigorously inform research and evaluation processes. However, definitional issues, data reliability and consistency must be addressed as part of a public health model through the acknowledgement and understanding of the strengths and benefits of each data source. This data becomes even more critical in considering evidence associated with evaluating outcomes and monitoring trends over time and across jurisdictions.

Public health practitioners in the field of child maltreatment must carefully consider, in addition to data rigour, the ethical and cultural challenges of conducting studies in such an area. It is essential that both factors be a consideration throughout all stages of research development, from planning, implementation and data reporting; weighing up the feasibility, potential harms and benefits of the various approaches outlined throughout this chapter.

References

Bates, S. C., & Cox, J. M. (2008). The impact of computer versus paper-pencil survey, and individual versus group administration, on self-reports of sensitive behaviors. *Computers in Human Behavior, 24*, 903–916.

Bhalla, K., Harrison, J., Shahraza, S., & Fingerhut, L. (2010). Availability and quality of cause-of-death data for estimating the global burden of injuries. *Bulletin of the World Health Organization, 88*, 831–838.

Butchart, A., Phinney Harvey, A., Kahane, T., Mian, M., & Fuerniss, T. (2006). *Preventing child maltreatment: A guide to taking action and generating evidence*. Geneva: World Health Organization.

Cadzow, S. P., & Armstrong, K. L. (2000). Rib fractures in infants: Red alert! The clinical features, investigations and child protection outcomes. *Journal of Paediatrics and Child Health, 36*(4), 322–326.

Child Family Community Australia (CFCA). (2015). *What is child abuse and neglect? Resource Sheet.* Retrieved from https://aifs.gov.au/cfca/publications/what-child-abuse-and-neglect

Child Family Community Australia (CFCA). (2017). *Child deaths from abuse and neglect. Resource sheet.* Retrieved from https://aifs.gov.au/cfca/publications/child-deaths-abuse-and-neglect

Dunne, M., Zolotor, J., Runyan, D., Andreva-Miller, I., Yuen Choo, W., Dunne, S., Gerbaka, B., Dipty-Jain, O., Kasim, S., Macfarlane, B., Mamyrova, N., Ramirez, C., Volkova, E., & Youssef, R. (2009). ISPCAN Child Abuse Screening Tools Retrospective version (ICAST-R): Delphi study and field testing in seven countries. *Child Abuse and Neglect, 33*(11), 815–825.

Fallon, B., Trocmé, N., Fluke, J., MacLaurin, B., Tonmyr, L., & Yuan, Y. Y. (2010). Methodological challenges in measuring child maltreatment. *Child Abuse & Neglect, 34*, 70–79.

Fantuzzo, J. W., Perlman, S. M., & Dobbins, E. K. (2011). Types and timing of child maltreatment and early school success: A population-based investigation. *Children and Youth Services Review, 33*(8), 1404–1411.

Finkelhor, D., Ormrod, R., Turner, H., & Hamby, S. (2005). The victimisation of children and youth: A comprehensive national survey. *Child Maltreatment, 10*(1).

Finkelhor, D., Turner, H., & Hamby, S. (2011). *Questions and answers about the National Survey of Children's exposure to violence* (OJJDP Juvenile Justice Bulletin – NCJ235163, pp. 1–4). Washington, DC: US Government Printing Office.

Fraser, J., Sidbotham, P., Frederick, J., Covington, T., & Mitchell, E. (2014). Learning from child death review in the USA, England, Australia, and New Zealand. *The Lancet, 384*(9946), 894–903.

Graham, A., Powell, M., Taylor, N., Anderson, D., & Fitzgerald, R. (2013). *Ethical research involving children.* Florence: UNICEF Office of Research – Innocenti.

Hamby, S. L., Finkelhor, D., Ormrod, R., & Turner, H. (2005). *The juvenile victimization questionnaire (JVQ): Administration and scoring manual.* Durham: Crimes Against Children Research Center.

Hill, R. (2004). Institutional racism in child welfare. *Race and Society, 7*(1), 17–33.

Krug, E., Dahlberg, L., Mercy, J., Zwi, A., & Lozano, R. (2002). *World report on violence and health.* Geneva: World Health Organization.

Livingston, M., Komro, K., & Wagenaar, A. (2015). The effects of survey modality on adolescents' responses to alcohol use items. *Alcoholism: Clinical and Experimental Research, 39*(4), 710–715.

MacMillan, H., Wathen, N., Barlow, J., Fergusson, D., Leventhal, J., & Taussig, H. (2009). Interventions to prevent child maltreatment and associated impairment. *The Lancet, 373*(9659), 250–266.

Mathews, B., Walsh, K., Dunne, M., Katz, I., Arney, F., Higgins, D., Octoman, O., Parkinson, S., & Bates, S. (2016). *Scoping study for research into the prevalence of child abuse in Australia: Report to the Royal Commission into Institutional Responses to Child Sexual Abuse. Sydney: Social Policy Research Centre* (SPRC Report 13/16). UNSW Australia in partnership with Australian Institute of Family Studies, Queensland University of Technology and the Australian Centre for Child Protection (University of South Australia).

McKenzie, K., & Scott, D. (2011a). Using routinely collected hospital data for child maltreatment surveillance: Issues, methods and patterns. *BMC Public Health, 11*, 7.

McKenzie, K., & Scott, D. (2011b). Reliability of routinely collected hospital data for child maltreatment surveillance: Issues, methods and patterns. *BMC Public Health, 11*, 8.

McKenzie, K., Scott, D., Fraser, J., & Dunne, M. (2012). Assessing the effectiveness of the child safety net: Linkage of hospital and child protection services data on 'maltreated' and 'unintentionally injured' children. *Injury Prevention, 18*, 50–57.

Nikolaidis, G., Petroulaki, K., Zarokosta Tsirigoti, A., Hazizaj, A., Cenko, E., Brkic-Smigoc, J., Vajzovic, E., Stancheva, V., Chincheva, S., Ajdukovic, M., Rajter, M., Raleva, M., Trpcevska, L., Roth, M., Antal, I., Ispanovic, V., Hanak, N., Olmezoglu-Sofuoglu, Z., Umit-Bal, I., Bianchi,

D., Meinck, F., & Browne, K. (2018). Lifetime and past-year prevalence of children's exposure to violence in 9 Balkan countries: The BECAN study. *Child and Adolescent Psychiatry and Mental Health, 12*(1).

O'Donnell, M., Nassar, N., Leonard, H., Mathews, R., Patterson, Y., & Stanley, F. (2010). Monitoring child abuse and neglect at a population level: Patterns of hospital admissions for maltreatment and assault. *Child Abuse and Neglect, 34*(11), 823–832.

O'Donnell, M., Nassar, N., Jacoby, P., & Stanley, F. (2011). Western Australian emergency department presentations related to maltreatment and intentional injury: Population level study utilising linked health and child protection data. *Journal of Paediatrics and Child Health, 48*(10), 57–65.

Osofsky, J. (2003). Prevalence of children's exposure to domestic violence and child maltreatment: Implications for prevention and intervention. *Clinical Child and Family Psychology Review, 6*(3), 161–170.

Parrish, J., Young, M., Perham-Hester, K., & Gessner, B. (2011). Identifying risk factors for child maltreatment in Alaska: A population based approach. *The American Journal of Preventive Medicine, 40*(6), 666–673.

Pinheiro, P. S. (2006). *World report on violence against children*. Geneva: UNICEF.

Putnam-Hornstein, E. (2011). Report of child maltreatment as a risk factor for injury death: A prospective birth cohort study. *Child Maltreatment, 16*(3), 163–174.

Putnam-Hornstein, E., & Needell, B. (2011). Predictors of child protective service contact between birth and age five: An examination of California's 2002 birth cohort. *Children and Youth Services Review, 33*(11), 2400–2407.

Richman, W. L., Kiesler, S., Weisband, S., & Drasgow, F. (1999). A meta-analytic study of social desirability distortion in computer-administered questionnaires, traditional questionnaires, and interviews. *Journal of Applied Psychology, 84*, 754–773.

Schnitzer, P. G. (2004). Child maltreatment in Missouri: Combining data for public health surveillance. *The American Journal of Preventative Medicine, 27*(5), 379–384.

Scott, D. (2012). *Improving the measurement and surveillance of child abuse in Queensland emergency departments*. Doctor of Health Science. Brisbane: Queensland University of Technology.

Scott, D. (2017). *Reporting of fatal neglect in NSW.* Retrieved from https://www.ombo.nsw.gov.au/news-and-publications/publications/reports/child-death-review-team/reporting-of-fatal-neglect-in-nsw

Scott, D., & Fraser, J. (2015). Mandatory reporting of child abuse and neglect by health professionals. In B. Mathews & D. Bross (Eds.), *Mandatory reporting laws and the identification of severe child abuse and neglect* (pp. 381–394). Denver: Springer.

Scott, D., Tonmyr, L., Fraser, J., Walker, S., & McKenzie, K. (2009). The use of ICD in child maltreatment research: Literature review. *Child Abuse and Neglect, 33*(11), 791–808.

Straus, M. A., Hamby, S. L., Finkelhor, D., Moore, D. W., & Runyan, D. (1998). Identification of child maltreatment with the Parent-Child Conflict Tactics Scales: Development and psychometric data for a national sample of American parents. *Child Abuse and Neglect, 22*(4), 249–270.

Tilbury, C., & Thoburn, J. (2009). Using racial disproportionality and disparity indicators to measure child welfare outcomes. *Children and Youth Services Review, 31*(10), 1101–1106.

Tonmyr, L., Li, Y. A., Williams, G., Scott, D., & Jack, S. M. (2010). Patterns of reporting by health care and nonhealth care professionals to child protection services in Canada. *Paediatrics & Child Health, 15*(8), E25–E32.

United Nations. (1989). *Convention on the rights of the child.* Retrieved from https://www.ohchr.org/EN/ProfessionalInterest/Pages/CRC.aspx

Walker, R., & Shepherd, C. (2008). *Strengthening Aboriginal family functioning: What works and why?* (AFRC Briefing 7). Melbourne: AIFS.

World Health Organization (WHO). (2016). *Child maltreatment.* Geneva: WHO. Retrieved from www.who.int/mediacentre/factsheets/fs150/en/

Chapter 17
Understanding the Neighbourhood and Community Factors Associated with Child Maltreatment

Paul Bywaters

17.1 Introduction

It is often said that it takes a village to raise a child. Over the years, a key debate in the field of child abuse and neglect has been whether community or neighbourhood has an independent effect on maltreatment rates in addition to the impact of poverty and wider socio-economic forces on individuals. Is it children, parents, households, groups or places that are the most appropriate focus of attention for those wanting to reduce maltreatment? While most research is clear in reinforcing the idea that neighbourhood as well as individual factors affect the incidence of maltreatment, exactly what the nature of that relationship is and what can be done as a consequence is less well evidenced (Minh et al. 2017; Sharkey and Faber 2014). This chapter discusses these issues and argues the need to struggle with their complexity, placing the discussion in the context of an inequalities perspective.

Population studies internationally have found very large inequalities in the proportion of children who experience child abuse or neglect associated with three key factors: identity – who they are; place – where they live; and community – to which group of people they may be said to belong (Gilbert 2011; Gilbert et al. 2012). As with inequalities in child health and education, inequalities in child maltreatment can be a matter of chance, but more commonly they reflect structural economic, social and environmental factors. As such, inequities in the incidence of maltreatment are a matter of social justice and human rights, as well as reflecting individual human suffering (Bywaters 2015; Davidson et al. 2017).

Responding to child maltreatment within a public health paradigm requires actions to address how economic, social and environmental factors influence not only the overall level of maltreatment but also the inequitable distribution of mal-

P. Bywaters (✉)
University of Huddersfield, Huddersfield, UK
e-mail: P.Bywaters@hud.ac.uk

B. Lonne et al. (eds.), *Re-Visioning Public Health Approaches for Protecting Children*, Child Maltreatment 9, https://doi.org/10.1007/978-3-030-05858-6_17

treatment between areas and between groups. This involves taking a whole population approach to analysing the fundamental causes of maltreatment and substantiated maltreatment rates within the central objective of reducing the incidence of abuse and neglect (Phelan et al. 2010; Sethi et al. 2013). Three key lessons emerge from the study of health inequalities (Graham 2007; WHO 2008):

- Reducing overall rates of maltreatment alone does not guarantee that maltreatment is more equally distributed;
- Without reducing inequity in the distribution of maltreatment, maximum reduction of maltreatment rates cannot be achieved; and
- Achieving greater equity is primarily a matter of addressing the underlying structural causes of maltreatment but reducing inequities in service responses to maltreatment is also important.

Effective action to reduce maltreatment, therefore, has to address the social structures that shape people's lives, the differential experience of particular communities and groups, and factors affecting individual children, parents and others. This will involve primary, secondary and tertiary prevention. Primary prevention means measures that are designed to prevent maltreatment occurring at the whole population level, for example, by legislation relating to corporal punishment or to redistribute income, wealth and other basic resources. Secondary prevention means action to reduce the greater likelihood of maltreatment affecting particular populations of children, for example, by focusing on groups at greater risk such as families in poverty, disabled children or indigenous peoples subject to institutional discrimination. Tertiary prevention means mitigating the consequences of maltreatment for children who experience it, for example, by providing services to enhance resilience, repair traumatic childhood experiences and prevent recurrence. A comprehensive approach to prevention involves actions at macro, meso and micro levels.

This deceptively simple position statement underpins this chapter which focuses on the role of place and community in child maltreatment. It presents recent evidence from the United Kingdom (UK) which explores structural relationships between neighbourhood deprivation, service supply, ethnicity and maltreatment rates. This evidence is used to illustrate some of the theoretical and methodological complexities involved in building clear evidence about the nature and direction of factors associated with maltreatment and some of the insights that result from taking a whole population approach. Finally, the chapter discusses recent evidence from the United States about patterns of neighbourhood and community factors that may affect children's chances and experiences of maltreatment.

17.2 Place, Community and Inequity: A UK Case Study

17.2.1 Neighbourhood, Community and Maltreatment: The Role of Deprivation

A recent study of the proportion of children with substantiated child protection concerns in the United Kingdom (UK), funded by the Nuffield Foundation (www.coventry.ac.uk/cwip) has revealed substantial differences between and within the four UK countries: England, Northern Ireland (NI), Scotland and Wales (Table 17.1). Child welfare policy is a devolved responsibility from the UK government to the four national governments, with crucial differences in legislation, service structures and the political context emerging increasingly clearly in the past two decades (Bunting et al. 2018; McGhee et al. 2018). Examining child maltreatment data at a population level raises profound questions about policy and practice and the four UK countries provide a form of 'natural experiment' for testing hypotheses about causation and intervention. This example is used here to illustrate key issues and complexities in disentangling the role of place and community in child maltreatment.

At first sight (Table 17.1, right hand column), rates per 10,000 children in England, Northern Ireland and Wales are very similar, with Scotland being the outlier. However, when the level of deprivation affecting children is taken into account a rather different picture emerges.

Deprivation is measured here using Index of Multiple Deprivation scores for small neighbourhoods containing up to 2000 people. These scores are based on two key indicators, the income and employment levels of households. Using these measures, every neighbourhood in the UK can be allocated a rank which can be converted into five equal groups from the least deprived 20% of neighbourhoods (column 1) to the most deprived 20% (column 5). Next, the total child (0-17) population in each neighbourhood – and therefore in each quintile – can be identified from mid-year estimates. Finally, by identifying the neighbourhoods in which children with substantiated protection concerns (children on child protection plans or registers) live, the proportion of such children in each quintile (the intervention rate per 10,000 children) can be calculated. This convoluted approach to linking deprivation to maltreatment at a population level is necessary in the UK in the absence of

Table 17.1 Proportion of children per 10,000 in the population who have substantiated child protection concerns by neighbourhood deprivation quintile, four UK countries, 2015

	Neighbourhood Deprivation Quintiles: 1 = least deprived					
	1	2	3	4	5	All
England	11	22	33	49	94	44
NI	[a]	14	23	37	68	43
Scotland	4	9	21	25	57	26
Wales	5	11	26	47	94	45

[a]Numbers of children too small for rates to be reliable

any systematic data about the socio-economic circumstances of individual families where child protection is an identified issue. Dividing the child population into five quintiles in this way quantifies the link between a child's chances of maltreatment and their socio-economic circumstances.

17.2.2 Neighbourhood, Community and Maltreatment: The Social Gradient in Maltreatment

Table 17.1 shows clear evidence of a social gradient in substantiated child maltreatment. In every UK country the rate of substantiated child protection concerns increases step by step as deprivation increases. This would be expected from widespread international evidence of a structural relationship between socio-economic circumstances and maltreatment (Bywaters et al. 2016; Slack et al. 2017). Rates in quintile 5 are between 8 and 19 times greater than in quintile 1 in the different countries. The steepness of the social gradient varies between countries but is present in all. This applies too in each local authority (LA) or Health and Social Care Trust area in the four countries.

The social gradient implies that prevention and service provision should be focused proportionately across the population and that two central objectives of policy should be, first, to reduce rates in higher deprivation neighbourhoods towards those in the least deprived and, second, to reduce the slope of the gradient so that each step increase in deprivation has a smaller impact on maltreatment levels (Marmot and Bell 2016). Applying the methodology of Asaria et al. (2016) for health inequalities, if all neighbourhoods in the UK had the substantiated child protection rates of the least deprived 20% of neighbourhoods, the numbers of children involved would be reduced by almost 75%.

This population level perspective also tells us (again unsurprisingly) that notified child maltreatment does not just occur in impoverished neighbourhoods but across all levels of neighbourhood deprivation from the most disadvantaged to the most affluent. In this example, because of the absence of systematic data on individual family circumstances, it may be that maltreated children in low deprivation neighbourhoods are from isolated households in poverty. But pressures on families (Conger and Elder 1994) exist across all levels of socio-economic status although they vary in nature and intensity. A focus on impoverished neighbourhoods alone would exclude many maltreated children. In the UK countries over 40% of substantiated cases are from households living outside the most deprived 20% of neighbourhoods. Like Rose et al. (2008) the approach suggested advocates for preventive measures that are not only targeted at the most disadvantaged populations, as many children who are maltreated are found across the social spectrum. However, as Rose's critics have argued (Frolich and Potvin 2008), unless prevention takes into account the differential impact of social inequality it can exacerbate inequities in maltreatment even if it is effective in reducing the overall incidence.

The social gradient in Wales is steeper than in the other three UK countries. The reasons for this are unknown. As yet, in child maltreatment discussions internationally, little focus has been placed on the gradient and potential measures to reduce its impact, by comparison with the gradient in health or educational attainment, through approaches such as proportionate universalism (Marmot 2010; Marmot and Bell 2016). More research is needed to identify the factors which influence the steepness of the slope, and policies which can effectively reduce it. These are likely to include both measures to reduce the scale of inequality in social conditions between and within neighbourhoods and the impact of those inequalities on maltreatment (Eckenrode et al. 2014).

17.2.3 Neighbourhood, Community and Maltreatment: Supply and Demand

Differential reported rates reflect the fact that known cases of maltreatment are a product of both 'demand' and 'supply' factors: the number of children being maltreated and the role of services in identifying them (Coulton et al. 2007; Bywaters et al. 2015). At its most extreme, where there are no services there can be no substantiated child maltreatment because there is no-one to identify and confirm its occurrence. More subtly, the availability, accessibility and perceived appropriateness of maltreatment services and the connections to allied service providers and community groups and organisations are all likely to influence the level of identification and substantiation of cases.

One aspect of this was exemplified in the UK study. This was the replication of a previous finding which we call the inverse intervention law (Bywaters et al. 2015, p. 98). The Inverse Intervention Law states that 'local authorities that were more affluent overall … were placing a significantly larger proportion of children on (child protection plans) … than more disadvantaged local authorities, if you compare neighbourhoods with equivalent levels of deprivation.' (Clearly it is not a 'law', but copies the language of the 'inverse care law', coined by Tudor Hart (1971) to describe inequalities in health services provision.)

Repeating the methodology from a pilot study in a nationally representative sample of 18 local authorities containing over 10% of all children in England in 2015, we found the same pattern, as Table 17.2 exemplifies.

Table 17.2 shows that overall rates (column headed 'All') are higher in high deprivation, than mid deprivation local authorities, which are higher than in low deprivation local authorities, as would be expected. But within each equivalent quintile of neighbourhoods (columns headed 1 to 5), this pattern is reversed in almost every instance. For example, in the most deprived 20% of neighbourhoods in England (column 5) the rate of substantiated child maltreatment is almost 70 per cent greater in low deprivation local authorities (128 per 10,000) than in high deprivation local authorities (76 per 10,000). This inverse relationship is statistically

Table 17.2 The Inverse Intervention Law: child protection plan rates per 10,000 children by neighbourhood deprivation quintile in high, mid and low deprivation local authorities in England, 2015

	Neighbourhood deprivation quintiles. 1 = least deprived.					
	1	2	3	4	5	All
High deprivation local authorities	2	10	18	35	76	51
Mid deprivation local authorities	14	22	29	44	116	48
Low deprivation local authorities	11	24	41	72	128	35
All	11	22	33	48	92	44

significant. In every column the differences in rates between high deprivation and low deprivation local authorities are large, more than double in quintiles 1 to 4, and two thirds greater in quintile 5. The inequities seen here are not a 'postcode lottery', just reflecting random variations in local practices, they are structurally related to local authority level deprivation. Something about patterns in the supply of services was interacting with demand factors in neighbourhood deprivation to cause this unexpected inverse relationship.

To investigate the reasons for this, we built into the research some in-depth case studies of child welfare policy and practice a small number of individual local authorities (four in England and two in Scotland). We analysed quantitative and qualitative data about practice patterns, such as pathways through the service provision, staffing, and expenditure; mapped local resources; observed social workers, meetings and case conferences; interviewed workers and managers at different levels in the organisations; and conducted focus groups with social workers, using case vignettes. The resultant data were analysed using a methodology derived from Ritchie and Spencer (1994).

The findings led to the conclusion that differences in intervention rates were primarily the result of the level of resources available to different local authorities: that although high deprivation local authorities had higher average expenditure per child than low deprivation ones, the additional expenditure was not sufficient to compensate for the higher level of demand they were facing. The main factor at work in producing the inverse intervention law was rationing in the face of excessive demand (Morris et al. 2017; Webb and Bywaters 2018). In high deprivation local authorities, expensive services, such as admitting a child to out-of-home care (at an average cost around £50,000 per year) or full-scale child protection interventions, had to be more tightly rationed than in low deprivation local authorities. As a result, in high deprivation local authorities more cases were deflected from high cost services into other forms of provision or none (see also Hood et al. 2016).

This brief example further demonstrates the potential value of population based analysis as an integral part of a public health approach. A child in a higher deprivation neighbourhood in the UK is much more likely than a child in a lower deprivation neighbourhood to be experiencing a child protection intervention. But a child in the fifth quintile in a high deprivation local authority has about the same chance of being on a child protection plan as a child in the fourth quintile in a low deprivation local authority. A positive correlation between family poverty – or, as a proxy measure, neighbourhood deprivation – and child protection interventions was entirely expected and resulted in higher demand in high deprivation neighbourhoods. But this structural inverse relationship between local authority level deprivation and patterns of intervention in equally deprived neighbourhoods showed that supply factors also influenced a child's chances of substantiated maltreatment.

17.2.4 Neighbourhood, Community and Maltreatment: Ethnicity and Maltreatment

In addition to deprivation, the social gradient and local authority expenditure levels, a fourth structural factor linked to inequity became apparent from this population level analysis: the impact of ethnicity. In the UK, as in many countries, children from different ethnic groups have been found to have profoundly different chances of a child protection intervention (Bilson et al. 2015; Owen and Statham 2009; Putnam-Hornstein et al. 2013). Because the proportion of children from minority ethnic groups is small in Northern Ireland, Scotland and Wales (less than 7% of the child population) the data presented here is based on England, where over 20% of children were from minority ethnic groups at the 2011 census.

The national information published on the ethnicity of children on child protection plans for 2015 only contains one set of data: the number of children on child protection plans at March 31st in each of five broad ethnic categories: White, Mixed, Asian, Black, Other. Estimates can be made of the child protection plan rates per 10,000 children using the latest population data, which has to be taken from the 2011 Census and therefore will be somewhat out of date. It is likely that the child population of minority groups will have risen faster than in the white population because of the age profile of the minority groups i.e. a larger proportion of women are of child bearing age.

It can be seen (Table 17.3) that there are some differences between the representative sample in the CWIP project and the nationally reported data for the whole of England. The broad pattern is similar with highest rates in children of Mixed

Table 17.3 Child protection plan rates per 10,000 children by ethnic category, 2015, based on 2011 population data

	National published Data, 2015	Nuffield Project Sample, 2015
White	42	45
Mixed	71	76
Asian	26	21
Black	48	43
Other	52	43
All	41	44

heritage and lowest for children of Asian heritage. Whether Black rates are significantly different to the rates for White children is uncertain from this evidence and more accurate population data than is available would be needed to create greater certainty.

A further consideration has to be taken into account to make sense of these apparent differences. It is necessary to control for the very different distribution of deprivation affecting children in these ethnic categories. Once comparing equally deprived children a clearer picture emerges (Table 17.4).

Although numbers were small in some instances, patterns emerge that are at odds with the general picture for the population. Although overall rates for Mixed heritage children were higher than those for White children, in quintile 5, where 35% of Mixed heritage children lived, rates were lower than for White children. Asian rates in quintiles 3 to 5 were substantially lower than White rates as were Black rates in quintile 5, where over half of Black children were living. The interaction of deprivation and ethnicity is the key factor in overall rates with children from minority ethnic categories much more likely to be disadvantaged in their socio-economic circumstances.

The reasons for these different patterns urgently require further examination but two main possibilities seem likely. First, some communities may look after their children more safely than others, at least in terms of the definitions used for maltreatment. Second, services may reach some communities more comprehensively than others – more children may be missed in some communities. In addition, an explanation is needed for the flatter or inconsistent gradient in the minority groups, either the results of greater stress or lower informal support when minority groups live in small numbers in low deprivation areas, or the result of differential scrutiny by referral or investigative agencies.

Once again, this population data cannot tell us anything about the quality of the communities concerned or the neighbourhoods in which they live. But without including ethnicity in the list of structural factors to be investigated important issues of equity with major implications for policy and practice will be invisible.

Table 17.4 Child protection plan rates per 10,000 children by ethnic category and deprivation quintile, 2015 CWIP sample, 2011 population data

	Neighbourhood deprivation quintiles. 1 = least deprived.				
	1	2	3	4	5
White	9	20	33	51	116
Mixed	42	47	59	81	107
Asian	[a]	23	15	21	30
Black	[a]	29	45	56	39
Other	42	49	33	18	65

[a]Child numbers less than 10; rate unreliable

17.2.5 Neighbourhood, Community and Maltreatment: A Complex Issue

Of the four UK countries, Northern Ireland, while being less unequal, has the highest levels of deprivation. For example, in England, Scotland and Wales around 25% of children live in the most deprived 20% of neighbourhoods in the UK as a whole, in Northern Ireland the proportion is almost 37%. In Northern Ireland less than 1% of children live in the least deprived quintile of neighbourhoods in the UK, compared to 7% in Wales and over 19% in England and Scotland. When maltreatment rates are compared in each of the five deprivation quintiles, Scotland is consistently the lowest because of differences in structures and practice. But Northern Ireland's rates are substantially lower than in England and Wales in quintiles 3, 4 and 5 where 87% of Northern Ireland children live, and these differences are statistically significant.

So, in Northern Ireland intervention rates are lower than in England and Wales in neighbourhoods of equivalent deprivation. Two hypotheses have been advanced locally for why this may be: the strength of communities (which may include levels of resistance to state intervention) and an integrated neighbourhood focused approach to service provision through local community based hubs. Both explanations suggest there may be something about communities or factors which operate at the level of neighbourhoods that affect child protection rates. But can we determine which of these or other explanations are the key factors?

As the preceding discussion illustrates, distinguishing the role of communities or neighbourhoods in child protection is a complex issue. A number of these complexities can be identified. First, there is the question of how child maltreatment is defined and measured. In studies of neighbourhood effects, different markers of child maltreatment are used: substantiated concerns, referrals to CP authorities, self-reports, or other measures of child outcomes such as child development profiles and this has to be taken into account when weighing the evidence and how it relates to policy objectives. In the UK example given, the measure is children who have come to the attention of state services and been judged to be at risk and placed on a child protection register or plan. This measure includes both children who have experienced abuse or neglect and others where the risk factors are such that intervention is considered necessary but who may not have experienced maltreatment, including newborn babies or the siblings of abused children. And, of course, the line between being maltreated or not is often a matter of judgement, especially in cases of neglect. The very large differences between countries in the proportions of child protection cases which are said to result from neglect (28 per cent in Australia to 88 per cent in Norway) are unlikely to reflect real differences in incidence (Bywaters et al. 2016). There is no gold standard.

Second, the UK measure does not include children who have been maltreated but have not come to the attention of services. It also does not include cases where risks were unknown or underestimated and so were unsubstantiated (false negatives) and it may include children who were wrongly assessed as being at risk, perhaps because of judgements resulting from prior assumptions about the neighbourhoods or families in which they lived (false positives). Retrospective self-reported rates of maltreatment tend to differ from rates produced from administrative data (NSPCC) but ensuring consistency of definitions between service providers and the general population is profoundly difficult.

Third, there is the issue of how neighbourhoods are defined. The term 'neighbourhoods' may mean a variety of things to different audiences in different places. In research, it is often used to describe geographical areas that have an administrative purpose, such as census tracts in the USA, or Lower Super Output Areas in England and Wales. These units may also reflect neighbourhoods as experienced by residents or by service providers, but this cannot be assumed. They may be of different size in different places: in England so-called Lower Super Output Areas have an average population of around 1600 people; data zones in Scotland contain around 600 people, and Super Output Areas in NI around 2000. Census tracts in the USA average around 4000 with a range from 1200 to 8000. So when reading across studies, it cannot be assumed that comparisons of neighbourhoods are like with like. Larger units are likely to contain greater diversity, for example, of household economic circumstances but, if average conditions are measured this may mask the presence of smaller pockets of affluence or deprivation.

Fourth, a measure of neighbourhood deprivation or disadvantage may tell us little about the strength of relationships, informal support or security in those areas. For example, the UK study used neighbourhood deprivation as a proxy for family socio-economic circumstances, in the absence of data about individual families. So it was not (and did not claim to be) a study of neighbourhood characteristics at all. The measures of deprivation available to create a UK wide index only include the proportion of households with low income or without employment, measures of individual wellbeing and not of the quality of neighbourhood relationships or assets. As we discuss below, quite substantial theoretical work has been done to suggest the multiple kinds of characteristics of neighbourhoods, such as aspects of the social and physical environments that might be relevant to particular factors affecting different kinds of child maltreatment.

A further dimension of complexity is the relationship between particular forms of child maltreatment and features of neighbourhoods or communities. It is not likely that neighbourhood factors relevant to the neglect of babies will be just the same as factors affecting sexual exploitation of teenagers, for example.

In addition, what neighbourhoods mean to residents – how neighbourhoods are experienced – may depend on who those residents are. A child's concept of and experience of neighbourhood may be quite different to that of other residents: parents, single adults or pensioners, for example (Sadler and Lafreniere 2017). Neighbourhood may be experienced differently by men and women, for example by reference to routinely accessed places or social support systems – such as work, transport hubs, schools, parks, shops or bars. Equally, some factors will transcend geographical boundaries: pollution, for example, will reflect major traffic routes or industrial plants which may be no respecter or administrative lines on a map.

A final issue is whether neighbourhood as a geographical space or community as a set of social relations is the appropriate focus of attention – or both. For example, in areas with high levels of physical segregation between groups of people – Protestants and Catholics; White, Hispanic and African Americans; majority and indigenous peoples – neighbourhoods as places may be coterminous with residents' communities of identity or interest. But for many, community will cut across place and the key reference points, models and sources of support will be people with similar identities who may not be geographically close.

17.3 Neighbourhood and Maltreatment: Where Are We Now?

The UK example has been used to make the case for examining contributory causal factors behind maltreatment through population studies focusing on place and community, as well as illustrating the complexities involved. The study illustrates the relevance of structural demand and supply factors and provides a vital counterpoint to and context for studies focusing solely on individual behaviours. However, this was not a study which focused on the influence of key characteristics of either neighbourhoods or communities. To explore these issues further we turn now to evidence from the USA.

In the USA, in particular, quite an extensive body of research has reached the broad conclusion that identifiable aspects of neighbourhoods and communities are associated with maltreatment over and above factors that operate at the level of the individual household or family (Coulton et al. 2007; Maguire-Jack and Font 2016, 2017). As Minh et al. (2017) put it, the key question is no longer whether neighbourhoods affect health or development but how, where and to whom the effects apply. In the context of maltreatment: what aspects of neighbourhoods or communities interact with what kinds of susceptibilities in children and/or families to increase (or reduce) the incidence of which types of maltreatment?

For example, Maguire-Jack and Font (2017) have shown that different kinds of neighbourhood characteristics may be associated with different types of maltreatment. They report an interaction between disadvantaged neighbourhoods, family incomes and physical abuse. Higher income families living in impoverished neighbourhoods were significantly less likely to use corporal punishment than low income families in the same neighbourhoods, and physical abuse was also less likely, although this did not reach statistical significance. As the authors suggest, this may operate through the greater stress placed on low income families when neighbourhoods do not offer good employment opportunities, affordable shops or other facilities. They also found that high turnover in a neighbourhood had a greater effect on rates of corporal punishment and abuse in low income than higher income families.

In a separate study, Maguire-Jack and Font (2016) found that neglect was more likely in low income families in high deprivation neighbourhoods than either when low income families were living in low deprivation neighbourhoods or high income families were living in high deprivation neighbourhoods. The combination of low income and neighbourhood impoverishment produced the most powerful effect but neighbourhood status had an effect that was independent of income level. They hypothesised that when most families in a neighbourhood were poor, there was less opportunity for mutual support as everyone's resources were greatly stretched.

17.3.1 Modelling Neighbourhood Causation

Many authors across a range of disciplines have developed models for explaining the role of neighbourhoods and/or communities in the aetiology of a range of social, health and educational issues including child development generally (Hertzman 2010; Minh et al. 2017) and child maltreatment, in particular (Coulton et al. 2007; Maguire-Jack and Font 2017; Molnar et al. 2016). While the language varies and different emphases are present, some common elements are found.

What I have called demand and supply was discussed by Coulton et al. (2007, p. 1120) as a distinction between behavioural influences and the definition, recognition, and reporting of child maltreatment. By behavioural influences Coulton et al. meant 'how neighborhood conditions influence behavior that leads to child maltreatment'. By definition, recognition and reporting they refer to 'neighborhood differentials in the reporting process'.

17.3.2 Supply Factors

While these reporting processes are crucial to an analysis of substantiated rates of maltreatment and one factor that contributes to inequities in maltreatment rates between groups of children, I would argue that the influence of service provision on maltreatment rates at the neighbourhood level goes beyond reporting processes alone. Decisions about the availability, accessibility and appropriateness of services and resources are all an important part of the picture. Institutional, reactive and political rationing decisions (Hastings 2009) made, usually, at a combination of national and local administrative levels may reflect the differential needs of different communities and neighbourhoods or may fail to do so, reinforcing disadvantage. As Hastings says, poor neighbourhoods may get poor services rather than the enhanced services that might contribute to reducing the gradient.

In this context, availability refers to the level of resources provided to particular communities. For example, Attar-Schwartz et al. (2011) reported that higher levels of poverty amongst Arab communities in Israel were combined with lower levels of service provision, resulting from their minority status. In England, although high deprivation local authorities spend more per head on child protection than low deprivation local authorities, there is growing evidence that the differential is insufficient to compensate for the higher level of demand (Ofsted 2016; Webb and Bywaters 2018). Accessibility refers primarily to the location of services coupled with factors such as the availability of transport networks, although the issues of disabled access are also important. As Morton et al. (2014) and others have demonstrated, services such as treatment facilities for substance use may be located at a distance from impoverished populations and neighbourhoods who need them most. Appropriateness means providing services in ways that meet the requirements of the people they are meant to serve. For example, services may not be established in ways that make them equally welcoming or effective in working with populations across a range of religious, ethnic or other identities.

A gap between levels of reported or substantiated maltreatment and the incidence of maltreatment in the population may also reflect differential levels of resistance to service involvement in different areas or communities, for example, based on religious (Katzenstein and Fontes 2017) or other factors such as racial or social class identities.

17.3.3 Demand Factors

Broadly speaking, two key kinds of demand factors been emphasised in the literature of child maltreatment. First, structural mechanisms in neighbourhoods and communities: socio-economic conditions and the physical environment. Second, the social and relational environment: factors affecting social capital. Such factors can act directly on children – for example, exposing them to greater chances of becoming involved in either positive or risky situations outside the home – or indirectly through their families. Families' capacities to successfully and safely bring up their children are influenced either positively or negatively both by their experience of the structural context and by social relations, and also by their perceptions of these factors (Maguire-Jack and Showalter 2016). Families' capacity to parent safely and effectively can be supported directly when neighbourhoods offer concrete material and social assets and indirectly when neighbourhood or community relations –and the wider social context, for example, societal attitudes expressed through social media – relieve rather than adding to parents' stress.

17.3.4 Structural Mechanisms in Neighbourhoods

Many studies show an association between neighbourhood impoverishment and poor outcomes for children either in terms of their general development or maltreatment (Freisthler and Maguire-Jack 2015; Maguire-Jack and Font 2017; Molnar et al. 2016). Molnar et al. categorised these structural mechanisms as 'social and physical disorder' but they could equally be described as reflecting social disadvantage. Disadvantaged neighbourhoods may show a high level of physical deterioration in the housing stock and the wider environment, with high levels of pollution, while lacking positive assets such as safe green spaces. They may also lack resources such as affordable but good quality shops for food and other supplies, community facilities, including schools, health facilities and banks, and good access to employment, while having an over-representation of fast food, alcohol and gambling outlets. Such conditions both make good parenting more difficult in practical terms and also more stressful, and may attract discriminatory and stigmatizing attitudes with material consequences, for example, for securing financial credit or insurance.

17.3.5 Social Capital

An increasing focus in recent research has been on the social and relational aspects of communities, which may be described as social capital. As Hertzman (2010, pp. 2–3) outlined it, for child development more generally, this

> … encompasses constructs such as informal social control (e.g., I can leave my door unlocked because the neighbourhood teenagers respect the citizens here), norms of reciprocity (e.g., I believe that something promised will be kept because the standards in my community are like that), social engagement, participation, cohesion and trust. The relational community is the group that gives children and families their identity and, often, how outsiders identify them. It is a primary source of social inclusion or exclusion, sense of self-worth, self-esteem and gender socialization.

The significant elements of the social aspects of communities are characterised differently by different authors. Molnar et al. (2016) identify collective efficacy (combining social control and social cohesion), intergenerational closure and social networks as the key dimensions. But perhaps the central twin elements that are most relevant here can be described as the availability of social support or social assets (Treanor 2016) and the presence of informal social control. Treanor, in the UK, found that high social assets are significantly associated for mothers with persistent low income with higher levels of social, emotional and behavioural wellbeing in their children. Molnar et al. (2016) found that the size of a parent's social network was protective against both abuse and neglect.

Maguire-Jack and Font (2017) identified that neighbourhood turnover was associated with increased odds of corporal punishment and severe assault among lower income families. They suggested that in more transient neighbourhoods it may be harder for families to secure support from neighbours, increasing isolation but long-term residence in a neighbourhood may only be beneficial if the neighbourhood itself can provide positive supports. However, they also found (p. 8) that 'informal social control was not protective against physical neglect (which) may suggest that physical neglect is primarily driven by ability, rather than willingness, of parents to provide for their children's basic needs.' As is the case with the capacity of people to make health related behavioural changes, having more resources makes change easier to achieve. They concluded that if neglect in poor families is primarily due to a lack of resources, informal social control cannot be expected to exercise much impact. Similarly, Maguire-Jack and Showalter (2016) found that social cohesion did affect lower level neglect, such as leaving a child alone or failing to provide sufficient regular food, but not neglect that reflected substance use or mental ill-health.

17.4 Conclusions

What conclusions can be drawn from this brief introduction to the implications of a focus on neighbourhoods and communities for a public health approach to chid protection? First, while the level of evidential sophistication shown in some the studies discussed is clearly necessary, taking into account different features of neighbourhoods, different characteristics of families and children and different types of maltreatment, controlling for all the variables potentially at play makes it difficult to get consistent findings at a scale which allows for clear policy and practice outcomes.

However, second, the evidence presented here supports the broad position that neighbourhoods and communities have an impact on both the incidence of maltreatment and substantiated maltreatment. A focus on neighbourhoods and communities, as well as on individuals and families, is necessary to understand patterns of child maltreatment as a basis for constructing population level responses to prevention, protection and remediation. Population level studies underpin understanding of the factors that lead to the occurrence of maltreatment and how service responses may inadvertently reinforce rather than reduce inequities in children's life chances.

Third, a further dimension here is to look behind the relevant characteristics of neighbourhoods and communities to the underlying social structures that create and maintain the social and economic hierarchies they reflect (Minh et al. 2017). Looking upstream, involves not only a shift of gaze from individuals to groups but to the fundamental causes (Phelan et al. 2010).

Overall in this chapter, I have argued that a population level gaze incorporating an inequalities perspective is crucial to understanding maltreatment and hence to constructing effective measures for primary, secondary and tertiary prevention. The pervasive international evidence of structural inequities in child protection intervention rates, the scale of the inequities and the profound long term effects on children and parents present a major ethical challenge to policy makers and practitioners, educators and researchers.

Acknowledgement The author wishes to acknowledge the support of the Nuffield Foundation which funded the UK research reported here. The Nuffield Foundation is an endowed charitable trust that aims to improve social well-being in the widest sense. It funds research and innovation in education and social policy and also works to build capacity in education, science and social science research. The views expressed are those of the author and not necessarily those of the Foundation. More information is available at www.nuffieldfoundation.org

The author also wishes to thank the large team of colleagues without whom the UK work would not have been successfully completed.

References

Asaria, M., Doran, T., & Cookson, R. (2016). The costs of inequality: Whole-population modelling study of lifetime inpatient hospital costs in the English National Health Service by level of neighbourhood deprivation. *Journal of Epidemiology and Community Health, 70*(10), 990–996. https://doi.org/10.1136/jech-2016-207447.

Attar-Schwartz, S., Ben-Arieh, A., & Khoury-Kassabri, M. (2011). The geography of children's welfare in Israel: The role of nationality, religion, socio-economic factors and social worker availability. *British Journal of Social Work, 41*(6), 1122–1139. https://doi.org/10.1093/bjsw/bcq134.

Bilson, A., Cant, R. L., Harries, M., & Thorpe, D. H. (2015). *A longitudinal study of children reported to the child protection department in western Australia.* (August 2013), pp. 771–791.

Bunting, L., McCartan, C. J., McGhee, J., Bywaters, P., Daniel, B., Featherstone, B., & Slater, T. (2018). Trends in child protection across the UK – A comparative analysis. *British Journal of Social Work, 48*, 1154–1175.

Bywaters, P. (2015). Inequalities in child welfare: Towards a new policy, research and action agenda. *British Journal of Social Work, 45*(1), 6. https://doi.org/10.1093/bjsw/bct079.

Bywaters, P., Brady, G., Sparks, T., Bos, E., Bunting, L., Daniel, B., Featherstone, B., Morris, K., & Scourfield, J. (2015). Exploring inequities in child welfare and child protection services: Explaining the "inverse intervention law". *Children and Youth Services Review, 57*, 98. https://doi.org/10.1016/j.childyouth.2015.07.017.

Bywaters, P., Bunting, L., Davidson, G., Hanratty, J., Mason, W., McCartan, C., & Steils, N. (2016). *The relationship between poverty, child abuse and neglect: An evidence review*. York: Joseph Rowntree Foundation.

Conger, R. D., & Elder, G. H., Jr. (1994). *Families in troubled times: Adapting to change in rural America*. New York: de Gruyter.

Coulton, C. J., Crampton, D. S., Irwin, M., Spilsbury, J. C., & Korbin, J. E. (2007). How neighborhoods influence child maltreatment: A review of the literature and alternative pathways. *Child Abuse & Neglect, 31*(11–12), 1117–1142. https://doi.org/10.1016/j.chiabu.2007.03.0.

Davidson, G., Bunting, L., Bywaters, P., Featherstone, B., & McCartan, C. (2017). Child welfare as justice: Why are we not effectively addressing inequalities? *British Journal of Social Work, 47*, 1641–1651.

Eckenrode, J., Smith, E. G., McCarthy, M. E., & Dineen, M. (2014). Income inequality and child maltreatment in the United States. *Pediatrics, 133*(3), 454–461. https://doi.org/10.1542/peds.2013-1707.

Freisthler, B., & Maguire-Jack, K. (2015). Understanding the interplay between neighborhood structural factors, social processes, and alcohol outlets on child physical abuse. *Child Maltreatment, 20*(4), 268–277. https://doi.org/10.1177/1077559515598000.

Frolich, K. L., & Potvin, L. (2008). The inequality paradox: The population approach and vulnerable populations. *American Journal of Public Health, 98*, 216–221.

Gilbert, N. (2011). A comparative study of child welfare systems: Abstract orientations and concrete results. *Children and Youth Services Review, 34*(3), 532–536. https://doi.org/10.1016/j.childyouth.2011.10.014.

Gilbert, R., Fluke, J., O'Donnell, M., Gonzalez-Izquierdo, A., Brownell, M., Gulliver, P., et al. (2012). Child maltreatment: Variation in trends and policies in six developed countries. *Lancet, 379*(9817), 758–772. https://doi.org/10.1016/S0140-6736(11)61087-8.

Graham, H. (2007). *Unequal Lives: Health and Socioeconomic Inequalities*. Maidenhead: Open University Press.
Hastings, A. (2009). Poor neighbourhoods and poor services: Evidence on the "Rationing" of environmental service provision to deprived neighbourhoods. *Urban Studies, 46*(13), 2907–2927. https://doi.org/10.1177/0042098009344995.
Hertzman, C. (2010). *Framework for the social determinants of early child development*. Encyclopedia on Early Childhood Development, (November), 1–9. Retrieved from http://child-encyclopedia.com/pages/PDF/HertzmanANGxp.pdf
Hood, R., Goldacre, A., Grant, R., & Jones, R. (2016). Exploring demand and provision in English child protection services. *British Journal of Social Work, 46*(April), 923. https://doi.org/10.1093/bjsw/bcw044.
Katzenstein, D., & Fontes, L. A. (2017). Twice silenced: The underreporting of child sexual abuse in orthodox Jewish communities. *Journal of Child Sexual Abuse, 0*(0), 1–16. https://doi.org/10.1080/10538712.2017.1336505
Maguire-Jack, K., & Font, S. A. (2016). Intersections of individual and neighborhood disadvantage: Implications for child maltreatment. *Children and Youth Services Review*, (October). https://doi.org/10.1016/j.childyouth.2016.10.015.
Maguire-Jack, K., & Font, S. A. (2017). Community and individual risk factors for physical child abuse and child neglect: Variations by poverty status. *Child Maltreatment*, 107755951771180. https://doi.org/10.1177/1077559517711806.
Maguire-Jack, K., & Showalter, K. (2016). The protective effect of neighborhood social cohesion in child abuse and neglect. *Child Abuse & Neglect, 52*(January), 29–37. https://doi.org/10.1016/j.chiabu.2015.12.011.
Marmot, M. (2010). *Fair society, healthy lives: Strategic review of health inequalities in England Post 2010*. Retrieved from www.marmotreview.org
Marmot, M., & Bell, R. (2016). Social inequalities in health: A proper concern of epidemiology. *Annals of Epidemiology, 26*(4), 238–240. https://doi.org/10.1016/j.annepidem.2016.02.003.
McGhee, J., Bunting, L., McCartan, C., Elliot, M., Bywaters, P., & Featherstone, B. (2018). Looking after children in the UK – convergence or divergence? *British Journal of Social Work, 48,* 1176–1198.
Minh, A., Muhajarine, N., Janus, M., Brownell, M., & Guhn, M. (2017). A review of neighborhood effects and early child development: How, where, and for whom, do neighborhoods matter? *Health & Place, 46*(November 2016), 155–174. https://doi.org/10.1016/j.healthplace.2017.04.012.
Molnar, B. E., Goerge, R. M., Gilsanz, P., Hill, A., Subramanian, S. V., Holton, J. K., Duncan, D. T., Beatriz, E. D., & Beardslee, W. R. (2016). Neighborhood-level social processes and substantiated cases of child maltreatment. *Child Abuse and Neglect, 51*(1), 41–53. https://doi.org/10.1016/j.chiabu.2015.11.007.
Morris, K., Mason, W., Bunting, L., Hooper, J., Mirza, N., Brady, G., Bunting, L., Hooper, J., Mirza, N., Scourfield, J., & Webb, C. (2017). Social work, poverty, and child welfare interventions. *Child and Family Social Work*, 1–9. https://doi.org/10.1111/cfs.12423.
Morton, C. M., Simmel, C., & Peterson, N. A. (2014). Neighborhood alcohol outlet density and rates of child abuse and neglect: Moderating effects of access to substance abuse services. *Child Abuse & Neglect, 38*(5), 952–961. https://doi.org/10.1016/j.chiabu.2014.01.002.
Ofsted. (2016). *Education, children's services and skills 2016/17*. Retrieved from https://www.gov.uk/government/uploads/system/uploads/attachment_data/file/666871/Ofsted_Annual_Report_2016-17_Accessible.pdf
Owen, C., & Statham, J. (2009). *Disproportionality in child welfare*. London: Institute of Education, University of London.
Phelan, J., Link, B., & Tehranifar, P. (2010). Social conditions as fundamental causes of health inequalities: Theory, evidence and policy implications. *Journal of Health and Social Behaviour, 51*(Special Issue), S28–S40.

Putnam-Hornstein, E., Needell, B., King, B., & Johnson-Motoyama, M. (2013). Racial and ethnic disparities: A population-based examination of risk factors for involvement with child protective services. *Child Abuse and Neglect, 37*(1), 33–46.

Ritchie, J., & Spencer, L. (1994). Qualitative data analysis for applied policy research. In A. Bryman & R. Burgess (Eds.), *Analysing qualitative data* (pp. 173–194). London: Taylor & Frances.

Rose, G., Khaw, K.-T., & Marmot, M. (2008). *Rose's strategy of preventive medicine*. Oxford: Oxford University Press.

Sadler, R. C., & Lafreniere, D. J. (2017). You are where you live: Methodological challenges to measuring children's exposure to hazards. *Journal of Children and Poverty, 0*(0), 1–10. https://doi.org/10.1080/10796126.2017.1336705.

Sethi, D., Bellis, M., Hughes, K., Gilbert, R., Mitis, F. and Galea, G. (2013). European report on preventing child maltreatment European report on preventing child maltreatment. WHO. http://www.euro.who.int/__data/assets/pdf_file/0019/217018/European-Report-on-Preventing-Child-Maltreatment.pdf?ua=1 Accessed August 2017

Sharkey, P., & Faber, J. W. (2014). Where, when, why, and for whom do residential contexts matter? Moving away from the dichotomous understanding of neighborhood effects. *Annual Review of Sociology, 40*(1), 559–579.

Slack, K. S., Berger, L. M., & Noyes, J. L. (2017). Introduction to the special issue on the economic causes and consequences of child maltreatment. *Children and Youth Services Review, 72*(November 2017), 1–4. https://doi.org/10.1016/j.childyouth.2016.11.013.

Treanor, M. (2016). Social assets, low income and child social, emotional and behavioural well-being. *Families Relationships and Societies, 5*(2), 209–228. https://doi.org/10.1332/204674315X14281323517164.

Tudor Hart, J. (1971). The inverse care law. *Lancet, 297*(7696), 405–412.

Webb, C., & Bywaters, P. (2018). Austerity, rationing and inequity: Trends in children's and young peoples' services expenditure in England between 2010 and 2015. *Local Government Studies, 44*(3), 391–415. https://doi.org/10.1080/03003930.2018.1430028.

WHO. (2008). *Closing the gap in a generation, final report of the commission on the social determinants of health*. Geneva: World Health Organisation.

Chapter 18
Framing Child Protection as a Public Health Law Issue

Donald C. Bross and Ben Mathews

18.1 Introduction

During their remarks for a University of Michigan symposium on "Rethinking Foster Care"[1] a variety of participants addressed foster care, or even rethinking child protection policy as a whole, from 'the ground up'. Several speakers referenced the model of public health as a useful framework for child welfare policy. During many formal and informal exchanges, many others alluded to public health, touching on themes such as the importance of promoting primary prevention over later intervention, reducing reliance on punitive models for intervention, and relying more on science as a foundation for child welfare policy development.

Given the role of public health as a touchstone[2] for these views, likely shared by many non-lawyers, this chapter revisits the nature of public health, and the related

[1] The meeting was held May 12–13, 2016, in Ann Arbor, Michigan, organized by the University of Michigan Law School, and supported in part by the Anne E. Casey Foundation.

[2] This essay supports the importance of more reliance on science in public policy, specifically related to child welfare. For that reason, it is of at least passing relevance to revisit the origin of the term "touchstone" since it is an example of an early 'probe' or 'test' of the nature of different physical elements and thus an example of evaluative scientific thinking very early in our understanding of the elements and physical chemistry. A touch stone was a mineral, commonly gneiss that could be used for a primitive assay of a substance offered as a precious metal, e.g. gold, silver,

D. C. Bross (✉)
University of Colorado School of Medicine, Aurora, CO, USA

Kempe Center for the Prevention and Treatment of Child Abuse and Neglect, Denver, CO, USA
e-mail: donald.bross@ucdenver.edu

B. Mathews
School of Law, Queensland University of Technology (QUT), Brisbane, Australia
e-mail: b.mathews@qut.edu.au

B. Lonne et al. (eds.), *Re-Visioning Public Health Approaches for Protecting Children*, Child Maltreatment 9, https://doi.org/10.1007/978-3-030-05858-6_18

field of public health law, before considering briefly a few examples that have been raised as embodying a public health application to child welfare.[3] A review of historic and recent public health practices and law cannot be comprehensive, but can be instructive for any who would apply public health to child welfare, and who need to be informed by the workings, achievements and weaknesses of the vast field of public health. Moreover, this can avoid oversimplification and maximize the utility of a public health perspective for child protection policy analysis.[4]

In this chapter, with a primary but not exclusive reliance on US experience, we revisit the definition of public health and trace its origin (Part II); chart its development to apply to contexts of personal violence and child abuse (Part III); explain the public health framing of child welfare from a prevention standpoint (Part IV); explore secondary prevention in the context of out of home care (Part V); consider questions of monitoring and measurement, using data and policy perceived from a scientific, public health or law perspective (Part VI); and observe the need for law and policy interventions to be subjected to scientific scrutiny (Part VII).

18.2 Revisiting the Definition of Public Health and the Expansion of the Public Health Tradition

For some, the original core concern of public health was to promote social justice, and for governments and societies to be responsible for preserving and protecting people's health and human rights (Krieger and Birn 1998; Krieger 2005). For others, the history of public health, or 'the population health approach,' is much more complex, including the beginning of the disease model, the relationship between economic

---

or copper, or an amalgam of alloy of more than one of these metals: yellow for gold, white for silver and red for copper. https://en.wikipedia.org/wiki/Touchstone_(assaying_tool)

[3] To his credit, Josh Gupta-Kagan has already reviewed the need for a public health law approach to child welfare and acknowledged a number of individuals who have also introduced the framework previously. Gupta-Kagan 2014 (Towards a Public Health Legal Structure for Child Welfare Nebraska L. Rev. 42(4), 897–965.) After criticizing infringements on the rights of families, Gupta-Kagan states that: "Many in the field now recognize that a public health model would more effectively support the parent–child relationship and protect children from maltreatment than the current paradigm. Despite much attention to such an approach, the field has yet to develop a clear vision for how the law could or should support a public health approach or shape the actions of individuals and institutions best suited to lead a public health response." Gupta-Kagan's example illustrates how different people can find solutions to perceived short-comings in child protection work in the promise of a 'public health model.'

[4] In the interest of transparency, some of the illustrations discussed are informed and biased by the perspective of Bross, a periodic public health practitioner (Rothenberg et al. 1980; Richards and Bross 2008) and his psychologist colleague, Edward Garrido. a researcher on foster care. (Garrido et al. 2011a, b, 2010). Additional related chapters on public health law and sexually transmitted diseases appear in all four editions of the leading international treatise on sexually transmitted infections (STIs), the last three revised with co-author Edward Richards, with the most recent chapter printed in 2008 (Richards and Bross 2008).

growth and its effects on different segments of a population, especially during the Industrial Revolution, and from its beginning, national defense. The expanded reach of public health philosophy and culture during the immediate past half century reveals a broadening search for answers to vexing problems of human health, behavioral health and safety. Turning to public health as a framework for so many issues suggests there is both growing recognition and concern about human conduct and conditions that were either not recognized or else formerly could not be examined sufficiently well, without applying the analytical perspectives and theories of modern science with its tools of population-based analysis and individualized, controlled clinical studies. By implication, a public health model for child welfare introduces and endorses seeking and hopefully relying on data and evidence-based interventions for addressing many politically contentious and demanding policy debates. Public health law and child protection law developed in parallel in the twentieth century in particular, each responding to and sometimes needing the other. Efforts to apply a public health framework to child maltreatment can succeed best when proponents can incorporate a thorough appreciation of the great variety of interactions between public health practice, public health policy and public health law.

The potential for broad public health approaches to problems of human health and safety is supported by many historical achievements. The most important impetus for modern public health systems was the challenge of illness and death due to communicable diseases. Once the work of Pasteur, Snow and others established a disease model as a matter of science during the second half of the nineteenth century, understanding of communicable diseases expanded to include recognition of specific bacterial agents, gradual recognition of the variety of possible vectors and reservoirs of disease, and the importance of physical environmental factors of clean water, sewage control and even 'bad air' (not only malaria but air pollution).

The appearance and application of the first widely effective antibiotic, penicillin, made treatment of a number of bacterial infections possible but did not eliminate the need for additional science and the careful implementation of each advance (Dubois 1959).[5] Communicable disease vaccination campaigns, investigation of chains of disease communication, chlorination of water to prevent gastrointestinal illnesses, and fluoridation of water to prevent dental decay, are examples of continuing public health efforts which even today remain controversial. Public health efforts can and sometimes do overlap with child welfare, as in the example of school immunizations[6] (Immunization & Health Checkup – *CalEdFacts. California Department of Education* 2016). More broadly, contamination of water, air and soil are a threat to public health, and most

[5] Dubois presciently anticipated the appearance of new and evolved infections such as HIV, SARS, MERS, Ebola, and others.

[6] Following outbreaks of preventable childhood infections, California state law now requires that children be immunized, following many years of a policy in which parents could 'opt out' of vaccination for their school children. Immunization & Health Checkup – *CalEdFacts. California Department of Education* (2016).

http://www.cde.ca.gov/ls/he/hn/cefimmunization.asp Checked July 25, 2016. Deaths due to measles at a Christian Science identified college are another example, discussed along with other situations of not providing medical care or prevention, in (Assner and Swan 1998).

specifically children's health is risked when they are exposed to toxins. Examples of toxins that are particularly damaging to the rapidly developing central nervous system of children are cadmium and lead. The presence of environmental hazards usually attracts more attention to harms in the environment that should be eliminated, compared to much less attention that is paid to regulations designed to add or improve what might be absent in the environment with negative health consequences. Examples of responses to the latter are adding vitamin D to milk, adding calcium to orange juice, and making iodized salt available so that adding flavor can also prevent iodine deficiency. These measures seem to offer simple solutions to health challenges compared to the problems faced when child welfare systems must address abuse and neglect, yet these examples remind us that many public health efforts were enforced as public health imperatives.

Before violence became a highly visible public health concern, non-intentional, 'non-inflicted' injury had attracted the attention of the public health tradition. 'Industrial hygiene', defined as 'the science of protecting man's health through the control of the work environment,'[7] began to develop as its own discipline early in the twentieth century.[8] The Occupational Safety and Health Administration was created within the Department of Labor in 1970,[9] Public Law 91–596 and the Act also created The National Institute for Occupational Safety and Health (NIOSH). In 1973 NIOSH was transferred to CDC from the Health Service & Mental Health Administration (NIOSH). Given that non-inflicted, non-intentional injury is the leading cause of death in the United States from the age one until 45, it deserves such elevated attention[10] (Centers for Disease Control and Prevention 2016).[11] The chapter on injury written by Runyan and Runyan, and found in this volume, comprehensively reviews this well developed and important area of science and policy.

Throughout the twentieth century, influenza epidemics, including at least one abortive epidemic (Swine flu), were identified, reported and managed through pub-

[7] Clayton, History of Industrial Hygiene. PDF. Page 1. Centers for Disease Control, National Institute for Occupational Safety and Health. https://www.cdc.gov/niosh/pdfs/74-177-b.pdf. Checked July 25, 2016. George D. Clayton, page 1

[8] Id. "The US Public Health Service has been a world leader in evaluation diseases of the working man and development of controls, as well as fostering an interest in occupational diseases by various state agencies, universities, management and unions. The US Public Health Service, and the US Bureau of Mines were the first federal agencies to conduct exploratory studies in the mining and steel industries, and these were undertaken as early in 1910," Clayton page 2. The same author identifies exposure to toxic gases and other substances a major early focus.

[9] Public Law 91–596, 84 STAT. 1590, 91st Congress, S.2193, December 29, 1970, as amended through January 1, 2004.

[10] "Injuries and violence affect everyone, regardless of age, race, or economic status. In the first half of life, more Americans die from violence and injuries – such as motor vehicle crashes, falls, or homicides – than from any other cause, including cancer, HIV, or the flu. This makes injury the leading cause of death among persons 1-44." Centers for Disease Control and Prevention. http://www.cdc.gov/injury/wisqars/overview/key_data.html.

[11] Note that directly related to child protection and neglect are laws enacted requiring seat belts and car seats for children, along with numerous laws and regulations ranging from the age at which minors can lawfully drive to more recent efforts to address distractions by drivers of all ages who try to text or phone while driving.

lic health measures. Later analyses detailed how the response to these epidemics developed and the many lessons learned (Kilbourne 2006). The abortive epidemic of Swine flu ultimately received close examination as to its necessity and wisdom (Sencer and Millar 2006)[12]; research began promptly on the vaccination campaign and its possible association with cases of Guillain-Barre syndrome (Schonberger et al. 1981). However, years later the extent of an actual association remains unclear[13] These examples illustrate the obvious: that science can be slow, doesn't always answer our questions nor necessarily lead initially to the right choices.

18.2.1 The Nature of Public Health Law Before and After Injury and Violence Drew Attention

If lawyers individually or together work with colleagues in the related field of child protection to endorse public health approaches to child welfare, then we are responsible for becoming sufficiently aware of the nature of laws and legal systems that have closely attended, supported and sometimes contained public health practice and policy. The antecedents of public health law are many and perhaps occasionally surprising. The foundations of public health law developed before the disease model was established, and in the eighteenth century in the part of America that became the United States, authorized interventions included isolation and quarantine for plagues, whose nature was poorly understood:

> The colonies were ravaged by communicable diseases such as cholera, yellow fever, and smallpox. Early state governments carried out draconian measures to control these diseases. The early and middle 1800s saw extensive state regulation of all aspects of life, including the core areas of public health and safety. Regulation of food and water, sanitation, and housing conditions, combined with communicable disease control measures such as mandatory vaccination laws and isolation of communicable disease carriers, raised the life expectancy in cities such as Boston by more than fifty years between 1850 and 2004 (Richards 2007).[14]

---

[12] The authors concluded that: "When lives are at stake, it is better to err on the side of overreaction than underreaction. Because of the unpredictability of influenza, responsible public health leaders must be willing to take risks on behalf of the public. This requires personal courage and a reasonable level of understanding by the politicians to whom these public health leaders are accountable. All policy decisions entail risks and benefits: risks or benefits to the decision maker; risks or benefits to those affected by the decision. In 1976, the federal government wisely opted to put protection of the public first."

[13] Sencer DJ and Millar JD (2006) Reflections on the 1976 Swine Flu Vaccination Program. *Emerg. Infect Dis* 12(1), 29–33.

[14] Within Richards' note there is a citation to the effect that: "the Shattuck Report found that the average age of death in Boston between 1840 and 1845 was 21.43 years. Lemuel, S et al. (1850) *Report of the Sanitary Commission of Massachusetts,*, Boston (Harvard Univ. Press 1948 at 194). Federal health statistics show that life expectancy in 2004 was 77.8 years. Nat'l Ctr for Health Statistics, Health, United States (2006) with chartbook on trends in the health of AMS 176 *available at* http://www.cdc.gov/nchs/hus.htm

The experience of the American Colonies was not unique as concerns about national defense were an early justification for the broad powers of public health law:

> Prior to the adoption of the Constitution, the colonies, and then the states under the Articles of Confederation, carried out administrative regulations based on the traditional right of the government to protect itself and its population from threats such as plagues and attacks by foreign invaders (Novak 1996). In this world, communicable diseases such as yellow fever and smallpox were as much a national security threat as a foreign invasion (Richards 2009).

In an accompanying foot note Richards states:

> This view was well grounded in fact. The Black Plague destabilized the feudal system in Europe, and measles helped destroy the Aztec civilization, allowing conquest by the Spanish[15] (McNeill 1976).

In the body of his analysis, Richards goes on to write:

> It is this common heritage that explains the broad reach of these administrative powers. What is surprising for many who encounter these powers today is that they were not limited by the criminal due process rights when the Constitution and Bill of Rights were drafted[16] (Richards 2009).

For Richards, all forms of administrative law are influenced by these precedents and as an example "Modern environmental law, the heart of many administrative law texts, is an extension of traditional public health law."[17] (Richards 2009).

Tracing back as early as Edwin Chadwick a student of Jeremy Bentham, health (and by implication public health) also has been seen as a human right (Gostin 2000; Susser 1993). Writing as an epidemiologist within the field of public health, Susser defines public health as he has practiced it. Health is a basic human right in his view and thus public health is also necessary to health as a human right whether or not public health is a human right in itself.

> Epidemiology is a basic science for those whose concern is the health of populations, but its roots are in its utility when applied to serving (and improving) the public health. First, I consider the idea of health as a human right: What are its origins? What is its content? And what does that entail? Second, I consider the approaches that have been taken to implement the idea, and the successes and failures of two exemplary attempts to institute the right"[18] (Gostin 2000; see also Susser 1993).

Susser proceeds to compare the effects of health policy broadly examined in Great Britain, Cuba, and Costa Rica and concludes that:

> The British experience yields two lessons. First, professional interests can be reconciled with the health interests of the people at large by reform, and equity in health care can be achieved by that means. Second, equitable service alone is insufficient to bring about equity in health states; in the face of enduring social, economic, and educational disparities, more is required[19] (Susser 1993).

---

[15] Citing McNeill, W.H. *Plagues and Peoples* (1976) at 160–65.

[16] Richards at 29

[17] Id. Again citing Novak.

[18] Id.

[19] Id.

Writing further, Susser discusses the types of structural changes that have enabled apparent improvements in the health of the populations of two smaller countries[20] (Susser 1993). Following Susser's example, recent improvements in life expectancy in the US that seem to be favoring the young over the very elderly also reveal that broad societal factors can make the effects of the child protection system appear to be more beneficial or detrimental than should be attributed to child welfare per se. It is possible to obscure the health experiences of a smaller population, e.g. children in foster care, in aggregate data suggesting substantial improvements in children's health (Currie and Schwandt 2016). In other words, society-wide improvements in children's health care might be more important overall at some points in history than the favorable or inimical effects of various child welfare placement decisions.

Classic public health law inheritance includes instances in which the 'greater good' has been cited as the basis for limiting individual freedom. In Jacobsen v. Common Wealth of Massachusetts[21] the US Supreme Court upheld mandatory vaccination for Reverend Jacobsen and also upheld a requirement that he should pay the five-dollar cost of the vaccination. Individual cases of extensive isolation to specific geographical areas are dramatized by the case of "Typhoid Mary" (Leavitt 1997). The role of individual rights in the face of epidemics is well-illustrated by the public health response to HIV/AIDS, which was accompanied by many conflicts between patients, physicians, and politicians related to the trade-offs between public health and individual autonomy (Shilts 1987). Specific individuals can be singled out based on suspicion of being a carrier of a sexually transmitted disease and placed under a health hold order pending testing and treatment if necessary (Potterat et al. 1978). At the same time, the legal basis for non-criminal detention or restriction, such as isolation or quarantine, must be based on current scientific understanding, notwithstanding political or public perception[22] (Bidgood and Phillipps 2014). Deliberate or reckless behavior by individuals related to public health violations can be punished criminally but these matters are commonly handled as an administrative law matter, as in the closing of a restaurant after a great many, and also often egregious, violations. While rare, criminal responses to some public health violations can be prosecuted. For example, large-scale or corporate level public health violations of a criminal nature fall under the jurisdiction of the Environmental Protection Agency[23] (US Environmental Protection Agency, Enforcement 2016).

If 'public health law' has many faces and a variety of legal 'tools in the tool kit,' its legal efforts tend to be better defined in practice as well as in theory by scientific

[20] Id.

[21] "This court has more than once recognized it as a fundamental principle that persons and property are subjected to all kinds of restraints and burdens, in order to secure the general comfort, health, and prosperity of the State; of the perfect right of the legislature to do which no question ever was, or upon acknowledged general principles ever can be made, so far as natural persons are concerned." (at 26) Jacobson v. Commonwealth of Massachusetts, 197 US 11 (1905).

[22] See Also: http://www.nytimes.com/2014/11/01/us/ebola-maine-nurse-kaci-hickox.html?_r=0. Checked July 27, 2016.

[23] See for example: Enforcement Annual Results for Fiscal Year (FY) 2015 https://www.epa.gov/enforcement/enforcement-annual-results-fiscal-year-fy-2015.

inquiry than is true for most related systems of behavioral health. Systems of behavioral health thought to be broadly related in this essay include mental health, chemical dependency and, especially for the purposes of discussion here, child protection. Within public health, whether a civil or legal intervention occurs, someone is usually responsible to scientifically evaluate the cumulative outcomes of public health policies as applied through legal interventions. This practice is not yet 'standard of care' in most aspects of child protection—and especially not in terms of the effects of law as a system. We do not ignore the reality that while scientific study takes time, legal resolution of conflict is often made with an urgency that does not allow appropriate science to be introduced, or even to have been developed. As discussed more extensively in Sect. 18.7 of this chapter, when health officials began to raise awareness of the possible bad effects of lead in the water at the beginning of the twentieth century, the courts of that time ruled that it was a personal not a civic responsibility. But legal decisions did bring closure for some time to the conflicts associated with contaminated water.

Another factor that affects the invocation of public health remedies, then as now, is that interventions are largely a discretionary function of public officials. As a specific example, public health officials in different American cities made different choices during the Spanish influenza of the early twentieth century (Markel et al. 2006). Municipal variations in the use of legal tools were studied well after the fact, with dramatic evidence of the power of public health and law interventions (the difference between saving and losing tens of thousands of lives), now usefully reported in a 2005 *JAMA* publication that by implication directly endorses the power of applied public health law)[24] (Markel et al. 2007).

In recent history, the response to HIV/AIDS as a sexually transmissible disease varied greatly as a function of the relative power of physicians, interest groups, politicians and public health officials (Shilts 1987). The 'final word' from the perspective of communicable disease policy was registered when the CDC policy returned to recommending contact tracing and notification for all states ultimately underlying the public health nature of STI's even when balanced against individual rights[25] (Potterat 2015). Creating a public health and law framework will not immunize the field of child welfare from both scientifically and non-scientifically supported criticism.

[24] See especially Figure 3 highlighting how tens of thousands of deaths might have been prevented in the United States by introduction of traditional public health law sanctioned measures in sophisticated US cities.

[25] It was argued most strongly at the beginning of the HIV epidemic that contact tracing was not justified without a cure. This position diverts attention from the historic reality that non-treatable diseases engendered policies such as quarantine and contact tracing for responding to epidemics, at a point in time when no treatment was available Once HIV was perceived much like more than 30 other STDs, the CDC's overall policy returned to classic identification and contact tracing.

18.2.2 The Emergence of Violence as a Public Health Concern

Violence and inflicted injury as a separate public health problem first began to be widely recognized by US public health authorities after the mid-twentieth century following the publication of the Battered Child Syndrome (Bross and Mathews 2012). Child abuse reporting laws (Runyan and Runyan 2014) are the most obvious marker for an early public health innovation related to violence, and the rapid, state by US state enactment of child abuse reporting laws (Paulsen 1967) developed directly from the work of a pediatric virologist, Dr. C. Henry Kempe, (Bross and Mathews 2012) who first had labored to end small pox world-wide and then promoted the elimination of smallpox vaccinations (Kempe 1972).

In the midst of efforts to determine the effects, good or bad, of mandatory reporting of child abuse and neglect, it is worth noting that classic public health has always been founded on an adequate definition of the condition or conduct that is the focus of attention, followed by efforts to measure its incidence and prevalence. Epidemiological identification, incidence and prevalence of the disease or hazard remains the *sine qua non* of modern public health, and the countries that have mandatory reporting of child abuse and neglect produce continuing reports to the public about success and failure in responding to child maltreatment. Nations with mandatory reporting yielded some of the earliest research on treatment of children and parents who were maltreated or themselves maltreated others, Countries with mandatory reporting have produced a continuing epidemiological picture of child maltreatment within their borders. Many challenges to mandatory reporting of severe child abuse and neglect have been addressed, and future challenges to the practice deserve research of equal or higher quality. (Mathews and Bross 2015).

Family violence of all forms became more visible with the creation of battered wives shelters and rape crisis centers, drawing attention to marital rape, child sexual abuse, and domestic violence, even though domestic violence has been approached differently and is usually not an activity that must reported. Domestic violence specifically became part of the formal national US public health agenda through the efforts of Surgeon General C. Everett Koop, who facilitated a crucial conference on domestic violence in 1985, when he also testified about it before a Congressional Committee (Senate Subcommittee on Children, Family, Drugs and Alcoholism, October 30, 1985). The subsequent development of domestic violence as a public health issue in the US is widely documented (Flitcraft 1993; Rosenberg and Fenley 1991).

Among others, these events demonstrate the degree to which 'modern child protection efforts' have, throughout the past five decades, been based at least to some degree not only on medical science but on a public health perspective supporting accurate and continuing identification and study of conditions and etiologies of harm to children's health.

18.2.3 Public Health and Child Abuse

Violence affecting children, whether through direct experience or witnessing violence, became a more focused priority as a public health issue in the early 1990s (Mercy et al. 1993). It is also true that child sexual abuse was first recognized specifically as a public health issue in the late 1980s, and has been consistently perceived as such (Djeddah et al. 2000; Koop 1989; Mercy 1999; Zimmermann and Mercy 2010). It is well to remember that, as discussed above, these 'formal' engagements of public health as an institution followed the already existing framework of child abuse and neglect reporting created following the publication of the battered child syndrome.

To treat child abuse and neglect as a public health issue requires applying its traditional tools to prevention, identification, and response (Hammond et al. 2006). Public health theory is concerned with the optimal ways to design, implement, and evaluate programs to prevent risk to children (Mercy and Saul 2009) at the population level but also to groups of children at higher risk. Adopting a public health approach to child abuse requires a multidisciplinary approach to the four dimensions of any public health response: defining and measuring the problem; identifying risk factors; developing and testing interventions; and implementing interventions (Hammond et al. 2006; Mercy et al. 1993).

This systematic public health approach – applied to primary prevention community-wide, to secondary prevention for high risk groups, and to tertiary prevention after the event – requires commitment to prevention, early intervention, responding to fundamental causes of violence, monitoring the efficacy of initiatives and ongoing refinement (Mercy et al. 1993). Also required is the coordinated implementation of responses by government and non-government agencies and communities, to foster widespread ownership of the problem and contribution to its solutions (Hammond et al. 2006).

Additionally, new measures should be considered (Hammond et al. 2006). Cooperative networks of organizations may be required to mobilize in order to respond effectively and proactively (Zimmerman and Mercy 2010). A major challenge for any public health strategy is to achieve coordinated implementation in different agencies and communities, with the full participation of communities. As will be discussed later, all such measures require rigorous planning, and scientific evaluation and refinement. The implementation of a rigorous scientific approach to the design and evaluation of policy and legal frameworks incorporating public health approaches to child welfare requires effective cooperation between government policymakers, researchers, and the service sector. A report commissioned by Australia's Royal Commission on "optimising implementation of reforms to better prevent and respond to child sexual abuse in institutions" provides a succinct but detailed example of how public health, public health law and regulatory theory can combine for a comprehensive approach to child sexual abuse in institutional settings.[26]

18.3 Public Health 'Framing' of Child Welfare

Sometimes public health and child welfare intersect naturally at the clinical level.[27]

At the same time, no one should carelessly use public health tradition or law as a mantra to justify any personal or particular view of child welfare. While *parens patriae* (legal protection authorized by 'paternalistic' or 'best interests' law) practice is uncommon in public health it is the basis on which most authorized child protection intervention occurs. Thus the 'public good' and the 'paternalistic' or 'best interests' view are sometimes overlapping but often disparate approaches to child welfare. To illustrate, an individual child might be ordered by a judge to receive medical treatment for a non-contagious illness, or an inoculation in the midst of an epidemic, over parental judgement. The first order would have to be based on a *parens patriae* foundation, while the second occurrence might be based either on public health or 'best interests of the child' (*parens patriae*) grounds. By the time that the United Nations Convention on the Rights of the Child (UNCRC) was enacted, both the child welfare law and the public health law of many nations had been developing for centuries.

Both classic child welfare and public health law recognize that the term 'rights' can be meaningless without provisions for enforcement of the 'rights'. It is the view of the authors, that the strength of the UNCRC lies not within its framework for enforcement but with its aspirational vision and advocacy for universal commitment to a world better managed to maximize the normal or even optimal development and

[26] Mathews, B. (2017) Optimising implementation of reforms to better prevent and respond to child sexual abuse in institutions: Insights from public health, regulatory theory, and Australia's Royal Commission *Child Abuse & Neglect* 74, 86–98.

[27] An STI clinical investigator in the late 1970's called Bross puzzled about several 'clusters' of children under five with gonorrhea, at a time when the reality of child sexual abuse especially to young children was in question. The puzzle wasn't that adults might have sex with children under five, however; it was that, since it appeared that males were likely sources of the infection why would symptomatic males have sex if they were positive for gonorrhea? This question arises against the background of standard symptomology in which the national epidemiology is that all but about 10% of males develop a drip from the penis after they acquire gonorrhea, and the question can still arise today. Further investigation revealed that all of the cases involved men who confirmed that they were acting as pimps. The known group consisted of 11 active pimps known to public health investigators in the middle-sized community in question, and further investigation revealed that all but one of the men in this group in the community studied were positive for asymptomatic gonorrhea (emphasis added). The public health lesson from this includes an observation that "all epidemiology" is local, meaning that careful attention to individuals and individual communities is essential for work similar to that of public health. This example also illustrates the detailed case work necessary in clinical public health.

well-being of children. If prevention fails will there be a commitment to upholding the rights of an individual child to not be abused or neglected, even if court ordered intervention is necessary? Primary, secondary and tertiary prevention together can improve children's chances for optimal development and safety.

18.3.1 Primary Prevention: An Example

In focusing more on traditional child welfare concerns, there are unique advantages to using the Nurse Family Partnership (NFP) as a specific touch stone and true model for discussing child welfare as a public health issue: NFP's strengths and limitations have been widely published by David Olds and his colleagues for anyone interested in attention to the details of highly nuanced and, especially for the nature of the subject matter, very rigorous research. Outcomes include five year improvements in health of mother and child, as much as an 80% reduction in physical child abuse, and cost-benefit effectiveness. The long-term effects of the NFP intervention include a reduction in rates of crime and delinquency for children and their mothers fifteen years after the intervention, a remarkable persistence achieved through a behavioral intervention (Olds et al. 1997). A further illustration of efficacy draws results from the second of the three randomized trials of the NFP model held in Memphis, Tennessee. Data for the nurse-visited mothers reveal reductions in both inflicted and non-inflicted injuries for their children. Both inflicted and non-inflicted injury were very prevalent in the lives of children whose mothers did not receive a nurse visitor, as indicated by the children's experience with hospitalizations before the age of two and as contrasted to the experience of the babies of mothers in the nurse-visited group. More startling, by age nine, the children of the non-visited mother-child dyads (those in the random control group) suffered more than a four times greater mortality than the children whose mothers accepted the visits.

Among many remarkable aspects of the work of Dr. Olds and his colleagues is the thoroughness of their dedication to science and the public health model. An essential element in the reputation for integrity of the model is its transparency with respect to limitations and caveats. The model is supported by NFP for dissemination only when clear criteria are met. Before being enrolled and supported, programs must show that they will maintain fidelity to NFP protocols. This allows continued evaluation of the NFP model when it is replicated to new settings in order to find out when previously unidentified factors interfere with program effectiveness. This continuing research might suggest, for example, that if domestic violence is present in the home positive NFP effects will be attenuated or lost unless the domestic violence is addressed. The program is not available through NFP for all new mothers but only for first-time mothers. It is not intended for mothers already identified as neglecting or abusing and enrolled by child protection, but only those identified as possibly benefiting from the nurse visitors before there is maltreatment. It is made available only as a voluntary program.

A distinctive finding is that some 25% or more of eligible women refuse the service (Donelan-McCall et al. 2009). Another finding is that women who accepted a nurse visitor but whose 'self-efficacy' was sufficiently high to begin with did not appear to benefit from the program (Olds, University of Colorado Department of Pediatrics Grand Rounds). Mothers are not charged for the service and no money is given to the mothers. Such findings challenge assumptions that should be evaluated more scientifically as to what role either law or poverty truly play in the provision of child welfare services and in what ways it can be empirically documented that the factors of poverty and law affect efforts to address child maltreatment.

18.3.2 Prevention within Child Welfare More Broadly

The limitations listed and the specificity of the NFP intervention, in addition to being exceptionally well stated and revealed are nearly unique in the field of child protection prevention. It is common for child welfare 'reforms' to be introduced with no claim of a research basis. Many programs are promoted with no limits or cautions against their misapplication. It is not uncommon to be presented with a focus on 'marketing' that cites only benefits and minimizes limitations if any are noted. Observers with many years of working with child protection as a field might have noticed that when agencies adopt programs the implementation, the new policies can be accompanied with implicit or explicit administrative penalties for staff who do not accept a new program despite the lack of research support. Merely associating NFP with a another prevention effort should not allow the other program to acquire a veneer of research respectability. It should also be acknowledged that while funding and political challenges are probable factors in the "slowness" of NFP adoption, the integrity of NFP probably also slows its dissemination. Other touted 'reforms' in the slogan-driven world of modern child welfare can proceed more quickly when there is no acknowledgement, and no reliable data is provided, as to possible limitations and cautions that should also be anticipated before and during implementation. Unfortunately, disappointment from cycles of reform that are not shown to be effective, risks delegitimization of child welfare policy and administrations.

Holding every new program to the standards of NFP's careful science is unrealistic because research at the highest level is very demanding in time, intellect and money. Programs can, however, inject a degree of rigor into their evaluation efforts even if the 'gold standard' is not achievable. A small number of other prevention programs have either conducted a randomized trial or have revealed a promising degree of sophistication in their evaluation (Chaffin et al. 2012; Prinz et al. 2009).

Finally, with all due attention to 'fully scientific' innovations emphasized here it must also be recogized that history demonstrates that not every successful public health effort will begin or even gain momentum only through science. The hygienic or sanitarian movement that started in the early 1800s, promoting clean water, clean air and clean hands, preceded in time the development of the disease model. It is now established that the greatest proportionate decreases in illness and death due to contagious diseases occurred in the 1800s as communities in different parts of the world adapted to new beliefs and behaviors[28] (Toms 2010; Barr 2015). As cited in the following paragraph, the work by the Meltons and their colleagues (also described in this volume) to promote 'Strong Communities' illustrates the potential for community reform of the conditions of childhood 'from the ground up'.

Eventually, historians might surmise that the attention to family violence in all of its forms beginning in the second half of the twentieth century changed cultures in some parts of the world, promoting attention to care giving and the need to reduce conflict beginning at the earliest formation of human life including child rearing and relationships between family members. Public awareness via information campaigns, schooling, and other means of publicizing these issues is still promoted from time to time. But projects such as the Strong Communities model, fostered by the Meltons and their colleagues, are much more than an advertising attempt to influence entire communities to reshape their own priorities in a way that will decrease preventable harm to children[29] (Melton et al. 2008). Their efforts involve on the ground and intensive interventions over an extended period of time.

18.4 Comparing Public Health and Child Protection Interventions After Prevention Fails: Children in Out of Home Placements

While public health is most visible with respect to its activities related to primary prevention, public health does operate at many different levels of understanding and action, with individual, organizational, and population research among the obvious domains. Although 'prevention' is generally thought to be 'the' model of public health, within the discussions of adherents of child welfare the term 'public health' remains curiously unevenly articulated and even subject to different interpretation and use. Perhaps, going forward, we can at least explain the sense in which we are using the terms.

For example, does public health do anything besides primary prevention? An example sphere of concern for public health that is somewhat analogous to child welfare placements of children is public health policy and administration related to hospitals. Hospitals are of course an aspect of public health in that the public's

---

[28] Note the great distinction between the control of biological contagions and the 'mental hygiene' developments of later years. Toms, J. (2010) Mind the Gap: MIND, the mental hygiene movement and the trapdoor in measurements of intellect. J Intellectual Disabilities Research 54(01), 16–27. It is a useful caution about borrowing words or concepts by analogy and without a fully explicated appreciation of how different the new application of the word or concept proposed is from the original understanding and application of the term or word borrowed.

[29] Melton, GB. et al. (Eds.) (2000). Strong Communities as Safe Havens for Children. Family & Community Health. 31(2)(April–June).

health is affected by the availability and capability of hospitals, just as out-of-home placements are an aspect of child welfare. The public health examination of the distribution, availability, and qualities of patient outcomes for different hospitals receives more attention today than ever (Wright et al. 2002; Barr 2015). Concerns about hospital safety are studied with great care as to the prevalence, definition and need for correction (Brennan 2000) and in ways that are well beyond current scientific discussion of foster care. It would be a rare discussion about hospitals presently that would fall back to 'it's not good and can even cause harm' or 'it's sometimes necessary and can even do good'. Additionally, while only in rare instances, certain special purpose public hospitals fall under the direct administrative authority of the Public Health Service (42 U.S.C. 22 § 2001). There are also visiting nursing services and public health investigators in areas as different as food services and sexual contacts that do draw upon specific case management training and skills.

In drawing an analogy to hospitals as they relate to public health as a system, an important opening comment about child welfare culture is to note the lack of strong, continuing, scientific epidemiology regarding one of child welfare's major concerns, i.e. children in out of home placements. Both in the US and world-wide, episodes of children's placement away from home for centuries are varied, are many and are recurrent. These displacements can occur within the most 'advanced' countries and can arise as a result of war, (Wicks 1988) campaigns to reduce populations of poor children,[30] (Canberra, Australia 2009) and policies to require indigenous populations to change their language, religion or culture to that of an invading majority. These policies have led not only to removals, but other cultural disruptions such as institutionalized residential schooling (Indian Child Welfare Act 1978). Even children in orphanages have not been free from whole sale 'distribution' to families interested in taking them 'on sight'[31] (Holt 1992). At any point in history, dislocations of children can create the need for out of home care, as in the US example of immigrant and refugee children,[32] (Taxin 2016) and the example of natural disasters.

[30] For example: "Canberra, Australia, Prime Minister Kevin Rudd apologized today to thousands of impoverished British children shipped to Australia in past centuries with the promise of a better life only to suffer abuse and neglect thousands of miles from home." The Denver Post, Monday, November 16, 2009, page 16A. (Associated Press 2009).

[31] Holt, I. M. (1992) *The Orphan Trains: Placing Out in America*. Lincoln: University of Nebraska Press; see also Bellows Summerford, B. The Orphan Trains: Did the Benefits Outweigh the Damage? Master of Arts Thesis 2011 Charlestown, W.Va. American Pubic University System. http://www.apus.edu/content/dam/online-library/masters-theses/Bellows-Summerford-2011.pdf https://www.pdffiller.com/63045562-Bellows-Summerford-2011pdf-The-Orphan-Trains-American-Public-University-System-apus-Various-Fillable-Forms

[32] Taxin, A.. Associated Press. April 19, 2016. A Freedom of Information Act request to the Department of Health and Human Services "provided data showing that 80 percent of the 71,000 mostly Central American Children placed between February 2014 and September 2015 were sent to sponsors who were not here legally" and only "In some cases, the department's Office of Refugee Resettlement conducts a home study to determine if the placement is safe." http://bigstory.ap.org/article/40acc163f5d245ce940e7571d0f54bd4/immigrant-kids-placed-adults-who-are-us-illegally

A decade after Hurricane Katrina there are many unanswered questions about the over 100,000 children displaced, and we rely on stories of remarkable achievement and unknown outcomes providing a mosaic of images but no complete epidemiological picture[33] (Barmore 2015). However, if someone asserts that there is a 'crisis' of foster care placements, what is the frame of reference? An example to be emulated in applying science to child protection is found in the article by Clare Huntington (2014) on Child Welfare and the Limits of Determinacy.[34] In her article, Professor Huntington uses 1980–2006 child maltreatment rates in the US to suggest "the possibility that an increase in child maltreatment drove the increase in foster care." She adds immediately: "It is hard to confirm this link in a definitive matter, because the relationship between child-maltreatment rates and foster-care placement is so complex (citations omitted)"[35] (Huntington 2014). This approach emulates the analysis of foster care rates as being loosely akin to the rise and fall of other conditions, such as occurs with communicable diseases.

In child protection, a quarter of a century ago, there were few treatment interventions with indications of effectiveness achieved through any degree of scientific rigor[36] (Oates and Bross 1995). The picture has brightened (Shipman and Taussig 2009), but specific treatment programs that do appear to be helpful, e.g. Trauma-Focused Cognitive Behavioral Therapy (TF-CBT), are sometimes used as the only therapy despite broader needs of the client. Such treatments are not yet available for many clients, given a political and economic environment in which psychotropic drugs appear to be favored for reimbursement over psychotherapy, despite evidence for the effectiveness of the latter for many situations (Shedler 2010). Careful study of which family dynamics or individuals cannot be treated sufficiently well in a way that will allow a child to have a chance for recovery and normal development during the reasonably foreseeable future are virtually absent from the literature. This is the recurrent issue of a lack of good triage science in child protection (Merkel-Holguin and Bross 2015). In the discussion of foster care that follows immediately, the problem is raised of the need for 'controlling' for the condition of children placed in foster care before one measures 'the effects' of foster care. Without control or comparison measures, much current foster care research might be suffering from the potentially 'fatal' limitation on the strength of the arguments both for and against foster car.

---

[33] Barmore, P. Hechinger Report 2015, http://hechingerreport.org/what-we-can-learn-from-the-katrina-children-who-thrived-after-disaster/

[34] 76 Law & Cont. Probs. 221–248 (2014)

[35] Id. 237.

[36] Oates, R.M. & Bross, D.C.. (1995). What Have We Learned about Treating Child Physical Abuse: A Literature Review of the Last Decade. Child Abuse & Neglect 19(4): 463–474.

18.4.1 The Example of Foster Care as an Intervention for Research Study

The details of which treatments are best evidenced and where the greatest questions remain cannot be evaluated in a thorough fashion within a single chapter on public health and child welfare. However, questions surrounding the placement of children away from their primary family and even their extended family are an enduring challenge and a useful example for discussion.

Although the factors that precipitate placing children into foster care often vary, typically in contemporary child protection practice in wealthier nations, there is either a history of maltreatment perpetrated by a caregiver, a history of a caregiver failing to protect a child from maltreatment by others, and/or a severely chaotic living environment (US Department of Health and Human Services 2014). Despite inconsistencies in the reasons youth are placed into foster care, over the past 15–20 years a question often raised is: what are the benefits and drawbacks associated with foster care placement? Those who are advocates of foster care point out that the prevention of further maltreatment to children is accomplished in the majority of cases (Arad 2001; Landsverk and Garland 1999) and that the likelihood of parental recidivism following a youth's reunification with their parent is significantly reduced (Landsverk and Garland 1999). Aside from outcomes associated with protecting a child from further harm, the question of whether foster care placement results in improved child well-being has recently been investigated in several studies, and some of these studies find foster care to be harmful.

Before beginning a discussion of whether placement into foster care results in better or worse outcomes for youth when compared to other types of placements, a methodological caveat should be noted. For obvious ethical reasons, it is not possible to perform a truly randomized controlled trial (RCT) where youth in need of out-of-home care are randomly assigned to different types of placements. Such a study of differences in outcomes associated with different types of placements would, through the process of random assignment to groups, equate youth on a variety of potential confounds such as, differences in the type of traumatic experiences they had been exposed to prior to placement, differences in the composition of the family from which the child is being removed and/or placed into, and demographic and psychosocial differences among the youth themselves. In the absence of the ability to perform a true RCT, researchers are, at best, left with having to statistically control for these potential confounds.

Among studies that have controlled for potential confounds, the empirical evidence in some appears to suggest that foster care placement is associated with worse outcomes when compared to placement with kinship providers. Winokur et al. (2008), for example, randomly selected a group of youth placed with kinship providers and a group placed in foster care and matched the two groups on a number of demographic factors including, gender, race/ethnicity, and age at entry into placement. Results of the study found that placement into foster care was associated with a greater number of subsequent placements, a greater amount of time remaining in care, a lesser likelihood of being reunified with parents, and greater odds of youth being involved in the juvenile justice system. A limitation of the Winokur et al. study was an inability to control for pre-placement behavioral and mental health functioning in the two placement groups. In a similar comparison study of youth placed in either foster or kinship care, Rubin et al. (2008) did statistically control for pre-placement levels of behavioral problems and placement instability in examining differences in behavioral problems after placement. Their findings were similar to those of Winokur and colleagues, with youth in foster care having significantly higher rates of behavioral problems 3 years after placement compared to youth placed with kin.

This evidence appears to suggest worse outcomes associated with foster care relative to other types of placement. There is other evidence, however, that maltreated youth who remain in foster care demonstrated better psychosocial functioning relative to youth who were reunified with their biological parents or who were never removed at all (Taussig et al. 2001; Taussig and Culhane 2005). Thus, the evidence is mixed as to the outcomes associated with different placement types for maltreated youth. What is consistent from previous studies is that youth who enter foster care placements have significantly higher levels of mental and behavioral health issues relative to youth placed with kinship providers or who remain at home.

Accordingly, it is imperative to review and discuss treatment programs that have been developed to address the needs of maltreated youth in foster care and the empirical evidence associated with these programs. Although we do not provide an exhaustive review of these programs, we do highlight those for which a significant amount of empirical evidence has been accumulated.

18.4.1.1 Early Childhood

The majority of early childhood interventions for children in foster care are designed around two primary developmental tasks: (1) the formation of secure and positive relationships with caregivers and (2) the development of emotional and behavioral regulation skills. One such example of an intervention designed specifically for young children in foster care is the *Attachment and Biobehavioral Catch-up* (ABC) program. The ABC program is a 10-session for parents of infants and toddlers aged 0–3. The intervention primarily focuses on helping caregivers provide nurturing care and the conditions necessary to promote emotional expression and recognition in children. The results of various RCTs have shown the program has benefits for children's cortisol levels (Dozier et al. 2006, 2008) internalizing and externalizing problems (Sprang 2009) and cognitive flexibility (Lewis-Morrarty et al. 2012).

A second program developed for young children in foster care is the Early Intervention Foster Care (EIFC) program. The EIFC program is designed for preschool-aged youth (3–6 years of age) and works to provide foster parents with specialized training in managing problem behavior and encouraging positive behavior prior to children being placed into their homes (Fisher et al. 1999). In addition to pre-placement training, foster parents receive ongoing support, supervision, and consultation from a foster parent consultant, an early interventionist, and a family therapist. An RCT conducted with 90 families found fewer failed placements for those receiving the EIFC program (Fisher et al. 2005).

18.4.1.2 Middle Childhood and Adolescence

Several programs have been developed for children in foster care in middle childhood and early adolescence. One example is the program Middle School Success (MSS). The MSS program is designed to help girls navigate the difficulty transition to middle school. As part of the program, parents receive group-based training in behavior management techniques, while the girls participate in group sessions prior to the start of middle school and then individual coaching sessions throughout the school year. Evidence from two rigorous studies has found evidence of the program's success. Intervention participants evidenced fewer mental health and behavior problems, less substance use, and greater prosocial behaviors up to 3 years post-baseline when compared to control group youth (Kim and Leve 2011; Smith et al. 2011).

The Fostering Healthy Futures (FHF) program is a second program that's been designed for early adolescents. The FHF program is a preventive intervention for maltreated youth, ages 9–11, who entered foster care over the prior year. The intervention provides one-on-one mentoring and skills groups to children over a 30-week period. Graduate students serve as mentors and spend 3–4 h per week with each child. Mentors also advocate for services to help youth overcome any challenges they may face and connect them with resources and activities to build on their strengths. Children attend a weekly skills group that consists of sessions on social skills, healthy coping strategies, and resisting peer pressure for risky behaviors. An RCT has demonstrated positive outcomes, including: (1) a reduction in mental health symptoms according to youth self-report, as well as reports from their caregivers and teachers 6-months post-intervention, (2) a reduction in mental health service utilization 6-months post-intervention, and (3) fewer placements changes, fewer placements in residential treatment centers, and increased permanency (Taussig et al. 2007, 2012; Taussig and Culhane 2010).

18.5 Data and Policy Perceived from a Scientific, Public Health or Law Perspective

As child welfare professionals, even lawyers, strive to support a public health framing of child welfare, they will bring the advantages of their various traditions of education and training to bear on the topic. This means there will be attention to detail, logical reasoning, respect for scientific research and legal precedent and belief in human rights to support the process. What risks are there in the greater engagement of the legal profession in this reframing of child welfare?

While lawyers are singled out in part of this discussion, the broad issue of 'confirmation bias' being discussed should be in the minds of every person trying to utilize science to establish policy. Completely normal behavior includes confirmation bias, a tendency to discount, diminish or even disregard information contrary to one's assumptions and beliefs, especially on issues for which we hold a strong emotional attachment. This tendency can have major personal, policy and political consequences (Nickerson 1998).

Moving the focus for the moment to lawyers, our purpose is to engage colleagues with the idea that legal training is akin to scientific training in the way that it tries to establish 'truth'. Legal training is indeed rigorous, and those with scientific training often do well in law school. At the same time, legal training is intended to produce a dedicated focus on client interests, client's views, and their representation. 'Discovery' in law is a step towards finding information that favors a client's position or, if it tends to undermine the client's position, find out so that it can be countered. Discovery of conflicting data is not rewarded as an end in itself as a general goal of law.[37] In contrast, data that is contrary or surprising to perceived wisdom is sought after and rewarded in science as 'discovery'. Original discoveries are valued as knowledge for its own sake. This form of 'discovery' is often rewarded as an end in itself.[38] Scientific training, as a general rule, attempts to reduce confirmation bias. Sooner or later, of course, scientifically trained individuals can make assumptions that limit or even blind scientific development until a 'scientific revolution' overturns the paradigm (Kuhn 1962). Unlike a dialectic process in which the new replaces the old—but makes the process sequential, and a step by step, scientific development is very often not sequential. Illustrations of confirmation bias can be found within child welfare on the part of many, but also to be found are overgeneralizations and exaggerations of hopeful effects without specifying the conditions in which fidelity to a protocol might yield replicable effects. Confidence in results is usually a prolonged process in science and often occurs as well in scientifically supported systems like public health.

---

[37] This not to say that legal scholars are not capable of performing highly objective and fact-based, objective briefing and proposals for possible solutions to complex human problems.

[38] Lawyers can consider whether their legal training has reinforced a natural human tendency, by emphasizing and rewarding the work of taking one view and presenting it in the most effective way possible as well as finding any way effective, even at some risk of ethical 'slips', to wish to prevail in an argument. Taking each client as a focus, even when it means taking on science, is appropriate in litigation. In policy work, who is the client? If the 'client' is the lawyer's staked-out academic or personal belief then data contrary to the position can be perceived as adverse to the interests of 'the client' within the culture of 'rights framing' of issues. Lawyers therefor are like others in needing to recognize their power to diminish the influence of a science-based culture of public health.

18.6 Subjecting Law and Its Interventions to Scientific Scrutiny and Validation

There is an additional consideration if public health and law are to advance understanding of and reduce child maltreatment and its sequelae through a relationship of engagement. Law reflects and sometimes codifies public policy but there must also be recognition for the separate role that law plays. Law itself is a variable of intervention and it should be studied as such[39] (Irueste-Montes and Montes 1988; Tjaden and Thoennes 1992; Wolfe et al. 1980). Knowing whether laws and legally sanctioned interventions have a negative or positive effect are most often debated within law based on almost no rigorous empirical research and without careful evaluation studies. Many non-lawyers shy away from court interventions and participation, perhaps to prevent their own 'secondary trauma' or because they believe families are unnecessarily traumatized, but they should do so based on more than personal comfort and impression. Research on involuntary treatment and conditions such as substance misuse and mental illness can produce interesting outcomes. For example, some men with Alcohol Use Disorder appear to respond more positively under court order than when they are not court ordered, but one study showed that it depended on whether or not they were also diagnosed with an antisocial personality disorder, (Daughters et al. 2008) and research on drug courts is reasonably promising (Gottfredson et al. 2006; Wilson et al. 2006). The most telling point to be made is that the money and time devoted to legal responses to problems of the public's health, mental illness, substance misuse, and family violence justify careful, and whenever possible, scientific evaluation.

If this is done, it will be an acknowledgement of expected standards of self-examination in the practice of public health and public health law. At the same time that the power and influence of public health as a factor in addressing violence is recognized, it is timely to point out that limitations of public health approaches are to a degree embedded in the nature of the precepts of public health itself. Public health and scientifically based efforts overall, generally derive much of their strength and reputation from the process of recognizing errors as a primary means of laying the foundation for discovery and progress. The errors can be real, and so can be their consequences. But it is often how errors and systems are reviewed that sets a scientifically-based practice apart from other well-intended efforts.

Neglect of children presents many problems including barriers to making its effects apparent, and failing to fully appreciate the nature of the problem or necessary solutions. The same has happened in public health. There is an example of recent exposure to lead-contaminated water supplies in Flint, Michigan, but the

[39] It is uncommon to discover research related to the possible effects of court interventions with child welfare populations. Yet the effects of legal policy changes can be described objectively. From the public health perspective, progress in public health depends on discovery of etiological and immunizing factors, among many other factors in health, and this can include examining rights-based clinical and legal practice as a value in itself justifying public health, but also a factor to be examined dispassionately for its contribution to public health.

problem is long-standing. By 1900, lead piping had been brought to 85% of large US cities as part of a massive effort to deliver indoor plumbing and clean water to residences with the goal of better public health. Only with time and in retrospect did the potential downside of fresh water delivery via lead piping become apparent.

> Meanwhile, late nineteenth century women trying to abort a baby would often take pills made of lead plaster. In towns with the worst lead problems, a woman could get the same dose of lead by drinking a glass of water (Renner 2007).

In Massachusetts and northern England:

> lead water pipes appeared to increase infant mortality rates and stillbirth rates by up to 25%. By any measure, this was one of the most serious environmental disasters of the past 200 years, and yet few people recognized it at the time."[40]

There were many reasons why evidence was ignored. Symptoms were not unique nor immediately dramatic (compared to cholera for example). Most doctors tended to focus on adults rather than the more-vulnerable children. Although wide-spread, the problem was not always associated with lead pipes. Municipalities were in denial. Lead pipes were an expensive improvement that brought pure water to homes, how could that be wrong? The doctrine of 'protective power' theorized that most lead pipes developed a protective interior coating. Finally, courts compounded the problem when judges ruled that customers not municipalities were responsible for any contamination that came from pipes installed by the cities.[41] Eventually lead contamination in water and air was regulated, but only after many years. A brief review of a another public health policy application that was followed with a 'quality review,' immunization against Swine Flu, is noted above. (See footnotes 11 and 12 and associated text, supra). These examples illustrate the obvious: that science can be slow and doesn't always answer our questions.

Even with the inevitable limitations of science, the legal or social science observer can think of many issues that might yield important information for child protection services through good scientific research. The role of law as a factor, not merely as a narrow negative or positive factor related to court proceedings, should become a greater matter of interest to the child protection community. Unlike studies of medical services, very few child protection agencies make it ordinary practice to ask parents, and children old enough, regarding their 'consumer satisfaction' with child protection workers and the 'system' more broadly. Nor are their routine 'check-ups' as to the degree to which current foster parents feel supported in their work. While not obvious, underlying such questions are the degree to which the existing legal frameworks are supportive or interfering in the protection of children.

How might science improve the response of the legal system, both in terms of policy and case management? Among questions that a 'public health and public health law' framework might recommend for research are the many issues related to placements (which are always subject to legal review or authority): Can we describe

[40] Id.

[41] Id.

the 'natural history' or the common developmental pathways of how introducing kin and guardianship arrangements in lieu of termination of parent-child legal relationships is working in practice? Can absolutely necessary out-of-home care be made more thoroughly safe and therapeutic? As only one example of neglected opportunities, the Adult Adolescent Parenting Inventory was used to compare parenting competencies of abusive parents, ordinary or 'control parents' and foster parents. Bavolek's (1980) largely ignored work on the different competencies found among statistically significant differences in measures of empathy, attitudes towards corporal punishment, and role reversal between these three categories of caregivers. His research comparing parents with no previous or current child welfare involvement, parents with current child welfare involvement, and foster parents might help identify potential foster parents who should be given extra education and support before having a child placed with them, recognizing that in many locations recruitment of foster parents is already difficult. Can we create conditions in which randomized trials involving placements of children might be contemplated, once shown to be ethical, necessary, and practical, by reforming state laws related to trials related to child welfare and family violence so as to permit appropriate research? Can we improve termination laws and parental representation to prevent wrongful terminations and, with other possible results, reduce the number of children who lose families wrongly or become 'kites without strings'?

18.7 Summary and Conclusions

Without an adequate legal framework, child protection efforts cannot have either the legitimacy that only law can provide nor the authorization and agreements that enable the coordinated implementation of responses by government and non-government agencies and communities, which in turn foster widespread ownership of the problem and contribution to its solutions. There are other good reasons to favor a public health framework for managing and setting policy related to child maltreatment. Perhaps the most important reason to support such an approach is that it might increase attention to and reliance on more scientific thinking about child abuse and neglect, as illustrated by the closing paragraph of the discussion just above. Continued application of public health policies and law to child welfare, not as a panacea but as a framework relying on more than two centuries of population health improvements based on science, should not only mobilize interest and engagement with the scientific tradition of public health but it might also serve to clarify and enrich legal discussions and even research about some of the trade-offs between individual rights and population well-being. Yet the law and its interventions must also be subjected to good scientific inquiry. Inevitably, and valuably, our understanding of when and how law is helpful or not must be informed by good science and not only good intentions.

References

Arad, B. D. (2001). Prenatal features and quality of life in the decision to remove children at risk from home. *Child Abuse and Neglect, 25*, 47–64.

Assner, S. M., & Swan, R. (1998). Child fatalities from religion-motivated medical neglect. *Pediatrics, 101*(4), 625–629.

Associated Press. (2009, November 16). Australian prime minister apologizes for treatment of child migrants. *The Denver Post*, A16.

Barmore, P. (2015, July 5). What we can learn from the Katrina children who thrived after disaster. *The Hechinger Report*. Retrieved from http://hechingerreport.org/what-we-can-learn-from-the-katrina-children-who-thrived-after-disaster/

Barr, P. (2015, April 14). Public partners in population health. *Hospitals and Health Networks*. Retrieved from http://www.hhnmag.com/articles/3576-public-partners-in-population-health

Bavolek, S. J. (1980). *Primary prevention of child abuse: The identification of high risk parents*. Educational Resources Information Center (ERIC).

Bidgood, J., & Philipps, D. (2014, November 1). Judge in Maine eases restrictions on nurse. *The New York Times*, A18.

Brennan, T. A. (2000). The Institute of Medicine report on medical errors: Could it do harm. *New England Journal of Medicine, 342*, 1123–1125.

Bross, D. C., & Mathews, B. (2012). The battered child syndrome: Changes in the law and child advocacy. In R. D. Krugman & J. E. Korbin (Eds.), *C. Henry Kempe: A 50 year legacy to the field of child abuse and neglect* (pp. 39–50). Amsterdam: Springer Scientific.

California Department of Education (2016). Immunization & Health Checkup – *CalEdFacts. California Department of Education*. Retrieved from http://www.cde.ca.gov/ls/he/hn/cefimmunization.asp

Centers for Disease Control and Prevention. (2016). *Web-based injury statistics query and reporting system (WISQARS)*. Retrieved from www.cdc.gov/ncipc/wisqars

Centers for Disease Control and Prevention (2011). *Notable milestones in NIOSH history*. National Institute for Occupational Safety and Health. Retrieved from http://www.cdc.gov/niosh/timeline.html

Chaffin, M., Hecht, D., Bard, D., Silovsky, J. F., & Beasley, W. H. (2012). A statewide trial of the SafeCare home-based services model with parents in child protective services. *Pediatrics, 129*(3), 509–515.

Clayton, G. D. (2000). Industrial hygiene: Retrospect and prospect. In R. Harris (Ed.), *Patty's industrial hygiene* (Vol. 1, 5th ed.). New York: Wiley.

Currie, J., & Schwandt, H. (2016). Inequality in mortality decreased among the young while increasing for older adults, 1990–2010. *Science, 352*, 708–712.

Daughters, S. B., Stipelman, B. A., Sargeant, M. N., Schuster, R., Bornovalova, M. A., & Lejuez, C. W. (2008). The interactive effects of antisocial personality disorder and court-mandated status on substance abuse treatment dropout. *Journal of Substance Abuse Treatment, 34*(2), 157–164.

Djeddah, C., Facchin, P., Ranzato, C., & Romer, C. (2000). Child abuse: current problems and key public health challenges. *Social Science & Medicine, 51*(6), 905–915.

Donelan-McCall, N., Eckenrode, J., & Olds, D. L. (2009). Home visiting for the prevention of child maltreatment: Lessons learned during the past 20 years. *Pediatric Clinics of North America, 56*(2), 389–403.

Dozier, M., Peloso, E., Lindhiem, O., Gordon, M. K., Manni, M., Sepulveda, S., & Levine, S. (2006). Developing evidence-based interventions for foster children: An example of a randomized clinical trial with infants and toddlers. *Journal of Social Issues, 62*, 767–785.

Dozier, M., Peloso, E., Lewis, E., Laurenceau, J. P., & Levine, S. (2008). Effects of an attachment-based intervention on the cortisol production of infants and toddlers in foster care. *Development and Psychopathology, 20*(03), 845–859.

Dubos, R. J. (1959). *Mirage of health: Utopias, progress, and biological change*. New York: Harper.

Fisher, P. A., Ellis, B. H., & Chamberlain, P. (1999). Early intervention foster care: A model for preventing risk in young children who have been maltreated. *Children services: Social policy, research, and practice, 2*(3), 159–182.

Fisher, P. A., Burraston, B., & Pears, K. (2005). The early intervention foster care program: Permanent placement outcomes from a randomized trial. *Child Maltreatment, 10*, 61–71.

Flitcraft, A. (1993). Physicians and domestic violence: Challenges for prevention. *Health Affairs, 12*(4), 154–161.

Garrido, E. F., Culhane, S. E., Raviv, T., & Taussig, H. N. (2010). Does community violence exposure predict trauma symptoms in a sample of maltreated youth in foster care? *Violence and Victims, 25*(6), 755–769.

Garrido, E. F., Culhane, S. E., Petrenko, C. L., & Taussig, H. N. (2011a). Psychosocial consequences of intimate partner violence (IPV) exposure in maltreated adolescents: Assessing more than IPV occurrence. *Journal of Family Violence, 26*(7), 511–518.

Garrido, E. F., Culhane, S. E., Petrenko, C. L., & Taussig, H. N. (2011b). Psychosocial consequences of caregiver transitions for maltreated youth entering foster care: The moderating impact of community violence exposure. *American Journal of Orthopsychiatry, 81*(3), 382–389.

Gostin, L. O. (2000). *Public health law: Power, duty and restraint*. Berkeley: University of California Press.

Gottfredson, D. C., Najaka, S. S., Kearley, B. W., & Rocha, C. M. (2006). Long-term effects of participation in the Baltimore City drug treatment court: Results from an experimental study. *Journal of Experimental Criminology, 2*, 67–98.

Gupta-Kagan, J. (2014). Towards a public health legal structure for child welfare. *Nebraska Law Review, 42*(4), 897–965.

Hammond, W., Whitaker, D., Lutzker, J., Mercy, J., & Chin, P. (2006). Setting a violence prevention agenda at the centers for disease control and prevention. *Aggression and Violent Behavior, 11*(2), 112–119.

Holt, M. I. (1992). *The orphan trains: Placing out in America*. Lincoln: University of Nebraska Press.

Huntington, C. (2014). The child-welfare system and the limits of determinacy. *Law and Contemporary Problems, 76*(221), 221–248.

Indian Child Welfare Act. (1978). 25 U.S.C. §§ 1901–1963.

Indian Hospitals and Health Facilities. 42 U.S.C. 22 § 2001.

Institute of Behavioral Science, University of Colorado Boulder (2015). *Blueprints for healthy youth development. Center for the Study and Prevention of Violence: Nurse-Family Partnership*. Retrieved from http://www.blueprintsprograms.com/evaluation-abstract/nurse-family-partnership

Irueste-Montes, A. M., & Montes, F. (1988). Court-ordered vs. voluntary treatment of abusive and neglectful parents. *Child Abuse and Neglect, 12*, 33–39.

Jacobson v. Commonwealth of Massachusetts, 197 US 11 (1905).

Kempe, C. H. (1972). The end of routine small pox vaccination in the United States. *Pediatrics, 49*(4), 489–491.

Kilbourne, E. D. (2006). Influenza pandemics of the 20th Century. *Emerging Infectious Disease, 12*(1), 9–14.

Kim, H. K., & Leve, L. D. (2011). Substance use and delinquency among middle school girls in foster care: A three-year follow-up of a randomized controlled trial. *Journal of Consulting and Clinical Psychology, 79*(6), 740–750.

Krieger, N. (2005). Researching critical questions on social justice and public health: An ecosocial perspective. In B. Levy & V. Sidel (Eds.), *Social injustice and public health* (pp. 460–479). New York: Oxford University Press.

Krieger, N., & Birn, A. (1998). A vision of social justice as the foundation of public health: commemorating 150 years of the spirit of 1848. *American Journal of Public Health, 88*(11), 1603–1606.
Kuhn, T. S. (1962). *The structure of scientific revolutions*. Chicago: University of Chicago Press.
Landsverk, J., & Garland, A. F. (1999). Foster care and pathways to mental health services. In P. A. Curtis & D. E. Grady (Eds.), *The foster care crisis: Translating research into practice and policy* (pp. 193–210). Nebraska: The University of Nebraska Press.
Leavitt, J. W. (1997). *Typhoid Mary: Captive to the public's health*. Boston: Beacon Press.
Lewis-Morrarty, E., Dozier, M., Bernard, K., Terracciano, S., & Moore, S. (2012). Cognitive flexibility and theory of mind outcomes among foster children: Preschool follow-up results of a randomized clinical trial. *Journal of Adolescent Health, 51*, S17–S22.
Markel, H., Stern, A. M., Navarro, J. A., & Michalsen, J. R. (2006). A historical assessment of nonpharmaceutical disease containment strategies employed by selected US communities during the second wave of the 1918–1920 influenza pandemic. *Emerging Infectious Disease, 12*(12), 1961–1964.
Markel, H., Lipman, H. B., Navarro, J. A., Sloan, A., Michalsen, J. R., Stern, A. M., & Cetron, M. S. (2007). Nonpharmaceutical interventions implemented by US cities during the 1918–1919 influenza pandemic. *JAMA, 29*(6), 644–654.
Mathews, B., & Bross, D. C. (Eds.). (2015). *Mandatory reporting laws and the identification of severe child abuse and neglect*. Amsterdam: Springer Scientific.
McNeill, W. H. (1976). *Plagues and peoples*. New York: Random House.
Melton, G. B., Holaday, B. J., & Kimbrough-Melton, R. J. (2008). Community life, public health, and children's safety. *Family & Community Health, 31*(2), 84–99.
Mercy, J. (1999). Having new eyes: Viewing child sexual abuse as a public health problem. *Sexual Abuse: A Journal of Research and Treatment, 11*(4), 317–321.
Mercy, J., & Saul, J. (2009). Creating a healthier future through early interventions for children. *JAMA, 301*, 2262–2264.
Mercy, J., Rosenberg, M., Powell, K., Broome, C., & Roper, W. (1993). Public health policy for preventing violence. *Health Affairs, 12*(4), 7–29.
Merkel-Holguin, L., & Bross, D. C. (2015). Commentary: Taking a deep breath before reflecting on differential response. *Child Abuse and Neglect, 39*(1), 1–6.
Nickerson, R. S. (1998). Confirmation bias: A ubiquitous phenomenon in many guises. *Review of General Psychology, 2*(2), 175–220.
Novak, W. J. (1996). *The people's welfare: Law and regulation in nineteenth-century America*. Chapel Hill: The University of North Carolina Press.
Oates, R. K., & Bross, D. C. (1995). What have we learned about treating child physical abuse: A literature review of the last decade. *Child Abuse & Neglect, 19*(4), 463–474.
Olds, D. L., Eckenrode, J., Henderson, C. R., Jr., Kitzman, H., Powers, J., Cole, R., & Luckey, D. (1997). Long-term effects of home visitation on maternal life course and child abuse and neglect. Fifteen-year follow-up of a randomized trial. *JAMA, 278*(8), 637–643.
Paulsen, D. M. (1967). Child abuse reporting laws: The shape of the legislation. *Columbia Law Review, 67*(1), 1–49.
Potterat, J. J. (2015). *Seeking the positives: A life spent on the cutting edge of public health*. North Charleston: Createspace.
Potterat, J. J., Rothenberg, R., & Bross, D. C. (1978). Gonorrhea in street prostitutes: Epidemiologic and legal implications, sexually transmitted diseases. *Journal of the American Venereal Disease Association, 6*(2), 58–63.
Prinz, R. J., Sanders, M. R., Shapiro, C. J., Whitaker, D. J., & Lutzker, J. R. (2009). Population-based prevention of child maltreatment: The US Triple P system population trial. *Prevention Science, 10*(1), 1–12.
Public Law 91–596, 84 STAT. 1590, 91st Congress, S.2193, (1970).
Renner, R. (2007). Plumb crazy. *Science, 315*, 1669.

Richards, E. P. (2007). Public health law as administrative law: Example lessons. *Journal of Health Care Law and Policy, 10*(1), 61–88.

Richards, E. P. (2009). Dangerous people, unsafe conditions: The constitutional basis for public health surveillance. *The Journal of Legal Medicine, 30*, 27–50.

Richards, E. P., & Bross, D. C. (2008). Legal and political aspects of STD control: Public duties and private rights. In K. K. Holmes, P. F. Sparling, P.-A. Mardh, et al. (Eds.), *Sexually transmitted diseases* (pp. 2039–2046). New York: McGraw-Hill.

Rosenfeld, A., Pilowsky, D., Fine, P., Thorpe, M., Fein, M., Simms, M., et al. (1997). Foster care: An update. *Journal of the American Academy of Child and Adolescent Psychiatry, 36*(4), 448–457.

Rothenberg, R., Bross, D. C., & Vernon, T. M. (1980). Reporting of Gonorrhea by private physicians: A behavioral study. *American Journal of Public Health, 70*(9), 983–986.

Rubin, D. M., Downes, K. J., O'Reilly, A. L. R., Mekonnen, R., Luan, X., & Localio, R. (2008). Impact of kinship care on behavioral well-being for children in out-of-home care. *Archives of Pediatric and Adolescent Medicine, 162*(6), 550–556.

Runyan, C. W., & Runyan, D. K. (2014). Applying a public health approach to child welfare. In D. Chadwick (Ed.), *Chadwick's child maltreatment* (pp. 579–594). Florissant: STM Learning.

Schonberger, L. B., Hurwitz, E. S., Katona, P., Holman, R. C., & Bregman, D. J. (1981). Guillain-Barré syndrome: Its epidemiology and associations with influenza vaccination. *Annals of Neurology Supplement: Guillain-Barré Syndrome, 9*, 31–38.

Senate Committee on Labor and Human Resources (1985). *Domestic violence and public health: Hearing before the Senate subcommittee on children, family, drugs and alcoholism*. Retrieved from https://www.ncjrs.gov/App/Publications/abstract.aspx?ID=102525

Sencer, D. J., & Millar, J. D. (2006). Reflections on the 1976 Swine Flu Vaccination Program. *Emerging Infectious Disease, 12*(1), 29–33.

Shedler, J. (2010). The efficacy of psychodynamic psychotherapy. *American Psychologist, 65*(2), 98–109.

Shilts, R. (1987). *And the band played on: Politics, people, and the AIDS epidemic*. New York: St. Martin's Press.

Shipman, K., & Taussig, H. N. (2009). Mental health treatment of child abuse and neglect: The promise of evidence-based practice. *Pediatric Clinics of North America, 56*(2), 417–428.

Smith, D. K., Leve, L. D., & Chamberlain, P. (2011). Preventing internalizing and externalizing problems in girls in foster care as they enter middle school: Impact of an intervention. *Prevention Science, 12*(3), 269–277.

Sprang, G. (2009). The efficacy of a relational treatment for maltreated children and their families. *Child and Adolescent Mental Health, 14*(2), 81–88.

Susser, M. (1993). Health as a human right: An epidemiologist's perspective on the public health. *American Journal of Public Health, 83*(3), 418–426.

Taussig, H. N., & Culhane, S. E. (2005). Foster care as an intervention for abused and neglected children. In K. A. Kendall-Tackett & S. M. Giacomoni (Eds.), *Child victimization: Maltreatment, bullying and violence, prevention and intervention* (pp. 20:1–20:25). Kingston: Civic Research Institute.

Taussig, H. N., & Culhane, S. E. (2010). Impact of a mentoring and skills group program on mental health outcomes for maltreated children in foster care. *Archives of Pediatrics & Adolescent Medicine, 164*(8), 739–746.

Taussig, H. N., Clyman, R. B., & Landsverk, J. (2001). Children who return home from foster care: A six-year prospective study of behavioral health outcomes in adolescence. *Pediatrics, 108*(1), e10.

Taussig, H. N., Culhane, S. E., & Hettleman, D. (2007). Fostering healthy futures: An innovative preventive intervention for preadolescent youth in out-of-home care. *Child Welfare, 86*(5), 113.

Taussig, H. N., Culhane, S. E., Garrido, E., & Knudtson, M. D. (2012). RCT of a mentoring and skills group program: Placement and permanency outcomes for foster youth. *Pediatrics, 130*(1), e33–e39.

Taxin, A. (2016, April 19). Immigrant kids and their guardians are mostly in the US illegally. *US News and World Report*. Retrieved from http://www.usnews.com/news/us/articles/2016-04-18/immigrant-kids-placed-with-adults-who-are-in-us-illegally

Tjaden, P. G., & Thoennes, N. (1992). Predictors of legal intervention in child maltreatment cases. *Child Abuse and Neglect, 16*, 807–821.

Toms, J. (2010). Mind the gap: MIND, the mental hygiene movement and the trapdoor in measurements of intellect. *Journal of Intellectual Disabilities Research, 54*(1), 16–27.

United States Department of Health and Human Services, Administration for Children and Families (2014, July). *The AFCARS report: Preliminary FY 2013 estimates*. Retrieved from http://www.acf.hhs.gov/sites/default/files/cb/afcarsreport21.pdf

United States Environmental Protection Agency (2016). Enforcement annual results for Fiscal Year (FY) 2016. Retrieved from https://www.epa.gov/enforcement/enforcement-annual-results-fiscal-year-fy-2015

Wicks, B. (1988). *No time to wave goodbye*. Toronto: Stoddart Publishing.

Wilson, D. B., Mitchell, O., & MacKenzie, D. L. (2006). A systematic review of Drug Court effects on recidivism. *Journal of Experimental Criminology, 2*, 459–487.

Winokur, M. A., Crawford, G. A., Longobardi, R. C., & Valentine, D. P. (2008). A matched comparison of child welfare outcomes between children in kinship care and foster care. *Families in Society, 89*, 338–346.

Wolfe, D. A., Aragona, J., Kaufman, K., & Sandler, J. (1980). The importance of adjudication in the treatment of child abusers: Some preliminary findings. *Child Abuse and Neglect, 4*, 127–135.

Wright, J., Franks, A., Ayres, P., Jones, K., Roberts, T., & Whitty, P. (2002). Public health in hospitals: The missing link in health improvement. *Journal of Public Health, 24*(3), 152–155.

Zimmerman, F., & Mercy, J. A. (2010). A better start: Child maltreatment prevention as a public health priority. *Zero to Three*, 4–10.

Chapter 19
Innovative Approaches to Improving Outcomes for Children Involved with Child Welfare: Youth Mentoring

Heather Taussig and Lindsey Weiler

19.1 Introduction

For the past 5 years, estimates of the number of youth in foster care in the US have held steady at approximately 400,000 on any given day (Child Welfare Information Gateway 2017). Nearly half live in non-relative foster homes, 30% in relative foster homes (referred to as 'kinship care'), 8% in institutions, 6% in group homes, and about 5% in other placements (e.g., pre-adoptive homes) or have run away. Many youth experience multiple placements while in care, and some move in and out of the system throughout their childhood. About 10% of youth who exit foster care 'age out' or emancipate, defined as reaching age 18 without achieving permanency, including adoption or reunification with their biological families (Child Welfare Information Gateway 2017).

The experience of substantial and traumatic adversity (e.g., abuse and neglect, exposure to substance use and violence, chronic disruptions in school and living situations, and abandonment) is linked to diminished physical and mental health, academic underachievement and school dropout, problematic substance use, poverty and homelessness, and incarceration (Felitti et al. 1998; Weiler et al. 2016). Despite all odds, however, some youth avoid this negative trajectory (Hass and Graydon 2008; Simmel 2007). While there are various perspectives on why and

H. Taussig (✉)
University of Denver Graduate School of Social Work, Denver, CO, USA

Kempe Center for the Prevention and Treatment of Child Abuse and Neglect, University of Colorado School of Medicine, Aurora, CO, USA
e-mail: Heather.Taussig@du.edu

L. Weiler
Institute for Translational Research in Children's Mental Health, College of Education and Human Development, University of Minnesota, Minneapolis, MN, USA
e-mail: lmweiler@umn.edu

B. Lonne et al. (eds.), *Re-Visioning Public Health Approaches for Protecting Children*, Child Maltreatment 9, https://doi.org/10.1007/978-3-030-05858-6_19

how youth exhibit resilience (i.e., the maintenance of positive adaptation despite experiences of significant adversity; Luthar et al. 2000), central to most empirical and theoretical frameworks is the presence of competent, caring adults in the lives of children. In fact, increasing the number and quality of significant figures of support (e.g., mentors) available to youth increases their chances of healthy development (Egeland et al. 1988; Masten et al. 2009).

This chapter reviews studies of mentoring for youth in foster care. With the influx of mentoring programs nationally, more empirical studies are beginning to examine the impact of mentoring for extremely vulnerable populations, including youth in foster care. Research in this area has focused on a wide range of outcomes including social skills, relationship quality, life skills, self-determination, self-confidence, academic functioning, educational outcomes, mental health functioning, delinquency, placement stability, and employment. Following a brief description of relevant theoretical models, this chapter reviews the evidence related to mentoring youth in foster care.

19.2 Conceptual Framework

Fundamentally, mentors can fill an important relational void in children's lives while facilitating the development of cognitive abilities, sparks and interests, prosocial behaviour, positive self-esteem and identity, and social relationships (Rhodes et al. 2006). Youth-centered relationships characterized by trust, consistency, mutuality, and respect can result in positive youth development which has been shown to buffer the impact of adversity on youth's life trajectories (Raposa et al. 2016). While there is great potential, mentoring youth in foster care also requires an understanding of the challenges that confront youth in care. Because mentoring-based interventions are relational in nature and youth in foster care often experience interpersonal difficulties, mentoring poses both opportunities and challenges.

Although not all children in foster care experience disruptions in early parent-child relationships, many do. Attachment theory states that early relationship experiences set the stage for future close relationships (Bowlby 1988). When children have positive, secure attachments with caregivers, they have appropriate "working models" (i.e., a set of expectations and beliefs about oneself, others, and the relationship between self and others) and glean benefits in the form of healthy relationships and positive youth outcomes across multiple domains (e.g., psychosocial, cognitive). When children lack secure attachments due, for example, to abandonment, maltreatment, or placement in foster care, their internal working models are more negative and distorted and they may be fearful of trusting others. Fortunately, these models are amenable to change via corrective relational experiences (Cassidy and Shaver 2016), such as ongoing, consistent, and meaningful relationships with adults. These nurturing relationships not only promote healthy attachments for children, but they may also prepare children to build stronger and safer relationships with their own children.

In healthy social contexts, children are provided guidance in developing relationships and positive support networks. When this support is absent, however, youth in foster care may view dependence on others as a personal weakness or failure (Samuels and Pryce 2008). Youth who age out of foster care without social guidance may experience what is referred to as "psychological homelessness" – that is, a longing for 'home' and enduring connections (Samuels 2008). Public health approaches and ecological theories emphasize the role adults play in modeling and facilitating social bonding across contexts, which increases social capital and the capacity for closeness (Aquilino 2006; Bronfenbrenner and Morris 2006; Overton 2010; Scharf et al. 2004). Over time, youth in foster care who experience positive relationships with adult mentors can learn to form, maintain, and benefit from other healthy relationships, thereby promoting health and wellbeing across the lifespan.

In addition to improving youth's relational capacity, there are other reasons to believe that mentoring may be a contextually-sensitive and efficacious intervention for youth in foster care (Hambrick et al. 2016). Many young people in foster care say that they are not interested in "doing more therapy," but they are open to a mentoring relationship. From a pragmatic perspective, mentoring does not require a stable caregiver to participate (as many youth interventions do), which enables the intervention to continue even after a child changes placement. Mentoring also may provide the young person opportunities to engage in activities that are often restricted by social services or logistically difficult to engage in due to issues with transportation, time, and financial resources. As most mentoring relationships are individualized, mentoring may work well as a strategy to intervene with youth in foster care who have heterogeneous challenges, including cognitive and learning disabilities and mental and physical health problems. Finally, when so much of the focus in social services is on identifying and ameliorating *family* problems, mentoring can focus on the *child*—fostering positive youth development among young people by nurturing their interests and talents. Interventions for high-risk youth often emphasize the reduction of risk, but a positive youth development (PYD) framework rejects this type of deficit model and focuses instead on fostering the development of competencies within multiple contexts (individual, family, school, and community) in order to help youth chart a future that will make them healthy, productive citizens (e.g., Gavin et al. 2010). A PYD perspective emphasizes the role of developmental assets in promoting positive development, and mentors – defined as caring, competent adults invested in the lives of youth people – are a crucial asset. This framework is consistent with a public health approach that focuses on prevention and empowerment of individuals (Herrenkohl et al. 2015).

Although mentoring holds great promise for youth in foster care, there are also some cautions. Youth who have experienced loss may have more adverse reactions to mentoring relationships that end prematurely and yet may be at particular risk for this, given their lack of stable living arrangements and high rates of emotional and behavioural problems. Mentors may interpret a lack of responsiveness or openness from their mentees as disinterest in the relationship without understanding the impact of their attachment history or the complicated lives that they lead. Young people in care discuss the importance of consistency and emotional closeness in mentoring relationships which may require more flexibility, persistence, and patience on the part of the mentors (Spencer et al. 2010).

19.3 Impact of Mentoring on Youth in Foster Care

19.3.1 Big Brothers Big Sisters Studies

Two studies examined the impact of Big Brothers Big Sisters (BBBS) programs on youth in foster care. The first study analysed data previously collected in a randomized controlled trial (RCT) of a national study of BBBS involving youth ages 10–15. This study examined the 90 youth participants who identified themselves as living in foster care and compared those randomized to the BBBS intervention to those assigned to the control group. Relative to youth in the control group, foster youth in the BBBS group demonstrated larger improvements in peer support 18-months after the start of the study (Rhodes et al. 1999). A more recent non-experimental pilot study examined the perceived impact of a BBBS program in North Texas involving youth in foster care, ages 5–16. Both youth and mentors were surveyed 4 and 10 months post referral to the BBBS program. The study encountered significant enrolment, retention, and fidelity problems, rendering the data collected difficult to interpret. Those study participants who were surveyed at the follow-up assessment, however, reported high rates of program satisfaction and retrospective improvements in 5 areas: school, employment, friendships, relationships with authority figures and self-confidence (Scannapieco and Painter 2013).

19.3.2 Mentoring Programs to Improve Educational Outcomes

Several studies have examined the outcomes of mentoring programs specifically focused on improving education-related outcomes for youth in foster care. In the first study, a child welfare agency partnered with 18 school districts to provide individual tutoring/mentoring during the academic year to maltreated youth in foster care in grades K-12. The tutors/mentors were certified teachers, but not the child's teacher. Most of the mentoring/tutoring activities were focused on academics and study skills. Although there was no comparison group in this study and fairly small subsets of the 206 participants completed assessments at later time points, results suggested that students had improved their academic skills (Mallett 2012).

A second educationally focused mentoring program, *TAKE CHARGE*, was tested in two RCT studies of older youth who were living in foster care and receiving special education services. The first study enrolled 69 youth ages 16–17 and the second study enrolled 133 youth ages 14–17. The youth in the intervention groups received individualized coaching by trained staff as well as group mentoring by "near-peer foster care alumni" over the academic year. Across the two studies, positive outcomes were noted in self-determination and mental health (as rated by youth and parents, but not by teachers), independent living activities, use of transition services, self-identified educational goals and accomplishments, educational planning knowledge and engagement, postsecondary preparation, and quality of life. There were no significant differences, however, between the intervention and control groups in GPA or school attitude (Geenen et al. 2013; Powers et al. 2012).

Finally, two small studies within schools of social work at universities provided mentoring programs to transitioning foster youth with the goal of increasing their awareness of and access to higher education. Although there were no comparison groups, participating youth reported increases in knowledge about post-secondary options and improvements in academic self-efficacy (Bruster and Coccoma 2013; Kirk and Day 2011).

19.3.3 Multicomponent Programs to Improve Mental Health and Behavioural Outcomes

Two studies evaluated multicomponent programs each with a manualized skills group and mentoring/coaching component that focused on improving mental health and behavioural functioning of children in foster care. The first study, *Fostering Healthy Futures (FHF),* enrolled 9- to 11-year-old children recently placed in foster care. The children attended 30 weeks of social skills groups and received individualized mentoring over the academic year. Mentors were graduate students in social work and psychology. Results of the RCT included improvements in mental health problems (including trauma symptoms) and quality of life, as well as a reduction in mental health services utilized, number of placement changes, and placement in residential treatment centers. There were no demonstrated effects on coping skills, social support or social acceptance (Taussig and Culhane 2010; Taussig et al. 2012). An adaptation of FHF for teens is currently being tested in another RCT. A preliminary pilot study of this adapted program, *Fostering Healthy Futures for Teens*, which uses mentoring without skills groups for older children with a history of foster care, demonstrated high rates of program engagement and satisfaction (Taussig et al. 2015).

Another intervention, *Middle School Success*, for girls in foster care was similar to FHF in that it was implemented over an academic year, although group sessions for girls and their caregivers occurred for 3 weeks (2×/week) prior to the start of the school year. Parents continued weekly group meetings and girls received individualized coaching by trained staff over the academic year. Short-term results of the RCT included improvements in internalizing and externalizing behaviours in the girls assigned to the intervention, relative to controls. At the 2-year post intervention follow-up, girls who were enrolled in the intervention had experienced fewer placement changes, demonstrated more prosocial behaviours, were less likely to be using substances and were less likely to be engaging in delinquent behaviours than girls assigned to the control group (Kim and Leve 2011; Smith et al. 2011).

19.3.4 System-Run Mentoring/Advocacy Programs

Some mentoring programs for youth in foster care were administered by social services, in which trained staff provided the mentoring/coaching. One study examined the impact of "therapeutic mentoring" for 262 children ages 6–15 who were at risk of placement disruption from their foster homes. Caseworker reports were used to evaluate the impact of the program using a quasi-experimental design in which clinicians referred some youth to therapeutic mentoring if they determined the child was "able to benefit" from a mentoring relationship. Those youth who were not referred to mentoring served as the comparison group. Mentored youth were reported by caseworkers to have fewer trauma symptoms than youth in the comparison group. Unfortunately, the small number ($n = 27$) of participants at follow-up limits our ability to understand the impact of the program (Johnson and Pryce 2013; Johnson et al. 2011).

In the *Massachusetts Adolescent Outreach Program*, outreach workers were matched with older youth (ages 15–20) to help them develop skills and engage in appropriate developmental tasks including applying for jobs and college. A RCT of the program found positive impacts on college enrollment and retention, obtaining important documents (e.g., birth certificate, license) and receiving assistance with education, employment, housing and financial management. There were no differences, however, between the control and intervention groups on several other target indices including employment, economic well-being, stable housing, delinquency, pregnancy, or preparedness for independence (Courtney et al. 2011; Greeson et al. 2015a, b).

An innovative British study reviewed case files of 181 participants across 11 mentoring programs for emancipating youth ages 15–23. Many of the mentoring programs were situated within departments of social services, as the program was mandated by the Prince's Trust Leaving Care Initiative. The case reviews found that over three-quarters of the young people achieved program goals, but that half the relationships evidenced "negative outcomes" including not meeting the goals and also having unplanned endings to the mentoring relationship (Clayden and Stein 2005).

Finally, youth in foster care are often paired with court-appointed special advocates (CASA). CASA volunteers are lay persons who receive specialized training to assist children through the court proceedings. They are typically assigned only a small number of children and can provide more time and attention to youth than attorneys or caseworkers are able (Litzelfelner 2000). One key difference between CASA volunteers and typical mentors is that CASA volunteers are charged with providing information to court officials to inform decision making. CASA volunteers are focused on the well-being of the child and may be one of the only sources of stability, as social workers, attorneys, and/or foster parents change (Youngclarke 2004). Evidence for the effectiveness of CASA volunteers is based mostly on quasi-experimental studies and is limited almost exclusively to outcomes related to permanency. A full review of CASA models is outside the scope of this chapter, but existing studies tentatively suggest that youth with a CASA volunteer may experience fewer placement changes, less time in care, greater likelihood of achieving permanency, greater access to services and resources, and more support through adult relationships (Caliber Associates 2004; Calkins and Millar 1999). It is important to note, however, that not all studies have replicated these findings (e.g., Tuff 2014), and few differences between those with a CASA volunteer and those without have been reported on measures of well-being and development (e.g., Caliber Associates 2004).

19.3.5 Natural Mentoring

While program-based mentors can certainly develop positive relationships with youth in foster care, naturally-forming mentoring relationships might be particularly impactful for this population, as these relationships typically involve mutual trust and a shared understanding of the youth's difficult background and associated emotional and behavioural problems. Because these relationships form naturally over time, there is less likelihood that they will terminate abruptly and a greater likelihood that they will last for many years, helping bridge important transitions for foster youth, especially the transition to independence (Greeson 2013).

Approximately 22,000 young people emancipate from foster care each year (Child Welfare Information Gateway 2017) many of whom lack the social capital that is available to most young adults making the transition to independence (Duke et al. 2017). The importance of close, meaningful relationships between foster youth and supportive adults during the transition to adulthood has been recognized at a policy level. The Fostering Connections to Success and Increasing Adoptions Act of 2008 (PL 110-351) provided states with enhanced opportunities to ensure that young adults do not exit foster care without having established connections to caring adults. This was based on research which suggests that identifying natural mentors is incredibly important when young people are emancipating from care.

Young adults who emancipate from care report high rates (over 70% in most studies) of non-parental natural mentorship, with relationships most likely to have begun before or during adolescence. Although most of these studies involved small samples of youth that were not necessarily representative of the larger foster care population, there were many consistencies in their findings. Non-parental natural mentors most often consist of relatives, friends of the family, caseworkers, former foster parents or staff at their former placements, therapists, and teachers. Young adults describe their relationship with their natural mentor as very close, using phrases such as "like a parent," or "trusted advisor"; in one study, over half of the respondents were in contact with their mentor nearly every day. The types of support that natural mentors are reported to provide include instrumental, informational, and emotional support, teaching social skills, providing advice, and "keeping them on track," which many young people described as key for preventing negative outcomes and most importantly supporting them in achieving positive outcomes (Ahrens et al. 2008, 2011; Collins et al. 2010; Duke et al. 2017; Greeson et al. 2016; Hass and Graydon 2008; Munson et al. 2010).

Studies have also empirically examined whether the presence of a natural mentor is associated with better functioning. In two studies of emancipating/emancipated youth, those with a natural mentor experienced more favourable outcomes than those without a mentor – they had lower levels of stress and higher life satisfaction, were more likely to complete high school or obtain a GED, and were less likely to be arrested or experience homelessness as a young adult. The presence of a natural mentor was, however, unrelated to employment or substance use (Collins et al. 2010; Munson and McMillen 2009). Two other studies used data from the National Longitudinal Study of Adolescent Health (Add Health) to examine the effects of a natural mentor. The Add Health study is a 6-year, multi-wave longitudinal study that enrolled several nationally representative cohorts of youth in grades 7 to 12. At Wave 3, when participants were between the ages of 18 and 26 (average age of 21.5), they were asked to retrospectively report whether a non-parental adult had made an "important positive difference in your life since you were 14 years old." Among study participants who reported they had lived in foster care, having a natural mentor was associated with several positive outcomes including participation in higher education, less suicidal ideation, lower rates of sexually transmitted infections, less physical fighting, better perceived general health, and a higher number of positive outcomes across domains. Natural mentorship was not, however, associated with self-esteem, depression, completion of high school, current employment, assets (including having a bank account or owning a car or home), physical activity, body-mass index, substance use, arrests, or gang membership (Ahrens et al. 2008; Greeson et al. 2010).

Although almost all studies of natural mentorship for youth in foster care examined the effects on adolescents or young adults, one study looked at whether the presence of a natural mentor in preadolescence was associated with better psychosocial functioning. This study found that children with natural mentors reported greater attachment to friends; however, having a natural mentor was unrelated to attachment to parents (either biological or substitute), social skills, or perceived future opportunities (Greeson et al. 2016).

19.4 Conclusions

Research on the impact of mentoring for youth in foster care is emerging. Mentoring appears to be highly acceptable to youth in foster care, and mentors are reported to provide life-changing informational, instrumental, and emotional support to young people who often lack consistent adults to help them navigate the many challenges they face. Available research suggests that mentoring for children in foster care (across a range of ages and mentoring formats) can have positive impacts on mental health, educational functioning and attainment, peer relationships, placement outcomes, and life satisfaction. Mentoring has demonstrated null or mixed results, however, for other outcomes, including social skills, attachment to adults, physical health, employment and financial assets, risky behaviours and associated negative life-course outcomes (e.g., substance use, delinquency, arrests) among this population. Because of the interpersonal vulnerability and high potential for adverse outcomes among youth in foster care, great care and coordination is required when implementing mentoring programs. If done well, however, the benefits of mentoring may be realized and youth in foster care may experience positive outcomes across a range of domains, thereby reducing health disparities and potentially disrupting the devastating cycle of violence.

References

Ahrens, K. R., DuBois, D. L., Richardson, L. P., Fan, M., & Lozano, P. (2008). Youth in foster care with adult mentors during adolescence have improved adult outcomes. *Pediatrics, 121*, e246–e252.

Ahrens, K. R., DuBois, D. L., Garrison, M., Spencer, R., Richardson, L. P., & Lozano, P. (2011). Qualitative exploration of relationships with important non-parental adults in the lives of youth in foster care. *Children and Youth Services Review, 33*, 1012–1023.

Aquilino, W. S. (2006). In J. J. Arnett & J. L. Tanner (Eds.),. *Emerging adults in America: Coming of age in the 21st century Family relationships and support systems in emerging adulthood* (pp. 193–217). Washington, DC: American Psychological Association.

Bowlby, J. (1988). *A secure base: Parent-child attachment and healthy human development*. New York: Basic Books.

Bronfenbrenner, U., & Morris, P. A. (2006). The bioecological model of human development. In W. Damon & R. M. Lerner (Eds.), *The handbook of child psychology. Vol. 1: Theoretical models of human development* (6th ed., pp. 793–828). Hoboken: Wiley.

Bruster, B. E., & Coccoma, P. (2013). Mentoring for educational success: Advancing foster care youth incorporating the core competencies. *Journal of Human Behavior in the Social Environment, 23*, 388–399.

Caliber Associates. (2004, January 20). "Evaluation of CASA Representation." *Evaluation of the Casa Representation.* Final Report: n. pag.

Calkins, C. A., & Millar, M. (1999). The effectiveness of court appointed special advocates to assist in permanency planning. *Child and Adolescent Social Work Journal, 16*(1), 37–45.

Cassidy, J., & Shaver, P. R. (Eds.). (2016). *Handbook of attachment: Theory, research, and clinical applications* (3rd ed.). New York: Guilford Press.

Child Welfare Information Gateway. (2017). *Foster care statistics 2015*. Washington, DC: US Department of Health and Human Services, Children's Bureau.

Clayden, J., & Stein, M. (2005). *Mentoring young people leaving care: 'Someone for me.'* York: Joseph Rowntree Foundation.

Collins, M. E., Spencer, R., & Ward, R. (2010). Supporting youth in the transition from foster care: Formal and informal connections. *Child Welfare, 89*, 125–143.

Courtney, M., Zinn, A., Johnson, H., & Malm, K. (2011). *Evaluation of the Massachusetts adolescent outreach program for youths in intensive foster care: Final Report*. OPRE Report #

2011–14. Washington, DC: Office of Planning, Research and Evaluation, Administration for Children and Families, US Department of Health and Human Services.

Duke, T., Farruggia, S. P., & Germo, G. R. (2017). "I don't know where I would be right now if it wasn't for them": Emancipated foster care youth and their important non-parental adults. *Children and Youth Services Review, 76*, 65–73.

Egeland, B., Jacobvitz, D., & Sroufe, L. A. (1988). Breaking the cycle of abuse. *Child Development, 59*, 1080–1088.

Felitti, V. J., Anda, R. F., Nordenberg, D., Williamson, D. F., Spitz, A. M., Edwards, V., Koss, M. P., & Marks, J. S. (1998). Relationship of childhood abuse and household dysfunction to many of the leading causes of death in adults. The Adverse Childhood Experiences (ACE) Study. *American Journal of Preventive Medicine, 14*, 245–258.

Gavin, L. E., Catalano, R. F., & Markham, C. M. (2010). Positive youth development as a strategy to promote adolescent sexual and reproductive health. *Journal of Adolescent Health, 46*(3), S1–S6.

Geenen, S., Powers, L. E., Powers, J., Cunningham, M., McMahon, L., Nelson, M., Dalton, L. D., Swank, P., Fullerton, A., & Consortium to Increase the Success of Youth in Foster Care. (2013). Experimental study of a self-determination intervention for youth in foster care. *Career Development and Transition for Exceptional Individuals, 36*, 84–95.

Greeson, J. K. P. (2013). Foster youth and the transition to adulthood: The theoretical and conceptual basis for natural mentoring. *Emerging Adulthood, 1*, 40–51.

Greeson, J. K. P., Usher, L., & Grinstein-Weiss, M. (2010). One adult who is crazy about you: Can natural mentoring relationships increase assets among young adults with and without foster care experience? *Children and Youth Services Review, 32*, 565–577.

Greeson, J. K. P., Garcia, A. R., Kim, M., & Courtney, M. E. (2015a). Foster youth and social support: The first RCT of independent living services. *Research on Social Work Practice, 25*, 349–357.

Greeson, J. K., Thompson, A. E., Evans-Chase, M., & Ali, S. (2015b). Child welfare professionals' attitudes and beliefs about welfare-based natural mentoring for older youth in foster care. *Journal of Social Service Research, 41*, 93–112.

Greeson, J. K. P., Weiler, L. M., Thompson, A. E., & Taussig, H. N. (2016). A first look at natural mentoring among preadolescent foster children. *Journal of Community Psychology, 44*, 586–601.

Hambrick, E. P., Oppenheim-Weller, S., N'Zi, A. M., & Taussig, H. N. (2016). Mental health interventions for children in Foster Care: A systematic review. *Children and Youth Services Review, 70*, 65–77. https://doi.org/10.1016/j.childyouth.2016.09.002.

Hass, M., & Graydon, M. (2008). Sources of resiliency among foster youth. *Children and Youth Services Review, 31*, 457–463.

Herrenkohl, T. I., Higgins, D., Merrick, M. T., & Leeb, R. T. (2015). Positioning and public health framework at the intersection of child maltreatment and intimate partner violence. *Child Abuse & Neglect, 48*, 22–28.

Johnson, B., & Pryce, J. M. (2013). Therapeutic mentoring: Reducing the impact of trauma for foster youth. *Child Welfare, 92*, 9–25.

Johnson, B., Pryce, J. M., & Martinovich, Z. (2011). The role of therapeutic mentoring in enhancing outcomes for youth in foster care. *Child Welfare, 90*, 51–71.

Kim, H. K., & Leve, D. L. (2011). Substance use and delinquency among middle school girls in foster care: A 3-year follow-up of a randomized controlled trial. *Journal of Consulting and Clinical Psychology, 79*, 740–750.

Kirk, R., & Day, A. (2011). Increasing college access for youth aging out of foster care: Evalution of a summer camp program for foster youth transitioning from high school to college. *Children and Youth Services Review, 33*, 1173–1180.

Litzelfelner, P. (2000). The effectiveness of CASAs in achieving positive outcomes for children. *Child Welfare, 79*(2), 179–193.

Luthar, S. S., Cicchetti, D., & Becker, B. (2000). The construct of resilience: A critical evaluation and guidelines for future work. *Child Development, 71*, 543–562.

Mallett, C. A. (2012). The school success program: Improving maltreated children's academic and school-related outcomes. *Children & Schools, 34*, 13–26.

Masten, A. S., Cutuli, J. J., Herbers, J. E., & Reed, M.-G. J. (2009). Resilience in development. In C. R. Snyder & S. J. Lopex (Ed.), *Oxford handbook of positive psychology* (pp. 117–131). Oxford: Oxford University Press.

Munson, M. R., & McMillen, J. C. (2009). Natural mentoring and psychosocial outcomes among older youth transitioning from foster care. *Children and Youth Services Review, 31*, 104–111.

Munson, M. R., Smalling, S. E., Spencer, R., Scott, L. D. S., Jr., & Tracy, E. M. (2010). A steady presence in the midst of change: Non-kin natural mentors in the lives of older youth exiting foster care. *Children and Youth Services Review, 32*, 527–535.

Overton, W. F. (2010). Life-span development: Concepts and issues. In R. M. Lerner & W. F. Overton (Eds.), *The Handbook of life-span development. Vol 1: Cognition, biology, and methods* (pp. 1–29). Hoboken: Wiley.

Powers, L. E., Geenen, S., Powers, J., Pommier-Satya, S., Turner, A., Dalton, L. D., Drummond, D., & Swank, P. (2012). My life: Effects of a longitudinal, randomized study of self-determination enhancement on the transition outcomes of youth in foster care and special education. *Children and Youth Services Review, 34*, 2179–2187.

Raposa, E. B., Rhodes, J. E., & Herrera, C. (2016). The impact of youth risk on mentoring relationship quality: do mentor characteristics matter? *American Journal of Community Psychology, 57*, 320–329.

Rhodes, J. E., Haight, W. L., & Briggs, E. C. (1999). The influence of mentoring on the peer relationships of foster youth in relative and nonrelative care. *Journal of Research on Adolescence, 9*, 185–201.

Rhodes, J. E., Spencer, R., Keller, T. E., Liang, B., & Noam, G. (2006). A model for the influence of mentoring relationships on youth development. *Journal of Community Psychology, 34*, 691–707.

Samuels, G. M. (2008). *A reason, a season, or a lifetime: Relational permanence among young adults with foster care backgrounds*. Chicago: Chapin Hall Center for Children at the University of Chicago. Retrieved from https://www.fosterclub.com/sites/default/files/docs/blogs/18916-A_Reason_a_Season_or_a_Lifetime-Relational_Permanence.pdf

Samuels, G., & Pryce, J. (2008). "What doesn't kill you makes you stronger": Survivalist self-reliance as resilience and risk among young adults aging out of foster care. *Children and Youth Services Review, 30*, 1198–1210.

Scannapieco, M., & Painter, K. R. (2013). Barrier to implementing a mentoring program for youth in foster care: Implications for practice and policy innovation. *Child and Adolescent Social Work Journal, 31*, 163–180.

Scharf, M., Mayseless, O., & Kivenson-Baron, I. (2004). Adolescents' attachment representations and developmental tasks in emerging adulthood. *Developmental Psychology, 40*, 430–444.

Simmel, C. (2007). Risk and protective factors contributing to the longitudinal psychosocial well-being of adopted foster children. *Journal of Emotional and Behavioral Disorders, 15*, 237–249.

Smith, D. K., Leve, L. D., & Chamberlain, P. (2011). Preventing internalizing and externalizing problems in girls in foster care as they enter middle school: Impact of an intervention. *Prevention Science, 12*, 269–277.

Spencer, R., Collins, M. E., Ward, R., & Smashnaya, S. (2010). Mentoring for young people leaving foster care: Promise and potential pitfalls. *Social Work, 55*, 225–235.

Taussig, H. N., & Culhane, S. E. (2010). Impact of a mentoring and skills group program on mental health outcomes for maltreated children in foster care. *Archives of Pediatric and Adolescent Medicine, 164*, 139–146.

Taussig, H., Culhane, S. E., Garrido, E., Knudtson, M. D., & Petrenko, C. L. M. (2012). Does severity of physical neglect moderate the impact of an efficacious preventive intervention for maltreated children in foster care? *Child Maltreatment, 18*, 56–64.

Taussig, H., Weiler, L., Rhodes, T., Hambrick, E., Wertheimer, R., Fireman, O., & Combs, M. (2015). Fostering healthy futures for teens: Adaptation of an evidence-based program. *Journal of the Society for Social Work and Research, 6*, 617–642.

Tuff, L. (2014). *Court appointed special advocates: Is their impact effectively evaluated by current research methodology?* Retrieved from https://digital.lib.washington.edu/researchworks/bitstream/handle/1773/25574/Tuff%20-%20Capstone.pdf?sequence=1

Weiler, L. M., Garrido, E. F., & Taussig, H. N. (2016). Wellbeing of children in the foster care system. In M. R. Korin (Ed.), *Health promotion for children and adolescents* (pp. 371–388). New York: Springer.

Youngclarke, D. (2004). Trends & developments in the juvenile court: A systematic review of the impact of court appointed special advocates. *Journal of the Center for Families, Children and the Courts, 5*, 109–169.

Chapter 20
Understanding Trauma and Child Maltreatment Experienced in Indigenous Communities

Deb Duthie, Sharon Steinhauer, Catherine Twinn, Vincent Steinhauer, and Bob Lonne

20.1 Introduction

This chapter outlines a conceptual framework for understanding and responding effectively to the primary causes of maltreatment affecting Indigenous children, and locates these within the historical and contemporary context of Colonization, intergenerational trauma and inequality. The Australian and Canadian situations are used as examples of child protection systems that are founded in Western worldviews which exacerbate continuing grief, loss and trauma in the lives of Indigenous peoples. While it is preferable to use the terms Aboriginal and Torres Strait Islander peoples in Australia, this paper will use the term Indigenous to include Aboriginal and Torres Strait Islanders and Canadian First Nations, Inuit and Métis peoples.

We take a systemic perspective and reject the individual and blaming focus characteristic of many contemporary examinations of child maltreatment. We argue that the spiritual foundation of Indigenous culture – "living out" Indigenous sacred laws – provides Indigenous families and communities with resilience, social capital

D. Duthie (✉)
School of Public Health and Social Work, Queensland University of Technology (QUT), Brisbane, Australia
e-mail: d.duthie@qut.edu.au

S. Steinhauer · V. Steinhauer
University nuhelot'įne thaiyots'į nistameyimâkanak Blue Quills, St. Paul, AB, Canada
e-mail: sharons@bluequills.ca

C. Twinn
Twinn Law, Edmonton, AB, Canada
e-mail: ctwinn@twinnlaw.com

B. Lonne
School of Health, University of New England, Armidale, NSW, Australia
e-mail: blonne@une.edu.au

B. Lonne et al. (eds.), *Re-Visioning Public Health Approaches for Protecting Children*, Child Maltreatment 9, https://doi.org/10.1007/978-3-030-05858-6_20

and the humane capacity to thrive and enable nurturing care for their children in otherwise hostile social, political and economic systems. As Navajo jurist and legal scholar Raymond Austin (2009) noted:

> American Indian peoples should realize that the potential solutions to their social, health, and educational problems may not lie in highly touted non-Indian methods, but in their own languages, philosophies, cultures and spiritual practices. In other words, use the local "tribal encyclopaedia", the wise Indian Elders and traditionalists for answers to Indian problems as our ancestors did. This is what I mean when I say, "Think like an Indian." (pp. xxii–xxiii)

We believe that substantial reform of child protection is required, and we call for the implementation of public health approaches with earlier prevention and intervention healing approaches that are:

- Comprehensive;
- Integrated;
- Family and community focused;
- Trauma informed;
- Culturally grounded;
- Indigenous controlled; and
- Evidence based.

We examine many instances where effective responses to the needs of children and struggling families are occurring within culturally-safe and empowering approaches. For Canadian peoples, the embedded use of ceremony is advocated, to support a deeply lived, spiritual mind set actualizing the seven sacred laws – love, respect, courage, honesty, wisdom, humility, and truth (Bouchard and Martin 2009). For Indigenous Australians, the focus must be upon the sense of community and kin within community-based and protective social care strategies that provide healing for Indigenous peoples experiencing ongoing interpersonal trauma and its impacts (Arney and Chong 2014).

20.2 A Framework for Understanding Indigenous Child Maltreatment

"God made me an Indian, but not a reservation Indian" Sitting Bull.

The gross over-representation of Indigenous children within many contemporary child protection systems is longstanding, and increasing in many jurisdictions (Vandna and Kozlowski 2013; Australian Institute of Health and Welfare (AIHW) 2017; Fluke et al. 2010; Lonne et al. 2016; Social Policy Evaluation and Research Unit (SPERU) 2016; US Department of Health and Human Services, 2017). The fact that conventional practice is founded in European or Western worldviews and values underscores the many, multi-layered causes and is critical to redressing the over-representation and injustices resulting from child protection practices. The picture of over-representation is complex and can be viewed as having three primary causes, namely:

- The longstanding historic and inter-generational impacts of Colonization of Indigenous peoples;
- Intergenerational trauma within Indigenous communities; and
- The social, political, legal and economic inequalities resulting from profound social inequity.

The plight of Indigenous people's regular contact with child protection authorities is driven, in different respects, by each of these three inter-related primary causes, stemming from deep-seated, historical, institutionalized racism that has evidenced itself in the unjust treatment of Indigenous peoples in Australia, Canada, New Zealand and the United States. These groups experienced forceful colonial powers that led to their social, legal, political and institutional subjugation. Despite the variable nature of their experiences, in our view, there is a remarkable consistency in these processes and outcomes, which have directly contributed to the gross over-representation of Indigenous children within child protection systems and other sorrow systems. Hence, the injustices continue, albeit in latter-day contexts, as noted by Justice Melvyn Green (2012):

> To the degree that law is an instrument of Colonialism (and it is), Canadians of Aboriginal descent remain as subject to its influence now as they were when European settlers and mercantile interests first invaded these shores and asserted their dominance some four to five hundred years ago. Indeed, to characterize Aboriginal Canadians as merely "marginalized" is more than charitable to those who occupy the centre of the page. Aboriginal Canadians have relatively little economic or political power. They have been alienated from their land, culture and history through physical and legal coercion, misguided paternalism and discriminatory laws (p. 362).

20.2.1 The Longstanding, Intergenerational Impacts of Colonization

> *The Stolen Generations never stopped. It's a continuation. They just changed the language of it* (Swan, cited in McQuire 2015).

In both Canadian and Australian contexts, centuries of cultural oppression manifest themselves in disproportionately high rates of physical and social pathology in every sphere of public concern: Alcohol and drug abuse; widespread poverty; limited access to clean water, decent housing, medical services and education; academic under-accomplishment; unemployment; high morbidity; early mortality; family instability and violence; and mental distress and suicide (Australian Indigenous HealthInfoNet 2018; Dyck 2007; Marmott 2011; Owler 2015; Starkes and Baydala 2014).

Since Colonization, policy has been deployed against Indigenous peoples through broader government policies such as Protectionism, Assimilation and

Integration. Aboriginal peoples and communities were tightly regulated, often forcibly placed in missions and reservations, had their livelihoods controlled, found their children systematically removed and placed into institutional care, and denied equality before and under the law, including the right to the equal protection and equal benefit of the law without discrimination. Legal conditions create social conditions that generate outcomes. The removal of children became known as the Stolen Generations in Australia and referenced as the Residential Schools era and the Sixties Scoop in Canada, a time of very aggressive apprehension practices following the closure of residential schools. In both Canada and Australia, a Pass or permit system was enforced whereby Indigenous peoples residing on reservations or missions were required to seek permission of government agents for every facet of their lives – hunting, visiting, economic activity, medical needs and even visiting their children at residential schools (Truth and Reconciliation Commission 2015) or dormitories and institutions (HREOC 1997). This persisted into the 1960s in Canada and the 1970s in Australia. Compounding this, were the Canadian Indian Act status rules which, from the 1860s to the present, split the status of family members. This statutory banishment, separated many from kin and community. Belonging, the most powerful need, was cannibalized.

In both countries, traditional lands were appropriated. Proud and self-sufficient peoples were reduced to states of dependency. Families and generations were divided. Language and ceremony were prohibited or expunged. Institutional discipline replaced parental nurturing, thereby dehumanizing children who learned to survive by the "don't talk, trust and feel" rules. Many children were abused by those charged with their moral education. Almost all were stripped of their language and identity, treated as inferior beings, and ultimately returned to their homes with few useful trades, and no parenting skills (Alston-O'Connor 2010). It is now generally recognized that programs like residential schools and institutions were part of a national policy of cultural and ethnic erasure, better understood as a strategy of cultural genocide or obliteration – one that has rightly become a source of national and international shame.

The program to "remove the Indian from the child" proved futile, but at enormous inter-generational cost to community self-sufficiency, traditional governance, cultural identity, psychological coherence and individual self-reliance. For Canadians, these recurring liabilities were compounded by the 'Sixties Scoop', whereby well-meaning but overzealous child welfare agencies apprehended thousands of children from their families, reserves and close-knit communities and, in most cases, placed them in non-Indigenous foster homes or institutions that repeated the cycle of cultural and personal disintegration (Alston-O'Connor 2010). Alongside Indian Residential Schools, were "Indian hospitals," repeating the same cycle. Similarly, Australian Indigenous children were removed at huge rates resulting in the 'Stolen Generations'. As Read (cited in Renes 2011) noted:

> In Australia today there may be one hundred thousand people of Aboriginal descent who do not know their families or communities. They are the people, or the descendants of people, who were removed from their families by a variety of white people for a variety of reasons. They do not know where they come from; some do not even know they are of Aboriginal

descent ... As they grew up, they were expected to think white, to act white, and in the end, to be white. (p. 36)

Such institutional practices enriched colonizing authorities through the sequestration of Indigenous lands which were promptly used for urban and agricultural economic development. This, in turn, led to increasing populations of non-Indigenous people emigrating to seek economic advancement, thereby expanding the spread of Colonization, and increasing dispersal and displacement of Indigenous peoples away from their homelands. Property rights were transferred to the colonizing force's leadership and privileged groups. Essentially, an all-powerful, politically-driven system was imposed which resulted in a culturally-hegemonic social order and power structure that led directly to the placing of power and control in the hands of the colonizers. The implementation of laws that engendered spiritual and existential devastation from loss of connection to the land, generated lifelong psychological and social trauma for Indigenous populations.

Colonization also led to the tragic deaths of countless Indigenous people through murder, violence, de-population and introduced diseases, such as small pox and measles, that destroyed many cultural groups on a catastrophic scope, scale and magnitude (Atkinson 2011; Butler 2007; Campbell 1985; Waratah 2007). Massacres, or 'the Frontier Wars' were commonplace in both Canada and Australia, as Indigenous peoples fought to retain their land, maintain connections, and basically survive (Frankland et al. 2010; The Truth Commission into Genocide in Canada 2001). Wesley-Esquimaux and Smolewski 2004) estimated that 90–95% of the Canadian Indigenous population died within two generations of contact between 1742 to the 1950s.

A reserved Australian estimate is that 20,000 Indigenous peoples were killed in Queensland, Australia alone (Daley 2014). However, according to Evans and Ørsted-Jensen (2014), the number is thousands more. Their research of Native Police records in Queensland suggests more than 41,000 Aboriginal people were killed during 3420 official frontier dispersals across almost 40 years of conflict, the figure being a statistical projection.

While some Australian critics might deny that genocide ever happened, Tatz (cited in Wesley-Esquimaux and Smolewski 2004) commented that:

Australia is guilty of at least, three, possibly four, acts of genocide: first the essentially private genocide, the physical killing committed by settlers and rogue police officers in the nineteenth century, while the state, the form of the colonial authorities, stood silently by (for the most part); second, the twentieth century official state policy and practice of forcibly transferring children from one group to another with the express purpose that they cease being Aboriginal; third, the twentieth century attempts to achieve the biological disappearance of those deemed "half-caste" Aborigines; forth, a prima facie case that Australia's actions to protect Aborigines in fact caused them serious bodily or mental harm. (p. 61)

Emotional and psychological trauma eventuated through witnessing institutional and racist violence and the loss of social roles, status, and cultural practices, which were critical to people's existential security and sense making (Aboriginal and Torres Strait Islander Social Justice Commissioner 2009). These events impacted far more than those directly affected – it undermined the social fabric. Wesley-Esquimaux and Smolewski (2004) identified five areas of impact – physical, economic, cultural, social and psychological – according to three waves of Colonization – cultural transition (early period), cultural dispossession (middle period) and cultural oppression (late period).

While some would argue that Australia and Canada are now in a post-colonial phase, statistics and research, particularly research conducted by Indigenous peoples, suggests that this is not the case. Trees (cited in Heiss 2014) stated that:

> In countries such as Australia where Aboriginal sovereignty, in forms appropriate to Aboriginal people, is not legally recognised, post-colonialism is not merely a fiction, but a linguistic manoeuvre on the part of some 'white' theorists who find this a comfortable zone that precludes the necessity for political action. Post-colonialism is a 'white' concept. (p. 2)

Some policy frameworks may be evolving, however, the administration of service delivery across a range of areas has been significantly problematic. From a policy level, ineffectiveness has been noted in Indigenous housing (Thompson et al. 2016) and child protection areas, with responses "yielding little", and with "little assistance for Aboriginal children and families to get help before parenting problems reach crisis point" (Arney and Chong 2014, para 8).

Hence, rather than protecting or progressing the well-being of Indigenous peoples, policies have left a legacy of continuing inter-generational trauma that, in economic and relational terms, impacts on many families and communities. Simultaneously, economic benefits accrue for non-Indigenous peoples "who thus benefit from the wealth that Colonialism brought …" (Watson cited in Koerner 2013, p. 30). Policy reconfiguration should incorporate Indigenous world views, values and legal norms about child protection systems and engender change in attitudes and behaviours at policy, organizational and practice levels (Thompson and Duthie 2016).

More recently, Australia's Northern Territory Emergency Response, now known as Stronger Futures was proposed to 'protect' Indigenous women and children from sexual abuse and violence by implementing paternalistic culturally inappropriate policy guidelines to specific Indigenous Australian communities including child health checks, welfare quarantining and alcohol restrictions without consultation with Indigenous peoples or communities (Department of Families, Housing, Community Services and Indigenous Affairs 2011). Rather than be praised as a 'fix the Aboriginal problem', this policy led to Indigenous peoples being stigmatised as dysfunctional and child abusers (Perche 2017). Additionally, concerns have also been raised of a second generation of stolen children currently emerging in Australia (Murphy 2017) with Pilger (2014) citing Indigenous children's removals at five times the number than when the Bringing Them Home Report was released in 1999. As such, it would appear that the Australian government continues to repeat history in terms of attempting to 'fix' Indigenous affairs.

20.2.2 Historic and Inter-Generational Trauma

Complex trauma has been defined as:

> a result of traumatic stressors that are interpersonal – premeditated, planned and perpetrated by one human being on another. It is particularly damaging if it occurs in childhood. These actions can be both violating and exploitative of another person. Complex, interpersonally generated trauma is severely disruptive of a person's capacity to manage internal states. (Mental Health Coordinating Council (MHCC) 2013, p. 8)

Atkinson (2011) noted that trauma:

> … leads to fragmented and fractured identities that in turn contribute to the escalation of violence between people. The future feels meaningless, and people articulate their felt sense of powerlessness and lack of life purpose in violent acts on themselves and others. Relationships are destroyed and communities fragment. These problems cascade down the generations, growing more complex over time. (p. 262)

Inter-generational trauma, combined with historic trauma (Aguiar and Halseth 2015), is embedded in Indigenous communities (Aboriginal and Torres Strait Islander Social Justice Commissioner 2009). It involves complex trauma "inflicted on a group of people who share a specific group identity or affiliation" (Calgary Collaborative Partnership 2012, n.p.) that is passed from one generation to the next through processes that entail the vicarious transmission of stressful emotional, psychological and spiritual pain and suffering from one generation to the next. This is often through ongoing exposure to child maltreatment, aggression, violence, mental health and substance abuse (Atkinson 2011). Yellow Horse Brave Heart (2016, n.p.) defined historic trauma as "cumulative emotional and psychological wounding over the lifespan and across generations, emanating from massive group trauma; historical unresolved grief accompanies that trauma" and suggested best practice for inter-generational healing involves four phases of recovery focusing on collective communal healing based on spirituality and traditional cultural practices, combined with trauma theory at the individual and community levels.

20.2.3 Social Inequity and Inequalities

The final primary cause is related to the outcomes of the first two, namely trans-generational social exclusion and poverty. Numerous economic, social and health indicators show that Indigenous peoples and communities are generally positioned well below other groups (SCRGSP 2016; Turnbull 2017). For example, Indigenous peoples experience higher unemployment, lower incomes, poorer housing and health, and die younger than their non-Indigenous counterparts (SCRGSP 2016, Chapter 4). While there are innumerable examples of highly successful and creative Indigenous peoples across nations and societies, gross inequality nonetheless remains. Many Indigenous communities, particularly rural and remote ones, are impoverished. This is despite significant policy, program and resource initiatives by governments of all political persuasions, such as Australia's Closing the Gap national agenda for improved health, education and well-being outcomes (Turnbull 2017).

Importantly, the social, economic, physical, psychological, emotional and relational impacts of Colonization and inter-generational trauma are exacerbated by this continuing social inequity and the impacts of inequality. In our view, this situation highlights the profound discrimination and social injustice that is endemic and long-standing. While there are no 'quick fixes', there are encouraging success stories which signpost the way forward, examined in the latter part of this chapter. Without significant policy reconfiguration and system transformation, the over-representation of Western worldviews, values and legal norms found in our child protection systems presents ongoing existential threats to Indigenous communities. Therefore a new approach is needed.

20.3 Over-Representation of Indigenous Children

Over-representation of Indigenous children in child protection systems is seemingly ubiquitous (AIHW 2017; Blackstock et al. 2004; Lonne et al. 2016; SPERU 2016). While this is partly explained by the cumulative harm from Colonization and inter-generational trauma, "it also reflects the insidious impacts of health and social inequalities on particular groups in society" (Lonne et al. 2016, p. 97).

The rate of Australian Indigenous children receiving child protection services has continued to escalate numerically and for rates per 1000 children, from 126.9 to 157.6 (24.2% ↑) in the four-year period 2012–2013 to 2015–2016, with children under orders growing from 13,268 to 18,409 (rates increasing from 46.1 to 61.9 per 1000) (AIHW 2017). Children in rural and remote communities, and from lowest socio-economic areas, were more likely to have substantiated outcomes to investigations of maltreatment than were their counterparts. Hence, it is unsurprising that Indigenous children were seven times more likely than non-Indigenous children to have maltreatment substantiated, with emotional abuse (39%) and neglect (36%) being the most common types of harm.

A third (36.3%) of all Australian children in out-of-home care (OOHC) in June 2016 were Indigenous, being 10 times the rate of non-Indigenous children nationally, but 14 times higher in the major cities (AIHW 2017). This over-representation was most evident in younger children. The numbers of all Australian children in OOHC has doubled over the past decade and "the steady rise in the rate of Indigenous children in out-of-home care has largely driven the rise in the overall rate of children in out-of-home care" (AIHW 2017, p. 62). Importantly, these alarming increases have occurred despite legislative, policy and procedural requirements for practice to be inclusive of Indigenous community participation and the Aboriginal and Torres Strait Islander Child Placement Principle which necessitates that Indigenous children in OOHC are to be placed with Indigenous family as the first priority, followed by other Indigenous community member.

Canadian statistics indicate similar findings. A recent report (Aboriginal Children in Care Working Group 2015) found that over-representation occurred across Canada, with rates of Indigenous children in government care ranging from 55% in the west to 34% in the east. While the Indigenous child population of Alberta was noted as 9%, 69% of children in care were Indigenous (Truth and Reconciliation Commission 2015). Similarly, the First Nations Canadian Incidence Study of Reported Child Abuse and Neglect (Sinha et al. 2011) found that First Nation investigations involving informal kinship care during the 3-month sampling period in 2008 was 11.4 times the rate for non-Indigenous investigations. The rate for investigations involving formal child welfare placement was 12.4 times the rate for non-Indigenous investigations. Like Australia, alarmingly, there are now more Indigenous children in care than there were during the Residential Schooling system.

Sinha et al.'s (2011) report also described the conditions of complex systems, driven by a mix of legislation, policy and standards developed by provincial, federal and Indigenous governments which are in transition towards more culturally appropriate services for Indigenous children and families, and more local decision making and governance over programs and services (for example, see Chap. 24 in this volume).

20.4 Consequences of Over-Representation of Western Worldviews

It is important to recognize that contemporary child protection systems experience almost continual reform and change processes (SPERU 2016). Although many governments have attempted policy reforms to reduce the over-representation of Indigenous children, these have not been successful and have entailed a focus upon:

- Legislative change to enable more intrusive authority into family privacy;
- Alteration to mainstream institutional arrangements and responsibilities, including organizational restructures;
- Increased utilization of risk management, safety discourses and proceduralism; and
- Professionalization of the protective workforce, which has often meant the exclusion of Indigenous staff from participating in significant ways (SPERU 2016).

In our view, policy makers have not properly recognized the three distinct, but inter-related primary causes outlined earlier and have ignored the over-representation of Western world views and values upon which laws, policies and practice are founded. Hence, this fundamental failure to either reduce child maltreatment in Indigenous communities or render the required support and assistance to address the inter-generational trauma and inequality require a roots and branch rethink because dominant current approaches are not working and are unworkable (Lonne et al. 2009).

Perhaps more to the point, the ongoing removal of Indigenous children entails the prospect of repeated grief, distress and trauma for future generations. It is no exaggeration to suggest that the situation is dire for many Indigenous families and communities. Yet, there are many examples of very successful Indigenous and other programs, and interventions, underpinned by sound principles.

20.4.1 Principles for Public Health Approaches

Suitable programs need to operate at primary, secondary and tertiary levels and to provide integrated macro-, mezzo- and micro-service responses (Williams 1999). Further, such programs need to capture, simultaneously, the complexity involved and address all three primary sources of the over-representation of Indigenous children and their impacts. An ethical, humane, multi-faceted and integrated systemic response is required. Moreover, robust data systems and systematic evaluations of the effectiveness of the formal and informal helping systems are required that address each of the primary sources and program efficacy for all groups of service users. Without these evaluative processes, there will, undoubtedly, be a continuation of the ongoing systemic failures identified earlier.

We do not advocate a one-size fits all approach but, rather, argue that the principles outlined below need to be applied in contextually and culturally-appropriate ways within the diverse array of cultures, communities, organizations and jurisdictions. A public health approach to prevent child maltreatment must be principle-based rather than rule-driven. They should form society-wide early interventions that provide timely, accessible supports and resources to address the three primary causes and their consequences. These integrated whole-of-government, community-based and Indigenous community-controlled responses will directly address the:

- Existential, spiritual and emotional impacts of Colonization;
- Psychological, health and relational consequences of inter-generational trauma; and
- Economic, social and community impacts of profound inequity and resultant inequalities.

These principles need to be applied across the landscape of public health approaches and levels that are outlined in this book and elsewhere (Scott et al. 2016). Importantly, when developing programs and services, agency personnel need to be armed with detailed knowledge of the historical and contemporary issues that impact on Indigenous peoples in their location and elsewhere. They also need to recognize the limitations of dominant Western approaches to child protection and the counterproductive and harmful outcomes from these systems (Lonne et al. 2009), and the over-representation of Western worldviews and values that shape and drive the discriminatory institutional arrangements, policy settings, processes and practices.

The key policy and program principles for public health approaches are as follows:

- Indigenous worldviews and cultural values are foundational to effective social care and protective responses that help families and communities address the impacts of the three primary sources upon children's and community health and well-being;
- Community-controlled organisations, and community members, are at the forefront of early intervention and prevention responses to family and community needs for support and resources, and therefore need to be skilled, trauma informed and resourced to provide the range of required programs and services;
- Culturally-safe practices and approaches need to be embedded within mainstream and community-controlled programs, and utilized by staff, including the use of ceremony and country and kinship protocols;
- Indigenous ways of being, doing and knowing should be recognized as an underpinning framework of Indigenous child protection work;
- Support should be accessible, timely and non-stigmatizing;
- The strengths of Indigenous child-rearing practices must be recognised and acknowledged;
- Formal support and assistance should build upon natural community-based helping/healing networks rather than supplant them;
- Caring for Indigenous children within their own families and communities that demonstrate, emphasise and practice proven trauma healing modalities;
- Indigenous people should be represented across all levels of the child protection workforce including leadership and executive levels in proportion to the over-representation of Indigenous children in the protective system;
- A collaborative approach between government, policy-makers and direct child protection workers must be implemented; and
- Reform of health, legal, protective, education, community and related systems must utilize collective impact processes, and western practices that align with and validate Indigenous healing modalities.

20.5 Reducing Over-Representation of Western Worldviews in Public Health Approaches to Reduce Child Maltreatment

Successfully managing programs and services for Indigenous peoples by Indigenous peoples has occurred since the 1970s in numerous local community and national representative bodies (Morley 2015). Commonalities for effectiveness (Morley 2015) include:

- Community ownership and control over decision-making;
- Culture being central to the program, including an understanding of the local context, history and community leaders;

- Local Indigenous staff working on the program or in the organisation, thereby harnessing existing capacity;
- Good corporate governance;
- Trusting relationships with partners being established; and
- Flexibility in implementation timelines.

Conversely, barriers to success focus on funding issues, particularly a lack of commitment from external funding bodies, uncertainty concerning ongoing funding, and onerous reporting requirements (Hoffman et al. 2012). Internally, a lack of strong Indigenous leadership, infrastructure gaps, community politics and difficulties of securing experienced staff have been problematic (Morley 2015). Despite perceived barriers, what has been successful in Australia, and continues to thrive, is the Aboriginal Community Controlled Services sector.

Aboriginal Community Controlled Health Services (ACCHS) has been one area funded by the Australian government to support the health and well-being needs of Indigenous peoples and communities. Established in the 1970s, ACCHS were initially operated by Indigenous and non-Indigenous volunteers who considered mainstream health services as lacking the ability to provide culturally-safe care and support to the Indigenous urban population. Commonwealth funding was provided in the early 1980s and, since then, has become a key Indigenous-specific primary health care strategy (Aboriginal Health & Medical Research Council 2015; AIHW 2016), reducing cultural, locational and financial barriers (Bell et al. 2000). ACCHSs are run by the Indigenous community for the Indigenous community and specifically cater to the holistic health, well-being and cultural needs of Indigenous Australians and their communities. It is estimated that approximately 60% of the Australian Indigenous population regularly access these services (Scrimgeour 2014), with the average number of clients at 2484 as opposed to 1451 for non-ACCHSs (AIHW 2016). While there may be criticisms of service delivery in specific locations, the overall system is widely recognized as performing well.

The Aboriginal and Torres Strait Islander Child Placement Principle was instigated in the 1970s in response to evidence suggesting that better outcomes would be achieved if Indigenous peoples participated fully in decisions that affected them, their families and their communities. However, Indigenous peoples still have limited opportunities to be involved in decisions regarding the removal of their children (Secretariat of National Aboriginal and Islander Child Care (SNAICC) 2017), even though decision-making participation of family and community has long been recognised as a basic right within Australia's child placement principle (Victorian Department of Human Services 2002). Poor compliance with implementing the Principle has been associated with a number of issues (Arney et al. 2015) including:

- The increasing over-representation of Indigenous children in the statutory child protection system;
- A shortage of Indigenous foster and kinship carers;
- Poor identification and assessment of carers;

- Inconsistent involvement of, and support for, Indigenous peoples and organisations in child protection decision making;
- Deficiencies in the provision of cultural care and connection to culture and community
- Practice and systemic issues impacting the operation of Indigenous child care agencies; and
- Inconsistent quantification, measurement and monitoring of the application of the Principle across jurisdictions.

These appear to be areas for system change that could be addressed with appropriate funding, recruitment, training and support for Indigenous foster and kinship carers and improved consultative frameworks between programs and organizations.

Over the years, many government-funded programs have been undertaken in Australia aimed at reducing the numbers of Indigenous children in child protection and OOHC. These emphasize the importance of family and community connections underpinned by five core elements of the Principle – prevention, partnership, placement, participation and connection (SNAICC 2017). However, “despite good intentions, the systems across Australia are failing to support the safety and well-being of our children” (SNAICC 2016, p. 3), and OOHC over-representation continues to increase alarmingly with projections of a tripling in the numbers by 2035. SNAICC has argued that policy responses are short term and reactive, rather than considered and holistic.

Hitherto, improving skills and abilities of staff working with Indigenous peoples and communities has placed emphasis on cultural competency training that provides a “set of congruent behaviours, attitudes and policies” aimed at preventing “negative effects” from ignorance of diversity (Braschi and Frasereirector, cited in Downing et al. 2011, p. 248). Yet, cultural competency can seem mechanistic and tokenistic (Furlong and Wight 2011), and focused on behavioural actions rather than being a nuanced approach entailing a critical analysis of power (Sakamoto 2007) and the maintaining of ‘otherness’ (Downing and Kowel 2011). In this sense, Indigeneity is then only perceived as ethnicity and race, which continues to relegate Indigenous peoples as the ‘other’, who have the problem to be fixed (Kumas-Tan 2007). Cultural competency training then, has limited effectiveness in understanding holistically, the historical and contemporary experiences of Indigenous peoples (Bainbridge et al. 2015; Downing et al. 2011). Importantly, making people aware of other cultural differences, does not necessarily mean they can effectively support Indigenous peoples and communities (van den Berg 2010).

Hence, the development of a more grounded, in-depth and meaningful method of cultural acknowledgement is required. Cultural safety was originally developed to increase the health and well-being of Māori peoples within the health system (Ramsden 1992). In our view, cultural safety is a far more appropriate concept, taking into consideration:

1. Practitioner reflection on their own culture rather than the cultures of ‘others’;

2. Recognizing and challenging personal and societal assumptions and stereotypes that suggest Indigenous peoples and communities need to be 'fixed' by enforcing inappropriate policy;
3. Understanding the impacts of historical policies and processes and their relationship to contemporary inter-generational trauma and trauma-based behaviour;
4. Possessing awareness of potential personal and institutional power imbalances; and
5. Challenging the notion of slavishly 'treating all people the same' regardless of their circumstances, and acknowledging that it is recipients of policies who will assess whether or not policies are culturally safe based on their experiences.

It can be seen that cultural safety is not about being respectful of ethnicity so much as it is about relational engagement that child protection and family support practitioners establish while honouring family voice and responsibility to determine their own indicators of well-being – determining cultural safety from their own experience.

In Australia, the importance of culturally-safe practice has been advocated for professional practice in areas such as nursing (Cox and Taua 2012) and child protection (Higgins 2010; Zon et al. 2004). Yet, there have been few recommendations of cultural safety within policy-making contexts apart from Thompson and Duthie's (2016) contention that "policy-makers engage in culturally safe practices and processes when engaged in decision making with Indigenous peoples and communities" (p. 58). Although consultation with Indigenous Australians is a regular policy-making catch-cry, it is more a rhetorical concept than a practice reality. Cultural safety requires policy makers to embrace the five key principles mentioned above (Kruske et al. 2006; Thompson and Duthie 2016).

The Australian historical policy context shares many aspects with Canadian policy, but it is also different in some important ways. In Canada, the responsibility for First Nation child welfare falls under provincial jurisdiction. Each province has evolved practice based on its own legislation and governance, with funding being provided by federal government directly to First Nation Agencies or reimbursed to Provincial governments. However, this has resulted in inconsistent funding, inefficiency, duplication and jurisdictional disputes with paradoxical gaps in programs and services. Success continues to be undermined by the social and economic realities for Indigenous peoples. For example, the Assembly of First Nations, in its 2011 report noted that neglect, rather than abuse, is the predominant reason for Indigenous children coming into care. Australia is similar. Neglect has been closely linked with poverty, caregiver substance abuse, social isolation and domestic violence; factors that impede a caregiver's abilities to meet children's needs.

Concurrent with these practice realities, in Alberta Canada there emerged an emphasis on outcomes-based service delivery, which shifted the focus of protection services to clearly identified expected outcomes of service provision. In 2014, Alberta implemented the Casework Intervention Practice Framework and Signs of

Safety. While these are not specifically targeted to Indigenous children, there has been a safe reduction of all children receiving intervention services, including Indigenous children (Council of the Federation Secretariat 2015). For a more in-depth overview of the Casework Intervention Practice Framework, see Chap. 24 in this volume.

Signs of Safety emerged in Australia in the 1990s through front line work with Indigenous and non-Indigenous communities, focusing on partnerships with families and their networks (natural and agency-based) to increase safety for children, reduce risks and danger, identify complicating factors and support the development of meaningful safety plans (Department for Child Protection 2011). Best outcomes occur when this approach is grounded in Indigenous circle practice, which holds everyone equal and determines collectively, the best interests of children. Parental rights and responsibility is a cornerstone of accountability. Safety Plans are the focus for collective decision making and building on family strengths, hence, Signs of Safety engages families in reclaiming knowledge and skills around relational safety. Thus, the approach is restorative and aligns with Indigenous social work practices.

Additionally, Alberta has taken a Children's First approach by legislating policy frameworks addressing the well-being of all children in Alberta, including strategic initiatives responsive to the unique needs of children with disabilities and children in government care. Alberta established cross-ministry partnerships to address family violence, through community-based networks across the province. A Prevention and Early Intervention Framework (Alberta Government 2012), along with a Children First Act (2013), proposed amendments to legislation to improve well-being, safety, security, education and health of children, and to develop processes impacting on how government and service providers deliver programs and services for children.

Research on adverse childhood events (ACEs) has been embedded in all provincial systems serving children, particularly health, education, and child intervention services. For Indigenous children, the colonial impacts have resulted in a legacy of unprecedented ACEs being experienced through intergenerational trauma. It is critical to approach child intervention services from preventative child-centred positions, providing supports and services for children in the home *before* removal into child protection services. The key to reducing the number of children in care is promoting the development of strong families (Auditor General of Alberta 2016, p. 11). This necessitates the development of strong communities, the decolonization of legislation (in particular Canadian, Indian Act reserve system), development of community systems based on a deep respect for human rights, and freedoms and recognition of the inherent dignity and needs of all members. This would return communities to the cultural practices that preceded Colonization, entailing a cohesive community where the well-being of a child is a whole-of-community responsibility.

In 2009, Australia's national policy framework embraced an early intervention and prevention framework (Council of Australian Governments 2009). Unfortunately, since this, there has been minimal follow up action (Scott et al. 2016), with Victoria being an exception (Lonne et al. 2015). This is despite the continual rapid escalation of children in OOHC, driven mostly by increased numbers of Indigenous children (AIHW 2017). Although statutory child protection approaches dominate, it is, nonetheless, encouraging that there are some signs of public health approaches being recognized as offering a better way forward, for Indigenous children, families and communities. For example, the 2017 report by the Royal Commission and Board of Inquiry into the Protection and Detention of Children in the Northern Territory recommended (39.1) that child protection approaches change to a public health model with community consultation, needs assessment, outcomes and evaluation identified as needed. But much more is required to address the situations outlined earlier concerning the gross over-representation and causes of Indigenous children.

In 2015, Canada's Truth and Reconciliation Commission published 94 Calls to Action. Its mandate was to gather stories from residential school survivors and bring the true history of Canada forward to all Canadians who have been mostly ignorant of colonial history and its impacts. Significantly, the first set of recommendations are directed at child welfare practices. Simultaneously, there is considerable evidence of Indigenous cultural resurgence emerging in Canada to dismantle colonial mind-sets and restore control to Indigenous peoples to build their own programs. Vincent Steinhauer, President of *University nuhelot'įne thaiyots'į nistameyimâkanak Blue Quills,* the first locally controlled Indigenous institute in Canada, offers his perspectives from that position of Indigenous governance:

> Europeans broke the first law of 'love' when they abducted Indigenous children into residential schools and caused loss of hope across generations. Indigenous people were given many spiritual laws to guide their relationships with all life. A child-rearing law is *opikinawasowin* (Cree word for nurturing our children well). Children are sacred gifts from the creator and ceremonies were embedded at each phase of their life – protocols to welcome a child into this world, embraced by community as spiritual beings, celebrated in ceremonies with each stage of development. So much has been lost in practice but remains in genetic memory and Elder wisdom which is still available for happy, healthy and sustainable futures.

20.6 Conclusions

The historical policy failures that have occurred in both Canada and Australia has significantly impacted Indigenous peoples over generations and today. As detailed above, the devastation wrought by Colonization has been inter-generational, and has left a legacy of profound trauma within Indigenous communities. The array of inequalities stemming from contemporary social inequity, is noted in the still high levels of disparity in the social determinants of health between Indigenous and non-Indigenous peoples, which continues to impact. We have used Australia and Canada as examples of this, but there are others around the world with their own devastating accounts.

Underlying these social determinants are the legal determinants which shape social conditions. The complexities of this history and, subsequently, within child protection matters, has not been addressed appropriately as can be seen in the continued trauma that child removal brings. Hence, we suggest that multiple integrated responses are required across economic, health, education and welfare systems and contexts. In our view, public health approaches to preventing maltreatment and supporting families and communities have much to offer. Earlier interventions and prevention strategies provide hope in what is otherwise a landscape characterized by gross over-representation of Indigenous children within statutory child protection systems underpinned by over-representation of Western world views. Until these systems and contexts are responded to in culturally safe and collaborative methods, child protection systems are doomed to continue to fail Indigenous children, peoples and communities.

References

Aboriginal and Torres Strait Islander Social Justice Commissioner. (2009). *2008 social justice report*. Canberra: Australian Human Rights Commission.

Aboriginal Children in Care Working Group. (2015). *Aboriginal children in care: Report to Canada's Premiers.* Retrieved from https://fncaringsociety.com/sites/default/files/Aboriginal%20Children%20in%20Care%20Report%20%28July%202015%29.pdf

Aboriginal Health & Medical Research Council. (2015). *Aboriginal communities improving Aboriginal health: An evidence review on the contribution of Aboriginal Community Controlled Health Services to improving Aboriginal health.* Sydney: AH&MRC. Retrieved from http://www.ahmrc.org.au/media/resources/research/298-aboriginal-communities-improving-aboriginal-health/file.html

Aguiar, W., & Halseth, R. (2015). *Aboriginal people and historic trauma: The process of intergenerational transmission*. Prince George: National Collaborating Centre for Aboriginal Health. Retrieved from http://www.nccah-ccnsa.ca/430/aboriginal-peoples-and-historic-trauma.nccah

Alberta Government. (2012). *Prevention and early intervention framework for children, youth and families*. Edmonton: Author.

Alston-O'Connor, E. (2010). The sixties scoop: Implications for social workers and social work education. *Critical Social Work, 11*(1), 53–61.

Arney, F. & Chong, A. (2014). Empowering Indigenous communities to prevent child abuse and neglect. *The Conversation*, October 30. Retrieved from https://theconversation.com/empowering-indigenous-communities-to-prevent-child-abuse-and-neglect-32875

Arney, F., Iannos, M., Chong, A., McDougall, S., & Parkinson, S. (2015). *Enhancing the implementation of the Aboriginal and Torres Strait Islander Child Placement Principle: Policy and practice considerations* (CFCA Paper No. 34). Melbourne: Australian Institute of Family Studies. Retrieved from https://aifs.gov.au/cfca/publications/enhancing-implementation-aboriginal-and-torres-strait-islander-child

Atkinson, J. (2011). *Trauma trails, recreating song lines: The transgenerational effects of trauma in Indigenous Australia*. North Melbourne: Spinifex.

Auditor General of Alberta. (2016). *A report on human services systems to deliver child and family services to Indigenous children in Alberta.* Retrieved from https://www.oag.ab.ca/webfiles/reports/July2016HSReport.pdf

Austin, R. (2009). *Navajo courts and Navajo common law: A tradition of tribal self governance*. Minneapolis: Minnesota University Press.

Australian Institute of Health and Welfare. (2016). Healthy futures: Aboriginal Community Controlled Health Services Report Card *2016*. Cat. No. IHW 171. Canberra: AIHW. Retrieved from http://www.aihw.gov.au/publication-detail/?id=60129557721

Australian Institute of Health and Welfare. (2017). *Child Protection Australia 2015–16*, Child Welfare series no. 66. Cat. no. CWS 60. ACT: AIHW.

Bainbridge, R., McCalman, J., Clifford, A., & Tsey, K. (2015). Cultural competency in the delivery of health services for Indigenous people. *Closing the Gap Clearinghouse Issues 13*, 1–44. Retrieved from http://www.aihw.gov.au/uploadedFiles/ClosingTheGap/Content/Our_publications/2015/ctgc-ip13.pdf

Bell, K., Couzos, S., Daniels, J., Hunter, P., Mayers N. & Murray, R. (2000). *Aboriginal community controlled health services. General Practice in Australia.* Retrieved from http://www.kooriweb.org/foley/resources/pdfs/120.pdf

Blackstock, C., Trocmé, N., & Bennett, M. (2004). Child maltreatment investigations among Aboriginal and non-Aboriginal families in Canada: A comparative analysis. *Violence Against Women, 10*(8), 901–916.

Bouchard, D. & Martin, J. (2009). *Seven sacred teachings: Niizhwaaswi gagiikwewin*. Retrieved from http://www.btgwinnipeg.ca/uploads/5/2/4/1/52412159/the_seven_sacred_teachings_.pdf

Butler, B. (2007). Perpetual grief. *In Reflections: 40 years on from the 1967 Referendum*. Adelaide SA: Aboriginal Legal Rights Movement Inc.

Calgary Collaborative Partnership. (2012). *Intervention to address inter-generational trauma: Overcoming, resisting and preventing structural violence.* Calgary: Collaborative partnership between University of Calgary, YMCA & Urban Society for Aboriginal Youth (USAY). Retrieved from https://www.ucalgary.ca/wethurston/files/wethurston/Report_InterventionToAddressIntergenerationalTrauma.pdf

Campbell, J. (1985). Small pox in Aboriginal Australia: The early 1830s. *Historical Studies, 21*(84), 336–358. https://doi.org/10.1080/10314618508595711.

Council of Australian Governments. (2009). *Protecting children is everyone's business: National Framework for Protecting Australia's Children 2009–2020*. Canberra: FaHCSIA. Retrieved from https://www.dss.gov.au/our-responsibilities/families-and-children/publications-articles/protecting-children-is-everyones-business

Council of the Federation Secretariat. (2015). *Aboriginal children in care: Report to Canada's Premiers.* Retrieved from http://canadaspremiers.ca/phocadownload/publications/aboriginal_children_in_care_report_july2015.pdf

Cox, L., & Taua, C. (2012). Cultural safety: Cultural considerations. In H. Forbes & E. Watt (Eds.), *Jarvis's physical examination and health assessment* (pp. 40–60). Chatswood: Elsevier.

Daley, P. (2014). Why the number of Indigenous deaths in the frontier wars matters. *The Guardian.* Retrieved from https://www.theguardian.com/commentisfree/2014/jul/15/why-the-number-of-indigenous-deaths-in-the-frontier-wars-matters

Department for Child Protection. (2011). *The signs of safety child protection practice framework.* East Perth: Department for Child Protection, Government of Western Australia. Retrieved from: https://www.dcp.wa.gov.au/Resources/Documents/Policies%20and%20Frameworks/SignsOfSafetyFramework2011.pdf

Department of Families, Housing, Community Services and Indigenous Affairs. (2011). *Northern Territory Emergency Response: Evaluation report 2011.* Canberra: Department of Families, Housing, Community Services and Indigenous Affairs.

Downing, R., & Kowal, E. (2011). A postcolonial analysis of Indigenous cultural awareness training for health workers. *Health Sociology Review, 20*(11), 5–15.

Downing, R., Kowal, E., & Paradies, Y. (2011). Indigenous cultural training for health workers in Australia. *International Journal for Quality in Health Care, 23*(3), 247–257. https://doi.org/10.1093/intqhc/mzr008.

Dyck, M. (2007). *Social determinants of Métis health*. Retrieved from http://www.naho.ca/documents/metiscentre/english/Research_SocialDeterminantsofHealth.pdf

Evans, R., & Orsted-Jensen, R. (2014). *"I cannot say the numbers that were killed": Assessing violent mortality on the Queensland frontier*. Retrieved from: https://doi.org/10.2139/ssrn.2467836

Fluke, J., Chabot, M., Fallon, B., MacLaurin, B., & Blackstock, C. (2010). Placement decisions and disparities among Aboriginal groups: An application of the decision making ecology through multi-level analysis. *Child Abuse and Neglect, 34*(1), 57–69.

Frankland, R., Bamblett, M., Lewis, P., & Trotter, R. (2010). *This is 'forever business': A framework for maintaining and restoring cultural safety in Aboriginal Victoria*. Melbourne: Victorian Aboriginal Child Care Agency: Victoria. Retrieved from https://www.researchgate.net/publication/265741954_'FOREVER_BUSINESS'_A_FRAMEWORK_FOR_MAINTAINING_AND_RESTORING_CULTURAL_SAFET_Y_IN_ABORIGINAL_VICTORIA

Furlong, M., & Wight, J. (2011). Promoting "critical awareness" and critiquing "cultural competence": Towards disrupting received professional knowledges. *Australian Social Work, 64*(1), 38–54.

Green, Justice M. (2012). *The Challenge of Gladue Courts*. Criminal Reports (Articles), 6th Series at 1.

Heiss, A. (2014). Post-colonial – NOT!! In A. Heiss, P. Minter, & N. Jose (Eds.), *Teaching guide for the Macquarie PEN anthology of aboriginal literature*. Retrieved from www.macquaripenanthology.com.au.

Higgins, D. (2010). *Community development approaches to safety and wellbeing of Indigenous children*. Close the Gap Clearinghouse. Available at: https://www.aihw.gov.au/reports/indigenous-australians/community-development-approaches-to-safety-and-wel/contents/table-of-contents

Hoffman, B., Roeger, S., Wise, P., Dermer, J., Yunupingu, B., Lacey, D., Yunupingu, D., Marika, B., Marika, M., & Panton, B. (2012). Achieving highly successful multiple agency collaborations in a cross-cultural environment: Experiences and lessons from Dhimurru Aboriginal Corporation and partners. *Ecological Management and Restoration, 13*(1), 42–50. https://doi.org/10.1111/j.1442-8903.2011.00630.x.

Human Rights and Equal Opportunity Commission (HREOC). (1997). *Bringing them Home: Report of the National Inquiry into the separation of Aboriginal and Torres Strait Islander children from their families*. Canberra: Commonwealth of Australia.

Indigenous HealthInfoNet. (2018). Child protection Australia 2016–17. Retrieved from https://www.aihw.gov.au/getmedia/66c7c364-592a-458c-9ab0-f90022e25368/aihw-cws-63.pdf.aspx?inline=true.

Koerner, C. (2013). Learning the past to participate in the future: Regional discourses of Australian colonial history. *International Journal of Critical Indigenous Studies, 6*(2), 29–40. Retrieved from http://www.isrn.qut.edu.au/publications/internationaljournal/documents/volume6_number2_13-Koerner.pdf

Kruske, S., Kildea, S., Verlie, L., & Barclay, M. (2006). Cultural safety and maternity care for Aboriginal and Torres Strait Islander Australians. *Women and Birth, 19*(3), 73–77.

Kumas-Tan, Z., Beagan, B., Loppie, C., MacLeod, A., & Frank, B. (2007). Measures of cultural competence: Examining hidden assumptions. *Academic Medicine, 82*, 548–557.

Lonne, B., Parton, N., Thomson, J., & Harries, M. (2009). *Reforming child protection*. London: Routledge.

Lonne, B., Brown, G., Wagner, I., & Gillespie, K. (2015). Victoria's Child FIRST and IFS differential response system: Progress and issues. *Child Abuse & Neglect, 39*, 41–49. https://doi.org/10.1016/j.chiabu.2014.08.003.

Lonne, B., Harries, M., Featherstone, B., & Gray, M. (2016). *Working ethically in child protection*. London: Routledge (Taylor & Francis).

Marmot, M. (2011). Social determinants and the health of Indigenous Australians. *Medical Journal of Australia, 194*(10), 512–513. https://www.mja.com.au/journal/2011/194/10/social-determinants-and-health-indigenous-australians

McQuire, A. (2015). They came for the Abbott spill and missed the only real story in town. *New Matilda*, 9 February. Retrieved from https://newmatilda.com/2015/02/09/they-came-abbott-spill-and-missed-only-real-story-town/

Mental Health Coordinating Council (MHCC). (2013). *Trauma-informed care and practice: Towards a cultural shift in policy reform across mental health and human services in Australia. A national strategic direction, position paper and recommendations of the national trauma-informed care and practice advisory working group*. Sydney: MHCC.

Morley, S. (2015). *What works in effective Indigenous community-managed programs and organisations*. CFCA Paper no. 32. Melbourne: Child Family Community Australia, Australian Institute of Family Studies. https://aifs.gov.au/cfca/publications/what-works-effective-indigenous-community-managed-programs-and-organisations

Murphy, K. (2017). Indigenous child removal rate risks 'second stolen generation', Kevin Rudd warns. *The Guardian,* 17 February. Retrieved from https://www.theguardian.com/australia-news/2017/feb/13/indigenous-child-removal-rate-risks-second-stolen-generation-kevin-rudd-warns

Owler, B. (2015, March). *The social determinants of health: The Australian perspective*. Paper presented at The Role of Physicians and National Medical Associations in Addressing the Social Determinants of Health and Increasing Health Equity, London. Retrieved from https://ama.com.au/media/social-determinants-health-australian-perspective

Perche, D. (2017). Ten years on, it's time we learned the lessons from the failed Northern Territory Intervention. *Social Policy Connections*, 3 July. Retrieved from http://www.socialpolicyconnections.com.au/?p=11763

Pilger, J. (2014). Another stolen generation: How Australia still wrecks Aboriginal families. *The Guardian,* 22 March. Retrieved from https://www.theguardian.com/commentisfree/2014/mar/21/john-pilger-indigenous-australian-families

Ramsden, I. (1992). *Kawa Whakaruruhau: Guidelines for nursing and midwifery education*. Wellington: Nursing Council of New Zealand.

Renes, M. (2011). The stolen generations, a narrative of removal, displacement and recovery. In M. Renes (Ed.), *Lives in migration: Rupture and continuity: Essays on migration* (pp. 30–49). Spain: Centre d'Estudis Australians, Universitat de Barcelona.

Sakamoto, I. (2007). An anti-oppressive approach to cultural competence. *Canadian Social Work Review, 24*(1), 105–118.

Scott, D., Lonne, B., & Higgins, D. (2016). Public health models for preventing child maltreatment: Applications from the field of injury prevention. *Trauma, Violence, & Abuse, 17*(4), 408–419. https://doi.org/10.1177/1524838016658877.

Scrimgeour, D. (2014). *The Aboriginal community-controlled health care model*. Retrieved from http://www.flinders.edu.au/medicine/fms/sites/southgate/documents/events/2014/David%20Scrimgeour.pdf

Sinha, V., Trocmé, N., Fallon, B., MacLaurin, B., Fast, E., Prokop, S., et al. (2011). *Kiskisik Awasisak: Remember the children.* Understanding the overrepresentation of First Nations children in the child welfare system. Ontario: Assembly of First Nations.

SNAICC National Voice for our Children. (2016). *The family matters report: Measuring trends to turn the tide on Aboriginal and Torres Strait Islander child safety and removal*. Retrieved from http://www.familymatters.org.au/wpcontent/uploads/2016/12/Family_Matters_Report_2016.pdf

SNAICC National Voice for our Children. (2017). Understanding and applying the Aboriginal and Torres Strait Islander child placement principle: A resource for legislation, policy and program development. Retrieved from http://www.qatsicpp.com.au/images/ATSICPP_book.pdf

Social Policy Evaluation and Research Unit (SPERU). (2016). *Modernising child protection in New Zealand: Learning from system reforms in other jurisdictions*. Wellington: SPERU.

Starkes, J. & Baydala, L. (2014). Health research involving First Nations, Inuit and Métis children and their communities. *Paediatric Child Health, 19*(2), 99–102. Retrieved from http://www.cps.ca/en/documents/position/health-research-first-nations-inuit-metis-children

Steering Committee for the Review of Government Service Provision (SCRGSP). (2016). *Overcoming Indigenous Disadvantage: Key Indicators 2016.* Canberra: Productivity Commission.

The Truth Commission into Genocide in Canada. (2001). *Hidden from history: The Canadian holocaust.* Accessed from http://canadiangenocide.nativeweb.org/genocide.pdf

Thompson, L., & Duthie, D. (2016). Towards culturally safe social policy processes for Aboriginal Australians. *The International Journal of Interdisciplinary Social and Community Studies, 11*(4), 48–62.

Thompson, L., Duthie, D., & Wadley, D. (2016). Well-being among Aboriginal Australians: Re-fashioning public housing policy. *Journal of Australian Indigenous Issues, 19*(3), 58–76.

Truth and Reconciliation Commission of Canada. (2015). *Calls to action.* Retrieved from http://www.trc.ca/websites/trcinstitution/File/2015/Findings/Calls_to_Action_English2.pdf

Turnbull, M. (2017). *Closing the gap: Prime Minister's report 2017.* Canberra: Department of Prime Minister and Cabinet, Australian Government.

US Department of Health & Human Services, Administration for Children and Families, Administration on Children, Youth and Families, Children's Bureau. (2017). *Child maltreatment 2015.* Retrieved from http://www.acf.hhs.gov/programs/cb/research-data-technology/statistics-research/child-maltreatment.

van den Berg, R. (2010). Cultural safety in health for Aboriginal people: Will it work in Australia? *Medical Journal of Australia, 193*(3), 136–137.

Vandna, S., & Kozlowski, A. (2013). The structure of aboriginal child welfare in Canada. *The International Indigenous Policy Journal, 4*(2). Retrieved from: https://ir.lib.uwo.ca/iipj/vol4/iss2/2. https://doi.org/10.18584/iipj.2013.4.2.2.

Victorian Government Department of Human Services. (2002). *Aboriginal child placement principle guide*. Victoria: Community Care Division. Retrieved from http://www.dhs.vic.gov.au/__data/assets/pdf_file/0006/580614/aboriginal-child-placement-principle-guide-2002.pdf

Waratah (2007). Sovereignty and survival. In *Reflections: 40 years on from the 1967 Referendum.* Adelaide: Aboriginal Legal Rights Movement Inc. https://trove.nla.gov.au/version/45106390

Wesley-Esquimaux, C., & Smolewski, M. (2004). *Historic trauma and Aboriginal healing.* Ottawa: Aboriginal Healing Foundation. Retrieved from http://www.ahf.ca/downloads/historic-trauma.pdf

Williams, R. (1999). Cultural safety – Wat does it mean for our work practice? *Australian and New Zealand Journal of Public Health, 23*(2), 213–214. Retrieved from http://onlinelibrary.wiley.com/doi/10.1111/j.1467-842X.1999.tb01240.x/epdf

Yellow Horse Brave Heart, M. (2016). *The mother of historical trauma.* Retrieved from http://discoveringourstory.wisdomoftheelders.org/resources/transcending-historical-trauma

Zon, A., Lindeman, M., Williams, A., Hayes, C., Ross, D., & Furber, M. (2004). Cultural safety in child protection: Application to the workplace environment and casework practice. *Australian Social Work, 57*(3), 288–298. https://doi.org/10.1111/j.1447-0748.2004.00147.x.

Chapter 21
Problems in Understanding Program Efficacy in Child Welfare

Melissa Jonson-Reid and Chien-Jen Chiang

21.1 Introduction

There are really two questions to be answered when faced with questions about program efficacy in child welfare. The first is a question about the efficacy of services already offered. Specifically, are we concerned with whether usual care approaches to intervention are having the intended (or unintended) effects. The second pertains to specific interventions. Here, the question is: Is a program or intervention mounted on top of usual care working? We need to understand the performance of current practices as the control or comparison condition for the added intervention that we hope will result in improved outcomes.

The combined need to understand current practices as well as new approaches to intervention is a fundamental methodological issue for research or evaluation in a setting in which all individuals must be served in response to a referral. In other words, child welfare cannot choose to randomize a family to no response for legal and ethical reasons, nor can public schools deny a child access to education, nor can crisis mental health agencies refuse existing treatment to someone who is suicidal. In many cases, these situations often limit research options to observational quasi-experimental designs at best. In some cases, the gold standard of an RCT can be used, but only when testing an added approach to what the agency normally provides. Even when they can be used, real world RCTs are unlikely to have the same rigorous controls as do drug trials or interventions developed for a laboratory set-

M. Jonson-Reid (✉)
Ralph and Muriel Pumphrey Professor of Social Work Research, The Brown School, Washington University, St Louis, MO, USA
e-mail: jonsonrd@wustl.edu

C.-J. Chiang
The Brown School, Washington University, St. Louis, MO, USA
e-mail: c.chiang@wustl.edu

B. Lonne et al. (eds.), *Re-Visioning Public Health Approaches for Protecting Children*, Child Maltreatment 9, https://doi.org/10.1007/978-3-030-05858-6_21

ting. This makes it difficult for organizations that are already serving a population to meet evidence-based practice standards for published RCT designs. Once a new approach shows promise, replication is necessary. However, replication can be difficult if regional or state policy variations guiding the system response continue to be the platform for a new approach.

Does this make the question of efficacy impossible to answer? No, but it requires thoughtful consideration of the aim of a given study and the degree to which results can be generalized without trials in different locations. Further, the very definition of 'what works' must be carefully contemplated. Does a program work if there is a statistically significant positive change or should we expect that any difference achieved must have some practically large effect? Is a program effective if it is successful for some but not all intended outcomes? Is a program effective if it is successful for certain populations but not others? How many replications should we expect before we have confidence that the program effects may generalize to a broad enough population to scale up? Although such questions impact many service sectors, we will explore these issues with a focus on child welfare in the following chapter.

21.2 Does Efficacy Mean Being Named an Evidence-Based Practice?

As standards of accountability in social welfare have increased, funders are increasingly looking to evidence-based lists (e.g., California-Based Clearinghouse). The metrics applied by the organizations hosting such lists may vary according to the number of published RCTs, type of effects found, or other factors. Generally, however the ability to achieve such status is complicated in cases where services are saturated (everyone known gets something) and/or it is not possible to have a 'no service' condition.

Agencies faced with this situation can seek out a comparison agency offering a different service to the same population- for example two different early childhood home visitation providers. One still has to account for potential variations in the population, for which there are some statistical methods available that will be discussed later. However, another more difficult problem arises in finding a willing partner for comparison given the fact that the agency attempting the study is hoping what they provide will be significantly better.

Other solutions exist but are problematic for agencies like child welfare organizations. For example, in some cases there are waitlist comparisons within an agency, but child welfare agencies cannot, by mandate, have people waiting to be served. Another option is to use program expansion as a possible tool- ideally randomly choosing a location to expand into first and comparing it to a similar location because one does not yet have sufficient funds to expand to that other location. In child welfare, this cannot happen for foundational functions like having some assessment response to a hotline call but may be possible for implementing new approaches to services to families. For example, when states began implementing differential response (i.e., some families being assigned to an assessment approach as compared to a traditional investigation), it was possible to implement this approach in certain regions rather than adopt it statewide while still providing traditional services in the other regions (Loman and Siegel 2012). The new Essentials for Childhood framework (see Chap. 13 by Klevens and colleagues in this volume) may offer a chance to research a collective impact prevention approach providing controls for state differences among those not part of the initial implementation cohort are available to create an adequate comparison condition.

Of course, not all agencies are concerned with being named an evidence-based practice. In this case, efficacy is more likely to be defined by policy outcomes. For child welfare, that would be safety, permanency (which includes keeping a child with their biological family if possible, reunifying if foster care is needed or a permanent exit to kin or adoption), and well-being (which is limited to children who receive services after a hotline and typically defined as attention to education, health and mental health needs) (US Department of Health and Human Services 2012). There are three primary issues to be addressed in this case: (1) Who comes to the attention of child welfare? (2) Which subgroups progress into differing levels of intervention? and, (3) What outcomes are obtained at what level of intervention for whom? For ease of discussion, we focus on the outcomes of safety (prevention of initial or further maltreatment) and permanency (either a child remaining with their family of origin or achieving a stable alternative home). We will also briefly address difficulties with the more recent addition of child well-being as an outcome for child welfare.

21.3 Who Is Served?

In any evaluation of program efficacy or effectiveness, it is important to define the population served. In the case of service systems, like child welfare however, the population characteristics are gated by eligibility set in state policy.

21.3.1 Discrepancies in the Definitions of Child Maltreatment Across States

Federal legislation (Child Abuse Prevention and Treatment Act of 1984, CAPTA) provides guidance to states by identifying a minimum set of acts or behaviors for major types of maltreatment (physical abuse, sexual abuse and neglect), but states are given significant latitude in adding other categories as well as defining subtypes or specific acts or behaviors to be included within the major categories. For example, in 1993 the National Research Council stated that child neglect "covers a range of behaviors including educational, supervisory, medical, physical and emotional neglect, and abandonment, often complicated by cultural and contextual factors" (National Research Council 1993, p. 60). Twenty years later, the adopted state definitions reflect diverse ideas as to what constitutes neglect (McSherry 2007; Renninger et al. 2002). The variation in definitions of child neglect, obtained from the Child Welfare Information Gateway (2016) across states, can be seen in Table 21.1. Some states identify emotional, medical neglect and exposure to substance abuse as a part of neglect. Some include educational neglect as maltreatment and others do not. Some states separate out 'abandonment' or 'medical neglect' from the definitions of child neglect and others do not. Additionally, some states include child exposure to domestic violence as a form of maltreatment while others do not and the response provided varies according to the type of exposure or harm demonstrated (Jonson-Reid and Drake 2018).

It is not clear how state variation in how maltreatment is defined impacts the population characteristics of those served. There is great diversity in thought about whether there are 'true' differences in risk and protective factors according to most types of maltreatment (i.e., excluding sexual abuse). Also known as the 'iceberg theory', is the idea that any given family may have a similar set of risks or propensity to certain behaviors as another family but this can manifest in different visible conditions and leads to differing types of maltreatment reported (Jonson-Reid et al. 2003). If this is true, then the state definitions for reporting may have less impact on population variations because eventually the family will fit within a reportable reason for maltreatment. If, on the other hand, certain types of risk factors and family characteristics are associated with specific forms of maltreatment then definitions may impact the population served in a significant way. For example, if families that experience domestic violence do not have a similar risk or behavioral patterns to families that are reported for physical or sexual abuse or neglect, then states that include domestic violence as maltreatment will be serving a quite different set of families.

The debate about exactly how to define maltreatment presents challenges for research and evaluation (Leeb et al. 2008). Researchers can and do use their own measures of maltreatment as seen across three large studies of child welfare involvement or reporting: LONGSCAN, NSCAW and the NIS-4 (see Dowd et al. 2002; English et al. 2005; Sedlak et al. 2010). However, when the base or target population is families that are eligible for a maltreatment report and investigation, this does not take care of the problem of who got into the sample. It merely provides an additional layer of explanation for what maltreatment looks like among those reported. In other words, if a child lives in a state that does not accept reports for emotional abuse, then a study that samples from reported children may be able to discern that emotional abuse exists within the group, but it will be combined with whatever other form of maltreatment actually triggered the investigated report.

Table 21.1 State statue in definitions of the child abuse and neglect

States/type of neglect	Physical	Emotional	Educational	Medical	Abandonment		Parent[a] substance abuse	Supervision	State or County
					Neglect	Separate			
Alabama	×			×				×	S
Alaska	×			×					S
Arizona	×			×		×	PA	×	S
Arkansas	×	×	×	×		×	PAS	×	S
California	×			×	×		U	×	C
Colorado	×		×	×	×		PM	×	C
Connecticut	×	×	×		×				S
Delaware	×	×	×	×			U	×	S
Florida	×	×		×		×	S		S
Georgia									S
Hawaii	×	×		×			S	×	S
Idaho	×		×	×					S
Illinois	×			×	×		PS		S
Indiana	×		×	×		×	PM	×	S
Iowa	×			×			PM	×	S
Kansas	×			×		×		×	S
Kentucky	×		×		×		U	×	S
Louisiana	×	×			×		P		S
Maine	×		×			×		×	S
Maryland	×	×		×				×	S
Massachusetts	×	×		×			P	×	S
Michigan	×			×					S
Minnesota	×		×	×	×		PSU	×	C
Mississippi	×		×	×				×	S

(continued)

Table 21.1 (continued)

States/type of neglect	Physical	Emotional	Educational	Medical	Abandonment		Parent[a] substance abuse	Supervision	State or County
					Neglect	Separate			
Missouri	×		×	×					S
Montana	×	×	×	×		×	M	×	S
Nebraska	×		×	×		×		×	S
Nevada	×		×	×	×				H
New Hampshire	×	×	×	×		×			S
New Jersey	×	×	×	×	×			×	S
New Mexico	×		×	×		×			S
New York	×	×	×	×		×	U	×	C
North Carolina	×			×	×			×	C
North Dakota	×	×	×	×		×	P		C
Ohio	×		×	×		×	MS		C
Oklahoma	×	×	×	×		×	PMU	×	S
Oregon	×			×			PM		S
Pennsylvania	×			×			M	×	C
Puerto Rico	×	×	×	×				×	S
Rhode Island	×			×	×		U	×	S
South Carolina	×		×	×				×	S
South Dakota	×		×	×	×		PM	×	S
Tennessee	×		×	×			M	×	S
Texas	×			×		×	SU		S
Utah	×			×	×				S
Vermont	×			×	×				S
Virginia	×			×	×		M		C
Washington	×			×			A		S
West Virginia	×		×	×	×		M	×	S

Wisconsin	×			×			P		H
Wyoming	×		×	×	×			×	C

[a]Parent Substance Abuse: Parental substance abuse is an element of the definition of child abuse or neglect in some States.
Prenatal **(P)** exposure of a child to harm due to the mother's use of an illegal drug or other substance (14 States)
Manufacture **(M)** of a controlled substance in the presence of a child or on the premises occupied by a child (12 States)
Allowing **(A)** a child to be present where the chemicals or equipment for the manufacture of controlled substances are used or stored (3 States): Arizona, Arkansas, and Washington.
Selling **(S)**, distributing, or giving drugs or alcohol to a child (7 states and Guam): Arkansas, Florida, Hawaii, Illinois, Minnesota, Ohio, and Texas.
Use **(U)** of a controlled substance by a caregiver that impairs the caregiver's ability to adequately care for the child (8 States).

21.3.2 Variations in State Populations

State populations vary significantly according to racial and immigrant composition as well as the relative urban compared to rural proportion of residents. This will, by definition, impact the demographics of child welfare caseloads. For example, in Alaska, a significant portion of children with substantiated reports of maltreatment are identified as Alaskan Native with few Hispanics whereas the proportion of indigenous peoples in California is less than 3% but nearly half are Hispanic (US DHHS 2017). Cultural factors have been found to be important for child maltreatment and intervention outcomes (Aarons and Palinkas 2007; Dettlaff and Johnson 2011; Molnar et al. 2016; Pelton 2015; Valentino et al. 2012). Relatively little attention to this has been paid in research on services outcomes.

The socio-economic conditions of communities in which children live are not equal and, in the U.S., communities can vary significantly by race as well as maltreatment type (Drake et al. 2009; Drake and Rank 2009; Jonson-Reid et al. 2013). The availability of funds for child welfare and other supportive programs varies greatly by state and region and may impact the broader range of supports available to families that come to the attention of child protective services (DeVooght et al. 2014; Harris and Hackett 2008). Structural issues like transportation also vary. For example, in the National Survey of Child Health, over 45% of Native American respondents reported that transportation was a barrier to accessing health care compared to between 0 and 6.6% for all other groups (Flores and Tomany-Korman 2008). Finally, communities vary in their access to things like alcohol outlets or likelihood of exposure to community violence (Freisthler and Maguire-Jack 2015; Valentino et al. 2012).

It remains unclear how these contextual factors combine with other child and family characteristics to influence outcomes of safety and permanency following child welfare involvement (IOM and NRC 2014). Therefore, it becomes difficult to know if findings based on results in one state or territory differ due to the services offered or because services might have differing impacts for subgroups based on local contexts (i.e. urban v. rural). This requires significant attention to the context of a study and commitment to replication of findings in different areas.

21.4 Usual Care Varies Across Regions

Before moving on to considerations of testing programs added to child welfare, a consideration of the comparison or control usual care condition is warranted. Generally, there has been less attention in research to describing how cases are screened and served (Jonson-Reid et al. 2017).

21.4.1 Screening Cases

States and counties have differing approaches to screened-in calls, in other words calls that result in some kind of assessment or investigation. At a minimum, screened in cases must meet the state's criteria for what is considered reportable maltreatment. Not only do these definitions vary, the metrics and process for screening cases assuming it meets the criteria for acceptance also varies. Among states that report screening rates to the national child abuse and neglect data system, screen out ranges from a low of 1.9% to a high of 84.4% (US DHHS 2018). Most recently, this has included the use of predictive risk modelling to augment traditional screening practice in one region in Pennsylvania (Vaithianathan et al. 2017), but it is too early and limited in scope to understand its potential effects.

Once a report is 'accepted' some determination of how to handle the report is made. Some states now employ a differential response (DR; also called alternative response) that sorts cases screened in into either an assessment or investigation track. Differential response was implemented statewide in 26 states and regionally or county-based in 7 states as of 2015 (US DHHS 2017). The basic idea is that less serious cases would be handled by a more supportive, family friendly approach (assessment track). There is, however, significant variation in how cases are sorted. In some areas most neglect cases are automatically sent to assessment while abuse cases typically remain in the traditional investigative track (Hughes et al. 2013). Yet research on neglect does not suggest a lower risk of harm in many these cases (Gilbert et al. 2009; Jonson-Reid and Drake 2018). Incorrect sorting of cases into track based on a label based on what category of maltreatment a case fits into rather than risk could result in poor safety outcomes. In other states, the process for differentiating cases by track is less clear (Piper 2016).

Differences also exist in screening among states that retain a traditional investigation model. Within the investigation track, about half of the states use some form of structured decision-making (Harbert and Tucker-Tatlow 2012) with the others using a variety of other methods (National Resource Center for Child Protective Services, n.d.). Much debate remains regarding the relative effectiveness of assessment approaches in predicting future risk (Van der Put et al. 2016). Generally actuarial methods are thought to perform better than consensus approaches (e.g., Loman and Siegel 2005; Van der Put et al. 2016), but outcomes of decision are also likely dependent on the quality of the information available, the experience of the worker and other factors (Maguire-Jack and Font 2014; Font and Maguire-Jack 2015a, b).

Workload may also impact early case decision-making. States vary considerably in the number of workers employed per case. Among the states that report workforce numbers, the complete reports per worker vary from mid-forties to more than 189 (US DHHS 2018). One new study found that the allocation of resources had a significant impact (albeit small) on how cases are screened (McLaughlin and Jonson-Reid 2017). Once screened in, the level of caseload burden may also impact the thoroughness of the risk assessment and service provision decision-making. This has not been well investigated, although one study found caseload to be non-significant in predicting recurrent maltreatment once other factors were controlled (Maguire-Jack and Font 2014).

So, after understanding who is in the initial sample pool of children potentially reported for maltreatment, studies of efficacy in child welfare services must consider the additional gate-keeping practices associated with whether a report is accepted and the type of assessment or investigation that follows. While this may seem a bit onerous, it is not that different from the sample flow charts expected for intervention trials that detail the process from recruitment to consent to participation.

21.4.2 What Is Included in Services Varies

At this point, the child welfare researcher has a sample that may or may not be eligible for services even though the children and families have received an initial response. Here again, there is state variation. Generally, services fall on a continuum from fully voluntary to mandated by the court. At the lowest level, families may be offered voluntary in-home services that are essentially a form of case management (rarely court supervised). A much smaller proportion of families who are considered at high risk of requiring a child be placed into foster care are offered more intensive family preservation or intensive in-home services (IIHS) for a short period of time. Finally, a child may be placed into foster care due to safety concerns or the unavailability of a caregiver after the report or after in-home services fail.

21.4.3 Eligibility

In some cases, the ability to provide a family services is dependent upon a decision after an investigation that results in substantiation, while other states may serve cases irrespective of their official disposition (US DHHS 2003, 1997). Interestingly the effect may be somewhat bidirectional in that workers who know that substantiation is required in order to provide services may be more likely to substantiate a case (Maguire-Jack and Font 2014). While the decision to substantiate a case or not is made by the worker, there are legal standards set by the state regarding the quality/quantity of evidence required. In 2012, 39 states required high evidentiary standards to substantiate (US DHHS 2003), but 2 years later this had dropped to 37 (Child Welfare Information Gateway 2016). Unfortunately, although substantiation may be required to provide services, research on substantiation suggests that the label is neither predictive of ongoing safety nor indicative of child well-being (Drake et al. 2003; Hussey et al. 2005).

What does this mean for research on outcomes? It means that while one would not expect the substantiation label to be highly predictive of outcomes, it may still be an important factor in reaching the point of receiving services. On a final note, eligibility for services may also be impacted by legal status. The policies regarding the ability to provide services for undocumented families through child welfare are unclear and there has been very little research on this issue (Križ and Skivenes 2012).

21.4.4 Services Content

Sometimes innovations are piloted in ways that do not reflect the reality of long-term implementation. For example, the earliest and most positively evaluated tests of the DR approach were enhanced by funds provided by a foundation that could be used to purchase services or meet material needs (Loman and Siegel 2015). This was not sustainable nor was it replicated in state approaches later. As mentioned earlier, how cases are sorted by track and what is provided following varies. For example, in one California county, DR includes provision of paraprofessional home visitation (Conley and Berrick 2010). This variation in implementation may help explain some of the more recent neutral (e.g., Fluke et al. 2016) or negative results of DR evaluations (e.g., Bartholet 2014) (See Chap. 12 in this volume). Without careful attention to such variation, one could imagine very different outcomes obtained even though the program has the same title. Federal child maltreatment data is limited to a single variable that indicates any in-home service which, as stated earlier, can mean anything from occasional visits by a case manager to mandated intensive in-home services.

21.4.5 Delivery Systems

Other policy shifts may impact not only what services are provided but by whom. For example, the Indian Child Welfare Act provides the ability for federally recognized tribes to operate all or part of child welfare services and specifically mandates attention to the tribes wishes in regard to foster care (Indian Child Welfare Act 1978). Where these systems exist, the cross-reporting of decisions and services to state agencies is often incomplete (Smith and Fox 2003). Several states have also moved to some level of privatization. This means that, in some cases, child welfare services are provided by private agencies under some type of contractual arrangement with the state (IOM and NRC 2014). Once again, the type of contract that provides oversight, the level of privatization (regional, statewide, foster care only, all services) varies (McCullough and Lee 2007). Although, hypothetically, the quality and/or content of services may vary under these circumstances, we know very little about such variation or the impact on outcomes obtained (Wells et al. 2014).

21.5 Do Services Work?

While all states are required to promote permanency and child safety, as the reader has no doubt recognized, there is significant variability in the populations served, eligibility for services after a report and content of those services that are provided if eligible. This may be one reason that the research on both safety and permanency following child welfare intervention is mixed.

21.5.1 Dosage of Services (Frequency of Contact)

Dosage of services is also a potential confounder, but less well studied. In an older study of child-welfare involved families receiving in-home services, only about two-thirds reported having seen their caseworker in the last month (Chapman et al. 2003). Of course, it is hard to know if caseworkers may be seeing higher functioning and more compliant families less and therefore outcomes might appear independent of the amount of contact.

21.5.2 Worker Preparation

States vary substantially in the training required for child welfare workers from having a bachelor's degree in any related discipline to requiring a master's level degree in social work or counseling (Jonson-Reid and Drake 2018). Worker preparation and training may impact the ability to engage with families. Generally, family satisfaction with child welfare services includes reference to both the compassion and the competency of the workers they interact with (De Boer and Coady 2007; Jonson-Reid and Drake 2018). This makes intuitive sense, but we have little understanding of how much this relates to the entry-level education required or the organizational culture of a given agency. In one study of maltreatment recurrence using NSCAW II data, higher training requirements were significantly associated with reduced recurrence at the bivariate level but this association was not significant once family risk factors were controlled (Maguire-Jack and Font 2014).

21.5.3 What is My Outcome of Interest?

In evaluation methodology, some sort of 'logic model' is commonly called for to better connect what one expects as outcome given the services provided (Besharov and Call 2016). For example, the Family Connections Model is a proactive program that provides in home services in their neighborhoods to help them meet the basic needs of their children and prevent child neglect. DePanfilis and Dubowitz (2005a, b) stated that this model was designed not only to reduce risk factors but also to strengthen protective factors associated with child maltreatment. Studies examining this model (Collins et al. 2015; DePanfilis and Dubowitz 2005a, b; Lindsey et al. 2009; Sharpe et al. 2009) found promise in areas of caregiver and child functioning but little impact on maltreatment reports. This is a similar finding to that reported in evaluations of various early childhood home visitation programs (Howard and Brooks-Gunn 2009). A number of explanations have been posited for such mixed and somewhat counterintuitive findings, such as surveillance bias (Drake et al. 2017), but in reality it is not always clear that we have sufficient knowledge to know exactly what interventions, or components of interventions, are tied to specific outcomes. Nor is it clear when a short-term outcome may be quite different (positive or negative) from a longer-term outcome.

This issue circles back around to an idea we mentioned earlier in relation to the meaning of success. It may be possible, for example, to successfully intervene to improve long-term child outcomes without having the hoped for effect on interim outcomes like reducing maltreatment reports in early childhood (Olds et al. 1998; Zielinski et al. 2009). On one hand, most studies of early childhood programs commonly implemented find that early developmental gains fade by about the third grade for children who participate (Copple and Bredekamp 2009). On the other hand, some longer-term follow-ups of children participating in at least one nurse home visiting model and the Chicago Child-parent Centers have found that reports of maltreatment in later childhood as well as later youth outcomes like graduation from high school and lower crime were better for those served (Reynolds and Robertson 2003; Temple and Reynolds 2007; Zielinski et al. 2009). So, from a child welfare safety outcome perspective a program could 'fail' during one period of development and yet have longer term protective benefits for later maltreatment and/or result in other positive developmental outcomes. Unfortunately, many studies are limited in their ability to follow cases for a long enough time to be able to tease out differences in program effects.

21.5.4 In-Home Case Management or Family Centered Services (FCS)

If a family receives services following a report of maltreatment, services will most likely be low intensity case management (hereafter family-centered services or FCS). One of the difficulties in assessing this type of service is that the services a family receives as a result of CPS case management are dependent on the availability and accessibility of services from agencies in the community. While studies indicate that families involved with child protection have multiple needs (Loman 2006; Millett et al. 2016; Saldana 2015), very little information is available on what services are obtained. In one study limited to public sector agencies, over 60% of families received income maintenance after a first report, but less than 5% of families received public agency funded mental health services after a first report (Jonson-Reid et al. 2010). To date, no known published work includes the range of non-profit and government funded services that may be included in a case plan. Here again, initiatives like the Essentials for Childhood collective impact approach discussed by Klevens and Metzler (See Chap. 13 in this volume) may provide a unique opportunity to help fill this gap-particularly if the evaluation can include family level data in addition to organizational collaboration information.

Relatively few studies exist that break out low intensity case management from family preservation services (reviewed next). Among families in one city in Maryland with substantiated reports of maltreatment, families known to have attended services as part of the case plan were less likely to have another report (DePanfilis and Zuravin 2002). In a Missouri study of families with a first report of maltreatment, families receiving FCS following a substantiated neglect case had a lower recidivism rate (Drake et al. 2003). A later study controlling for a range of factors, including additional services outside child welfare (e.g., public mental health, special education, poverty, substantiation, other services, service refusal, etc.) found that FCS was associated with reduced risk of recurrence (Drake et al. 2006). Obviously, the resources available for meeting a family's needs will vary by location as we discussed earlier in this chapter. To our knowledge, no published studies of FCS specific to rural areas have been done. Yet significant literature suggests problems in services availability in rural areas (Child Welfare Information Gateway 2012).

21.5.5 Intensive In-Home Services (IIHS) Models

Intensive in-home services are provided to families deemed to be at high risk of having a child placed into foster care. Services are shorter term than FCS but very intense (often 24/7). The debate on the effectiveness of this approach has long been waged (e.g., Littell and Shuerman 1995). Interestingly, evidence-based lists have played a role in this debate. For example, the California Evidence Based Clearinghouse (n.d.) on Child Welfare (http://www.cebc4cw.org/) rates Homebuilders (a program with significant number of studies), as 'supported by research evidence' – a lower level than 'well supported by research evidence'. This means the research is mixed. A recent meta-analysis by Al et al. (2012) found that these programs did not appear effective for child-welfare involved families but may be effective for multi-problem families that are not involved in child welfare. This is of course very problematic when IIHS is viewed as an intervention within the child welfare system.

21.5.6 Foster Care

Foster care, except in the case of residential treatment facilities, is really not a service in the sense of an intervention designed to impact behaviors or outcomes of the child. For the child, it is designed to be a safe and ideally nurturing place while the family of origin either complies with service plans for reunification or a new permanent home can be found. While there are a fair number of studies looking at permanency within foster care (i.e., the number of times a child moves), there is much less attention to safety and permanency following an exit from care. When reunification is the goal, the family of origin often continues to receive some form of in-home services in addition to whatever external services are required. There is some indication that such services may reduce re-entry (Carnochan et al. 2013; Lee et al.

2012), but few studies of this exist and it is difficult to know in the latter study cited what exactly the parents received. Another study suggested that repeated engagement with child welfare over time ultimately resulted in lower re-entry after reunification (Barth et al. 2008). This may indicate that it takes more than one episode of intervention for some families to benefit (Millett et al. 2016), but clearly more investigation is needed. Three studies examined recurrent maltreatment after reunification and found that about a third of these children experienced a subsequent report (Connell et al. 2007; Fuller 2005; Jonson-Reid et al. 2003).

21.6 Testing an Additional Program in Child Welfare? Some Additional Considerations When Thinking About Usual Care

To our knowledge, nearly all innovations with the exception in screening changes like DR are implemented as additions to the usual care process of decision-making in child welfare. As stated earlier, a better understanding of usual care and related outcomes can also help inform implementation of evidence based interventions as the context of agencies and the systems in which they are embedded can facilitate or impede innovations in new settings (Damschroder et al. 2009; Glisson et al. 2008). This context may include the impact of broader societal shifts in policy or economic context that may impact usual care even though the changes are not part of child welfare per se.

Sometimes broader, unforeseen, changes occur in politics or economics or both that may alter the operation of a service system. In a recently completed study of engaging child welfare involved families in home visitation, both the policies gating child welfare services and the funding for home visitation services shifting dramatically at the start of the study due to the advent of the recession (Stahlschmidt et al. 2018). This required a rapid redesign of the study and completely eliminated the possibility of replication as planned in the region. Generally, we have not paid attention to policies and allocation impacts outside child welfare, despite their potential import. For example, Klevens et al. (2015) argued there is a dearth of research that examines how public policies prevent child maltreatment, especially neglect. They applied multilevel modeling to explore the effects of 11 policies, including housing, child care, pre-K programs, children's health care insurance, and parents' health insurance policies. They found states' continuity of eligibility for Medicaid/children's health care insurance (SCHIP) were significantly associated with decreased child maltreatment, but there were significant limitations in the measurement of the implementation of policies. The absence of policy effects could come from other contributing factors, such as poor implementation, reduced or inequitable coverage, a time lag, competing policies, or simply ineffective policies. While the impact of policies or funding may not always be known, when changes occur that have broad effects, researchers should consider whether or not these may confound the results of a study or replication.

21.6.1 How Big an Effect Size Is Reasonable?

One way to think about outcomes, as presented earlier, is whether or not something "worked." As we have discussed this depends on your definition of success. A second consideration, however, is how strong an effect is when you find one. Here again, it is important to ask, compared to what? Studies have found that SafeCare can decrease self-reported parental stress (Tiwari et al. 2017), home safety issues (Gershater-Molko et al. 2003; Rostad et al. 2017), and improve parenting engagement (Carta et al. 2013; Damashek et al. 2011; Silovsky et al. 2011). Some of these studies had radically different sample sizes and comparisons. For example, in some early studies of SafeCare the comparison group was intensive in-home services (Edwards and Lutzker 2008), but most families are not deemed at sufficient risk to warrant this level of usual care intervention. Tiwari and colleagues conducted a small pilot where mothers were recruited based on risk factors for maltreatment not child welfare involvement (2017). Another study included families reported for maltreatment, but lost over half to attrition (Gershater-Molko et al. 2003). A third study included families with maltreatment report histories, families with just a current investigated report, and those currently receiving child welfare services (Damashek et al. 2011). On one hand, the replication across populations and regions is exactly in line with our recommendations so far. On the other hand, while these varied replications are occurring it is hard to summarize findings until sufficient numbers of studies with similar populations occur. This means that when one has a program like this, it is important to consider what a reasonable effect size may be given the population you are comparing it to. Analyses testing an intervention within a higher risk population may well have stronger effects than the same intervention in a relatively low risk sample. Further when studies move from efficacy to effectiveness, the effect size may be reduced (Littell 2008).

21.6.2 Who Stayed in the Intervention?

Attrition is also likely to be a significant concern. Many program effects are predicated on longterm participation in a given intervention (e.g., Chicago Child-Parent Centers – Reynolds and Robertson 2003). Child welfare involved families have been noted as highly mobile and chaotic (Coulton et al. 2012). In at least one study of an early childhood intervention with this population, several consenting families did not complete baseline interviews because they were gone (moved) by the time the interview was scheduled (Stahlschmidt et al. 2018). Home visitation studies, outside the early highly controlled studies of the Olds model, are plagued with very high attrition rates (Gershater-Molko et al. 2003; Olds 2003). This does not mean we should toss them to the side, but it does bring us back to questions of what works with whom. While one can examine similarities and differences between families who remain in a program until the end with those who exit early, there may be unmeasured differences that are important to questions of replication and scalability. This is an important part of building prevention and intervention science. We can identify a program that works for certain populations and then turn our attention to what else is needed for those that dropped out or for whom the program did not impact.

21.6.3 How Long Does the Effect Remain?

Researchers have pointed out the disconnect between the crisis-based theory approach that suggests a brief service will return someone to positive functioning (Staudt and Drake 2002) as compared to the multi-problem families that come to the attention of child welfare. It is perhaps not surprising that research finds that over time families who were once served by child welfare are eventually re-reported (Bae et al. 2010; Jonson-Reid et al. 2010). It is possible that renewed contact and services to meet new or continuing need may, in part, explain the findings that families with prior services increasingly do better (Jonson-Reid et al. 2010; Barth et al. 2008). As yet, it is not clear how much additional programming increases the ability to maintain a positive trajectory over time. It is, however, an important consideration when designing studies. It may be that at one point in time the findings regarding an added intervention are not impressive because the protective benefits of usual care may still be in play while later when any such usual care effects wear off, the added benefit of the additional intervention may appear.

21.7 Suggestions for Moving Ahead

By now the reader may have a sense of the complexity involved in attempted to understand effectiveness in public sector systems like child welfare. Difficult, however, is not the same as impossible and we would argue that continued pursuit of understanding of such effects is imperative from a policy and moral standpoint. In other words, public sector services are not likely to avoid the increasing demands for accountability that tend to be tied to funding. Of course having a positive effect does not guarantee funding by any means, but not showing worthwhile effects leaves programs with little defense in regards to budget cuts. From a moral standpoint, the recipients of services from systems like child welfare are among the most vulnerable in our country. The outcomes for children impacted by maltreatment are serious and often persist across the life course (e.g., Currie and Widom 2010; Fang et al. 2012; Gilbert et al. 2009; Jonson-Reid et al. 2012). It is therefore important that we are offering the best possible services to prevent and intervene. We conclude with some suggestions going forward. As a caveat, there are many excellent texts on evaluation and analytic approaches and clearly a strong grounding in such methods is key. We do not attempt to offer a crash course on research methods here but merely highlight some of the more critical issues specific to the question(s) at hand.

21.7.1 Thorough Description of Usual Care Practices and Target Population

Often in services research, the goal is to compare one service or screening condition to another, but the need to serve all cases that fit certain criteria make it impossible to create a randomized, non-served group at the point of initial referral. Understanding the baseline (usual care) expected trajectory of cases allows for a better understanding of treatment group effect sizes and potential costs. Sometimes adequate descriptions of practices may be available through state or regional program descriptions. Where such data are not available already, intervention researchers can help add to the knowledge base by thoroughly documenting the usual care context (e.g., Chaffin et al. 2011). In either case, studies seeking to evaluate existing usual care approaches or those mounting additional intervention on usual care platforms need to provide a thorough description of the population and the service for the consumer of the study.

There are three layers of the description of the population that should be a part of all research designs. First, one has to consider the population of the region in which a program is offered. If a given area is racially/ethnically homogenous, for example, one cannot expect racial or ethnic variation in the child welfare system serving that region. Second, one has to consider gatekeeping mechanisms that may limit the characteristics of families that can enter the sample pool from this population. Here we refer to issues like differing definitions of maltreatment and screening mechanisms that lead to entry into child welfare. Third, is the population included in the particular study being conducted the same as the population eligible for services? In other words, within the child welfare involved population, what group of families are actually consenting to the study. All three levels of population description are key to future replication, as well as considering whether or not a program needs to be adapted if the target population is different than the population in initial studies (e.g., Chaffin et al. 2012).

The collection of all the population, policy and services variables may well be some of the most time consuming and tedious aspects of thinking through research on child welfare services. While it is unlikely that studies will be able to perfectly describe every detail, it is a worthy endeavor. It is, we think, absolutely key to advancing science in this area. One of the authors often instructs their students to think about a methods section like a recipe for cookies, if some of the ingredients or processes are left out it may be impossible to duplicate the cookie desired. And, because the person trying to make the cookies later does not know if something was left out, they may not be able to explain why the resulting cookie does not look or taste the same.

21.7.2 Analytic Techniques to Enhance Comparability of Groups

As mentioned earlier, in most cases research on services like child welfare requires the use of comparison groups rather than being able to randomize. Although this is generally thought to be a weakness, there are a number of cogent criticisms of randomized trials in relation to relevance to the real world, selection bias, and the common flaws in implementation (Grossman and MacKenzie 2005; Landsverk et al. 2011; Stewart-Brown et al. 2011; Sullivan 2011). Increasingly statistical approaches like propensity score analysis, regression discontinuity design, instrumental variable approaches, and directed acyclic graph methods are endorsed as means of very closely approximating the level of control of randomization (Guo 2014; Guo and Fraser 2014; Imbens and Woolridge 2009; Knight and Winship 2013). Of course, not all of these are equally applicable across situations. Instrumental variables are theoretically derived based on the presence of an outside factor that influences a behavior, which then impacts the outcome (see for example, Doyle 2013). Such variables can be difficult to identify in practice. Generally, the use of some form of propensity score adjustment has been the favored and most common choice in child welfare research (e.g., Guo et al. 2006; Guo and Fraser 2014; Jonson-Reid et al. 2007; Ryan et al. 2008). As methods become more accessible and easy to implement in commonly available software, we suspect the variety of approaches in child welfare will increase. For example, more recently, predictive risk modeling has been employed in child welfare (Vaithianathan et al. 2013, 2017). This may provide promise as a new way of developing comparisons. For example, if we can predict with high certainty that a given outcome will occur for families with a set number of characteristics, then we may be able to use this as a baseline for comparing outcomes following policy or program innovations.

Because of the variability in implementation of child welfare services by regional and state policy, analyses also need to be methodologically appropriate to different geographic levels. Techniques like multilevel modelling, interrupted time series designs and other approaches capable of adjusting for influences on outcomes that included nested levels of data need to be employed (e.g., Allison 2010; Lawrence et al. 2011; Luke 2005).

These advanced techniques are increasingly employed by research teams without having to rely on advanced statistical consultation due to the increasing applied documentation of their use (e.g., Allison 2010). These techniques are also accessible to researchers through a variety of statistical packages (SAS, R, and others) and technological advances in computing have largely enabled the desktop computer to become sufficient for even complex and large scale analyses.

21.7.3 Defining the Outcome

Not only are there potentially a range of outcomes expected from a given service or intervention, but also a range of measures of such outcomes. For example, researchers have pointed out that most child neglect intervention programs fail to address the primary goal of the intervention, reducing the recidivism of child neglect (Allin et al. 2005; Hearn 2011; MacMillan et al. 2009). But many such programs target risk factors associated with child neglect as their major aim (e.g., mental health problems, substance abuse, material hardship, underdeveloped parenting skills, and a disconnection between family and the community). Intervention programs such as Health Families America (HFA), and Family Connections have shown promising results in reducing risk factors for maltreatment and some self-reported aggressive or neglectful parenting behaviors, but mixed results were found in reducing an official report of child abuse or neglect (Cullen et al. 2010; DePanfilis and Dubowitz 2005a, b; Harding et al. 2007). While addressing risk factors is important, in many cases we do not yet understand what factors are comorbid as compared to causally related to maltreatment or recurrence (IOM and NRC 2014). Studies of program efficacy need to include system relevant measures of the behavior to be prevented in addition to measuring risk or self-reported parenting behaviors to begin to close this gap in our understanding. It is important to understand the underlying similarities and differences in the outcomes themselves and what that means for children's safety and well-being.

Whenever possible, consideration of longer and shorter term outcomes should be included. There is growing evidence that not all successes at one stage lead to continued positive outcomes and not all failures at one stage lead to negative outcomes. We have much to learn about what outcomes are obtained at what point, for how long and whether or not this predicts longer term hoped for behaviors or events. In other words, we want to prevent recurrent maltreatment in the short term to prevent immediate harm and system burden. However, it is not always clear that a repeat report signals new harm and it is not clear how or why services may fail to address that immediate outcome and yet apparently positively impact developmental outcomes for a child. Nor is it clear that we have the right model in mind for intervening in multi-problem families. It may be that multiple points of intervention are to be expected not because a first attempt failed but merely because of the time it takes to address the complex issues involved. These questions can only be answered by studies that can measure longer term effects. We realize this is not always possible, but even shorter term studies can build in mechanisms like consent forms that ask a family if they are willing to be recontacted in the future that help facilitate the ability to revisit outcomes later when new funding may become available. It may also be possible to gain permission to link studies to administrative data over time that can track some outcomes of interest at a lower cost.

21.7.4 Should We Only Research "Evidence-Based Practices"?

We will not belabor the obvious bias toward a belief in the necessity of continued usual care research whether or not this is in the service of studying the effects of an additional intervention (Jonson-Reid et al. 2017). So in regard to this aspect of the question the answer is 'no'. There is however an additional part to this question in regard to intervention research. In other words, should we evaluate or continue to develop new approaches or should we be looking to the listings of evidence-based practices alone to target our efforts?

There has been increasing attention to the implementation of evidence-based services in child welfare and other systems. Various compilations of such programs exist like the Child Welfare Evidence-based Clearinghouse (CEBC), and the ways in which programs are rated as evidence-based varies. For example, the CEBC uses a five-point scale from 'concerning' to strongly supported by research (http://www.cebc4cw.org/ratings/). Other organizations like the Promising Practices Network divides programs into 'promising' or 'proven' depending on the strength of effect size and evaluation design (http://www.promisingpractices.net/criteria.asp). In some cases, various funding opportunities in research have limited the selection of potential interventions based on such listings (e.g., https://www.acf.hhs.gov/opre/research/project/early-head-start-university-partnership-grants-buffering-children-from).

On one hand, it makes sense to provide the most efficacious approach. On the other hand, limiting research to services listed on evidence-base repositories alone assumes that we have sufficient knowledge of effective programs that are appropriate across populations and that the effect sizes obtained warrant confidence in turning away from intervention development and focusing more solely on implementation. We have already noted how much variation exists in formal child welfare responses to maltreatment and how little we actually know. We would argue that both greater attention to the replicability and portability of effective programs is needed along with attention to innovative or understudied approaches that may continue to enhance effect sizes or address issues not addressed by a given EBP. For example, a therapeutic approach like cognitive behavioral therapy may be perfectly suited to addressing a given behavior but does not include attention to the material needs or social isolation that may also be contributing to maltreatment.

In all cases, it is critical that a thorough description of the additional or new program being evaluated is provided. For example, even when evidence-based practices are being tested in the field, they are often adapted in some way due to issues of cost, or context or population. Aarons et al. (2012) provide a more detailed discussion of this issue as well as offer a framework for assessing the adaption being made in a given setting.

21.7.5 Replication Across Sites with Differing Policy Gatekeeping Mechanisms

Given the considerable variation between states, it is important that this undertaking, at a minimum, be at the state as compared to national level. For states that have county administered systems, any analysis should incorporate multilevel modeling adjusting for county level policy variation. When planning a study, the research team should not only look for the existence of prior studies but where they were done and how child welfare policy guides screening and intervention in that region.

Useful policy-relevant research must also be a dynamic process. To the extent possible, prior outcomes found in research should be linked to the policies that guided reporting and service during the study period so that the process can be replicated over time to see how and when more recent policy shifts result in practical differences in system outcomes of interest. Administrative data that accurately captures the intensity and duration of services provided through child protection that is linked to data from agencies in the health, mental health and educational domains (at a minimum) is needed to accurately measure what services a child and family are receiving over time. In other words, a study of usual care in the 1990s needs to be repeated no matter how rigorous the original approach simply because the policies and practices, and perhaps the population in a given region itself, will no longer be the same.

21.8 Conclusion

Mapping out this landscape of policies, services and outcomes provided within child welfare is a necessary step for the advancement of evidence-based policies and programs. Understanding the trajectories through stages of CPS decision making and the relationship or lack thereof to outcomes obtained is a necessary backdrop not only for implementation of new policies but also for efforts to add or connect evidence-based interventions to the existing CPS platform. We have attempted to highlight both the difficulties and barriers inherent in this type of work while emphasizing the importance and offering suggestions for advancing the knowledge base in this area. While the present chapter largely focused on legislative goals of safety and permanency, the same attention needs to be made to the newer goal of child well-being that includes health, mental health and educational outcomes. Integrated data systems are increasingly common, making such research more feasible (Jonson-Reid and Drake 2008; Putnam-Hornstein et al. 2013). The continued development of and research using these resources at the state and county levels is needed. As these resources are developed, we believe that it will become increasingly feasible to both evaluate usual care and track outcomes associated with the added intervention. Services research is complex but complexity is not the enemy of research. There are millions of children and families that are in need of preventive intervention and understanding what is provided and to what end is critical to addressing this need.

References

Aarons, G. A., & Palinkas, L. (2007). Implementation of evidence- based practice in child welfare: Service provider perspectives. *Administration and Policy in Mental Health and Mental Health Services Research, 34*, 411–419.

Aarons, G. A., Green, A. E., Palinkas, L. A., Self-Brown, S., Whitaker, D. J., Lutzker, J. R., Silovsky, J. F., Hecht, D. B., & Chaffin, M. J. (2012). Dynamic adaptation process to implement an evidence-based child maltreatment intervention. *Implementation Science, 7*(1), 32.

Al, C. M., Stams, G. J. J., Bek, M. S., Damen, E. M., Asscher, J. J., & van der Laan, P. H. (2012). A meta-analysis of intensive family preservation programs: Placement prevention and improvement of family functioning. *Children and Youth Services Review, 34*(8), 1472–1479.

Allin, H., Wathen, C. N., & MacMillan, H. (2005). Treatment of child neglect: A systematic review. *The Canadian Journal of Psychiatry, 50*(8), 497–504.

Allison, P. (2010). *Survival analysis using SAS: Theory and application*. SAS Institute.

Bae, H. O., Solomon, P. L., Gelles, R. J., & White, T. (2010). Effect of child protective services system factors on child maltreatment re-reporting. *Child Welfare, 89*(3), 33.

Barth, R. P., Weigensberg, E. C., Fisher, P. A., Fetrow, B., & Green, R. L. (2008). Reentry of elementary aged children following reunification from foster care. *Children and Youth Services Review, 30*(4), 353–364.

Bartholet, E. (2014). Differential response: A dangerous experiment in child welfare. *Florida State University Law Review, 42*, 573.

Besharov, D. J., & Call, D. M. (2016). Using logic models to strengthen performance measurement. In D. Besharov, K. Baehler, & J. Klerman (Eds.), *Improving public services: International experiences in using evaluation tools to measure program performance*. Oxford: Oxford University Press.

California Evidence Based Clearinghouse on Child Welfare. (n.d.). *Homebuilders*. Retrieved from http://www.cebc4cw.org/

Carnochan, S., Rizik-Baer, D., & Austin, M. J. (2013). Preventing re-entry to foster care. *Journal of Evidence-Based Social Work, 10*(3), 196–209.

Carta, J. J., Lefever, J. B., Bigelow, K., Borkowski, J., & Warren, S. F. (2013). Randomized trial of a cellular phone-enhanced home visitation parenting intervention. *Pediatrics, 132*(Supplement 2), S167–S173.

Chaffin, M., Bard, D., Hecht, D., & Silovsky, J. (2011). Change trajectories during home-based services with chronic child welfare cases. *Child Maltreatment, 16*(2), 114–125.

Chaffin, M., Bard, D., Bigfoot, D. S., & Maher, E. J. (2012). Is a structured, manualized, evidence-based treatment protocol culturally competent and equivalently effective among American Indian parents in child welfare. *Child Maltreatment, 17*(3), 242–252.

Chapman, M. V., Gibbons, C. B., Barth, R. P., & McCrae, J. S. (2003). Parental views of in-home services: What predicts satisfaction with child welfare workers. *Child Welfare*, (5), 82.

Child Abuse Prevention and Treatment Act of 1984. (1985). P.L. 45 CFR § 1340, *14*(e), 93–247.

Child Welfare Information Gateway. (2012). Rural child welfare practice. Washington, DC: US Department of Health and Human Services, Children's Bureau.

Child Welfare Information Gateway (2016, February). Definitions of child abuse and neglect. *State Statutes*. Retrieved from https://www.childwelfare.gov/pubPDFs/define.pdf

Collins, K. S., Freeman, P. A. C., Strieder, F. H., Reinicker, P., & Baldwin, C. (2015). A pilot study examining the reduction of trauma symptomatology in families to prevent child abuse and neglect: Trauma adapted family connections. *Journal of Public Child Welfare, 9*(5), 506–527.

Conley, A., & Berrick, J. D. (2010). Community-based child abuse prevention: Outcomes associated with a differential response program in California. *Child Maltreatment, 15*(4), 282–292.

Connell, C. M., Bergeron, N., Katz, K. H., Saunders, L., & Tebes, J. K. (2007). Re-referral to child protective services: The influence of child, family, and case characteristics on risk status. *Child Abuse & Neglect, 31*(5), 573–588.

Copple, C., & Bredekamp, S. (2009). *Developmentally appropriate practice in early childhood programs serving children from birth through age 8*. Washington, DC: National Association for the Education of Young Children.

Coulton, C. J., Theodos, B., & Turner, M. A. (2012). Residential mobility and neighborhood change: Real neighborhoods under the microscope. *Cityscape: A Journal of Policy Development and Research, 14*, 55–90.

Cullen, J. P., Ownbey, J. B., & Ownbey, M. A. (2010). The effects of the Healthy Families America Home Visitation Program on parenting attitudes and practices and child social and emotional competence. *Child and Adolescent Social Work Journal, 27*(5), 335–354.

Currie, J., & Spatz Widom, C. (2010). Long-term consequences of child abuse and neglect on adult economic well-being. *Child Maltreatment, 15*(2), 111–120.

Damashek, A., Doughty, D., Ware, L., & Silovsky, J. (2011). Predictors of client engagement and attrition in home-based child maltreatment prevention services. *Child Maltreatment, 16*(1), 9–20.

Damschroder, L., Aron, D., Keith, R., Kirsh, S., Alexander, J., & Lowery, J. (2009). Fostering implementation of health services research findings into practice: A consolidated framework for advancing implementation science. *Implementation Science, 4*(1), 50–65.

De Boer, C., & Coady, N. (2007). Good helping relationships in child welfare: Learning from stories of success. *Child & Family Social Work, 12*(1), 32–42.

DePanfilis, D., & Dubowitz, H. (2005a). Family connections: A program for preventing child neglect. *Child Maltreatment, 10*(2), 108–123.

DePanfilis, D., & Dubowitz, H. (2005b). Family connections: A program for preventing child neglect. *Child Maltreatment, 10*(2), 108–123.

DePanfilis, D., & Zuravin, S. J. (2002). The effect of services on the recurrence of child maltreatment. *Child Abuse & Neglect, 26*(2), 187–205.

Dettlaff, A. J., & Johnson, M. A. (2011). Child maltreatment dynamics among immigrant and US born Latino children: Findings from the National Survey of Child and Adolescent Well-being (NSCAW). *Children and Youth Services Review, 33*(6), 936–944.

DeVooght, K., Fletcher, M., & Cooper, H. (2014). Federal, state, and local spending to address child abuse and neglect in SFY 2012. *Child Trends*. Retrieved from http://www.childtrends.org/?publications=14383

Dowd, K., Kinsey, S., Wheeless, S., Thissen, R., Richardson, J., & Mierzwa, F. (2002). *National Survey of Child and Adolescent Well-being (NSCAW): Introduction to the wave 1 general and restricted use releases*. Ithaca: Cornell University, National Data Archive on Child Abuse and Neglect.

Doyle, J. J. (2013). Causal effects of foster care: An instrumental-variables approach. *Children and Youth Services Review, 35*(7), 1143–1151.

Drake, B., & Rank, M. R. (2009). The racial divide among American children in poverty: Reassessing the importance of neighborhood. *Children and Youth Services Review, 31*(12), 1264–1271.

Drake, B., Jonson-Reid, M., Way, I., & Chung, S. (2003). Substantiation and recidivism. *Child Maltreatment, 8*(4), 248–260.

Drake, B., Jonson-Reid, M., & Sapokaite, L. (2006). Re-reporting of child maltreatment: Does participation in other public sector services moderate the likelihood of a second maltreatment report? *Child Abuse & Neglect, 30*, 1201–1226.

Drake, B., Lee, S. M., & Jonson-Reid, M. (2009). Race and child maltreatment reporting: Are Blacks overrepresented? *Children and Youth Services Review, 31*(3), 309–316.

Drake, B., Jonson-Reid, M., & Kim, H. (2017). Surveillance bias in child maltreatment: a tempest in a teapot. *International Journal of Environmental Research and Public Health, 14*(9), 971.

Edwards, A., & Lutzker, J. R. (2008). Iterations of the SafeCare model: An evidence-based child maltreatment prevention program. *Behavior Modification, 32*(5), 736–756.

English, D. J., Upadhyaya, M. P., Litrownik, A. J., Marshall, J. M., Runyan, D. K., Graham, J. C., & Dubowitz, H. (2005). Maltreatment's wake: The relationship of maltreatment dimensions to child outcomes. *Child Abuse & Neglect, 29*(5), 597–619.

Fang, X., Brown, D. S., Florence, C. S., & Mercy, J. A. (2012). The economic burden of child maltreatment in the United States and implications for prevention. *Child Abuse & Neglect, 36*(2), 156–165.

Flores, G., & Tomany-Korman, S. C. (2008). Racial and ethnic disparities in medical and dental health, access to care, and use of services in US children. *Pediatrics, 121*(2), e286–e298.

Fluke, J. D., Harlaar, N., Heisler, K., Darnell, A., Brown, B. & Merkel-Holguin, L. (2016, June). *Differential response and the safety of children reported to child protective services: A tale of six states.* Retrieved from https://aspe.hhs.gov/sites/default/files/pdf/204981/DifferentialResponse.pdf

Font, S. A., & Maguire-Jack, K. (2015a). Reprint of "Decision-making in child protective services: Influences at multiple levels of the social ecology". *Child Abuse & Neglect, 49*, 50–62.

Font, S. A., & Maguire-Jack, K. (2015b). Reprint of "Decision-making in child protective services: Influences at multiple levels of the social ecology". *Child Abuse & Neglect, 49*, 50–62.

Fox, K. A. (2003). Collecting data on the abuse and neglect of American Indian children. *Child Welfare, 82*(6), 707–726.

Freisthler, B., & Maguire-Jack, K. (2015). Understanding the interplay between neighborhood structural factors, social processes, and alcohol outlets on child physical abuse. *Child Maltreatment, 20*(4), 268–277.

Fuller, T. L. (2005). Child safety at reunification: A case-control study of maltreatment recurrence following return home from substitute care. *Children and Youth Services Review, 27*(12), 1293–1306.

Gershater-Molko, R. M., Lutzker, J. R., & Wesch, D. (2003). Project SafeCare: Improving health, safety, and parenting skills in families reported for, and at-risk for child maltreatment. *Journal of Family Violence, 18*(6), 377–386.

Gilbert, R., Widom, C. S., Browne, K., Fergusson, D., Webb, E., & Janson, S. (2009). Burden and consequences of child maltreatment in high-income countries. *The Lancet, 373*(9657), 68–81.

Glisson, C., Landsverk, J., Schoenwald, S., Kelleher, K., Hoagwood, K. E., Mayberg, S., & Green, P. (2008). Assessing the organizational social context (OSC) of mental health services: Implications for research and practice. *Administration and Policy in Mental Health and Mental Health Services Research, 35*(1–2), 98–113.

Grossman, J., & Mackenzie, F. J. (2005). The randomized controlled trial: Gold standard, or merely standard? *Perspectives in Biology and Medicine, 48*(4), 516–534.

Guo, S., Barth, R. P., & Gibbons, C. (2006). Propensity score matching strategies for evaluating substance abuse services for child welfare clients. *Children and Youth Services Review, 28*(4), 357–383.

Guo, S. (2014). Shaping social work science: What should quantitative researchers do? *Research on Social Work Practice, 25*, 370–381.

Guo, S., & Fraser, M. W. (2014). *Propensity score analysis: Statistical methods and applications* (Vol. 11). Thousand Oaks: Sage Publications.

Harbert, A., Tucker-Tatlow, J. (2012). *Review of child welfare risk assessments. Southern area consortium of human services.* Retrieved from http://theacademy.sdsu.edu/programs/SACHS/literature/SACHS_Risk_Assessment_Report_and_Appendices_11_2012.pdf

Harding, K., Galano, J., Martin, J., Huntington, L., & Schellenbach, C. J. (2007). Healthy Families America® Effectiveness: A comprehensive review of outcomes. *Journal of Prevention & Intervention in the Community, 34*(1–2), 149–179.

Harris, M. S., & Hackett, W. (2008). Decision points in child welfare: An action research model to address disproportionality. *Children and Youth Services Review, 30*(2), 199–215.

Hearn, J. (2011). Unmet needs in addressing child neglect: Should we go back to the drawing board? *Children and Youth Services Review, 33*(5), 715–722.

Howard, K. S., & Brooks-Gunn, J. (2009). The role of home-visiting programs in preventing child abuse and neglect. *The Future of Children, 19*(2), 119–146.

Hughes, R., Rycus, J., Saunders-Adams, S., Hughes, L., & Hughes, K. (2013). Issues in differential response. *Research on Social Work Practice, 23*(5), 493–520.

Hussey, J. M., Marshall, J. M., English, D. J., Knight, E. D., Lau, A. S., Dubowitz, H., & Kotch, J. B. (2005). Defining maltreatment according to substantiation: Distinction without a difference. *Child Abuse & Neglect, 29*(5), 479–492.

Imbens, G. W., & Wooldridge, J. M. (2009). Recent developments in the econometrics of program evaluation. *Journal of Economic Literature, 47*(1), 5–86.

Indian Child Welfare Act of 1978. (25 U.S.C. §§ 1901–63).

IOM (Institute of Medicine) and NRC (National Research Council). (2014). *New directions in child abuse and neglect research*. Washington, DC: The National Academies Press.

Jonson-Reid, M., & Drake, B. (2008). Multi-sector longitudinal administrative databases: An indispensable tool for evidence-based policy for maltreated children and their families. *Child Maltreatment, 13*(4), 392–399.

Jonson-Reid, M., & Drake, B. (2018). *After the cradle falls: What child abuse is, how we respond to it and what you can do about it*. Oxford: Oxford University Press.

Jonson-Reid, M., Drake, B., Chung, S., & Way, I. (2003). Cross-type recidivism among child maltreatment victims and perpetrators. *Child Abuse & Neglect, 27*(8), 899–917.

Jonson-Reid, M., Chance, T., & Drake, B. (2007). Risk of death among children reported for nonfatal maltreatment. *Child Maltreatment, 12*(1), 86–95.

Jonson-Reid, M., Emery, C. R., Drake, B., & Stahlschmidt, M. J. (2010). Understanding chronically reported families. *Child Maltreatment, 15*(4), 271–281.

Jonson-Reid, M., Kohl, P., & Drake, B. (2012). Child and adult outcomes of chronic child. *Maltreatment Pediatrics, 129*(5), 839–845. NIHMS 436968.

Jonson-Reid, M., Drake, B., & Zhou, P. (2013). Neglect subtypes, race and poverty: Individual, family, and service characteristics. *Child Maltreatment, 18*(1), 30–41.

Jonson-Reid, M., Drake, B., Kohl, P., Guo, S., Brown, D., McBride, T., Kim, H., & Lewis, E. (2017). What do we really know about usual care child protective services? *Children and Youth Services Review, 82*, 222–229.

Klevens, J., Barnett, S. B. L., Florence, C., & Moore, D. (2015). Exploring policies for the reduction of child physical abuse and neglect. *Child Abuse & Neglect, 40*, 1–11.

Knight, C. R., & Winship, C. (2013). The causal implications of mechanistic thinking: Identification using directed acyclic graphs (DAGs). In *Handbook of causal analysis for social research* (pp. 275–299). Dordrecht: Springer.

Križ, K., & Skivenes, M. (2012). How child welfare workers perceive their work with undocumented immigrant families: An explorative study of challenges and coping strategies. *Children and Youth Services Review, 34*(4), 790–797.

Landsverk, J., Brown, C. H., Reutz, J. R., Palinkas, L., & Horwitz, S. M. (2011). Design elements in implementation research: A structured review of child welfare and child mental health studies. *Administration and Policy in Mental Health and Mental Health Services Research, 38*(1), 54–63.

Lawrence, C. N., Rosanbalm, K. D., & Dodge, K. A. (2011). Multiple response system: Evaluation of policy change in North Carolina's child welfare system. *Children and Youth Services Review, 33*(11), 2355–2365.

Lee, S., Jonson-Reid, M., & Drake, B. (2012). Foster care re-entry: The role of foster care placement experiences, child welfare and cross sector services. *Children and Youth Services Review, 34*(9), 1825–1833.

Leeb, R. T., Paulozzi, L., Melanson, C., Simon, T., & Arias, I. (2008). *Child maltreatment surveillance: Uniform definitions for public health and recommended data elements, Version 1.0.* Atlanta: Centers for Disease Control and Prevention, National Center for Injury Prevention and Control.

Lindsey, M. A., Hayward, R. A., & DePanfilis, D. (2009). Gender differences in behavioral outcomes among children at risk of neglect: Findings from a family-focused prevention intervention. *Research on Social Work Practice, 20*(6), 572–581.

Littell, J. H. (2008). Evidence-based or biased? The quality of published reviews of evidence-based practices. *Children and Youth Services Review, 30*(11), 1299–1317.

Littell, J. H., & Schuerman, J. R. (1995). *A synthesis of research on family preservation and family reunification programs*. Chicago: Chapin Hall Center for Children at the University of Chicago.

Loman, L. (2006). *Families frequently encountered by child protection services: A report on chronic child abuse and neglect*. Missouri: Institute for Applied Research. Available from http://www.iarstl.org/papers/FEfamiliesChronicCAN.pdf

Loman, L. A., & Siegel, G. L. (2005). *Alternative response in Minnesota: Findings of the program evaluation. Differential response: A common sense reform in child welfare*. St Louis: Institute for Applied Research.

Loman, L. A., & Siegel, G. L. (2012). Effects of anti-poverty services under the differential response approach to child welfare. *Children and Youth Services Review, 34*(9), 1659–1666.

Loman, L. A., & Siegel, G. L. (2015). Effects of approach and services under differential response on long term child safety and welfare. *Child Abuse and Neglect, 39*, 86–97.

Luke, D. A. (2005). Getting the big picture in community science: Methods that capture context. *American Journal of Community Psychology, 35*(3–4), 185–200.

MacMillan, H. (2000). Child maltreatment: What we know in the year 2000. *Canadian Journal of Psychiatry, 45*, 702–709.

MacMillan, H. L., Wathen, C. N., Barlow, J., Fergusson, D. M., Leventhal, J. M., & Taussig, H. N. (2009). Interventions to prevent child maltreatment and associated impairment. *The Lancet, 373*(9659), 250–266.

Maguire-Jack, K., & Font, S. A. (2014). Predicting recurrent maltreatment among high-risk families: Applying the decision-making ecology framework. *Children and Youth Services Review, 43*, 29–39.

McCullough, C., & Lee, E. (2007). *Program and fiscal design elements of child welfare privatization initiatives (Topical paper # 2)*. The Urban Institute for the Office of the Assistant Secretary for Planning and Evaluation, US Department of Health and Human Services. Retrieved from http://aspe.hhs.gov/hsp/07/CWPI/models/index.shtml

McLaughlin, M., & Jonson-Reid, M. (2017). The relationship between child welfare financing, screening, and substantiation. *Children and Youth Services Review, 82*, 407–412.

McSherry, D. (2007). Understanding and addressing the "neglect of neglect": Why are we making a mole-hill out of a mountain? *Child Abuse & Neglect, 31*(6), 607–614.

Millett, L. S., Ben-David, V., Jonson-Reid, M., Echele, G., Moussette, P., & Atkins, V. (2016). Understanding change among multi-problem families: Learnings from a formative program assessment. *Evaluation and Program Planning, 58*, 176–183.

Molnar, B. E., Goerge, R. M., Gilsanz, P., Hill, A., Subramanian, S. V., Holton, J. K., Duncan, D. T., Beatriz, E. D., & Beardslee, W. R. (2016). Neighborhood-level social processes and substantiated cases of child maltreatment. *Child Abuse & Neglect, 51*, 41–53.

National Research Council. (1993). *Understanding child abuse and neglect*. National Academies Press.

National Resource Center for Child Protection Services (n.d.). *Decision-making tools library.* Retrieved from: http://nrccps.org/information-dissemination/1249-2/

Olds, D. (2003). Reducing program attrition in home visiting: What do we need to know? *Child Abuse & Neglect, 27*(4), 359–361.

Olds, D., Henderson, C. R., Jr., Cole, R., Eckenrode, J., Kitzman, H., Luckey, D., Pettitt, L., Sidora, K., Morris, P., & Powers, J. (1998). Long-term effects of nurse home visitation on children's criminal and antisocial behavior: 15-year follow-up of a randomized controlled trial. *JAMA, 280*(14), 1238–1244.

Pelton, L. H. (2015). The continuing role of material factors in child maltreatment and placement. *Child Abuse & Neglect, 41*, 30–39.

Piper, K. A. (2016). Differential response in child protection services: A comparison of implementation and child safety outcomes. *APSAC Advisor, 28*(2), 23–28.

Putnam-Hornstein, E., Needell, B., & Rhodes, A. E. (2013). Understanding risk and protective factors for child maltreatment: The value of integrated, population-based data. *Child Abuse & Neglect, 37*(2), 116–119.

Renninger, S. M., Veach, P. M., & Bagdade, P. (2002). Psychologists' knowledge, opinions, and decision-making processes regarding child abuse and neglect reporting laws. *Professional Psychology: Research and Practice, 33*(1), 19.

Reynolds, A. J., & Robertson, D. L. (2003). School–based early intervention and later child maltreatment in the Chicago longitudinal study. *Child Development, 74*(1), 3–26.

Rostad, W. L., McFry, E. A., Self-Brown, S., Damashek, A., & Whitaker, D. J. (2017). Reducing safety hazards in the home through the use of an evidence-based parenting program. *Journal of Child and Family Studies*, 1–8.

Ryan, J. P., Marshall, J. M., Herz, D., & Hernandez, P. M. (2008). Juvenile delinquency in child welfare: Investigating group home effects. *Children and Youth Services Review, 30*(9), 1088–1099.

Saldana, L. (2015). An integrated intervention to address the comorbid needs of families referred to child welfare for substance use disorders and child neglect: FAIR pilot outcomes. *Child Welfare, 94*(4), 167–186.

Sedlak, A., Mettenberg, J., Basena, M., Petta, I., McPherson, A., & Li, S. (2010). *Fourth National Incidence Study of child abuse and neglect (NIS–4): Report to Congress.* Washington, DC: US Department of Health and Human Services, Administration for Children and Families.

Sharpe, T. L., DePanfilis, D., Strieder, F., & Gregory, G. (2009). Replication of family connections: Lessons learned from grandparents. *Protecting Children, 24*(3), 59–69.

Silovsky, J. F., Bard, D., Chaffin, M., Hecht, D., Burris, L., Owora, A., Beasley, L., Doughty, D., & Lutzker, J. (2011). Prevention of child maltreatment in high-risk rural families: A randomized clinical trial with child welfare outcomes. *Children and Youth Services Review, 33*(8), 1435–1444.

Stahlschmidt, M., Jonson-Reid, M., Pons, L., Constantino, J., Kohl, P., Drake, B., & Auslander, W. (2018). Trying to bridge the worlds of home visitation and child welfare: Lessons learned. *Evaluation and Program Planning, 66*, 133–140. NIHMSID 917550.

Staudt, M., & Drake, B. (2002). Intensive family preservation services: Where's the crisis? *Children and Youth Services Review, 24*(9–10), 777–795.

Stewart-Brown, S., Anthony, R., Wilson, L., Winstanley, S., Stallard, N., Snooks, H., & Simkiss, D. (2011). Should randomised controlled trials be the "gold standard" for research on preventive interventions for children. *Journal of Children's Services, 6*(4), 228–235.

Sullivan, G. M. (2011). Getting off the "gold standard": Randomized controlled trials and education research. *Journal of Graduate Medical Education, 3*(3), 285–289.

Temple, J. A., & Reynolds, A. J. (2007). Benefits and costs of investments in preschool education: Evidence from the Child–Parent Centers and related programs. *Economics of Education Review, 26*(1), 126–144.

Tiwari, A., Self-Brown, S., Lai, B. S., McCarty, C., & Carruth, L. (2017). Effects of an evidence-based parenting program on biobehavioral stress among at-risk mothers for child maltreatment: A pilot study. *Social Work in Health Care*, 1–27.

US Department of Health and Human Services, Administration for Children, Youth and Families. (2012). *Children's Bureau: Child and family services review fact sheet.* Retrieved from https://www.acf.hhs.gov/sites/default/files/cb/cfsr_factsheet.pdf.

US Department of Health and Human Services, Administration for Children, Youth and Families, Children's Bureau and Office of the Assistant Secretary for Planning and Evaluation. (2003). *National study of child protectives services systems and reform efforts.* Washington, DC: US Government Printing Office.

US Department of Health and Human Services, Administration for Children, Youth and Families (2012). Children's Bureau: Child and family services review fact sheet. Retrieved from https://www.acf.hhs.gov/sites/default/files/cb/cfsr_factsheet.pdf

US Department of Health and Human Services. (2013). *Child maltreatment 2012*. Author. Retrieved from https://www.acf.hhs.gov/sites/default/files/cb/cm2012.pdf

US Department of Health and Human Services. (2017). *Child maltreatment 2015*. Author. Retrieved from http://www.acf.hhs.gov/programs/cb/research-data-technology/statistics-research/child-maltreatment

US Department of Health and Human Services. (2018). *Child maltreatment 2016*. Author. Retrieved from https://www.acf.hhs.gov/sites/default/files/cb/cm2016.pdf.

Vaithianathan, R., Maloney, T., Putnam-Hornstein, E., & Jiang, N. (2013). Children in the public benefit system at risk of maltreatment: Identification via predictive modeling. *American Journal of Preventive Medicine, 45*(3), 354–359.

Vaithianathan, R., Putnam-Hornstein, E., Jiang, N., Nand, P., & Maloney, T. (2017). Developing predictive models to support child maltreatment hotline screening decisions: Allegheny County methodology and implementation. Retrieved from https://www.alleghenycountyanalytics.us/wp-content/uploads/2017/04/Developing-Predictive-Risk-Models-package-with-cover-1-to-post-1.pdf

Valentino, K., Nuttall, A. K., Comas, M., Borkowski, J. G., & Akai, C. E. (2012). Intergenerational continuity of child abuse among adolescent mothers authoritarian parenting, community violence, and race. *Child Maltreatment, 17*(2), 172–181.

Van der Put, C. E., Assink, M., & Stams, G. J. J. (2016). The effectiveness of risk assessment methods: Commentary on "Deciding on child maltreatment: A literature review on methods that improve decision-making". *Child Abuse & Neglect, 59*, 128–129.

Wells, R., Jolles, M. P., Chuang, E., McBeath, B., & Collins-Camargo, C. (2014). Trends in local public child welfare agencies 1999–2009. *Children and Youth Services Review, 38*, 93–100.

Zielinski, D. S., Eckenrode, J., & Olds, D. L. (2009). Nurse home visitation and the prevention of child maltreatment: Impact on the timing of official reports. *Development and Psychopathology, 21*(2), 441–453.

Chapter 22
Re-visioning Education and Training for Child Protection Using a Public Health Approach

Kerryann Walsh

22.1 Introduction: A Public Health Approach to Education and Training for Child Protection

One of the most famous verses from the Tao Ti Ching, "the journey of a thousand miles starts under one's feet", is sometimes also translated as "a journey of a thousand miles begins with a single step". This, of course, does not refer to educating and training professionals for child protection in the twenty-first century. Yet the entire verse (Verse 64) offers instruction on laying solid foundations, preventing problems before they arise, and responding to challenges with patience rather than hastening to premature solutions. This chapter uses the metaphor of 'a journey of small steps' to identify what is known about educating and training professionals in cognate systems about how to best respond to child maltreatment.

Worldwide, the need for education and training of professionals in child protection is widely acknowledged. As part of the Sustainable Development Goals (SDGs), world leaders have committed to ending all forms of violence against children by 2030 (United Nations 2015). It is an ambitious undertaking that will require the participation of *every* country, *every* community, and *every child-serving professional.* Population-based strategies are required, along with a shift in thinking towards a public health approach to child maltreatment prevention (Klika et al. 2018). Education and training is required for a diverse and constantly evolving child protection workforce with varying levels of knowledge and skills, diverse professional qualifications and experiences, and pluralism in identities, cultures, and values. Emboldened by the scope of this challenge, this chapter offers commentary on how a public health

K. Walsh (✉)
Faculty of Education, Queensland University of Technology (QUT), Kelvin Grove, QLD, Australia
e-mail: k.walsh@qut.edu.au

B. Lonne et al. (eds.), *Re-Visioning Public Health Approaches for Protecting Children*, Child Maltreatment 9, https://doi.org/10.1007/978-3-030-05858-6_22

approach to professional education and training can be used to build capacity in the child protection workforce and thereby enhance child protection.

Recognition of child maltreatment as a public health issue has progressed in earnest for almost 30 years, led by the work of organizations such as the International Society for Prevention of Child Abuse and Neglect, and the World Health Organization in recognising violence generally, and child maltreatment specifically, as significant public health issues (Krug et al. 2002; Meddings et al. 2005). At its core, a public health approach is about prevention. It aims to stop problems from occurring in the first place by introducing proven prevention measures to whole populations. A public health approach is conceptualised in four steps, beginning with understanding the extent of the problem, followed by identifying modifiable risk and protective factors, then developing and empirically testing prevention initiatives, and promoting widespread adoption of evidence-based programs and practices (Hammond 2003; Klika et al. 2018). These four steps are used as a framework for this chapter's four sections: (i) understanding education and training for child protection; (ii) identifying barriers and facilitators to education and training for child protection; (iii) developing and empirically testing education and training initiatives; and (iv) promoting widespread adoption of education and training initiatives.

In this chapter, *the child protection workforce* is conceptualised broadly, as more than statutory or front-line child protection workers. It embraces all child-serving professionals including, but not limited to, professionals in agencies having direct contact with children and families, such as teachers, school counsellors, educare workers, doctors, nurses, allied health professionals, lawyers, and judicial officers, and social workers; those intervening at times of crisis such as statutory child protection workers, police, paramedics, emergency department and mental health service staff; along with those working in agencies with key advocacy roles such as policy makers, and program advisors (Besharov 1990). Although not a comprehensive list, it gives a sense of the wide range of affiliates well placed to intervene on behalf of children. Magnified to a global scale, there are millions of professionals who fulfil these roles, and potentially millions more who will do so in future. Ensuring they are appropriately prepared for their roles in child protection is a public health priority that nations, institutions, communities, and individuals must embrace if efforts to prevent violence against children generally, and child maltreatment specifically, are to succeed.

22.2 Understanding Education and Training for Child Protection

22.2.1 Defining Education and Training for Child Protection

How can education and training for child protection be defined? Definitional issues abound in the field of child maltreatment (Feerick et al. 2006) and the education and training domain is no exception. There is currently no unifying definition of education and training in the context of child protection. This is significant because absence of an agreed definition may contribute to absence of a collective vision for the optimal ways to design, develop, and implement education and training initiatives for child protection, and may lead to inequity in learning opportunities available to particular professional groups. An agreed definition would need to reflect a common set of descriptors, and be generalizable to multiple professional groups.

In fields other than child protection, numerous terms have been used to denote professional education and training. For example, *pre-service education*, *in-service education/training*, *pre-qualifying education/training*, *post-qualifying education/training*, *initial preparation programs/courses*, *continuing education*, *continuing professional education*, *professional development*, and *staff development*. A robust discussion of the origins of and dimensions to these terms and their definitions is beyond the scope of this chapter, as are the philosophical and political debates surrounding the use of the terms education and training. Suffice to know that debates exist and are discussed elsewhere (e.g., Buysse et al. 2009; Gomez et al. 2015; Rhodes and Huston 2012).

Constructing a tentative working definition within which to frame a proposal for a public health approach to education and training for child protection is a difficult task on account of the proliferation of terms and associated definitions. In the health education discipline, for example, the United States (US) Centers for Disease Control and Prevention (2016) defined *professional development* as:

> the systematic process used to strengthen the professional knowledge, skills, and attitudes of an organization's staff. Professional Development is consciously designed to actively engage learners and includes the planning, design, marketing, delivery, evaluation, and follow-up of professional development offerings (events, information sessions, and technical assistance) (p. 1).

The American Medical Association defines *continuing medical education* as:

> educational activities which serve to maintain, develop, or increase the knowledge, skills, and professional performance and relationships that a physician uses to provide services for patients, the public or the profession. (Davis et al. 2008, p. 652)

Opting for brevity, the British Association of Social Workers (2017) defined *continuous* (rather than continuing) *professional development* as "the process by which professionals maintain and develop their knowledge and skills throughout their career" (para 1). Hinting at the types of delivery methods preferred, the National Professional Development Center on Inclusion (2011) defined *professional development* as:

> facilitated teaching and learning experiences that are transactional and designed to support the acquisition of professional knowledge, skills and dispositions as well as the application of this knowledge in practice. (p. 3)

Common to these few randomly-selected definitions is a sense that post-qualifying education and training is a continuum of intentional learning experiences leading to improvements in professionals' knowledge, skills, and practices (with attitudes or dispositions sometimes mentioned). Hence, the type of experiences that are the subject of this chapter can be distinguished from basic information sharing and mass media campaigns. In a broad sense, education and training for child protection can be seen as a public health intervention with predisposing, enabling, and inhibiting factors.

22.2.2 *Models for Education and Training for Child Protection*

What models exist for conceptualising education and training for child protection? The literature is far from awash with models for education and training. Some years ago, UK scholars conceptualised the content of education and training for child protection, developmentally, as a "broadening wedge of content" (Taylor 1997, p. 66; see also Taylor and Hodgkinson 2001). It begins narrowly with basic "survival" content early in pre-qualification courses, broadening through these courses by embedding incrementally deeper levels of content, and extending into post-qualification professional development where "reflexive" decision making on the best available evidence is learned (Taylor 1997). This "wedge" model provides a developmental heuristic for considering education and training for child protection as more than a single block that is "bolted on" to pre-qualification education and training (Taylor and Hodgkinson 2001). It illustrates that pre- and post-qualification education and training are both important and necessary, and comprise a process of incremental gains, somewhat like a "journey of small steps". Figure 22.1 shows an adapted version of the original model.

Another, more recent, example of a model or framework, this time applied to education and training for qualified health professionals, is the United Kingdom's (UK) Royal College of Paediatrics and Child Health (2014) *Safeguarding children and young people: roles and competences for health care staff*, which clarifies and sets out minimum training requirements for different categories of staff. This guidance lists five levels with examples of staff groups at each level as shown in Box 22.1, and details corresponding core competencies, knowledge, skills, attitudes and values for each level. Minimum durations for education and training at each level are also specified.

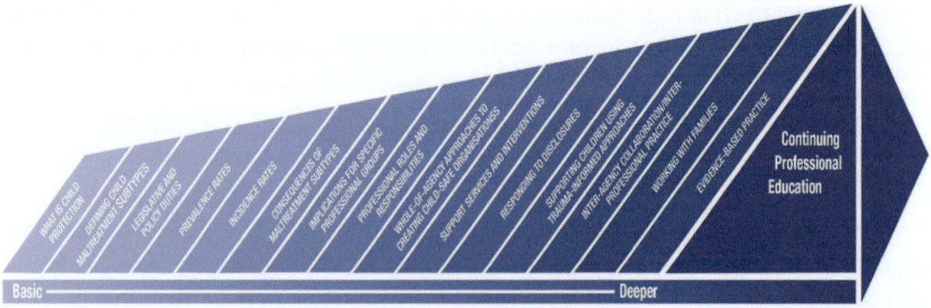

Fig. 22.1 Developmental model of education and training for child protection. (Adapted from Taylor 1997, pp. 66–68; Taylor and Hodgkinson 2001, pp. 82–84)

Box 22.1 Continuing Education Framework for UK Health Care Staff

Level 1	All staff including non-clinical managers and staff working in health care settings (includes senior managers such as Chief Executive Officers, Chairs, Board Members) (2 h)
Level 2	Minimum level required for non-clinical and clinical staff who have some degree of contact with children and young people and/or parents/carers (3–4 h)
Level 3	Clinical staff working with children, young people and/or their parents/carers and who could potentially contribute to assessing, planning, intervening and evaluating the needs of a child or young person and parenting capacity where there are safeguarding/child protection concerns (core = 8 h plus 2 h annual refresher training; specialist = 16 h)
Level 4	Named professionals who provide advice and expertise for fellow professionals and promote good practice within their organization (24 h)
Level 5	Designated professionals who take a professional and strategic lead on all aspects of the health service contribution to safeguarding children (24 h)
	Source: Royal College of Paediatrics and Child Health (2014, p. 10)

Despite the dearth of models available, together the two selected for mention above provide a pathway towards a public health approach to education and training, in which the goal (or collective vision) is to have professionals from a vast array of disciplinary backgrounds with a common base of knowledge and skills. This common base could be termed *child protection literacy*, that is, the full range of knowledge, skills, attitudes, and dispositions that determine the capacity of individuals to access, understand, and use information to promote child protection. Ideally, this foundation must be built using education and training programs with proven efficacy. But, as will be shown below, what is known about education and training efficacy is quite limited.

Borrowing from Zimmerman and Mercy (2010), re-visioning education and training for child protection from a public health perspective requires an "infrastructure" or architecture. Figure 22.2 depicts the way in which professional education and training for child protection can be conceptualised according to a public health approach that incorporates primary, secondary, and tertiary education and training interventions, provided differentially and with increasing complexity based on the nature and intensity of professionals' direct contact with children in their daily work. To be true to a public health approach, this would require the largest education and training component and the most substantial investment to be located in universal or primary education and training initiatives. The content would progressively increase in complexity and intensity from primary, through secondary, to tertiary components of the education and training system.

Hence, universal education and training (or child protection literacy) for *all* professionals who will work with children will begin in preservice (pre-qualifying) courses and extend through to in-service (post-qualifying) education and training

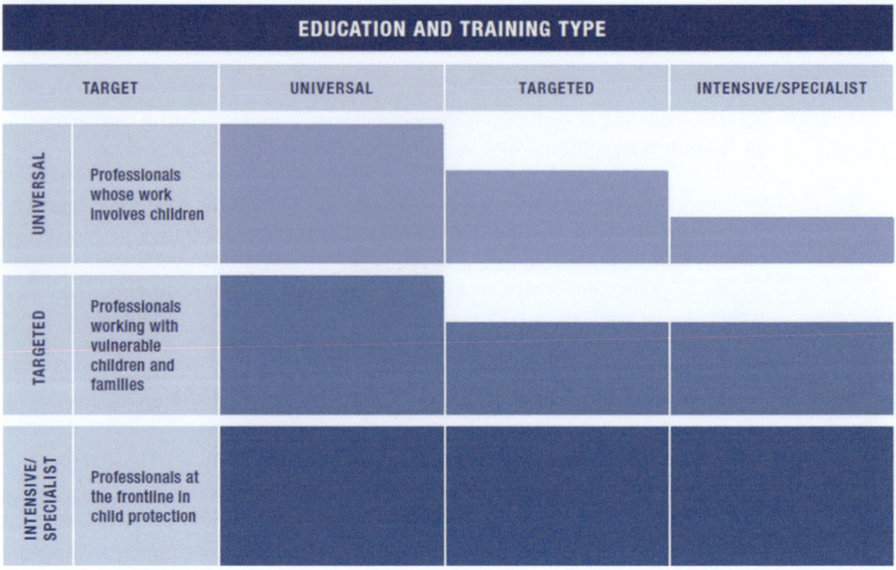

Fig. 22.2 A public health approach applied to education and training types and targets

programs including agency orientation programs. Targeted education and training for professionals working with vulnerable children and families will also begin in pre-service courses but will cover additional content in more intensive ways, again extending through to in-service programs where some material will be refreshed and new understandings gained. Intensive or specialist education and training for professionals at the front line in child protection will begin in pre-service and extend to in-service education and training reinforced and supported by professional supervision, and mentoring and coaching programs. Full participation will be essential to child maltreatment prevention.

22.2.3 Measuring Education and Training for Child Protection

What is known about the extent and nature of education and training for child protection? It is paradoxical that despite the rhetoric surrounding the importance of child protection (e.g., claims that it is a "shared responsibility" and "everyone's business"), in reality, education and training initiatives have been neglected and poorly measured. To begin with, little is known about the characteristics of child protection learners: who receives and does not receive education and training, by whom, when, and to what effect. Gaining evidence about who participates in education and training is a crucial first step in designing effective programs as this information sheds light on the alignment between education and training offerings and professionals' needs. This alignment is a key feature of education and training initiatives that take adult learning seriously (Bryan et al. 2009; Weber-Mayrer et al. 2015). Adult education theories posit that there may be causal associations between adult learner characteristics and education and training effectiveness (Merriam 2001, 2008).

Although there is very little data available on the often large-scale offerings of education and training for child protection and the features of learners, it remains the duty of employers to ensure that their employees clearly understand their child protection role within the employing organization, and hold the requisite knowledge, skills and dispositions to take up their roles. It is the obligation of employers to enable access to education and training which, in turn, enables the organization to fulfil its child protection duties. To this end, further data are required, especially on the features of large-scale training initiatives and the characteristics of participating learners. Organizations should routinely collect data on:

- Who attends what type of education and training (i.e., characteristics of those participating such as backgrounds, qualifications, positions, workplaces, baseline knowledge, and attitudes);
- When and how much education and training is delivered (e.g., number of sessions, duration, spacing, intensity or dose);
- Education and training procedures, materials, and delivery modes; and
- The qualifications and backgrounds of trainers.

Additionally, in an ideal world further steps could be taken to record and make available data on the extent to which education and training initiatives were delivered as planned and to document tailoring, adaptation, or modification for specific groups (i.e., exactly what was tailored and why) (Hoffmann et al. 2014). Useful education and training offerings can then be faithfully replicated. Finally, assessment of education and training costs can be part of a more rigorous, comprehensive and transparent approach to measuring education and training for child protection.

22.3 Identifying Barriers and Facilitators to Education and Training for Child Protection

Notwithstanding the barrier of appropriate measurement, what are other barriers and facilitators to education and training for child protection? Understanding the barriers and facilitators for education and training helps identify where additional effort is needed. A barrier is a characteristic or variable that increases the likelihood of education and/or training failures. A facilitator is a characteristic of variable that decreases the likelihood of education and training failures and simultaneously enables success.

Child protection system inquiries and child fatality reviews worldwide are replete with recommendations for more and better education and training for all relevant professionals (e.g., Cummins et al. 2012; Munro 2011; Palusci and Covington

2014). However, offering more or better education and training, in and of itself, may not lead to more successful outcomes unless it is acceptable to participants, its implementation is planned, and conducted with fidelity (Fixsen et al. 2009, 2013). In Australian research assessing the implementation of recommendations from 79 child protection system inquiries, professional education and training recommendations were found to be seldom followed through (Parenting Research Centre 2015). In fact, of all recommendations made in all of the inquiries studied, those relating to education and training were the *least* likely to be implemented. Strategies to address implementation barriers were identified as: greater investment in the child protection workforce; initial professional preparation and ongoing professional development in evidence-based practices; resource sharing across sectors and disciplines; greater emphasis on innovation; professional secondments between and across agencies; professional codes of conduct that include commitment to ongoing education and training; robust oversight of education and training; and rigorous evaluation (Albers and Mildon 2016; Parenting Research Centre 2015). These findings indicate that, in terms of maximising education and training outcomes, addressing barriers in implementation may be just as important as the substantive education and training initiative itself (Fixsen et al. 2009).

22.4 Developing and Empirically Testing Education and Training Initiatives

What is known about the effectiveness of education and training for child protection? Collectively there is a paucity of empirical literature on the effectiveness of education and training initiatives (i.e., programs, curricula, models) for child protection. Numerous registries or databases of evidence-based programs in child welfare and violence prevention exist; the most well-known of these are, in the US, the *Blueprints for Health Youth Development*; *National Registry of Evidence-based Programs and Practices*; the *Model Programs Guide*; and *What Works Clearinghouse*, and in the UK, the *Education Endowment Foundation's Promising Projects*. Effective program registries serve as a type of quasi-regulatory mechanism for the quality of interventions (Centers for Disease Control 2017; Dodge 2006). Inclusion in these registries typically requires more than one gold standard program evaluation, undertaken via experimental methods, assessing immediate and long-term program outcomes and harmful effects. No education and training initiatives have, so far, met the standards required for inclusion in any of these databases.

The most reliable and comprehensive way to decide education and training effectiveness is to take a bird's-eye view of the field by synthesising and appraising all available evidence using systematic review approaches. The only systematic review of education and training for child protection was published over a decade ago (Carter et al. 2006). That review critically appraised the published evidence of training and procedural interventions for health professionals for improving child protection. Of the 22 studies meeting the review's inclusion criteria, most were of poor quality, only one included long-term follow up, and none were conducted with a randomised controlled trial methodology (Carter et al. 2006). Outcomes measured in the studies included self-reported improvements in knowledge, confidence, general awareness, and training satisfaction. The studies had not assessed the relationship between education and training and actual child protection outcomes. On the upside, some interventions made use of adult learning theories, were interactive, and included e-learning components. The reviewers observed that an "unquantifiable amount of effort and resource" (Carter et al. 2006, p. 742) may have been wasted in poor program evaluation research.

More recent evaluations of single training programs have shown promising results. In the US, a rigorous single-blind test-retest randomised controlled trial of the *iLookout for Child Abuse – Online Learning Module for Early Childcare Providers* conducted in one state, showed large and significant increases in knowledge of reporting duties, and medium and significant enhancement in attitudes towards reporting in the 762 participants. Gains were sustained after follow up at 4 months (Mathews et al. 2017). Also in the US, a three-state independent multi-site randomised controlled trial of the 2.5-h *Stewards of Children* training in child sexual abuse prevention with childcare professionals ($n = 352$) showed that participants retained child sexual abuse knowledge immediately after program participation and at 3-month follow up, and endorsed more frequent preventive actions. The study found in-person and web-based delivery were equally effective (Rheingold et al. 2015). A further study assessed the training's effect on actual reporting practices by comparing child sexual abuse reporting rates between counties participating and not participating in *Stewards of Children* training over an 11-year period. The study found significant increases in allegation rates over time, and between-group differences in reporting trends for participating and non-participating counties (Letourneau et al. 2016).

In the Netherlands, a randomised controlled trial of the *Next Page* e-learning training to improve recognition of child maltreatment with nurses in emergency departments ($n = 38$) revealed that those who completed training had higher levels of self-efficacy and performed better on an in vivo case-simulation test (Smeekens et al. 2011). In Vietnam, a comparison of knowledge, attitudes and practices before and after introduction of the *Safe Children* 2-day interactive workshop (along with presentations, a DVD, and take-home workbook), showed that training increased knowledge, attitudes and child maltreatment reporting intentions of emergency staff ($n = 116$; Flemington and Fraser 2017). In Ireland, a retrospective survey and interviews with a sample of professionals whose work involved regular and direct contact with children who had attended either the *Children First Basic Level Training* or the *Keeping Safe* training ($n = 195$), found general agreement that the training achieved its aims and was relevant, and identified the need for more advanced and refresher trainings (Devaney and McGregor 2016).

No single education or training program can deliver all the capabilities and expertise required for child protection, nor make participants instant experts (Besharov 1990). However, we need to know more about the science underpinning education and training for child protection, the features of interventions and participating learners, and we need more rigorous evaluations to determine specific program's effectiveness.

22.4.1 *The "What" and "How" of Education and Training*

Professional education and training should be based on *evidence* (Puddy and Wilkins 2011) and be underpinned by a *theory of change* (Funnell and Rogers 2011). *Evidence* is conceptualised by Puddy and Wilkins (2011) as comprising three overlapping spheres: the best available empirical evidence; experiential evidence (e.g., professional knowledge, insights and expertise); and contextual evidence (e.g., setting-level factors). *Theory of change* is explained by Funnell and Rogers (2011) as an explicit description of how an intervention, in this case a curriculum intervention, produces its desired effects. It can be thought of in this way:

- The *evidence* is the "what" of education and training comprising the curriculum, content, and concepts that should be taught; and
- The *theory of change* is the "how" of education and training comprising the process or methods, that is, the teaching and learning methods, and delivery modes that should be employed.

22.4.1.1 The 'What'

Identifying contents that are hallmarks of effective education and training programs can only be determined in a rigorous, comprehensive and transparent systematic review. However, the only systematic review undertaken in this field, mentioned above (Carter et al. 2006), did not extract education and training intervention contents or methods. The question of what content should be learned in education and training for child protection was taken up some time ago by the Executive Committee of the Section on Child Maltreatment of the American Psychological Association's Division 37. Over a period of several years, the committee developed a curriculum guide on the topic of child maltreatment cutting across undergraduate and postgraduate university-level programs incorporating introductory to advanced resources on seven topics: (i) definitions of child maltreatment; (ii) incidence an prevalence; (iii) causes of child maltreatment; (iv) consequences associated with child maltreatment; (v) treatment issues; (vi) prevention; and (vii) legal issues (American Psychological Association 2006; Miller-Perrin and Malloy 2006). To some extent, this constellation of topics resembles the curriculum content suggested earlier in Fig. 22.1.

A non-systematic review of the literature reveals that curriculum content could be considered to comprise some universal elements (what was referred to earlier as "child protection literacy") such as: definitions of maltreatment subtypes; prevalence; criminality; consequences; who experiences child maltreatment, of what types and at what ages; who inflicts it; warning signs and indicators; dealing with disclosure and children's veracity; children's typical responses after victimization and the hallmarks of trauma-informed practice; legal and ethical duties to report child maltreatment, and guidelines or procedures for reporting (Besharov 1990; Crosson-Tower 2010; Mathews 2017; Miller-Perrin and Malloy 2006; Taylor 1997; Taylor and Hodgkinson 2001).

Drawing attention to the need for effective education and training for child protection in paediatrics, Bannon and Carter (2003) wrote that "child protection should be viewed as ... of equivalent importance to Advanced Life Support" (p. 561). Reflecting the unsustainable increases in reports to child protection authorities and lamenting the absence of universal education and training guidelines, Canadian researchers, Wolfe and McIsaac (2010) argued that education and training "should ensure that all community professionals can reliably distinguish acts requiring child protection investigations from those requiring family or parent-support services" (p. 20).

22.4.1.2 The "How"

From a public health perspective, the 'process' of professional education and training can be viewed as a "means to effect performance change and to improve practice outcomes, thereby achieving translation of knowledge into practice" (Davis et al. 2013, p. 165). Theory of change is central to understanding how education and training should be and can be delivered. In a protocol for a Cochrane systematic review, yet to be completed, Mathews et al. (2015) proposed a theory of change for training interventions for mandatory reporters thus:

> as an application of adult learning ... child protection training for professionals is an educational intervention through which professionals develop knowledge, skills, attitudes, and behaviours. By raising awareness, providing information and resources, developing skills and strategies, and fostering dispositions, training may change professionals' ability and willingness to engage in decision-making processes that lead to improved reporting (p. 3).

The way in which education and training should be delivered necessarily involves consideration of adult learning, which contributes to the science underpinning the process of education and training for child protection. There are several theories that describe how adults learn (Knowles 1980; Knowles et al. 2014; Merriam 2001, 2008) and there is general consensus on several key adult learning principles: (i) adults need to know why they are learning; (ii) adults are motivated to learn by their need to problem solve; (iii) adults prior experiences should be respected and used; (iv) adults require learning approaches appropriate to their backgrounds and diversity; and (v) adults need to be actively involved in learning processes (Bryan et al. 2009).

Adult learning principles can inform the design and development of education and training initiatives for child protection. Additionally, adult learning principles can be integrated with theories of behavior change, particularly those used in health research. For example, the *Intervention Mapping Approach* (Bartholomew et al. 2011) incorporates six steps, beginning with a needs analysis aligning with the third adult education principle above and sets the context in which adult learners' prior knowledge can be integrated with new knowledge. Further steps include: creating a theory of change (known as 'matrices of change' in this particular approach; selecting behavior-change theories to be used; designing the scope and sequence of program components; planning for program adoption, implementation and sustainability; and developing an evaluation plan (Bartholomew et al. 2011).

Adult learning principles can also be assimilated with the PRECEDE-PROCEDE planning framework (Green and Kreuter 1990, 2005), which provides a structure for designing program scope and sequence so that methods can be deployed at the time when adult learners most need these. Based on the concept that predisposing, reinforcing and enabling factors act as determinants of adults' education and training outcomes, the framework can be used to identify strategies for each. For example, predisposing strategies are those that can be a catalyst for change (such as didactic lectures, conferences, and print materials). Enabling strategies are those that facilitate change (these tend to be more interactive such as small group activities, communities of practice, and structured decision-making tools). Reinforcing strategies are those that help to embed changes already made (such as reminders, refreshers, self-assessment, and practice audits) (Davis et al. 2013; Hutchinson and Estabrooks 2013). The literature suggests that ubiquitous large-group information delivery sessions (e.g., with a speaker and presentation slides), when used alone, have limited effectiveness. Yet this education and training mode can be made more effective by conducting needs assessments prior to delivery, increasing opportunities for interactivity, and planning modules with varied, interactive, multi-modal learning experiences (Forsetlund et al. 2009).

22.5 Promoting Widespread Adoption of Empirically Supported Education and Training Strategies

What is known about the strategies that should be adopted and implemented, widely, in education and training for child protection? Congruent with a public health approach, when education and training initiatives have been proven effective, these can be implemented more widely. Once initiatives are in place, organizations can evaluate their delivery in different contexts, with different groups, as a way of monitoring their relevance and validity, and engaging in continuous program improvement. In further evaluations, it is critical to attend to the implementation process, that is, the way in which the program is delivered in the 'real world'.

The field of education and training for child protection should now be able to faithfully replicate education and training programs that have been found effective via rigorous experimental studies. However, it is worth noting what may lie ahead in terms of implementation challenges. The field of implementation science has identified several factors that are necessary to ensure education and training programs are delivered as intended. These include: (i) adherence to education and training models as specified by the developer; (ii) exposure or dosage; (iii) delivery quality; (iv) participant engagement and responsiveness; and (v) cognisance of program elements that can and cannot be subject to variation (Carroll et al. 2007). It has been shown that implementation matters: it affects program outcomes, profoundly, and is influenced by five categories of variables: (i) community level characteristics (e.g., policy, funding); (ii) program provider characteristics (e.g., self-efficacy, skills); (iii) characteristics of the program (e.g., relevance to local needs, adaptability); (iv) characteristics of the program delivery system (e.g., organizational capacity); and (v) characteristics relating to the program support system (e.g., ongoing technical support) (Durlak and Dupre 2008). In the 'real world' of implementation, these five categories interact to create conditions that can enhance or impede full scale implementation of education and training programs. Hence, implementation must be sustained via policy and appropriate resource allocation. Ideally, effective education and training for child protection should sit alongside supervision and workplace cultures that value and promote children's safety and wellbeing.

In some countries, such as the United Kingdom (UK), statutory inquiries into child abuse incidents and government policies have advocated that if professionals in the child protection workforce are to work together effectively, they should be trained together (Carpenter et al. 2010; Charles and Horwath 2009). This introduces the notion of interagency or multidisciplinary training involving collective participation in professional education and training of more than one agency or discipline. While comprehensive review of this education and training approach is beyond the scope of this chapter, readers may be familiar with some common examples including: the *International Training Program of ISPCAN* (ISPCAN 2008) which began in the 1990s with a focus on training child abuse and neglect professionals in developing countries; the *Keeping Children Safe: A Toolkit for Child Protection* (Keeping Children Safe Coalition 2014) used by agencies in many countries; and in the UK, the NSPCC Safeguarding Training (NSPCC 2017). Education and training specifically on child sexual abuse; *Stewards of Children®*, a US program developed by the advocacy group Darkness to Light, offered nationwide, that teaches adults how to prevent, recognise, and respond to child sexual abuse. The latter initiative has been evaluated using a randomised controlled trial (as noted in Sect. 2.4) (Letourneau et al. 2016; Rheingold et al. 2012, 2015). Finally, *Teach VIP-2* (World Health Organization 2015) has been available since 2005 and has a broader remit to teach adults worldwide about injury prevention (of which child maltreatment is part), preventive policies and programs design, surveillance system and data collection functions, and intervention program evaluation.

Although multi-agency or inter-professional education and training is a common training approach, a report reviewing education and training for interagency working in safeguarding in the UK concluded that both single-agency and multi-agency trainings were required (Long et al. 2006). In a very useful review of training approaches for the mental health workforce, US researchers concluded that interprofessional learning is a promising practice, but research findings are mixed, with rigorous studies emerging only recently (Lyon et al. 2011). Again, the most rigorous way of identifying exemplar programs would be via a systematic review. A systematic review could also extract the contents and methods used in effective interagency or multidisciplinary programs.

22.6 Conclusions and Thoughts and a Research and Practice Agenda

Developing a suite of high-quality education and training initiatives is essential to addressing the problem of child maltreatment within a public health approach. However, despite the mounting number of policy initiatives promoting child protection and safeguarding, education and training have not kept pace. At the center of the problem is a lack of coherent aligned professional development systems. Writing about the challenge of closing systematic gaps in professional development for the early childhood workforce, US researchers propose that at the heart of it, closing such gaps requires addressing fundamental issues in the field about professional purpose and identities (Winton et al. 2015; Goffin and Washington 2007). For example, the child protection field is comprised of multiple disciplines, with their own agencies and organizations, accreditation and credentialing systems, professional and practice standards, histories, cultures, professional development terminologies, delivery traditions, and funding arrangements. Their views of their responsibilities may differ and education and training may be contested in an industry that is jurisdictionally fragmented (Mathews 2017) with varying legal and policy commitments to prevention. Consequently, what is even considered as education and training may diverge. It seems overly predicable that one of the conclusions of this commentary shall be to suggest that more research is required, however, that is a precondition. As a starting point, researchers should begin with systematic reviews of education and training for child protection generally, and for multi-agency training specifically.

Informed by such research, at a high level, greater coordination of education and training is required, and universal guidance could be developed. Describing future directions and recommendations in a report into child protection training in Western Australia, Penter et al. (2005) concluded there would be merit in having an education and training infrastructure characterised by: (i) a coherent overarching strategic framework for provision of education and training for child protection; (ii) dedicated child protection education and training units; (iii) training programs with evidence-based curriculum and resources; (iv) multi-agency and inter-professional education and training models, (v) education and training quality control, minimum standards, and accreditation. These recommendations are re-offered here as possible future steps for enhancing education and training for child protection. Finally, somewhere in the world, could we aspire to establishing a centre for research excellence in education and training for child protection? The journey of small steps requires us now in the era of the Sustainable Development Goals to commit to thinking big and taking larger and bolder steps towards harnessing the enormous potential of education and training for child protection.

References

Albers, B., & Mildon, R. (2016). *Implementation best practice: A rapid evidence assessment*. Sydney: Commonwealth of Australia. Retrieved from http://www.childabuseroyalcommission.gov.au/policy-and-research/our-research/published-research/implementation-best-practice.

American Psychological Association. (2006). Announcement: New curriculum guide on child maltreatment now available. *Child Maltreatment, 12*(1), 106.

Bannon, M. J., & Carter, Y. H. (2003). Paediatricians and child protection: The need for effective education and training. *Archives of Disease in Childhood, 88*(7), 560–562.

Bartholomew, L. K., Parcel, G. S., Kok, G., Gottlieb, N. H., & Fernández, M. E. (2011). *Planning health promotion programs: An intervention mapping approach* (3rd ed.). San Francisco: Jossey-Bass.

Besharov, D. J. (1990). *Recognizing child abuse: A guide for the concerned*. New York: The Free Press.

British Association of Social Workers. (2017). *Continuous professional development*. Retrieved from https://www.basw.co.uk/cpd/

Bryan, R. L., Kreuter, M. W., & Brownson, R. C. (2009). Integrating adult learning principles into training for public health practice. *Health Promotion Practice, 10*(4), 557–563.

Buysse, V., Winton, P. J., & Rous, B. (2009). Reaching consensus on a definition of professional development for the early childhood field. *Topics in Early Childhood Special Education, 28*(4), 235–243.

Carpenter, J., Hackett, S., Patsios, D., & Szilassy, E. (2010). *Outcomes of Interagency Training to Safeguard Children: Final Report to the Department for Children, Schools and Families and the Department of Health*. Retrieved from http://dera.ioe.ac.uk/809/1/DCSF-RR209.pdf

Carroll, C., Patterson, M., Wood, S., Booth, A., Rick, J., & Balain, S. (2007). A conceptual framework for implementation fidelity. *Implementation Science, 2*(1), 40. https://doi.org/10.1186/1748-5908-2-40.

Carter, Y. H., Bannon, M. J., Limbert, C., Docherty, A., & Barlow, J. (2006). Improving child protection: A systematic review of training and procedural interventions. *Archives of Disease in Childhood, 91*(9), 740–743.

Centers for Disease Control and Prevention [CDC]. (2016). *Professional development practices inventory*. Retrieved from https://www.cdc.gov/healthyschools/trainingtools.htm

Centers for Disease Control and Prevention [CDC]. (2017). *Registries of programs effective in reducing youth risk behaviors*. Retrieved from https://www.cdc.gov/healthyyouth/adolescenthealth/registries.htm

Charles, M., & Horwath, J. (2009). Investing in interagency training to safeguard children: An act of faith or an act of reason? *Children & Society, 23*(5), 364–376.

Crosson-Tower, C. (2010). *Understanding child abuse and neglect* (8th ed.). Boston: Allyn & Bacon.

Cummins, P. D., Scott, D., & Scales, B. (2012). *Report of the protecting Victoria's vulnerable children inquiry*. Melbourne: Department of Premier and Cabinet. Retrieved from http://www.childprotectioninquiry.vic.gov.au/report-pvvc-inquiry.html.

Davis, N., Davis, D., & Bloch, R. (2008). Continuing medical education: AMEE education guide no. 35. *Medical Teacher, 30*(7), 652–666.

Davis, D., Davis, N., & Johnson, N. (2013). Formal education interventions. In S. E. Straus, J. Tetroe, & I. Graham (Eds.), *Knowledge translation in health care: Moving from evidence to practice* (pp. 163–175). Chichester: Wiley.

Devaney, C., & McGregor, C. (2016). A review of children first and keeping safe training in Ireland: Implications for the future. *Child Care in Practice, 22*(2), 166–182.

Dodge, K. A. (2006). Professionalizing the practice of public policy in the prevention of violence. *Journal of Abnormal Child Psychology, 34*(4), 475–479.

Durlak, J. A., & DuPre, E. P. (2008). Implementation matters: A review of research on the influence of implementation on program outcomes and the factors affecting implementation. *American Journal of Community Psychology, 41*(3–4), 327–350.
Feerick, M. M., Knutson, J. F., Trickett, P. K., & Flanzer, S. M. (2006). *Child abuse and neglect. Definitions, classifications, and a framework for research.* Baltimore: Paul H. Brookes Publishing Company.
Fixsen, D. L., Blase, K. A., Naoom, S. F., & Wallace, F. (2009). Core implementation components. *Research on Social Work Practice, 19*(5), 531–540.
Fixsen, D., Blase, K., Metz, A., & Van Dyke, M. (2013). Statewide implementation of evidence-based programs. *Exceptional Children, 79*(2), 213–230.
Flemington, T., & Fraser, J. (2017). Building workforce capacity to detect and respond to child abuse and neglect cases: A training intervention for staff working in emergency settings in Vietnam. *International Emergency Nursing, 34*, 29–35. https://doi.org/10.1016/j.ienj.2017.03.004.
Forsetlund, L., Bjørndal, A., Rashidian, A., Jamtvedt, G., O'Brien, M. A., Wolf, F. M., Davis, D., Odgaard-Jensen, J., & Oxman, A. D. (2009). Continuing education meetings and workshops: Effects on professional practice and health care outcomes. *Cochrane Database of Systematic Reviews, 2*. Art. No.: CD003030. https://doi.org/10.1002/14651858.CD003030.pub2
Funnell, S., & Rogers, P. (2011). *Purposeful program theory effective use of theories of change and logic models* (1st ed.). San Francisco, CA: Jossey-Bass.
Goffin, S. G., & Washington, V. (2007). *Ready or not: Leadership choices in early care and education.* New York: Teachers College Press.
Gomez, R. E., Kagan, S. L., & Fox, E. A. (2015). Professional development of the early childhood education teaching workforce in the United States: An overview. *Professional Development in Education, 41*(2), 169–186.
Green, L. W., & Kreuter, M. W. (1990). Health promotion as a public health strategy for the 1990s. *Annual Review of Public Health, 11*(1), 319–334.
Green, L. W., & Kreuter, M. W. (2005). *Health promotion planning: An educational and ecological approach* (4th ed.). New York: McGraw-Hill.
Hammond, W. R. (2003). Public health and child maltreatment prevention: The role of the centers for disease control and prevention. *Child Maltreatment, 8*(2), 81–83.
Hoffmann, T. C., Glasziou, P. P., Boutron, I., Milne, R., Perera, R., Moher, D., & Lamb, S. E. (2014). Better reporting of interventions: Template for intervention description and replication (TIDieR) checklist and guide. *British Medical Journal (BMJ), 348*, g1687.
Hutchinson, A. M., & Estabrooks, C. A. (2013). Educational theories. In S. Straus, J. Tetroe, & I. D. Graham (Eds.), *Knowledge translation in health care: Moving from evidence to practice* (pp. 298–307). Chichester: John Wiley & Sons.
ISPCAN. (2008). Special report: International training program of ISPCAN (ITPI): For training of CAN professionals in developing countries. *ISPCAN, 2008*(1), 1–12.
Keeping Children Safe Coalition. (2014). *Keeping children safe: A toolkit for child protection.* Retrieved from https://resourcecentre.savethechildren.net/library/keeping-children-safe-toolkit-child-protection
Klika, J. B., Lee, S., & Lee, J. Y. (2018). Prevention of child maltreatment. In J. B. Klika & J. R. Conte (Eds.), *The APSAC handbook on child maltreatment* (4th ed., pp. 235–251). Thousand Oaks: Sage.
Knowles, M. S. (1980). *The modern practice of adult education: From pedagogy to andragogy* (2nd ed.). New York: Cambridge Books.
Knowles, M. S., Holton, E. F., III, & Swanson, R. A. (2014). *The adult learner: The definitive classic in adult education and human resource development.* London: Routledge.
Krug, E. G., Dahlberg, L. L., Mercy, J. A., Zwi, A. B., & Lozano, R. (2002). *World report on violence and health.* Geneva: World Health Organization. Retrieved from http://apps.who.int/iris/bitstream/10665/42495/1/9241545615_eng.pdf.
Letourneau, E. J., Nietert, P. J., & Rheingold, A. A. (2016). Initial assessment of stewards of children program effects on child sexual abuse reporting rates in selected South Carolina counties. *Child Maltreatment, 21*(1), 74–79.

Long, T., Davis, C., Johnson, M., Murphy, M., Race, D., & Shardlow, S. M. (2006). Standards for education and training for interagency working in child protection in the UK: Implications for nurses, midwives and health visitors. *Nurse Education Today, 26*(1), 11–22.

Lyon, A. R., Stirman, S. W., Kerns, S. E., & Bruns, E. J. (2011). Developing the mental health workforce: Review and application of training approaches from multiple disciplines. *Administration and Policy in Mental Health and Mental Health Services Research, 38*(4), 238–253.

Mathews, B. (2017). Optimising implementation of reforms to better prevent and respond to child sexual abuse in institutions: Insights from public health, regulatory theory, and Australia's Royal Commission. *Child Abuse & Neglect, 74*, 86–98. https://doi.org/10.1016/j.chiabu.2017.07.007.

Mathews, B., Walsh, K., Coe, S., Kenny, M. C., & Vagenas D. (2015). Child protection training for professionals to improve reporting of child abuse and neglect (Protocol). *Cochrane Database of Systematic Reviews, 6*. Art. No.: CD011775. https://doi.org/10.1002/14651858.CD011775

Mathews, B., Yang, C., Lehman, E. B., Mincemoyer, C., Verdiglione, N., & Levi, B. H. (2017). Educating early childhood care and education providers to improve knowledge and attitudes about reporting child maltreatment: A randomized controlled trial. *PLoS One, 12*(5), e0177777.

Meddings, D. R., Knox, L. M., Maddaleno, M., Concha-Eastman, A., & Hoffman, J. S. (2005). World Health Organization's TEACH-VIP: Contributing to capacity building for youth violence prevention. *American Journal of Preventive Medicine, 29*(5), 259–265.

Merriam, S. B. (2001). Andragogy and self-directed learning: Pillars of adult learning theory. *New Directions for Adult & Continuing Education, 89*(1), 3–14.

Merriam, S. B. (2008). Adult learning theory for the twenty-first century. *New Directions for Adult and Continuing Education, 2008*(119), 93–98.

Miller-Perrin, C. L., & Malloy, L. C. (2006). *Curriculum guide for instruction in child maltreatment*. Retrieved from http://www.apadivisions.org/division-37/sections/2017_Curriculum_Guide.pdf

Munro, E. (2011). *The Munro review of child protection final report: A child-centred system*. Retrieved from https://www.gov.uk/government/publications/munro-review-of-child-protection-final-report-a-child-centred-system

National Professional Development Center on Inclusion [NPDCI]. (2011). *The big picture planning guide: Building cross-sector professional development systems in early childhood* (3rd ed.). Chapel Hill: The University of North Carolina/FPG Child Development Institute/Author. Retrieved from http://community.fpg.unc.edu/npdci.

NSPCC. (2017). *CPD workshops and courses*. Retrieved from https://cpduk.co.uk/directory/profile/nspcc

Palusci, V. J., & Covington, T. M. (2014). Child maltreatment deaths in the US National child death review case reporting system. *Child Abuse & Neglect, 38*(1), 25–36. https://doi.org/10.1016/j.chiabu.2013.08.014.

Parenting Research Centre. (2015). *Implementation of recommendations arising from previous inquiries of relevance to the Royal Commission into Institutional Responses to Child Sexual Abuse: Final report*. Sydney: Commonwealth of Australia. Retrieved from http://www.childabuseroyalcommission.gov.au/policy-and-research/our-research/ensuring-a-positive-impact.

Penter, C., Cant, R., Clare, B., & Peaty, A. (2005). *Child protection training: Project report for the ministerial advisory council on child protection*. Perth: Government of Western Australia.

Puddy, R. W., & Wilkins, N. (2011). *Understanding evidence part 1: Best available research evidence. A guide to the continuum of evidence of effectiveness*. Atlanta: Centers for Disease Control and Prevention/National Center for Injury Prevention and Control, Division of Violence Prevention.

Rheingold, A. A., Zajac, K., & Patton, M. (2012). Feasibility and acceptability of a child sexual abuse prevention program for childcare professionals: Comparison of a web-based and in-person training. *Journal of Child Sexual Abuse, 21*(4), 422–436.

Rheingold, A. A., Zajac, K., Chapman, J. E., Patton, M., de Arellano, M., Saunders, B., & Kilpatrick, D. (2015). Child sexual abuse prevention training for childcare professionals: An independent multi-site randomized controlled trial of stewards of children. *Prevention Science, 16*(3), 374–385.

Rhodes, H., & Huston, A. (2012). Building the workforce our youngest children deserve. *Society for Research in Child Development Social Policy Research Brief, 26*(1), 1–32.

Royal College of Paediatrics and Child Health. (2014). *Safeguarding children and young people: Roles and competences for health care staff: Intercollegiate document*. London: Royal College of Paediatrics and Child Health. Retrieved from https://www.rcpch.ac.uk/sites/default/files/page/Safeguarding%20Children%20-%20Roles%20and%20Competences%20for%20Healthcare%20Staff%20%2002%200%20%20%20%20(3)_0.pdf

Smeekens, A. E. F. N., Broekhuijsen-van Henten, D. M., Sittig, J. S., Russel, I. M. B., Ten Cate, O. T. J., Turner, N. M., & van de Putte, E. M. (2011). Successful e-learning programme on the detection of child abuse in emergency departments: A randomised controlled trial. *Archives of Disease in Childhood, 96*(4), 330–334.

Taylor, A. S. (1997). From survival to reflection: Locating child protection in teacher education. In J. Davies & P. Garner (Eds.), *At the crossroads: Special education needs and teacher education* (pp. 61–74). London: David Fulton Publishers.

Taylor, A. S., & Hodgkinson, K. (2001). Subjecting the initial teacher training curriculum for England and Wales to the test of child protection. *Teacher Development, 5*(1), 75–86.

United Nations. (2015). *Sustainable development goals*. Retrieved from http://www.un.org/sustainabledevelopment/sustainable-development-goals/

Weber-Mayrer, M. M., Piasta, S. B., & Yeager Pelatti, C. (2015). State-sponsored professional development for early childhood educators: Who participates and associated implications for future offerings. *Journal of Early Childhood Teacher Education, 36*(1), 44–60.

Winton, P. J., Synder, P. A., & Goffin, S. G. (2015). Rethinking professional development for early childhood teachers. In L. J. Couse & S. L. Recchia (Eds.), *Handbook of early childhood teacher education* (pp. 54–68). London: Routledge.

Wolfe, D. A., & McIsaac, C. (2010). *Distinguishing between poor/dysfunctional parenting and child emotional maltreatment*. Ottawa: Public Health Agency of Canada. Retrieved from https://www.canada.ca/content/dam/phac-aspc/migration/phac-aspc/sfv-avf/sources/nfnts/nfnts-dysfnct-parent/assets/pdf/archive-nfnts-dysfnct-parent-eng.pdf

World Health Organization [WHO]. (2015). *Preventing youth violence: An overview of the evidence*. Geneva: World Health Organization.

Zimmerman, F., & Mercy, J. A. (2010). A better start: Child maltreatment prevention as a public health priority. *Zero to Three, 30*(5), 4–10.

Chapter 23
A Good Fit? Ireland's Programme for Prevention, Partnership and Family Support as a Public Health Approach to Child Protection

John Canavan, Carmel Devaney, Caroline McGregor, and Aileen Shaw

23.1 Introduction

The global quest continues for fit-for-purpose child protection systems that keep children safe in an effective and efficient manner: systems that neither over-include children and families, subjecting them to unnecessary and intrusive assessments without providing substantive help, nor under-include them, running the risk of failing to identify abuse entirely, or providing supportive responses when protective ones are required. This system needs to be at one and the same time inclusive of children, young people and parents' voices and responsive to need and risk for certain children and families. The focus of this collection is the promise of public health approaches to child protection system development and delivery, and this chapter is a case study of what such an approach could look like in practice. Specifically, it is built on the experience of a programme of action developed in the Republic of Ireland that brings together a constellation of strategies based on Prevention, Partnership and Family Support (PPFS). While not a specific Public Health model, the PPFS programme aligns very well with a public health approach. The chapter begins by considering the main theoretical strands informing the programme of action that is represented in the case study before setting the programme in its social and policy context. The programme and attendant research and evaluation study are then outlined. The case study is then reimagined as a public health programme, using Scott et al.'s (2016) framework as a guide. Following this, an account is given of the learning thus far from the research study and the implications for a public health approach to child protection and welfare.

J. Canavan · C. Devaney · C. McGregor (✉) · A. Shaw
UNESCO Child and Family Research Centre, National University of Ireland (NUI), Galway, Ireland
e-mail: john.canavan@nuigalway.ie; carmel.devaney@nuigalway.ie; caroline.magregor@nuigalway.ie; aileen.shaw@nuigalway.ie

B. Lonne et al. (eds.), *Re-Visioning Public Health Approaches for Protecting Children*, Child Maltreatment 9, https://doi.org/10.1007/978-3-030-05858-6_23

23.2 Prevention, Early Intervention, Partnership and Family Support

This case study focuses on the experience of the development, implementation and evaluation of a programme of action focused on prevention, early intervention, partnership and family support within the child protection and welfare services in the Republic of Ireland. As in many other jurisdictions the Irish system entails a forensic approach that investigates and manages risk in a proceduralized way. This is coupled with a formal family support system positioned alongside a range of community based and voluntary support services. The programme of action is an attempt to embed prevention, early intervention, partnership and family support within this system in an overall effort to improve outcomes for children and young people.

This orientation fits well within a public health approach as it is adopting a multidisciplinary, in-part population wide, multi-level, evidence-based systematic method to addressing the social problem of children, young people and their families who are in need of additional support and interventions to prevent harm and abuse. In Ireland as elsewhere there is growing evidence of child maltreatment and neglect in society. Such knowledge along with an understanding of the long-term societal costs associated with unresolved difficulties in childhood has led to the development of a wide range of diverse interventions aiming to improve child welfare (Mason et al. 2016).

The concept of prevention is not a new one, and has its origins in the public health field. Allen (2011) reminded us of the old adage: "prevention is better than cure" (p. 3). Barlow and Schrader McMillan (2010) emphasised a focus in universal service provision on preventing difficulties arising in the first instance. Moreover, the role of prevention is not only viewed as a way to combat risk factors but also to enhance and promote the positives and opportunities for child development by maximising protective factors and processes (Allen 2011; Frost and Parton 2009). This promotion model is considered proactive because it assumes that all people have existing strengths and capacity to achieve and be competent (Dunst 2000).

There is an increasing recognition of the need to intervene early in the life of children and also early in the stage of a difficulty so as to improve outcomes in later life (Devaney and Dolan 2014; Harvey 2014). In the Irish context specifically, *Growing up in Ireland*, a national, longitudinal study of children, found that between a fifth and a quarter of children experience poor economic, social and educational outcomes that need to be responded to promptly (Dishion et al. 2008; Harvey 2014; Olds 2006). It is generally accepted that improving children's outcomes requires the integration of prevention and early intervention into children and young people's services. Dunst (2000) defined early intervention as:

> the provision of support and resources to families of young children from members of informal and formal social support networks, that both directly and indirectly influence child, parent and family functioning. (p. 99)

This definition highlights the need for a holistic approach including the child as the centre but also looking at their families, communities and environments as potential providers of support and provision of their needs; as well as drivers for the prevention of these needs in the first place. In the past, the response to children who were having difficulties involved direct work with the particular child (adopting an individualized and deficit-orientated approach) whereas current models take a broader view of the social environment in which the child is living and focus on different aspects of this (adopting a strengths-based ecological approach). This includes their relationship with their parents with an acceptance that this relationship is a key factor in fostering positive social, emotional and psychological development in children and young people (Devaney 2017; Sneddon and Owens 2012). As Bronfenbrenner (1979) highlighted, the developing child, his/her parents, and the wider family unit are influenced by events in settings beyond the family which directly and indirectly affect behaviour and functioning.

Prevention and early intervention has shown capacity to improve secure attachments, social and emotional development, protective relationships, language development, child health and welfare. Research also indicates that parenting (and poor parenting in particular) is a public health issue (Arkan et al. 2013; Mason et al. 2016) and that inadequate parenting practices have significant negative long-term impact on children's behaviour (Griffith 2008). It is also suggested that the provision of accessible parenting and family supports requires the collaboration of a range of services and a large pool of multi-disciplinary practitioners (Shapiro et al. 2015).

At a broader level, prevention and early intervention can be understood from the perspective of social investment. Understanding welfare from an 'investment' perspective emphasizes human potential, reducing the level of dependency on the state and instead investing in children, young people and their families as active contributors to society (Gray 2014). Understanding prevention and early intervention as a social investment requires the implementation of proactive, empowered and partnership relationships between service providers and children, young people and families that have access to or are referred into these services. Current tendencies in child protection and welfare and family support also advocate for inter-agency and multi-agency responses that can effectively enhance service effectiveness. Churchill and Fawcett (2016) described the case of Australia where local governments are now investing in more universal and family targeted services towards preventing child maltreatment and also promoting child welfare. From a universal perspective, one can argue that the more prevention that can occur the better and the ideal model within which to intervene at the universal level is via a public health model.

23.3 The Irish Context

To set the case study in context, the Republic of Ireland is geographically a small state of just over 70,000 square kilometres, with a population of 4,761,865, of which 1,251,796 are children. At the time of writing, there were 6258 children in the care of the state, with approximately 90% of these in either relative or general foster care arrangements. The average monthly rate of referral to child protection and welfare services was just under 4000 (61% of which are classified as child welfare concerns) with 'no further action' recorded in just over 50% of these referrals. The modern Irish Child Protection and Welfare system emerged as part of the overall health system in the 1970s, located within seven regional health boards, and subsequently as part of the Health Services Executive (HSE) national service delivery system. In 2014, a dedicated agency, known as Tusla, the Child and Family Agency was created and the main Child Protection and Welfare functions and associated staff migrated into the new agency. A number of other functions were also added, including Educational Welfare services, and a network of community-based cross generational Family Support services. The new child and family agency, for the first time, placed child welfare and protection on its own organisationally with a dedicated budget and independent governance structure. It also places a stronger emphasis on the rights of children and on their participation in decision making.

Although a rigorous account of the rationale for and pathway to the new agency remains to be researched and written, most would agree that Tusla was created following on a series of systems failures and consequent public inquiries and associated Reports on their findings and recommendations for change (e.g., Commission to Inquire into Child Abuse 2009; HSE 2010). One view was the Child Protection and Welfare priorities were not being met within a large Health Service Executive that carried a range of statutory functions, mostly health related. Although not articulated in any official accounts, it could be argued that the risk of losing interdisciplinary and inter-professional connections (e.g., with Public Health Nursing) was seen as less significant than the continuing risk of child protection being a low priority within a larger medically dominated state agency, already struggling to deliver services within budget. It was certainly the case that while child welfare and protection was housed within a broad Health and Social Services Framework, this did not translate to the service being framed within an ethos of health promotion or public health model as it is understood here. Conversely, child welfare services have been, until recently, piecemeal, reactionary, under-resourced, and individual deficit-orientated. Nonetheless, the separation of the Public Health nursing system (HSE) from the child welfare system (Tusla) from an organisational perspective does run the risk of limiting the potential for a stronger public health approach into the future.

Two other contexts are significant in locating this case study. First, is the status of children in Ireland. Historically, the social policy approach to children reflected the principle of family autonomy in which children's needs were perceived as a matter of private responsibility with the state adopting a minimalist approach to intervention (see Chap. 9). What Murphy (1996) referred to as the familialist nature of Irish State policy – upheld by the 1937 Constitution by a predominance of the rights of the family over the rights of children – meant that children were to a degree invisible. However, from the enactment of the 1991 Child Care Act onwards (Government of Ireland 1991), a shift in orientation has occurred that has led to a progressive set of children-focused policy developments. These changes took place within a wider context of rapid social, cultural and demographic change in Ireland, yet received specific prompting by a number of Child Protection failures and the commentary on these issues from the UN Committee on the Rights of the Child. Among the related developments were the appointment of a Junior Minister for Children (1996) and the creation of Ireland's first National Children's Strategy in 2000 (Government of Ireland 2000). This strategy sought for the first time to present Irish child welfare policy within an explicit children's rights framework. It was followed in 2011 by the setting up of a full department of State, the Department of Children and Youth Affairs (DCYA) and the second national children's strategy, Better Outcomes, Brighter Futures, 2014–2020 (Department of Children and Youth Affairs 2014). Legislatively, one key development has been the passing of the 31st Constitutional Referendum in 2012 (known as the Children's Rights Referendum) which has resulted in children and their rights receiving specific reference outside of those of their parents and the inclusion constitutionally of the duty to pay due regard to the voice of the child and to act in their best interests in matters of care, education and protection.

The second context is the wider development of state services for children. While there have been various innovations and attempts to improve the service delivery system for children led from within child protection and welfare, education, juvenile justice, family support, youth work and community development sectors, the period 2006 through to 2014 is notable for the significant programme of investment in children. The Programme for Early Intervention and Prevention, created as a joint initiative between the state and the philanthropic sector, in particular, the Atlantic Philanthropies Ireland, sought to drive the development of evidence-based, rigorously designed and evaluated services for children. It resulted in investment in a number of geographically-based sites in disadvantaged communities as well as funding to extant service providing organisations to undertake service design and to commission robust evaluations. Overall, the focus of the investment was in services operated by the community and voluntary sector rather than in mainstream services. Within the children and youth sector in Ireland, the culmination of this period of investment resulted in a degree of expertise in, commitment to, and capacity for developing and implementing evidenced-formed services and practices for children and families.

The programme of action explored in this case study emerged in the context of an ongoing relationship between the university in which the authors are based (the National University of Ireland (NUI), Galway) and Tusla. In the context of a formally agreed research and evaluation support partnership, a suite of work developed focused on strengthening the Family Support dimensions of the Tusla's work. Under the HSE, Family Services included the range of services traditionally understood in terms of Child Protection and Welfare including an Alternative Care provision. Prevention and Family Support services, while in place, had developed in an ad hoc manner and lacked any clear organisational mandate. Thus, Family Support services was a generic label covering a variety of services, projects and actions, some operated directly by the HSE and some contracted to the community and voluntary sector. In 2012, the university, through the UNESCO Child and Family Research Centre (UCFRC) received a grant to develop a set of guidance materials for the newly planned agency Tusla. The outputs included guidance documentation on establishing an early intervention process and interagency structure, guidance on family support as a practice orientation, children's participation, supporting parents and evidence-based commissioning.

23.4 The Case Study: The Development and Mainstreaming Programme for Prevention, Partnership and Family Support

In 2014, the philanthropic investment by The Atlantic Philanthropies in what became known as the Development and Mainstreaming Programme for Prevention, Partnership and Family Support (PPFS) represented one of the final grants made by the organisation prior to closing its Irish office in 2016. The investment of €10,185,202 in PPFS over three and a half years (2015–2018) comprised over €8 M to Tusla to support the nationwide implementation of the programme to embed early intervention and prevention within the agency and over €2 M to the UCFRC at NUI, Galway to support its research and evaluation. The specific context of the investment outlined above – the wider programme of investment in children's services, the creation of the new agency, and the pre-investment-increased the potential for significant change to take place.

At an overarching level, the emphasis on mainstreaming and the targeting of investment to statutory provision, can to some degree, be seen as an acknowledgement that to be effective, change must be embedded in the state systems and structures. In practice, this approach, characterised as 'strategic' philanthropy, adopts a public policy orientation and seeks engagement with the state (Anheier 2005). Sandfort (2008) and others argued that private investment in human services can only be effective when foundations craft their actions in relation to government and that a concerted and conscious positioning within the broad-based environment in which government dominates is essential. The genesis of the PPFS, developed in partnership with the Department of Children and Youth Affairs (DCYA), and targeted at core reform in statutory services, typifies this approach.

The PPFS programme resulted from a negotiated process between The Atlantic Philanthropies, the DCYA, Tusla and NUI, Galway that sought to address a series of problems relating to the unmet needs of children in Ireland and weaknesses in the service infrastructure that serves them. Tusla developed a detailed corporate plan to enable full implementation of the programme over six main work packages: Public Awareness; Parenting support; Participation; Meitheal (a national practice model aimed at ensuring that the needs and strengths of children and their families are effectively identified, understood and responded to in timely way) and Child and Family Support Networks; and Commissioning and Information (see Fig. 23.1).

The approach and its attendant research and evaluation plan at the UCFRC is designed to produce a key set of outcomes by 2018, namely that:

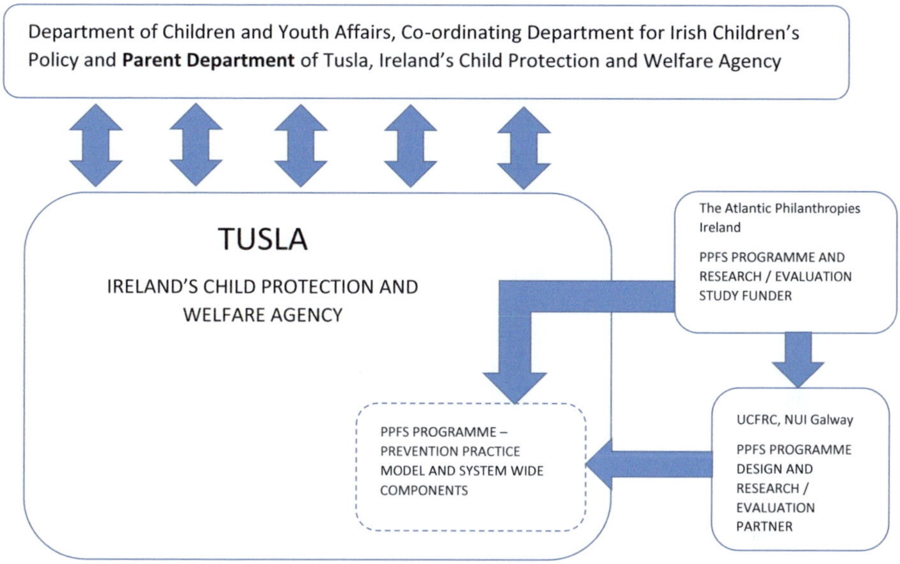

Fig. 23.1 The PPFS programme in context

1. Tusla's prevention and early intervention system is operating effectively, delivering a high quality, standardised and consistent service to children and families in each of the country's 17 management areas;
2. Tusla service commissioning is increasingly rigorous and evidence-informed and privileges prevention and early intervention;
3. A strategic approach to parenting is increasingly delivering cost-effective better practice and better outcomes for parents and children, thus reducing inequalities;
4. Children and families are increasingly aware of available supports and are less likely to fall through gaps, as all relevant services are working together in Tusla's prevention and early intervention system; and
5. The participation of children and parents is embedded in Tusla's culture and operations.

At the outset, the core structures, processes and roles associated with the programme were already Tusla policy. The PPFS programme provided the extra impetus to support the delivery of the system change envisaged, buttressing Tusla's capacity in key areas and increasing the prospects for full implementation and critically, sustainability. At the end of the programme, it is intended that these structures and processes will all be functioning effectively as a result of intensive workforce development, with ongoing capacity retained within Tusla's Workforce Development function. Staff working on the programme will have been recruited from within Tusla and commissioned agencies and will return to the system (within Tusla or commissioned agencies), bringing their knowledge, skills and experiences. Also anticipated is that the wider staff body of child serving agencies will have been trained, have participated in the Meitheal model, and will have the capacity to engage effectively with the commissioning process.

23.4.1 Research Plan and Objectives

The research and evaluation study is focused on the implementation and outcomes of Tusla's PPFS programme. It is founded on a partnership model between Tusla and the UCFRC to develop appropriate information and monitoring systems, so that data can be used to steer the implementation process. It involves a full assessment of the programme's implementation and outcomes, both at sub-programme level in each of the activity areas (Work Package) developed to operationalize the component streams and at an overall programme level. The overarching evaluation question can be expressed as:

> Is the organisational culture and practice of Tusla and its partners changing such that services are more integrated, preventative, evidence informed and inclusive of children and parents and, if so, is this contributing to improved outcomes for children and their families?

In terms of design, the study can be described as mixed, multiple methods involving a series of sub-studies on various programme elements. Most of these involve cross-sectional, point-in-time designs, but there are also longitudinal designs with studies focusing on outcomes from the application of the Meitheal process, capacity building with Tusla staff and on public awareness. The full range of methods includes individual interviews (face-to-face and telephone), focus-group interviews, surveys (including some standardised measures), observation and documentary analysis. While a range of theoretical perspectives infuse the different aspects of the research and evaluation study, a Systems Theory orientation underpins our approach to understanding the nature of change wrought by the programme. Ethical approval for the study comes from both the University and from Tusla with separate ethical approval sought and received for each sub-study. The study began in 2015 and ended in mid-2018.

23.5 Reframing the PPFS as a Public Health Model

Scott et al. (2016) concluded their consideration of public health models of prevention of child maltreatment by referring to the fact that "child protection is everyone's business" (p. 415). The same guidance is reflected in the opening sections of the Irish child protection guidelines for professionals and lay persons called Children First 2011. This mantra evidenced the philosophy that underpinned the Task Force on the Family support Agency (2012) which set out the blueprint for the establishment of Tusla.

The overall intention of Tusla, as an independent Child and Family Agency, is to move child welfare in Ireland from the predominance of an investigatory and reactionary system to a more holistic and proactive one that places the prevention of harm and promotion of parenting and family support as part of the overall package of child protection and welfare services for families and children. The principles of the PPFS approach in many ways reflect that of a public health model even though it is not explicitly stated as such. For example, both are based on partnership, the use of science and evaluation with an emphasis on multi-disciplinarity. In Ireland, the Institute of Public Health Ireland – an all-Ireland body – sets out an agenda that is very complementary to the PPFS agenda. They state that their aims are to: strengthen public health intelligence (in PPFS terms, to increase public awareness and intelligence), build public health capacity (in PPFS terms, to build system capacity to work in a preventative manner), and to develop a programme of policy development and evaluation (in PPFS terms through academic-agency partnership in implementation and review of a new PPFS programme for Ireland).

Specific similarities between public health and the PPFS model to note in particular include:

1. A Public Health model, be it related to health or social issues – is framed within the context of universal, secondary and tertiary services. In a similar way, the Prevention, Partnership and Family support model also differentiates interventions between universal (Level 1), targeted (Level 2 and 3) and focused on risk management and abuse prevention (Level 4) (see Hardiker et al.1991);
2. A public health model has prevention of disease, infection or related negative health outcomes as central to its mantra. Likewise, and as stated by Tusla, the PPFS approach is underpinned by an assumption that the 'best way to improve outcomes for children is to intervene at an early stage to resolve problems and prevent harm' (www.tusla.ie); and
3. A public heath model uses a range of strategies that map onto a PPFS approach. Using the work of Scott et al. (2016, p. 409), six core features are particularly notable and summarised in Table 23.1.

While the similarities between Public Health and PFFS strategies are clearly evident, there are also some challenges in developing PPFS as a public health strategy. The main considerations are as follows:

1. It must be acknowledged that while public health models are applied to both health and social related issues, it is the former that is most well established. Indeed, as the significant history of public health from a medical perspective written in the 1950s and updated recently shows (Rosen 2015), the medical profession have in many ways been engaged in broad public health practices for centuries (e.g., tackling major contagious diseases) whereas a public health approach to child welfare and child maltreatment is arguably a more recent phenomena;
2. The public health model is based on the triangulation of the idea of the HOST, AGENT and ENVIRONMENT when developing a strategy (Scott et al. 2016).

Table 23.1 Alignment of public health features and PPFS strateiges

Public health features	PPFS strategies
Population based	Tusla is designed to deliver population based services from universal parenting support (e.g., parenting 24/7) to targeted interventions (e.g., Meitheal)
Multi-disciplinary	Multi-disciplinarity is central to PPFS practice approach (e.g., Meitheal guidance)
Evidence based	The PPFS approach is based on evidence and research from national and international perspectives; commissioning as emphasising evidence – On outcomes from services, on making funding decisions on an evidence-informed basis
Subject to cyclical processes of review, intervention and evaluation	The PPFS model has been introduced to be delivered and evaluated in tandem to ensure cyclical review and evaluation
Relies on the identification of specific risk and prevention factors	A family support practice approach is likewise underpinned by this strategy
Puts in place population-level strategies to reducing risk and increase protective factors	A unique feature of the PPFS programme is a commitment to public awareness and education to ensure population-based level strategies can be developed to improve outcomes for children and families. Making child and family support networks and Meitheal as virtually universal easy and early access to help

While this can be translated to social issues such as child welfare and family support, the 'agent' - i.e. the cause of the problem on the host – is more nebulous and difficult to define. Often the cause of a family problem or child welfare concern is a mix of intrinsic and extrinsic factors that may need more differentiation beyond the notion of 'agent';

3. The use of the ecological model, a layered approach to looking at the environment, has potential beneficial contribution to make to the theorisation of the environment within the public health sphere; and
4. There is more reluctance in society to put matters considered more private to family life into public sphere in same way as individual and family health or maternal health has been.

23.6 Progress and Learning for Public Health Approaches to Child Protection

It is arguably through the public awareness strand of the PPFS programme that a strong public health dimension will develop through PPFS. We know that public health strategies and public awareness strategies are to some extent similar. Public awareness campaigns, for example, are a way for governments to impact public attitudes, values and behaviours towards the achievement of specific outcomes. Public awareness campaigns also have the potential to influence goals such as agenda setting and raising awareness in the wider society. As in the case of public health activity, public awareness have been targeted at a variety of issues including suicide prevention (Hoven et al. 2009; Pirruccello 2010); child maltreatment prevention (MacMillan et al. 2009), mental health promotion (Patel et al. 2008; Jorn 2012), enhanced well-being (Buila 2009), domestic violence prevention (Cismaru and Lavack 2011), sexual abuse prevention (Wurtele 2009), and to reduce stigma (Kakuma et al. 2010) and promote positive parenting (Prinz et al. 2009). Studies have also identified young people as a vulnerable sector in need of information about evidence-based services available (Hickey et al. 2007). Campaigns have been specifically targeted at young people's mental health literacy (Kubacki et al. 2015; Morgan and Jorm 2009), help seeking behaviours (Collin et al. 2011) and suicide prevention (Wasseman et al. 2012; Jenner et al. 2010). Reports of these interventions generally agree that public awareness campaigns can improve knowledge and awareness in the population (Dumensil and Verger 2009), reduce the occurrence of incidents such as child abuse (Jones and Finkelhor 2003) and can also increase the rates of referral and diagnosis (Maughan et al. 2005). The public can benefit from knowing which actions they can take for prevention, early intervention and treatment of issues and disorders (Jorn 2012).

The evidence informing the development of public awareness activity can be enhanced further through a framing within a public health model as described above. The emphasis on population based approaches is particularly pertinent. From the findings of the baseline survey of the Irish population (n = 1,000), some very interesting findings have emerged to inform current thinking in relation to how child welfare, family support and child maltreatment can be addressed through population based approaches.

Briefly, the population survey of public awareness of family support, prevention and early intervention services has found a low level of awareness overall of parenting, prevention and family support services. In most instances, families and their informal networks provide the majority of necessary support to families and children who need help and support. When families were not able to cope through their own informal support network, the next most likely point of call was found to be the local community nurse (Public Health Nurse PHN) or the General Medical Practitioner (GP). Only a very small number showed awareness of more specialist parenting, prevention and Family Support Services. The findings show the significance of the public health services - GP and PHN - as a source of general family support beyond traditional health needs (McGregor and NicGabhainn 2016). They point to the importance of greater awareness raising within the health professions about services for children and families in order that they can advise and direct families and children in need to the correct universal, secondary or tertiary service required. They also point to the importance of greater public education about family support, prevention and partnership for the general public.

The findings also offer some interesting themes to discuss with regard to the potential for PPFS to progress a strong public health agenda.

1. It is clear from considering PPFS within a broad public health context that any population -based public awareness campaign should be informed by the broad principles that underpin this long-established strategy derived primarily from the health sciences;
2. Public Health models and discourses could be developed through integration of some of the core concepts underpinning the PPFS approach especially the focus on partnership, multi-layered ecological and environmental analysis, and delivery of services across a spectrum of need from universal to targeted;
3. In order for a PPFS agenda to have a stronger public health approach, there is a need for stronger engagement between the traditional 'social services' (e.g., child and family services) and 'health services' (e.g., the GP, PHN and primary care community health sector). In other words, health professions seem to be crucial population-based personnel who are ideally placed to take on population based messaging in relation to parenting and family support. The public rely more on the generic services, and more promotion of family support, partnership and prevention services for child welfare through the Health sector may help raise awareness and thus help-seeking in the general population; and
4. Both PPFS and Public Health strategies generally need to continue to work on strategies that can engage effectively with the population diversity especially with regard to marginalized populations and those most likely to need services.

The interim findings of the experience of participating in the Meitheal model suggest it too can also be framed within the public health model. This model, based on the principles of being needs led and strengths based, is offered to families where there is a potential risk of maltreatment and also to families who have required a child protection response in the past (because of maltreatment) but where the level of risk has reduced and a supportive response is now required. As reflected in primary prevention universal services families can self-refer to Meitheal and the model can be used to respond to a range of needs. In line with public health models the model also recognizes that there is a continuum of need which is not static and that families may require secondary or even tertiary level services for a period of time to support or address specific issues (Higgins 2015). Participants in the Meitheal research have highlighted the potential for the model to support earlier intervention for families in need. This is in part due to a changed perception in families as to what Tusla as an agency can offer and also an increased awareness of the benefit of accessing support at an earlier stage than they may have done in the past (Rodriguez et al. 2017). The multidisciplinary nature of the supports available to families is also a key component of the findings on the Meitheal model which aligns well with public health approaches addressing social problems including child maltreatment which use strategies that are population based and multidisciplinary (Scott et al. 2016). Going forward a key consideration for Tusla and its partner organisations will be the mainstreaming of the Meitheal model as an integrated primary level preventative measure and as a secondary level 'step-down' support for families. The associated Child and Family Networks which are currently at various stages of implementation nationwide are also a promising preventative framework that can potentially help respond to the needs of families at an earlier stage in a co-ordinated manner.

The parenting support work package is another package of the approach with potential to be framed with a public health context. Parenting support is situated as a primary prevention model and can most certainly be described as similar to public health approaches in that it is equitable, cost effective, accessible and non-stigmatizing (Scott et al. 2016). A range of universally available initiatives are in place including: parenting 24/7, web-based information and advice on general parenting and for parenting in specific contexts or with particular challenges; designated parenting support champions at a local level who are trained and supported to be the 'go to' people within their own area to offer advice and guidance on parenting; and a number of parental participation initiatives aimed at both parents and relevant practitioners to encourage and supports parents involvement in all areas of their children's lives. Preliminary findings suggest that these projects are becoming increasingly visible within communities with a rising awareness of their purpose and function amongst the general population (Crosse and Devaney 2017).

Alongside this, the participation and commissioning packages are likewise underpinned by the overall aim of delivering better outcomes for children and families through partnership working with children and families, community groups, voluntary, private and statutory bodies. Collectively, they are underpinned by an ethos of devolved authority, consultation and partnership. In addition the commissioning package has the potential to inform the development of evidence- and outcomes-based approaches. Outcome-based approaches are broadly welcomed for focusing attention on the results of an intervention rather than on associated activities and outputs (Bovaird and Davies 2011). As the projects progress, the potential of the models to inform other public health/social strategies using well-developed practices and processes or partnership working becomes increasingly evident.

23.7 Discussion and Conclusions

One of the core differences between child welfare as a public health issue compared to more mainstream health related public health issues such as immunisation, disease control, smoking campaigns is the extent to which the public view it as a public rather than a private matter. While more open about family life and less tolerant of families who harm or neglect their children in Irish society and services, the public still have a different attitude to matters relating to family life and child care than they do to general health issues like contagious disease control and road safety for example. Moreover, most families are not at risk of harming their children or needing family support. In fact, only a very small number of children proportionately come to the attention of the child and family agency. This differs from public health issues where a wide sector of the population could be at risk where an infection is contagious (for example, childhood measles or chicken pox). And yet, a public health rather than an individual deficit approach to child welfare could literally transform how we view, interpret and intervene where a child is deemed to be at risk of harm or where a family is clearly in need of external help and support. It can also open up greater potential to engage with the views and perspectives of young people and their families. Greater public population wide responsibility for child welfare – i.e., the achievement of evidence that child protection and welfare is indeed considered and believed to be 'everybody's business' – has the potential to remove the stigma often associated with admitting and receiving help as a parent /carer and improve overall outcomes for children and families in Ireland. The PPFS programme is in essence an attempt to do just this; the programme aims to prevent risks to children and young people arising or escalating through sustainable interagency multidisciplinary early intervention work.

However, the findings from the Public Awareness work to date indicates the need for greater public education for families requiring support and better understanding about the possible supports available for children and families. More opportunities to hear from the public in general and service users (children and adults) in particular is crucial. In addition, greater partnership in training and practice between health and social service practitioners is necessary to help build on and develop the clear potential of the PPFS programme. The work of the Parenting Support Package will contribute to these developments into the future. Findings from the Meitheal model highlight very strongly that the challenges from a public health perspective lie in the need to address broader underlying inequalities which contribute to escalating need among children and families. The evidence is clear that many of the constraints on parents and their children lie in their environmental and social contexts. Issues in relation to health, housing, poverty and mental health services in particular are noted as significantly exacerbating the difficulties experienced by families. Arguably the PPFS programme, framed as a public health approach to child protection and welfare needs to consider how it can begin to address the inadequacies and inequalities within the wider environment in which families live in order to realise this potential. This issue was echoed in the most recent UN committee on the Rights of the Child report for Ireland noted that a major agenda for Ireland (and elsewhere) was to ensure that all public services - not just those specifically charged with child welfare and protection – need to ensure they are operating from a children's rights ethos and approach. In moving forward, investment across the system in the universal (e.g., housing, education, social welfare), secondary (e.g., mental health services, substance abuse/addiction support, services for those experiencing family violence) and tertiary services (e.g., child welfare and protection system, parent and family support investment, child and adolescent mental health services) is essential to enable the PPFS model to achieve a public health approach. If this were to be achieved, major obstacles to positive outcomes for children and families such as homelessness, poverty, parental mental ill-health, and inadequate disability support could be addressed from a broad public health approach which must, by instinct, also embrace an overt children's rights ethos.

References

Allen, G. (2011). *Early intervention: The next steps. An Independent report to her majesty's government*. London: Cabinet Office and Department for Work and Pensions. https://www.gov.uk/government/publications/early-intervention-the-next-steps%2D%2D2

Anheier, H. (2005). *Nonprofit organizations: Theory, management, policy*. London and New York: Routledge.

Arkan, B., Üston, B., & Guvenir, B. (2013). An analysis of two evidence-based parent training programmes and determination of the characteristics for a new programme model. *Journal of Psychiatric and Mental Health Nursing, 20*(2), 176–185. https://doi.org/10.1111/j.1365-2850.2012.01876.x.

Barlow, J., & Schrader McMillan, A. (2010). *Safeguarding children from emotional maltreatment: What works*. London: Jessica Kingsley.

Bovaird, T., & Davies, R. (2011). Outcome-based service commissioning and delivery: Does it make a difference? In S. Groeneveld & S. Van De Walle (Eds.), *New steering concepts in public management*. Vol. 21: Research in public policy analysis and management (pp. 93–114). Bingley: Emerald Group Publishing. Retrieved from https://www.emeraldinsight.com/doi/full/10.1108/S0732-1317%282011%290000021011

Bronfenbrenner, U. (1979). *The ecology of human development: Experiments by nature and design*. Cambridge: Harvard University Press.

Buila, S. (2009). Using the media to enhance well-being and mental health. *Rural Society, 19*, 363–367.

Churchill, H., & Fawcett, B. (2016). Refocusing on early intervention and family support: A review of child welfare reforms in New South Wales, Australia. *Social Policy and Society, 15*(2), 303–316. https://doi.org/10.1017/S1474746416000038.

Cismaru, M., & Lavack, A. M. (2011). Campaigns targeting perpetrators of intimate partner violence. *Trauma Violence and Abuse, 12*(4), 183–197.

Collin, P. J., Metcalf, A. T., Stephens-Reicher, J. C., Blanchard, M. E., Herrman, H. E., Rahilly, K., & Burns, J. M. (2011). ReachOut.com: The role of an online service for promoting help-seeking in young people. *Advances in Mental Health, 10*(1), 39–51. https://doi.org/10.5172/jamh.2011.10.1.39.

Commission to Inquire into Child Abuse. (2009). *Report of the Commission to inquire into child abuse*. Dublin: Commission to Inquire into Child Abuse. Retrieved from http://www.childabusecommission.ie/rpt/pdfs/

Crosse, R., & Devaney, C. (2017). *Parenting support and parental participation, parenting support champions questionnaire report*. Galway: UNESCO Child and Family Research Centre, NUI Galway.

Department of Children and Youth Affairs. (2014). *Better outcomes, brighter futures: The national policy framework for children and young people 2014–2020*. Retrieved from https://www.dcya.gov.ie/viewdoc.asp?fn=/documents/cypp_framework/BetterOutcomesBetterFutureReport.pdf

Devaney, C. (2017). Promoting children's welfare through family support. In P. Dolan & N. Frost (Eds.). *A global reader in child welfare* (pp. 99–109). London: Routledge. https://www.routledge.com/The-Routledge-Handbook-of-Global-Child-Welfare/Dolan-Frost/p/book/9781138942752

Devaney, C., & Dolan, P. (2014). Voice and meaning: The wisdom of family support veterans. *Child and Family Social Work, 22*(S3), 10–20. https://doi.org/10.1111/cfs.12200.

Dishion, T., Connell, A., Weaver, C., et al. (2008). The family check-up with high-risk indigent families: Preventing problem behaviour by increasing parents' positive behaviour support in early childhood. *Child Development, 79*, 1395–1414. https://doi.org/10.1111/j.1467-8624.2008.01195.x.

Dumensil, H., & Verger, P. (2009). Public awareness campaigns about depression and suicide: A review. *Psychiatric Services, 60*, 1203–1213.

Dunst, C. J. (2000). Revisiting "rethinking early intervention". *Topics in Early Childhood Special Education, 20*(2), 95–104. https://doi.org/10.1177/027112140002000205.
Frost, N., & Parton, N. (2009). *Understanding children's social care politics, policy and fractice*. London: Sage.
Government of Ireland. (1991). *The child care Act, 1991*. Dublin: Stationery Office.
Government of Ireland. (2000). *National children's strategy*. Dublin: Stationery Office.
Gray, M. (2014). The swing to early intervention and prevention and its implications for social work. *British Journal of Social Work, 44*(7), 1750–1769. https://doi.org/10.1093/bjsw/bct037.
Griffith, A. K. (2008). *An evaluation of boys town's common sense parenting behavioural parent training program*. University of Nebraska, Lincoln: ProQuest Dissertations Publishing.
Hardiker, P., Exton, K., & Barker, M. (1991). *Policies and practices in preventive child care*. Aldershot: Avebury.
Harvey, B. (2014). *The case for prevention and early intervention: Promoting positive outcomes for children, families and communities*. Dublin: Prevention and Early Intervention Network.
Hickey, I. B., Luscombe, G. M., Davenport, T. A., Burns, J. M., & Highet, N. T. (2007). Perspectives of young people on depression: Awareness, experiences, attitudes and treatment preferences. *Early Intervention in Psychiatry, 1*(33), 333–339. https://doi.org/10.1111/j.1751-7893.2007.00042.x.
Higgins, D. J. (2015). A public health approach to enhancing safe and supportive family environments for children. *Family Matters, No.96*. Australian Institute of Family Studies.
Hoven, C. W., Wasserman, D., Wasserman, C., & Mandell, D. J. (2009). Awareness in nine countries: A public health approach to suicide prevention. *Leg Med (Tokyo), 11*, 13–17. https://doi.org/10.1016/j.legalmed.2009.01.106.
HSE. (2010). *Report of the task force for children and families social services*. Dublin: HSE.
Jenner, E., Woodward, L., Metthews-Sterling, M., Butts, J. K., & Evans Williams, T. (2010). Awareness effects of a youth suicide prevention media campaign in Louisiana. *Suicide and Life-Threatening Behaviour, 40*, 394–406. https://doi.org/10.1521/suli.2010.40.4.394.
Jones, L. M., & Finkelhor, D. (2003). Putting together evidence on declining trends in sexual abuse: A complex puzzle. *Child Abuse & Neglect, 27*, 133–135.
Jorm, A. F. (2012). Mental health literacy: Empowering the community to take action for better mental health. *American Psychologist, 67*, 231–243.
Kakuma, R., Kleintjes, S., Lund, C., et al. (2010). Mental health stigma: What is being done to raise awareness and reduce stigma in South Africa? *African Journal of Psychiatry, 13*, 116–124.
Kubacki, K., Rundle-Thiele, S., Pang, B., & Buyucek, N. (2015). Minimizing alcohol harm: A systematic social marketing review (2000-2014). *Journal of Business Research, 68*, 2214–2222.
MacMillan, H., Wathen, N., Barlow, J., Fergusson, D. M., Leventhal, J. M., & Taussig, H. M. (2009). Interventions to prevent child maltreatment and associated impairment. *Lancet, 373*(9659), 250–266. https://doi.org/10.1016/S0140-6736(08)61708-0.
Mason, A., January, S. A., Fleming, C. B., Thompson, R. W., Parra, G. R., Haggerty, K. P., & Snyder, J. J. (2016). Parent training to reduce problem behaviours over the transition to high school: Tests of the indirect effects through improved emotion regulation skills. *Children and Youth Services Review, 16*, 176–183.
Maughan, B., Iervolino, A., & Collinshaw, S. (2005). Time trends in child and adolescent mental disorders. *Current Opinion in Psychiatry, 18*, 381–385.
McGregor, C., & NicGabhainn, S. (2016). *The development and mainstreaming programme for prevention, partnership and family support.* Work Package 2, Public Awareness, Baseline Population Report 2016. Galway: UNESCO Child and Family Research Centre, The National University of Ireland Galway.
Morgan, A. J., & Jorm, A. F. (2009). Recall of news stories about mental illness by Australian youth: Associations with help-seeing attitudes and stigma. *Australian and New Zealand Journal of Psychiatry, 43*, 866–872.
Murphy, M. (1996). From prevention to "family support" and beyond: Promoting the welfare of Irish children. *Administration, 44*(2), 73–101.

Olds, D. L. (2006). The nurse–family partnership: An evidence-based preventive intervention. *Infant Mental Health Journal, 27*, 5–25.
Patel, V., Flisher, A. J., Nikapota, A., & Malhotra, S. (2008). Promoting child and adolescent mental health in low and middle income countries. *Journal of Child Psychology and Psychiatry, 49*, 313–334. https://doi.org/10.1111/j.1469-7610.2007.01824.x.
Pirruccello, L. (2010). Preventing adolescent suicide. *Journal of Psychosocial Learning, 48*, 34–41.
Prinz, R. J., Saunders, M. R., Shapiro, C. J., Whitaker, D. J., & Lutzker, J. R. (2009). Population-based prevention of child maltreatment: The US triple P system population trial. *Prevention Science, 10*, 1–12.
Rodriguez, L., Cassidy, A., & Devaney, C. (2017). *Interim report on the Meitheal process and outcomes study, Galway*. Galway: UNESCO Child and Family Research Centre, National University of Ireland, Galway.
Rosen, G. (2015). *A history of public health*. Baltimore: John Hopkins University Press.
Sandfort, J. (2008). Using lessons from public affairs to inform strategic philanthropy. *Nonprofit and Voluntary Sector Quarterly, 37*(3), 537–552.
Scott, D., Lonne, B., & Higgins, D. (2016). Public health models for preventing child maltreatment: Applications from the field of injury prevention. *Trauma, Violence, & Abuse, 17*(4), 408–419.
Shapiro, C. J., Prinz, R. J., & Sanders, M. R. (2015). Sustaining use of an evidence-based parenting intervention: Practitioner perspectives. *Journal of Child and Family Studies, 24*, 1615–1624. https://doi.org/10.1007/s10826-014-9965-9.
Sneddon, H., & Owens, S. (2012). *Prevention and early intervention in young people's services – Parenting*. Dublin: The Centre for Effective Services.
The Task Force on the Child and Family Support Agency. (2012). *Final report to the Minister For Health*. Dublin: Stationery Office.
Wasserman, C., Hoven, C. W., Wasserman, D., et al. (2012). Suicide prevention for youth – a mental health awareness program: Lessons learned from the Saving and Empowering Young Lives In Europe (SEYLE) intervention study. *BMC Public Health, 12*, 776. https://doi.org/10.1186/1471-2458-12-776.
Wurtele, S. K. (2009). Preventing sexual abuse of children in the twenty-first century: Preparing for challenges and opportunities. *Journal of Child Sexual Abuse, 18*, 1–18.

Chapter 24
Collaborative Service Delivery: Catalyst to Innovation in Policy and Practice in Alberta, Canada

Rhonda Barraclough, Kim Spicer, Joni Brodziak, Kassidy Green, and Bruce MacLaurin

24.1 Introduction

Since the 1990s, Canadian child welfare jurisdictions have endeavoured to address the needs of children and families at risk in a manner that keeps pace with the changing Canadian population and context. Over this period, there was a significant increase in the number of children referred for investigation and the number of children in care (MacLaurin et al. 2003; Trocmé et al. 2010), as well as a dramatic increase in the costs of child welfare intervention in most Canadian provincial and territorial jurisdictions (McKenzie 2011). Waldfogel (1998) highlighted key system capacity concerns, specifically the question of which children and families were

R. Barraclough (✉)
ALIGN Association of Community Services, Edmonton, AB, Canada
e-mail: rhondaB@alignab.ca; rbarraclough@aascf.com

K. Spicer
Child and Youth Services Division, Ministry of Human Services, Calgary, AB, Canada
e-mail: kimberly.spicer@gov.ab.ca

J. Brodziak
Policy, Practice and Program Development, Ministry of Children's Services, Calgary, AB, Canada
e-mail: joni.brodziak@gov.ab.ca

K. Green
MacEwan University, Edmonton, AB, Canada

Intern with the Policy, Practice and Program Development for Child Intervention, Ministry of Children's Services, Edmonton, AB, Canada
e-mail: kassidy.green@gov.ab.ca

B. MacLaurin
Faculty of Social Work, University of Calgary, Calgary, AB, Canada
e-mail: bmaclaur@ucalgary.ca

B. Lonne et al. (eds.), *Re-Visioning Public Health Approaches for Protecting Children*, Child Maltreatment 9, https://doi.org/10.1007/978-3-030-05858-6_24

truly in need of child welfare investigation and which interventions were best designed to serve their needs. This critique challenged the continued use of a single practice orientation requiring all families and children referred to undergo a fairly authoritarian investigation process (Waldfogel 1998). These issues resonate with the experiences of a number of Canadian child welfare jurisdictions which have led to new policy and practice initiatives designed to ensure safety, and support the well-being of Canadian children and families at risk in the twenty-first Century (MacLaurin et al. 2014; Prilleltensky et al. 2001; Provincial and Territorial Directors of Child Welfare & Rogers 2003; Trocmé et al. 2014).

Since 2000, Alberta, a Western Canadian province, has been an active leader in addressing these legislative, policy and practice challenges. Collaborative Service Delivery (CSD) is one recent, and well-documented example of practice change developed in Alberta, and this initiative will be the primary focus of this chapter (Brodziak 2010; Gardiner and Hachkowski 2011; Gardiner et al. 2014). This chapter will review the historical legislation, policy and practice in Canada and Alberta, emerging and promising child intervention initiatives in Alberta, the larger context of the child intervention practice framework, and the lessons learned from policy and practice changes in Alberta.

24.2 The Context of Child Welfare in Canada

24.2.1 Provincial and Territorial Child Welfare Legislation

The protection of children from maltreatment is a relatively recent phenomenon in Canada. Legislation designed to protect children and youth was first enacted in 1888 and was informed by the 'child saving' and 'child rescue' movements initiated in North America (MacLaurin 2002). Canada has ten provinces and three territories, spanning a large and diverse geographical area, and Canadian child welfare is organized at this jurisdicational level (Bala 2004). While this organizational approach supports the development of legislation and services to meet the unique needs of children and families in each provincial and territorial jurisdiction, it also provides significant challenges to the development of a systematic national response to child maltreatment. For example, provincial/territorial differences are noted in definitions of maltreatment by legislation, funding levels for prevention, access to services, as well as the age limits of the child (Federal Provincial Working Group on Child and Family Services Information 2002; Trocmé et al. 2001).

24.2.2 Swinging Pendulum of Child Welfare Change

Canadian legislation and practice highlights a lack of consensus regarding the role of the state in the lives of children and families in Canada (MacLaurin and Bala 2004). Different value orientations are closely related to the ideologies and social and political climate of the time and suggest alternative approaches to meet the best interests of the child. These shifting orientations have a critical impact on the decisions that are made, as well as outcomes for children (Fernandez 1996; Spratt 2001). Shifts in child welfare legislation, policy and practice have been described as the swing of a pendulum – the shift from a less interventionist to a more interventionist approach highlights the delicate balance between ensuring the safety of the child while supporting parental and family rights (Bala 1999; Dumbrill 2006; Trocmé 1997).

24.2.3 Disentangling the Best Interests of the Child

The principle of best interest of the child is identified as a critical marker in legislation and policy for provincial child welfare legislation in Canada and also in the international context for the United Nations Convention on the Rights of the Child (Alberta Government 2004a, b; British Columbia Government 1996; Ontario Government 1996, 2000; United Nations Committee on the Rights of the Child 1990). This concept has long been criticized however, as lacking specific guidelines to assist decision-makers in the process of determining the best outcome for children at risk. In addition, the concept adopts different meanings during shifts in child welfare policy and services in Canada during the twentieth century. Child welfare perspectives on how best to meet the best interests of the child highlight the debate between the level of intervention (interventionist versus non-interventionist models) (Armitage 1993), the location of intervention (family versus out-of-home placement) (Altstein and McRoy 2000), and the paramount concerns of legislation (child safety versus family integrity) (Bala 1999). Historically the momentum for the pendulum shifts were too frequently driven by inquests or provincial/territorial fatality reviews rather than by foundations of evidence and knowledge (Gove 1995a, b; Hughes 2006; Panel of Experts on Child Protection 1998).

24.2.4 Historical Context of the Over-Representation of Indigenous Children

There is a significant over-representation of Indigenous children reported, investigated and placed in child welfare in Canada (Blackstock et al., 2003; MacLaurin et al. 2010; Sinha et al. 2013; Trocmé et al. 2010). This current overrepresentation is a result of an extended history of colonial policy and legislation intended to assimilate Indigenous peoples into Canadian society (Milloy 1999). This policy began with the residential school initiative that contributed to the systematic removal of Indigenous children from their homes over more than a century, and continued under the provincial and territorial child welfare systems which placed Indigenous children in out-of-home care at much higher rates during the noted child welfare 60's scoop (Blackstock 2011; Milloy 1999). These policies have had an ongoing impact upon the health and well-being of Indigenous peoples (LaBoucane-Benson et al. 2017), and communities and current services are further challenged by the inequitable on-reserve funding for Indigenous children as noted by the Truth and Reconciliation Commission of Canada (Milloy 2009; Truth and Reconciliation Commission of Canada 2015).

24.2.5 An Evolving Evidence Base for Child Welfare Practice

In 1993, Trocmé and colleagues conducted the first provincial incidence study of reported child abuse and neglect in the province of Ontario, Canada, establishing a strong foundation to inform child welfare policy and practice. Building on that success, there have been subsequent national cycles conducted in 1998, 2003 and 2008 led by a diverse academic research team and funded by Public Health Agency of Canada (Trocmé et al. 2010). As well, ongoing provincial incidence studies of reported child abuse and neglect, funded by their specific provinces and territories, were conducted in British Columbia, Alberta, Saskatchewan, Northwest Territories, Ontario, Quebec, and First Nations in Canada. The incidence studies were designed to provide reliable estimates of the scope and characteristics of child abuse and neglect investigations in each jurisdiction. Specific objectives of these studies include: determine rates of physical abuse, sexual abuse, neglect, emotional maltreatment, and exposure to intimate partner violence; investigate the severity of maltreatment regarding duration and harm; examine selected determinants of health associated with maltreatment; monitor short-term investigation outcomes; and compare selected characteristics of maltreatment over the different cycles of the study (Trocmé et al. 2010).

These data have proven to be useful in understanding the complexities of child welfare practice in Canada and supports analyses on characteristics of different types of maltreatment, alleged maltreatment compared to risk of maltreatment, worker characteristics, organizational characteristics, placement characteristics, investigations for Indigenous children, and urgent response versus chronic or ongoing investigation concerns (Black et al. 2008; Blackstock et al. 2003; Fallon and Trocmé 2011; Fallon et al. 2011; MacLaurin et al. 2003; Sinha et al. 2013; Trocmé et al. 2005, 2006).

24.2.6 Shift to an Outcomes Orientation to Services

There is agreement that children and youth in all Canadian provinces and territories deserve timely access to effective resources to promote optimal well-being and development. The question of how well children and families are served by systems of care however has historically been overshadowed by this urgency to help children at risk (Trocmé et al. 2000). Over recent years there has been growing consensus about the value of measuring outcomes for children and youth experiencing child welfare concerns as outcome measurement can clearly demonstrate which interventions are most useful for which populations and for what presenting concerns (Trocmé et al. 2000, 2009).

The National Child Welfare Outcomes Indicator Matrix (NOM) is one framework for tracking outcomes for children, youth and families involved in child welfare in Canada (Trocmé et al. 2000, 2009). The NOM was developed through a series of consultations initiated by the provincial and territorial Directors of Child Welfare and Human Resources Development Canada and provides a framework for tracking outcomes for children and families receiving child welfare services. The elements of NOM reflect the complexity and challenge experienced by child welfare authorities in ensuring a balance between maintaining a child's immediate need for protection, long-term requirement for a nurturing and stable home, a family with potential for growth, and, the community's capacity to meet a child's needs. The NOM includes four nested domains: child safety, child well-being, permanence, and family and community support. A total of ten outcome indicators were chosen based on select criteria determined according to whether or not the data was generally available on information systems, could be clearly defined, and was most useful to stakeholders. This framework has been adopted by the several Canadian provincial governments for reporting on indicators of child welfare success.

24.3 Foundations of Child Intervention in Alberta

24.3.1 The Alberta Response Model

In Alberta, child welfare is called Child Intervention Services and it first began over 15 years ago when Alberta, in line with child welfare service delivery across North America, was faced with increasing numbers of children coming into government care, budget pressures and a lack of relationship with critical partners, stakeholders and clients. Alberta began to redesign Child Intervention services with an enhanced emphasis on the effectiveness of services provided to children, youth and families through a focus on the outcomes of involvement with clients and the benefit of strong partnerships with partners and stakeholders.

The evolution of a strong strategic direction and shift in the way services were provided to children youth and families within the Ministry of Children's Service occurred through a series of critical, progressive organizational changes. The evolution began with an internal policy document 'Kids First: Building Alberta's Capacity to Support Children – A Strategic Framework for Change'. Drafted in 2002 by Alberta Children's Services Ministry, this policy document identified the need to shift to child-centred outcomes and family-centred services. These values were used as a foundation for the development of the Alberta Response Model (ARM) (Anselmo et al. 2003). ARM was built on the tenets of differential response, outcomes focus and community engagement. This model proposed two approaches that would decrease the likelihood that vulnerable children would need further child protection services. These included:

1. Developing an available and comprehensive system of community-based supports; and
2. Encouraging early permanency by promoting a variety of care options to give children safe, nurturing, and permanent homes.

Following the introduction of the Alberta Response Model in 2001, attempts were made to focus on differential response (determining how to approach initial contact with a family), early intervention, community partnerships, permanency planning, family involvement, evaluation and measurement (Anselmo et al. 2003). The principles established in the Alberta Response Model provided a strategic direction for the province's Child Intervention system over the last decade (Alberta Government 2004a, b).

24.3.2 The Child, Youth and Family Enhancement Act (CYFEA)

The key principles of the Alberta Response Model were embedded in legislation with the enactment of the Child, Youth and Family Enhancement Act (The Act or CYFEA) in 2004 (Alberta Government 2004a, b). Section 2 of the Act, 'Matters to Be Considered' outlines principles that call for an evidence-based orientation to practice. The CYFEA affirmed the importance of the family and the role of child intervention in supporting the family, and recognized that children need stable, permanent, nurturing relationships. The Act directs that children should be informed of their rights and that all services should be provided with the least disruption to the child. The legislation also acknowledged the importance of engaging with children and their families and ensuring that their opinions are heard and signaled intent, however staff struggled with how to operationalize several of the elements of CYFEA in their work. With the proclamation of this legislation, there was a critical need to align practice with the key principles and tenants of the Child, Youth and Family Enhancement Act. This led to the development and implementation of a research-based model of practice called the Casework Practice Model (CWPM).

24.3.3 The Casework Practice Model

The Casework Practice Model, a collaborative, decision-based orientation to practice, was developed in 2006 to provide a consistent process for a differential response in practice (Spicer 2016). The model identified assessment, engagement and collaboration as the key pillars of effective casework practice and assisted workers to use evidence-based practice to achieve optimal outcomes for children. This approach embraced a family-centred orientation to practice with child-centred outcomes (Alberta Children's Services 2006). The Alberta Response Model, The Child, Youth and Family Enhancement Act and the Casework Practice Model were all key initiatives contributing to the foundation that led to the development of Outcome-based Service Delivery (OBSD).

24.4 Current Innovations in Alberta

24.4.1 Outcomes-Based Service Delivery

In Alberta, services that a family or a child receives are primarily provided through a contractual agreement with a community-based agency. In this approach, most contracted agencies carve out a service niche, and provide the specific services that are required. In 2007 and 2008, as the Outcomes-Based Service Delivery (OBSD) model was first being conceived, agencies were experiencing great frustration. While contracted agencies wanted to make a true difference in the lives of the families that they served, their efforts were challenged in a number of ways. This included funding models that meant contract agencies did not receive flexible funding thus limiting their ability to shift staffing and services to meet changing needs; and staff attrition, with agencies spending time training and supporting the career development of staff, who subsequently left for higher paid government positions. A solution was established with the development of a governance structure that included a contract agency advisory committee which worked with Ministry executives, and concurrently staff from contracted agencies began to work side by side with staff from the Ministry to lead the way forward.

In 2008, OBSD was formally launched as an initiative to improve the effectiveness and measurability of services children and families receive and experience as they move in and out of the Child Intervention system (Brodziak 2010). Alberta's OBSD Initiative established an active and meaningful partnership between the contracted agency sector, the Child Intervention system and the Ministry of Children's Services. This relationship was based upon the values of collaboration and shared practice; and the measurement of specific as well as common outcomes for success. OBSD moved the focus of serving at-risk children and families away from identifying what specific services were provided and towards identifying what the results of the service should be. The ongoing process resulted in greater service flexibility and broader mandates for contracted agencies in terms of their roles and the services leading to the development of collaborative practice. Essentially, this evolved into shared practice and decision making. Contracted agency staff were always actively involved in effecting change with children and families, however OBSD initiatives placed increasing emphasis on the collaborative process between contracted agency staff and child intervention staff as they partnered to develop plans to reduce safety risks and increase the well-being of the children and families involved with Child Intervention. These grass roots practice shifts began to give energy and created the possibility of re-imagining the work with the organizations involved to improve the quality of the work and to produce better outcomes for families.

In May of 2009, Alberta sponsored a provincial forum, 'Improving Outcomes for Children, Youth and Families', which brought together academic and practice experts from across North America to present leading research on the topic of outcomes-based service delivery. This forum was the start-up of OBSD for the province of Alberta and highlighted current Canadian research in child intervention, trends regarding children, youth, and families involved in Child Intervention, and leading practice and research in providing Child Intervention services. Using the learning generated at the 2008 forum, as well as a thorough and critical review of the work accomplished in other jurisdictions on OBSD, the Ministry of Children's Services adopted a number of principles to guide the initial start-up of OBSD in Alberta. Brodziak (2010) provided a summary of the key underlying principles of OBSD, which include:

- Lead Agency Model: one agency provides a continuum of services to the family;·
- Outcomes Focused: outcomes are clearly articulated and defined;
- New Contracting Model: financial contracting is tied to outcomes, not outputs, and the contracting methods allow greater flexibility for service delivery to achieve outcomes; and
- Evaluation: clearer data-tracking and evaluation systems are established to measure achievement of outcomes.

The first implementation sites were launched in the Edmonton and Calgary regions in 2009. In 2017, all 7 of the Alberta regions have experience in delivering services under the model.

24.4.2 A Shift to Collaborative Service Delivery (CSD)

In 2016 the OBSD initiative was rebranded Collaborative Service Delivery (CSD) to support a focus on the core components of the model (collaborative practice, flexible funding, data) rather than the structural elements that had been anticipated to be key at the initial launch of the initiative. Practice evolved and new relationships between government, agencies, families, children and youth began to emerge. While outcomes were established as the targets for service, flexibility in service delivery was developing and collaborative practice was being established. It is the belief of those involved in policy, practice and service that collaborative practice has made the most significant impact on changing the trajectory of child intervention in Alberta.

From an agency sector perspective, child intervention services were historically provided to families in a menu driven manner. The caseworker would decide the family needed X-Y-Z services and then sought that service from a service provider. The providers had very little input into the development of a plan, or input into the treatment of a child or family. Agency staff did their part of the work well, and other individuals did another part of the care. Unless a child was in a residential situation, the agency staff always performed their activities as requested. Children in residential care, which could include foster or group care, may have had a key worker or someone who was following the lead of the caseworker and, in those circumstances, may have more input into the well-being of the child. With the implementation of OBSD, agencies took the opportunity to become co-responsible for better outcomes and began working with families early on in their journey in the child intervention assessments. They are able to wrap services around the families and children and strive for collective and innovative ways to create healthy, well families.

In its current state, there are three main components to CSD:

- Collaborative Practice: a collective shift in practice toward a collaborative and strengths-based way of working with children and families. Focused conversations about practice have been the area of greatest impact and enthusiasm from the field. The development of a Practice Framework has become an integral next piece for Child Intervention and agency staff in connecting philosophy, legislation and policy to practice;
- Data: a collective focus on client-centred outcomes for vulnerable children and their families between service delivery agencies and the Ministry. CSD sites are demonstrating success in key outcomes areas; and
- Flexible Contracting and Funding: funding flexibility for service delivery agencies to address pressures and allocate resources in a way that is adaptive continues to evolve in CSD.

The intended outcome of CSD is to create and sustain a collaborative approach to service delivery and to facilitate the achievement of five key provincial Child Intervention Outcomes:

- Supporting vulnerable children to live successfully in the community;
- Children in temporary care will be reunited quickly with their family and community;
- Children in permanent care will be placed in permanent homes as quickly as possible;
- Youth will be transitioned to adulthood successfully; and
- Aboriginal children will live in culturally appropriate placements.

24.4.3 The Child Intervention Practice Framework

The flexible natures of OBSD and then CSD led to the Regions having flexibility in their implementation plans, with a specific focus on what outcome the services were provided to achieve. Some regions chose to use this model with children and families who are newly referred to Child Intervention, while other regions chose to implement this approach with children and families when a file was opened to a legal status, or for those who were already in the system. This flexibility in model implementation provided unique opportunities for reflective practice for Child Intervention workers and service providers in a shared practice approach. It also opened the door to innovative thinking across the province and the participating staff began to understand that they needed to work from a common principle base. The practice that began to emerge led the way by beginning to work from intentional and principle based approaches. Figure 24.1 provides a visual representation of the organizational alignment and components of the Child Intervention Practice Framework.

The journey to building organizational principles was grounded in:

- Establishing partnerships with contracted agencies and community;
- Supporting Child Intervention staff to utilize various approaches in working with families;
- Consistent processes;
- Robust assessments; and
- Building empowering relationships with children, youth and families.

Each of these initiatives highlighted the importance of having clear principles to apply this work to support consistency in the day to day decisions and behaviors of Child Intervention staff (Alberta Government 2014). Through this feedback process, it became apparent to government and agency partners that although structural and financial elements supported the work, a principled foundation was needed. The

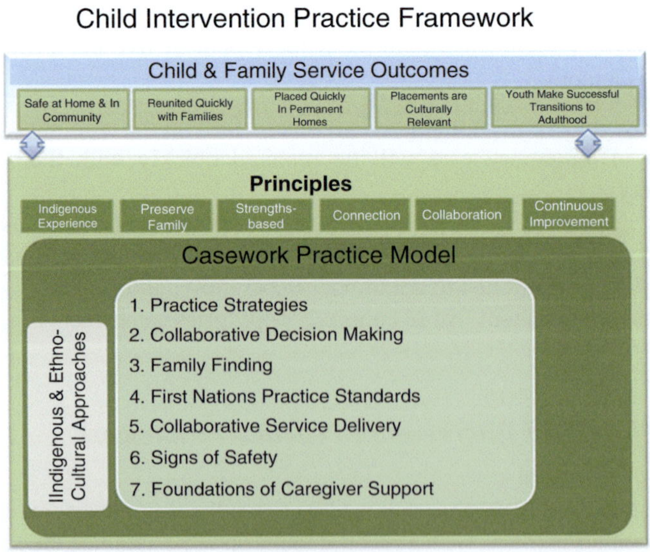

Fig. 24.1 Child Intervention Practice Framework

development of a framework was critical to articulate the core values and principles that support and guide child intervention work with children and families. This was the foundational aspect that was missing from the initial development and implementation of OBSD. The Child Intervention Practice Framework (CIPF) is the culmination of more than a decade of child intervention reform and legislation in Alberta. The Ministry of Children's Services held a Think Tank event in 2012 to launch the development of CIPF – a testament to feedback from frontline staff that leading practice includes elements of principles to support Child Intervention. Leading practice and staff-led initiatives, such as the Harm Reduction Approach to high risk youth, Signs of Safety and supports for family based care, were presented and the common elements of these initiatives were discussed. Participants agreed that a CIPF was required to support the movement towards staff-led, principle-based practice (Spicer 2016).

The development of the CIPF over the past 5 years has been an intentional, robust process led by the Ministry of Children's Services to engage Child Intervention staff in the development of organizational principles. The goal of the CIPF is to support staff and agencies involved with Child Intervention service delivery to address the ongoing challenges of their work by clearly articulating core principles to guide the organization and the actual practice. Specifically, to practice in a balanced way that addresses the critical need for child safety, while at the same time building meaningful relationships and partnerships with families, agencies and communities in order to support the long-term change needed for children to be cared for safely within their own families. Using organizational principles in critical thinking is a key aspect of the implementation of the CIPF. Historically, Child Intervention has tended to become risk adverse in the turbulent social and political climate of this decade. Tragic events such as child fatalities and serious injury of children involved in the Child Intervention system have resulted in numerous inquiries, expert panel reviews and recommendations to the Child Intervention system that tend to be reactive and focus on short term solutions, such as more restrictive policies and procedures. This heightened scrutiny results in an anxious workforce focused on singular child safety that is characterized by significant process and policy, and increased managerialism. As a result, staff struggle to engage in authentic partnerships as they are focused on their perceived sole responsibility for the safety of children and lack the support to share this work with family or agency and community partners (Turnell et al. 2013).

The next step in the development of a meaningful set of working principles was the completion of the meta-analysis of past consultations in government using a thematic research model. Consultations and reports from a broad spectrum were used to provide insight into what Albertans, partners, Child Intervention staff, clients and formal systemic reviews have suggested about Child Intervention practice. Forty reports representing the input from 20,000 Albertans were collected, reviewed and used to inform the principles. The outcome of the meta-analysis confirmed that further consultation was not required and the analysis that Child Intervention staff, clients and other stakeholders had all been indicating the need to move towards principle based practice. The completion of this meta-analysis supported the

Ministry of Children's Services to assess potential gaps in feedback from a broad stakeholder group regarding the expectation of Children's Services in engaging, assessing and interacting with children, youth, families, communities and agency partners. The information from the meta-analysis highlighted that there were no gaps in stakeholder feedback, and that there was consensus in what Albertans collectively wanted to see from Children's Services. From a strategic position, the meta-analysis provided intentional, robust and far reaching information from various viewpoints that will be used to inform strategic direction, policy, training, recruitment and retention processes and practice development within Children's Services.

Using this source of data and information as a foundation for the organizational redesign of Children's Services was unique, as history suggests that system reform is too often based upon system reviews or investigative expert reports initiated by a tragic event such as the death of a child receiving services. While systems reviews address the immediate tragedy, they lack the depth or scope of information to inform meaningful recommendations for the Ministry to use in prioritizing areas to focus improvements.

Six principles were drafted and reviewed by government and agency leadership. There was consensus that the principles should be tested in the practice field to determine if they resonated with those front-line staff who would be responsible for implementing the principles in practice. The principles were tested and validated with over 700 internal Child Intervention, First Nations, and agency staff in 19 communities before being affirmed by Child Intervention leadership.

The current principles are:

- Indigenous Experience: Indigenous peoples have always had their own ways of ensuring that vulnerable members, including children, are safe, protected, and nurtured. We honour this by recognizing their expertise in matters concerning their children, youth, and families.
- Preserve Family: We believe children and youth should be safe, healthy, and live with their families; therefore, we focus on preserving and reuniting families and building on the capacity of extended family and communities to support children, youth, and families.
- Strengths-based: Our approach is reflective, culturally responsive and strengths-based. Because all families have strengths and resources, we recognize and support the right and responsibility of parents to share in the decision-making process for them and their children.
- Connection: Children and youth are supported to maintain relationships that are important to them, be connected to their own culture, practice their religious or spiritual beliefs and, for those with involvement, have a plan for their care where they are included in the decision making process.
- Collaboration: We are child-focused and family-centered. We collaborate with families, community agencies, and other stakeholders in building positive, respectful partnerships across integrated multidisciplinary teams and providing individualized, flexible, and timely services to support these efforts.

- Continuous Improvement: Our casework is transparent and we share information appropriately. Our approach is outcome-oriented and evidence-based; therefore, we support innovative practice, evaluate our performance, and strive for continuous improvement.

24.5 Key Learning and Future Directions

24.5.1 From Collaboration to Innovation

The process of developing and launching OBSD and later CSD in unique areas across Alberta opened the door to innovation in Child Intervention. The successful creation of collaborative relationships with contracted agency partners, and the range of opportunities for staff to creatively engage with children, youth and families established a ground-level commitment to adapt Child Intervention services delivery. Child Intervention had spent a number of years attempting to shift service delivery resulting in progressive organizational steps to develop formal partnerships with the contracted agency sector, to develop organizational principles and establish consistent processes to guide staff in this work. CSD was able to expand on these accomplishments and strengthen the understanding of the organizational requirements to fully realize this strategic goal.

24.5.2 The Value of the Child Intervention Practice Framework

The area offices that became involved in CSD collaborative partnerships highlighted the need for formal organizational principles, which lead to the development of the Child Intervention Practice Framework to guide the collective work of Child Intervention staff as well as agency partners at all levels of each organization. The CIPF built on previous knowledge and utilized feedback from community, partners and staff in a way that supported staff to lead the process of developing and implementing the principles. This success can be attributed in part to a staff group who were engaged and invested in the principles, practice approaches and process of organizational change.

24.5.3 Leadership Support for Front-Line Staff

There was significant leadership support for staff to think creatively, experiment with different clinical approaches with children, youth and families and collaborate with partners. This lead to an energized ground level workforce that began to seek out leading practice approaches and tools and then try them in their work. These grassroots efforts to improve the relationships between Child Intervention staff, agency partners and clients led to local use of practice approaches such as Signs of Safety, which was subsequently adopted provincially.

24.5.4 The Impact of Collaborative Service Delivery

The impact of CSD on Child Intervention practice continues today in two significant areas. First, the continued implementation of intentional local collaborative partnerships between Child Intervention delivery offices and contracted agency partners continues to showcase the effectiveness of the core CSD elements (collaborative practice, flexible contracting and data) in action with children, youth and families. Second, at a strategic level, the learnings from the three core elements of CSD continue to influence and impact broad organizational shifts within the Child Intervention system. Leveraging the common focus and strategy direction that the CIPF has provided both government and the contracted agency sector has resulted in much collaborative work on further systemic change in several key areas. These include, work underway to support the Ministry of Children's Services becoming a trauma informed organization through embedding the foundational pillars of child development, trauma, and loss and grief through the organization with a significant focus on strengthening caregiver's capacity to improve positive outcomes for infants, children and youth.

The organization has also leveraged the successes of flexible contracting highlighted in the CSD initiative through embedding the elements of flexible contracting throughout the organization. In the Child Intervention area specifically, the CSD elements of outcomes focus, flexibility of service provision and collaborative work has been embedded throughout all contracts. The Ministry has embraced the learnings from using outcomes and data and utilizes this evidence to inform the continuous improvement of the system.

24.5.5 Using Evidence to Inform Practice

CSD utilized the National Child Welfare Outcomes Indicator Matrix (NOM) to guide the data collection, outcomes and analysis of the effectiveness of the collaborative work being completed with children, youth and families at the service delivery sites (Trocmé et al. 2009). Today, the NOM is well utilized in Children's Services by service delivery, policy, program and agency staff to inform program and policy development decisions, track trends and evaluate the impact of programs and policies.

24.5.6 Enhancing Collaborative Relationships

In terms of leveraging the learnings for practice enhancements Children's Services has continued to deepen the collaborative relationship between government and the agency sector through supporting collective training, use of common practice approaches and tools that support staff's collective work and improve the experience of children, youth and families involved with the system. These common practice approaches and tools include, the Signs of Safety practice approach which guides Child Intervention staff to work in partnership with families and children to increase safety and reduce risk and danger by focusing on strengths, resources and networks the family have. Alberta developed the Practice Strategies practice approach which utilizes the CIPF principles in action to support reflective practice and critical thinking at key decision points, explicit actions and behaviors of staff when interacting with clients and the intentional involvement of extended family and community in supporting children, youth and families. Currently Children's Services is supporting staff to learn and utlize the Family Finding tools to support them in engaging with extended family and community to develop a strong network to support children, youth and families in building long term capacity.

24.5.7 A Long-Term Commitment to the Process of Change

Child abuse or maltreatment for many people is a highly sensitive and emotive issue that is not easily discussed either privately or publicly. Investment in child abuse and neglect is challenged by the demand for immediate return on public investment, or at least a notable return within a political cycle. It often takes years to produce intended results in early intervention and prevention programs (World Health Organization 2006). There needs to be the availability of political support and advocacy that transcends political parties, government entities, and other policy-related priorities.

Evolving a child intervention system takes a long time, and requires continued focus. This approach to child intervention, like other public health approaches is vulnerable to changes in government or leadership (Sanders 2008). In addition, this way of working is complicated, challenging, multi-layered, and filled with many opinions and perspectives. However, early service provision seems to provide families with early support and a decreased need for their children to come into care or be in care for long periods of time. With families, agencies and caseworkers collaborating in a meaningful fashion, families can develop protective and preventable plans for themselves. This structure also provides clear and concise roles and responsibilities for the provision of services that ensures the work with families is efficient and relevant to the uniqueness of every individual family, child or youth.

In conclusion, Alberta continues to implement the core elements of CSD throughout the Children's Services organization. As Children's Services practice continues to evolve with a strengthened understanding of the benefits of using a principle based approach, and intentional redesign of all aspects of the organization to ensure the concepts of CSD and the CIPF principles are instilled in all child intervention practice.

References

Alberta Children's Services. (2006). *A new casework practice model*. Retrieved from http://www.assembly.ab.ca/lao/library/egovdocs/2006/alchs/155959.pdf

Alberta Government. (2004a). *Child, Youth and Family Enhancement Act, Revised Statutes of Alberta 2000, Chapter C-12*. Edmonton: Government of Alberta.

Alberta Government. (2004b). *Overview of changes to the child, youth and family enhancement act, August, 2004*. Edmonton: Queen's Printer.

Alberta Government. (2014). *Alberta children's services: Alberta's child Intervention system*. Retrieved from http://humanservices.alberta.ca/abuse-bullying/15403.html

Altstein, H., & McRoy, R. (2000). *Does family preservation serve a child's best interests?* Washington, DC: Georgetown University Press.

Anselmo, S., Pickford, R., & Goodman, P. (2003). Alberta response model: Transforming outcomes for children and youth. In N. Trocmé, D. Knoke, & C. Roy (Eds.), *Community collaboration and differential response: Canadian and international research and emerging models of Practice*. Ottawa: Centre of Excellence for Child Welfare, Child Welfare League of Canada.

Armitage, A. (1993). The policy and legislative context. In B. Wharf (Ed.), *Rethinking child welfare in Canada* (pp. 37–63). Toronto: McClelland and Stewart, Inc.

Bala, N. (1999). Reforming Ontario's child and family services act: Is the pendulum swinging back too far? *Canadian Family Law Quarterly, 17*, 121–173.

Bala, N. (2004). Child welfare law in Canada: An introduction. In N. Bala, M. K. Zapf, R. J. Williams, R. Vogl, & J. P. Hornick (Eds.), *Canadian child welfare law* (pp. 1–26). Toronto: Thompson Educational Publishing Inc.

Black, T., Trocmé, N., Fallon, B., & MacLaurin, B. (2008). The Canadian child welfare system response to exposure to domestic violence investigations. *Child Abuse and Neglect, 32*, 393–404.

Blackstock, C. (2011). Wanted: Moral courage in Canadian child welfare. *First Peoples Child and Family Review, 6*(2), 35–46.

Blackstock, C., Trocmé, N., & Bennett, M. (2003). *Child welfare response to aboriginal and non-aboriginal children in Canada: A comparative analysis*. International symposium on family violence, Montreal, QC.

British Columbia Government. (1996). *Child, family and community services act*. Victoria: Queen's Printer.

Brodziak, J. (2010). Outcomes-based·service delivery – On the ground. *Alberta Association of Services for Children and Families Journal, 3*, 19–25.

Dumbrill, G. (2006). Ontario's child welfare transformation: Another swing of the pendulum? *Canadian Social Work Review, 23*(1/2), 5–19.

Fallon, B., & Trocmé, N. (2011). Factors associated with the decision to provide ongoing services: Are worker characteristics and organization location important? In K. Kufeldt & B. McKenzie (Eds.), *Child welfare: Connecting research, policy, and practice* (pp. 57–73). Waterloo: Wilfrid Laurier University Press.

Fallon, B., Trocmé, N., & MacLaurin, B. (2011). Should child protection services respond differently to maltreatment, risk of maltreatment, and risk of harm? *Child Abuse & Neglect, 35*(4), 236–239.

Federal Provincial Working Group on Child and Family Services Information. (2002). *Child welfare in Canada 2000: The role of provincial and territorial authorities in the provision of child protection services*. Ottawa: Minister of Supply and Services Canada.

Fernandez, E. (1996). *Significant harm: Unravelling child protection decisions and substitute care careers of children*. Brookfield: Ashgate Publishing Company.

Gardiner, S., & Hachkowski, A. (2011). Outcome based service delivery: Launching, learning and looking forward. *Journal for Services to Children and Families, 4*(Spring), 16–21.

Gardiner, S., MacLaurin, B., & Reeves, J. (2014). Outcome-based service delivery (OBSD): The process and outcomes of collaboration. In D. Badry, D. Fuchs, H. Montgomery, & S. McKay (Eds.), *Reinvesting in families: Strengthening child welfare practice for a brighter future: Voices from the prairies*. Regina: University of Regina Press.

Gove, T. J. (1995a). *Report of the Gove inquiry into child protection in British Columbia: Mathew's story – Volume 1*. Victoria: British Columbia Ministry of Services to Children and Families.

Gove, T. J. (1995b). *Report of the Gove inquiry into child protection in British Columbia: Mathew's legacy – Volume 2*. Victoria: British Columbia Ministry of Services to Children and Families.

Hughes, E. N. (2006). *BC children and youth review: An independent review of BC's child protection system*. Victoria: Minister of Children and Family Development.

LaBoucane-Benson, P., Sherren, N., & Yerichuk, D. (2017). *Trauma, child development, healing and resilience: A review of literature with focus on aboriginal peoples and communities*. Edmonton: PolicyWise for Children & Families.

MacLaurin, B. (2002). *Historical and contextual factors associated with child welfare decisions in Canada*. Calgary: University of Calgary.

MacLaurin, B., & Bala, N. (2004). Children in care. In N. Bala, M. K. Zapf, R. J. Williams, R. Vogl, & J. P. Hornick (Eds.), *Canadian child welfare law* (pp. 111–138). Toronto: Thompson Educational Publishing Inc.

MacLaurin, B. J., Trocmé, N., & Fallon, B. (2003). Characteristics of investigated children and families referred to out-of-home placement. In K. Kufeldt & B. McKenzie (Eds.), *Child welfare: Connecting research policy and practice*. Waterloo: Wilfred Laurier Press.

MacLaurin, B., Trocmé, N., Fallon, B., & Sinha, V. (2014). *Urgent response in Alberta: Understanding the implications of 85/15 on policy and practice*. Calgary: University of Calgary.

McKenzie, B. (2011). Differential response in child welfare: A new early intervention model. In K. Kufeldt & B. McKenzie (Eds.), *Child welfare: Connecting research, policy and practice* (2nd ed.). Waterloo: Wilfred Laurier Press.

Milloy, J. S. (1999). *A national crime: The Canadian government and the residential school system* (pp. 1879–1986). Winnipeg: University of Manitoba Press.

Ontario Government. (1996). *Child and family services act*. Toronto: Queen's Printer of Ontario.

Ontario Government. (2000). *Child and family services act*. Toronto: Queen's Printer of Ontario.

Panel of Experts on Child Protection. (1998). *Protecting vulnerable children*. Toronto: Ontario Ministry of Community and Social Services.

Prilleltensky, I., Nelson, G., & Peirson, L. (Eds.). (2001). *Promoting family wellness and preventing child maltreatment: Fundamentals for thinking and actions*. Toronto: University of Toronto Press.

Provincial and Territorial Directors of Child Welfare, & Rogers, J. (2003). New directions in child welfare. In N. Trocmé, D. Knoke, & C. Roy (Eds.), *Community collaboration and differential response: Canadian and international research and emerging models of practice* (pp. 1–13). Toronto: Centres of Excellence in Child Welfare.

Sanders, M. (2008). Triple P-positive parenting program as a public health approach to strengthening parenting. *Journal of Psychology, 22*(3), 506–517.

Sinha, V., Trocmé, N., Fallon, B., MacLaurin, B., Fast, E., & Thomas-Prokop, S., et al. (2011). Kiskisik awasisak: *Remember the children. Understanding the overrepresentation of First Nations children in the child welfare system*. Ontario: Assembly of First Nations.

Sinha, V., Trocmé, N., Fallon, B., & MacLaurin, B. (2013). Understanding the investigation-stage overrepresentation of first nations children in the child welfare system: An analysis of the first nations component of the Canadian incidence study of reported child abuse and neglect 2008. *Child Abuse & Neglect, 37*, 821–831.

Spicer, K. (2016). *Child intervention practice framework implementation: Executive leadership needs assessment.* Retrieved from: http://dspace.library.uvic.ca:8080/bitstream/handle/1828/7366/Spicer_Kim_MPA_2016.pdf?sequence=1&isAllowed=y

Spratt, T. (2001). The influence of child protection orientation on child welfare practice. *British Journal of Social Work, 31*, 933–954.

Trocmé, N. (1997). Staying on track while the pendulum swings: Commentary on canadian child welfare policy trends. *OACAS Newsmagazine*, (Winter), 13–14.

Trocmé, N., McPhee, D., Tam, K. K., & Hay, T. (1994). *Ontario incidence study of reported child abuse and neglect (1993).* Toronto: Institute for the Prevention of Child Abuse.

Trocmé, N., MacLaurin, B., & Fallon, B. (2000). Canadian child welfare outcomes indicator matrix: An ecological approach to tracking service outcomes. *Journal of Aggression, Maltreatment, and Trauma, 4*(1), 165–190.

Trocmé, N., MacLaurin, B., Fallon, B., Daciuk, J., Billingsley, D., & Tourigny, M. (2001). Canadian incidence study of reported child abuse and neglect: Methodology. *Canadian Journal of Public Health, 92*(4), 259–263.

Trocmé, N., Fallon, B., MacLaurin, B., & Neves, T. (2005). What is driving increased child welfare caseloads in Canada? Analysis of the 1993 and 1998 Ontario incidence studies of reported child abuse and neglect. *Child Welfare, 84*(3), 341–363.

Trocmé, N., MacLaurin, B., et al. (2006). *Mesnmimk Wasatek – Catching a drop of light: Understanding the overrepresentation of first nations children in Canada's child welfare system: An analysis of the Canadian incidence study of reported child abuse and neglect (CIS-2003).* Toronto: Centres of Excellence for Child Welfare.

Trocmé, N., MacLaurin, B., Fallon, B., Shlonsky, A., Mulcahy, M., & Esposito, T. (2009). *National child welfare outcomes indicator matrix (NOM).* Montreal: McGill University: Centre for Research on Children and Families.

Trocmé, N., Fallon, B., MacLaurin, B., Sinha, V., Black, T., Fast, E., & Holroyd, J. (2010). Rates of maltreatment-related investigations in the CIS-1998, CIS- 2003, and CIS-2008. In Public Health Agency of Canada (Ed.), *Canadian incidence study of reported child abuse and neglect – 2008: Major findings*. Ottawa: Public Health Agency of Canada.

Trocmé, N., Kyte, A., Sinha, V., & Fallon, B. (2014). Urgent protection versus chronic need: Clarifying the dual mandate of child welfare services across Canada. *Social Sciences, 3*, 483–498.

Truth and Reconciliation Commission of Canada. (2015). *Honouring the truth, reconciling the future: Summary of the final report of the truth and reconciliation commission.* Ottawa: Truth and Reconciliation Commission of Canada.

Turnell, A., Munro, E., & Murphy, T. (2013). Soft is hardest: Leading for learning in child protection services following a child fatality. *Child Welfare, 92*(2), 199–216.

United Nations Committee on the Rights of the Child. (1990). *United nations convention on the rights of the child.* Geneva: Office of the United Nations High Commissioner for Human Rights.

Waldfogel, J. (1998). *Future of child protection: How to break the cycle of abuse and neglect.* Cambridge: Harvard University Press.

World Health Organization. (2006). *Preventing child maltreatment: A guide to taking action and generating evidence*. Geneva: WHO press.

Chapter 25
Building Research Capacity in Child Welfare in Canada: Advantages and Challenges in Working with Administrative Data

Nico Trocmé, Tonino Esposito, Barbara Fallon, Martin Chabot, and Ashleigh Delaye

25.1 Introduction

Child maltreatment is a major public health issue. Over 200,000 children are investigated by child welfare authorities because of maltreatment-related concerns (Trocmé et al. 2010) and on any 1 day approximately 62,000 children are living in out-of-home care (Jones et al. 2015). Although the number of investigations and children in care have reached historic highs across Canada, we know surprisingly little about the service trajectory of children through child welfare systems, and even less about the outcomes of child welfare services. In reviewing the literature on the efficacy of child welfare services, a Royal Society of Canada panel concluded that

> … despite consistent evidence of the severe and long-lasting effects of child maltreatment, research on how best to intervene to prevent maltreatment and its recurrence is surprisingly limited (Boivin and Hertzman 2012, pp. 102–103).

This conclusion has been echoed across many jurisdictions (See for example: Flynn and Bouchard 2005; Jones et al. 2017; MacMillan et al. 2009; Thyer et al. 2017).

N. Trocmé (✉) · M. Chabot · A. Delaye
Centre for Research on Children and Families, McGill University, Montreal, QC, Canada
e-mail: nico.trocme@mcgill.ca; Martin.chabot@mcgill.ca; Ashleigh.delaye@mail.mcgill.ca

T. Esposito
School of Social Work, University of Montreal, Montreal, QC, Canada
e-mail: Tonino.esposito@umontreal.ca

B. Fallon
Factor-Inwentash Faculty of Social Work, University of Toronto, Toronto, ON, Canada
e-mail: barbara.fallon@utoronto.ca

B. Lonne et al. (eds.), *Re-Visioning Public Health Approaches for Protecting Children*, Child Maltreatment 9, https://doi.org/10.1007/978-3-030-05858-6_25

One method of growing the evidence base for child maltreatment service efficacy is to use administrative data to understand service trajectories, and there is growing pressure from government funders to use such data as outcome performance measures before these data are fully understood by child welfare agencies themselves. One of the consequences of the limited evidence-base in child welfare is that service providers and policy makers do not have the tools needed to develop evidence-based programs. Although governments and agencies increasingly like to refer to policies and services as evidence-based, in practice there is little to suggest that the development of new child welfare programs are in fact evidence-based. In a survey of a sample of directors from public child welfare agencies across the United States, Horwitz et al. (2014) found that less than a quarter of new programs or practices were evidence-based. On a more hopeful note, using a self-report Research Evidence Use (REU) measure in a survey of 463 executives, managers, supervisors, and caseworkers in 26 private child welfare agencies, Wulczyn et al. (2015) found that agencies with higher REU scores moved children to permanency significantly quicker than agencies with lower REU scores. While the authors caution that these exploratory findings could be explained by a number of other factors, the results nevertheless add impetus to the movement towards greater use of evidence-based and evidence-informed practices in child welfare.

25.1.1 Building Research Capacity in Canadian Child Welfare

Over the past decade our research unit has been working with local, provincial, and federal agencies in an effort to encourage a stronger commitment to evidence informed policy and practice and to support the development of research capacity (Fallon et al. 2017; Gough et al. 2010; Trocmé et al. 2014, 2016). Most recently, through a Social Sciences and Humanities Research Council (SSHRC) funded knowledge mobilization and capacity development partnership between academic researchers affiliated with McGill's Centre for Research on Children and Families and a mix of mainstream and First Nations child welfare organizations. *Building Research Capacity with First Nations and Mainstream Youth Protection Services in Quebec* (BRC) was developed to support child welfare organizations' capacity to use clinical, administrative, and population statistics to better understand the service trajectories and outcomes for the children, youth and families they serve (Esposito et al. 2016; Trocmé et al. 2014). The BRC model rests on the assumption that by placing the university's research infrastructure at the service of community agencies, robust research partnerships are developed, access to agency-based research is significantly enhanced and community agencies make better use of research findings, leading to greater research utilization and research capacity building. Graduate students (BRC trainees), supported by a team of university researchers, work as knowledge brokers with community agencies by providing a range of support services, from accessing and summarizing studies from academic journals, to designing questionnaires for internal client or staff surveys, to developing data capture tools, to analyzing data, to writing proposals and reports. In most instances these information-gathering, analyzing and synthesizing projects remain the intellectual property of the community agencies and are used for their quality assurance and improvement purposes.

One of the priorities of the BRC initiative is to support the use of child welfare agency service statistics as program planning and management tools. To do so, the BRC initiative capitalizes on the untapped potential of administrative datasets in Quebec, which contain detailed service information on over 450,000 children who have been involved with child welfare agencies since 1989. Combining various clinical, administrative, and financial payment information systems, we are able to go beyond the usual descriptive, cross-sectional analyses to link profiles of children and families, including types and severity of maltreatment, family structure, and selected child and parent characteristics, to descriptions of services provided, types and durations of placements, and court involvement. In addition, by further linking these data to census track, community-level characteristics we are able to examine these case characteristics in the context of other public health data, including neighbourhood level socioeconomic indicators, and health and social service expenditures (Esposito et al. 2015, 2017a).

Although these initiatives have yielded some very positive results and policy relevant data, to our surprise, we have found that the more complex methodological issues that we anticipated were in fact not the day-to-day challenges we faced. The purpose of this chapter is to document and discuss some to the practical issues that arise and must be addressed in adapting longitudinal and spatial analysis tools to support quality assurance and program planning for child welfare organizations, implementation monitoring, and policy development for government funders.

Although the BRC initiative focused on research capacity in the child welfare sector, many other health, social service, and education sectors face the same expectation to incorporate evidence-based approaches with limited access to the tools and resources to develop an appropriate evidence base. In a policy context where access to funding is increasingly determined by service and outcome indicators, it is more important than ever for service providers to appropriate their own data and learn to use public health data to ensure that public resources are focused on those who need them the most.

25.2 The Challenges of Building Research Capacity in Canadian Child Welfare

Canadian child welfare jurisdictions have a very limited data use and research tradition. Other than some of the most basic service volume indicators (e.g., number of substantiated investigations on any given day), very few jurisdictions report publicly on service outcome indicators, such as recurrence of maltreatment, placement stability, or educational outcomes. Unlike the USA, data gathering and reporting mandates are strictly provincial or territorial and there is no national child welfare service organization with data analytic capacity, with the exception of the Public Health Agency of Canada's child maltreatment surveillance program, which has funded our team's national maltreatment incidence study (Trocmé et al. 2001, 2005, 2010). The lack of a national data collection infrastructure in child welfare is compounded by limited data management capacity in child welfare agencies, and a relatively weak tradition of data use in the field of social work (Flynn and Bouchard 2005; Rothwell et al. 2015). Child welfare administrative data are a potentially rich source of untapped information, including information about child and family characteristics, as well as the tracking of child welfare service activities, such as case opening and closing, new reports, placement in out-of-home care, and court activities (Fallon et al. 2017; Trocmé et al. 2014).

These large datasets can be used to track changes in services over time, to examine specific sub-populations, or compare services in across regions, and because they include the full-service population, are not subject to biases typical of smaller clinical or research samples. Through postal codes or anonymized case matching, these child welfare administrative data can be linked to Census statistics as well as a broad array of other administrative datasets, including economic, health, education, and police datasets (Brownell and Jutte 2013; Esposito et al. 2017a).

However, making use of the rich potential of these datasets requires an investment into a specialized analytic infrastructure and a shift in administrative cultures. In this chapter we discuss nine key challenges that we have encountered in accessing administrative datasets and developing analytic approaches that support use by administrators, policy makers and researchers. These include: (1) lack of researcher experience in working with administrative data; (2) coding and variable interpretation issues; (3) legal, ethical and cost issues related to data access; (4) the process to selecting meaningful indicators; (5) clarifying the difference between cross-sectional and longitudinal analyses; (6) when to use population rates or service event rates; (7) how to interpret comparisons between organizations; (8) determining when and how to share data publicly; and (9) caution about over-interpreting indicators based on service events.

25.2.1 Structure of Administrative Data is a Challenge for Traditional Social Scientists

One of the first challenges that we encountered in working with administrative data was our own lack of experience in working with administrative data architectures. As social science researchers we are trained to use research data systems but have less grounding in the use of administrative data systems. Research datasets are typically built around what is known as a primary 'unit of analysis' representing a 'case' such as an individual, which is structured in a data file with one case per row and variables (e.g., case characteristics, observations, and event counts) in columns. Research datasets can include several hundred columns, but the core structure remains a 'flat' file with one case per row.[1] In contrast, administrative datasets are built around administrative activities, where the unit of analysis is an activity as opposed to an individual and the data systems are composed of multiple system platforms, tables and records connected through a network of client, resource, staff, event, and payment identifiers. The core structure is a 'relational' web of files, and these data are referred to as 'relational datasets'. In a such a structure a child's trajectory in out-of-home care, for example, could involve at least three different types of tables, collated as a relational file: (1) a child table with first and last name, date of birth, sex, and some kind of child case identifier; (2) a placement event table describing each placement episode with the child identifier, a resource identifier, and a start and end date; and (3) a table describing each resource.

To track a child's trajectory in out-of-home care, a program has to be written to find all placement events associated with that child, to organize them sequentially, and then find the resources used for each placement event. Therefore, the number of tables that have to be linked expands rapidly as we track information about: the child's family; the investigation that led to their involvement with child welfare; the social workers who provided services; the foster parents or group home workers who interacted with the child; home visits; therapy sessions; and so on, all stored in different data platforms and tables using different units of analysis. The datasets produced by linking these tables can require extensive coding scripts and generate enormous amounts of information. The child welfare service dataset that we have developed in Quebec, for instance, produces a data file with 5.6 million lines of data requiring thousands of lines of programming.

Most social scientists are not trained to work with relational datasets. Not only does graduate research training not include the programming languages needed to work with relational datasets, but we also find that even experienced researchers struggle with conceptualizing research questions that are answerable by using these types of data. Conversely, programmers working in child welfare service agencies are not accustomed to extracting data for research purposes that will require statistical analyses. Most data requests from agency administrators are for aggregated point-in-time descriptions of service activity, not for case-level data. Although this may appear to be a relatively minor technical distinction between different file structures, in our experience it is a very significant barrier to integrating social science research and child welfare practice.

---

[1] Longitudinal datasets (multiple observations over time) or concatenated datasets (e.g. children nested within families within organizations) require more complex dataset structures, built, nevertheless from "flat" datasets.

25.2.2 Data Coding and Interpretation

Unlike research datasets, administrative datasets are not developed to answer specific research questions and can vary considerably with respect to data quality and completeness. The first task is for researchers to verify the definitions of relevant data fields and to develop comprehensive codebooks and data maps that reflect variations from one set of users to the next, and changes over time. We have found that as a result of the perceived complexity of customizing or making changes to the structure of an administrative data system, child welfare data users often develop their own internal definitions to adapt the information system to their specific needs. We find that at this initial stage it is useful for the research team to work closely with a small team comprising the child welfare agency's technical data management staff, a front-line user, and a mid-level administrator, each potentially having a different understanding of the meaning of specific data fields. Once identified, variations in the meaning of specific fields may then need to be mapped onto a new set of codes. These teams can also provide helpful interpretation of factors associated with missing data. For example, school grade level may be left blank simply because it does not apply to pre-school children, whereas for school-aged children a blank field is truly missing.

A similar collaboration between the research team and child welfare technical, front-line and administrative staff is also needed to build research datasets from administrative tables. Linking data elements from various tables and combining them into a single variable requires multiple coding and programming decisions that require input from agency staff to ensure that information is being assembled in a clinically-meaningful way. Tracking children in out-of-home care, for example, requires a series of decisions that are best made in consultation with agency staff to sort out what types of moves, over what period of time, should be counted to ensure that a weekend home visit, an overnight hospital stay, or a 2-week summer camp experience are not confused with a move from one placement to another. These decisions are further complicated if one considers temporary moves to a respite foster home or to a crisis mental-health center.

We have found that an effective method to support this level of consultation is to establish from the outset agency-researcher working groups. Entitled *Service Statistics Interpretation Groups* (SSIG), these groups guide the analytical process from the selection of questions, to developing operational definitions, to interpreting findings and reporting results within their organizations. The SSIGs include two or three members of the university research team, child welfare agency managers who are the end users of administrative data, clinical staff who understand the relationship between client characteristics and service events, and an agency data administrator who understands the structure of the administrative data systems. The SSIGs guide the analytic process, attending meetings approximately every 6 weeks to define and refine research questions, develop definitions, interpret and contextualize results, and identify additional avenues for analysis. Between meetings, the research team and the agency's data administrator develop definitional and analytic options that are then brought back to the SSIG for discussion.

25.2.3 Data Access: Costs, Legal and Ethical Issues

The time and costs associated with adapting administrative data systems to develop databases that can be used for research purposes are extensive. In Quebec, building a longitudinal data system from a province-wide, single information system, took us 5 years and over CA$900,000 in programming costs. In Ontario, the investment in time and resources was even greater, where we had to map eight different systems across 48 different agencies over 10 years with a team of two programmers and three researchers at a cost of approximately CA$2,000,000 (cost estimates do not include our time as the academic researchers developing and directing these initiatives).

Time and costs were nevertheless kept relatively low because the initiatives were developed as collaborations with child welfare agencies who provided in-kind support for their staff, and no-cost access to their administrative data. Developed as technical support initiatives where academic researchers were initially engaged to assist the agencies in making better use of their data, these initiatives avoid many of the hurdles involved in requesting data for academic research purposes. The agencies maintain full ownership of the data and control over the analyses. Quebec's research ethics framework governing access to 'clinical-administrative' data for program management and administrative purposes is much simpler than what is required for university-based researchers requesting access for academic purposes. This model functions very well during the developmental phases, which requires extensive work to extract and clean data, define and build variables, and build analyzable datasets. However, in later phases attention needs to be given to developing legal and ethical frameworks that eventually allow university-based researchers to make use of the data for scholarly purposes. Such frameworks are best negotiated at the outset of partnerships.

One of the most complex issues we have had to address with respect to the construction of research datasets using administrative data has been delineating Intellectual Property (IP) for the extensive programming required to construct analyzable datasets. The ownership of the administrative data remains with child welfare agencies, however, the coding scripts required to re-structure the data involve thousands of lines of programming, representing several years of development using university resources. Although the IP for these coding scripts remains with the university-based researchers, we have found that coding scripts and datasets are easily confused. Unlike traditional research datasets where data are more rigidly structured by the sample design and the data collection instruments, the datasets developed using administrative data have greater variability and tend to require programming specific to each set of analyses. Although the child welfare agency retains ownership of the original administrative data and directs the analyses produced for them, the programming expertise and the coding scripts are owned by the university researchers. In the long-term, developing programming and analytic expertise within the agency is the best way to help the agency fully appropriate their data; however, that is only possible if the agency can hire an analyst dedicated to this type of work.

Issues related to data access are particularly clearly delineated in working with First Nations agencies thanks to the Ownership, Control, Access, and Possession (OCAP) ethical framework that some First Nations communities and organizations work with across Canada (First Nations Centre 2007). OCAP principles were developed by First Nations people to "bring self-determination into the realm of research and information management" (First Nations Centre 2007, p. 4). Data held by First Nations or mainstream agencies about First Nations children or families is governed by a concept of ownership that recognizes that the data is not only owned individually by each child and parent, but also by the community more generally. Through OCAP, First Nations communities have legal possession of their data, and access to such data is obtained through a mechanism developed by individual communities. The questions, analyses, findings, and dissemination of research based on First Nations data are controlled, but not stifled, by the community. Working within this framework we have successfully partnered with First Nations organizations in Quebec to examine the over-representation of First Nations children and youth in child welfare to produce the most comprehensive longitudinal portrait of placement and service trajectories published to date in Canada (De La Sablonnière-Griffin et al. 2016).

25.2.4 Selecting Meaningful Service and Population Indicators

Administrative child welfare agencies' data systems track many types of activities that are relevant for administrative purposes, but are not necessarily meaningful in understanding client outcomes. Faced with a plethora of data, it is essential to focus on a manageable number of meaningful service and population health indicators, keeping in mind the risk of distortion given that what gets measured gets done (Knopf et al. 2007). We used a core framework of 10 indicators, developed on the basis of an iterative series of national consultations: the *National Child Welfare Outcomes Indicator Matrix* (NOM) (Trocmé et al. 2000, 2009). Designed to reflect the complex balance that child welfare agencies seek to maintain between a child's immediate need for protection, long-term requirement for a nurturing and stable home, the family's potential for growth, and the community's capacity to meet a child's needs. The NOM includes four nested domains: child safety, child well-being, permanence, and family and community support. There are 10 indicators within these domains that were selected on the basis of information that could be feasibly extracted from administrative data. These indicators represent service events, such as recurrence of a report, reunification delay, and culturally-matched placements, that are assumed to be associated with client outcomes, but are at best indirect outcome measures. Greater placement stability, for example, is assumed to be a positive outcome, as documented in several correlational studies (Barth et al. 2007; Price et al. 2008; Unrau et al. 2008); however, placement stability does not directly measure sense of belonging or well-being at the level of the child. In fact, overemphasizing stability could lead to unintended negative outcomes if a child or youth is left in an inappropriate placement.

Although socio-economic disadvantage is a key indicator to consider in analyzing and interpreting child welfare data, it is poorly documented in child welfare administrative information systems. Postal codes, however, provide an opportunity to measure socio-economic conditions in a family's immediate neighbourhood, an area including 400 to 700 families (Pampalon et al. 2012). We use a community-level index specifically developed to reflect factors associated with family socio-economic disadvantage (Esposito et al. 2017a), on a combination of five indicators: unemployment, individual, family and household median income, and post-secondary education.

25.2.5 Cross-Sectional Vs. Longitudinal

Administrative data systems designed for efficient data entry lend themselves well to point-in-time cross-sectional counts. Child welfare agencies, for example, are able to keep accurate count of how many cases are open for service on a specific day, how many children are in out-of-home care at month end, or how many cases have court orders at year end. However, most of these agencies cannot report the proportion of investigations that receive on-going services, the proportion of children who are investigated and admitted to out-of-home care, or the proportion of cases require a court ordered intervention. To describe service trajectories, agencies must be able to track case events over time using the child or the family as the unit of analysis. The current method of tracking obscures service trajectories, as agencies are only able to use day-end counts of the children in their care to report a total annual days in care. This method of counting does not distinguish between the same child in care over the year versus multiple different children over the year, so trajectories of individual children are unknown.

Not only do cross-sectional counts fail to describe service trajectories, but they also provide a distorted picture of service populations. A basic indicator like the proportion of children in out-of-home care yields two dramatically different counts as cross-sectional versus longitudinal measures. On March 31st 2010, 55% of children receiving child welfare services were in out-of-home care (46.5% excluding kinship care), however, when tracked longitudinally only 23.2% (19% excluding kinship care) of children investigated by child welfare services in 2010 were placed in out-of-home care. The representation of short- and long-term care placements is also biased by cross-sectional counts. On any 1 day, close to half (depending on whether you include kin or not) of all children in out-of-home care may be in long-term (3 or more years) or permanent care. Yet when tracked longitudinally, we find that less than one-third of children are placed long-term, and 52.6% end up returning home within 3 years. Of those returning home, more than half return within the first 6 months of being placed.

The biasing effect of cross-sectional data is also problematic in combination with retrospective counts. Duration and various repeated events are often represented in child welfare agency reports through a point-in-time retrospective count. For instance, at year end, an agency may report how long cases still receiving services on December 31 had been open. This measure of duration is very difficult to interpret since it is not measured in a consistent fashion nor does it correspond to a specific event, such as the provision of service. Recurrence measures are also typically reported in a confusing fashion by counting the proportion of investigations that had been previously investigated; a measure that tends to over-represent individual children with multiple reports. The recurrence figure reported in retrospective data from Quebec was in the range of 49%, while when measured prospectively the proportion of closed cases that are re-investigated within a year is significantly lower, in the range of 9.8%, and within 2 years: 15.4%, or 3 years: 18.6%.

The process of moving to a longitudinal representation of data requires the development of a method for organizing data in terms of meaningful clinical, legal, and administrative considerations. Longitudinal analyses follow cohorts defined by an entry or exit event within a specific timeframe. As with codebooks, defining and organizing data is ideally done in collaboration with a mix of agency data, front-line staff, and administrators. We've experimented with both entry and exit cohorts and have found that administrators and front-line staff find entry cohorts easier to interpret. In the context of Quebec's child welfare system we've focused on three types of cohorts: (1) a "service cohort" of all children investigated during the fiscal year and followed forward for 36 months; (2) a "placement cohort" of all children placed in care during the fiscal year and followed forward for 36 months; and, (3) a "recurrence cohort" of all cases that had received services that were closed during the fiscal year and followed for 12 months to determine whether there are any new child welfare investigations as shown in Fig. 25.1.

After experimenting with longer and shorter follow-up timeframes, 36 months was determined to be ideal for capturing most of the relevant clinical and legal considerations shaping service trajectories, whereas a 12-month post-service recurrence cohort captures the potentially most concerning reinvestigated cases. In addition to setting timeframes and defining the key service indicators to be tracked, a range of case selection criteria must be set. For instance, to avoid having children counted in two different placement cohorts, only those children who had not been placed in the previous 12 months were included in a placement cohort; this filtered out children returning to care after a recently failed reunification, while including children coming back into care several years later under new circumstances. Alternatively, one could only include 'first ever' placements. Youth over the age of 14 at the time of initial referral were also excluded from the service cohort as they

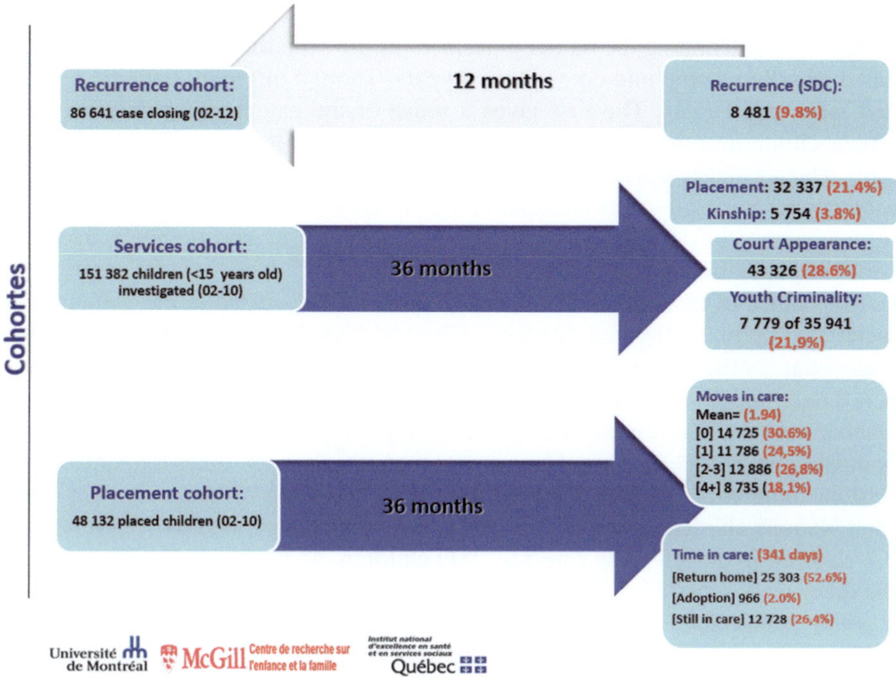

Fig. 25.1 Service outcomes tracking cohorts. (Reproduced from Esposito et al. 2017b)

would have reached the age of 18 before the end of the 36-month monitoring period. Children over the age of 17 who were too old to be subject to a new report during the follow-up period of 12 months were excluded from the recurrence cohort. These are the types of decisions that are best made through an iterative process in collaboration with child welfare agency staff who can set parameters that are most likely to describe meaningful client trajectories.

25.2.6 Population Incidence Rates Vs. Service Event Rates

Another issue needing to be considered is how maltreatment incidence rates and service rates are expressed. For certain purposes, rates are best presented relative to the general population and for other purposes rates should be offered relative to the service population. For agencies that have primarily focused on case counts – for example number of investigations during a month and number of children in care at month's end – there has been limited focus on the use and interpretation of rates and therefore the selection of denominators. With respect to placement, the incidence of placement is calculated as the number of children in care relative to the total child population. This method of comparison results in a very different picture than calculating the rate of placement as the proportion of children investigated who then come into care within 3 years. Though different, both are helpful and meaningful rates. The first gives a sense of the extent to which placement affects children in the general population (i.e., an overall maltreatment incidence rate). The second is a method for ascertaining the rate of out of home placement used as an intervention for children receiving child welfare services; that is, the service population (i.e., a service rate). It's a matter of appropriately deciding between population denominators.

The choice of denominators has been extensively discussed in the literature on racial disproportionality and disparity (Child Welfare Information Gateway 2016; Fluke et al. 2010; Lee et al. 2016; Sinha et al. 2011). The difference between incidence rates and service rates is clearly illustrated in a recent study we completed in Quebec on the overrepresentation of First Nations children in child welfare. At the population level, rates of out-of-home care were nearly eight times higher for First Nations children, with 25.2 First Nations children in out-of-home care per 1000 First Nations children, compared to the non-Aboriginal population which rests at 3.2 children in out-of-home care per 1000 children. At the service level, however, the difference is less dramatic, although highly significant from both a clinical and a policy perspective, with 35% of First Nations children being placed in out-of-home care compared to 21% of non-Aboriginal children. The difference between the two is that the disparity in placement rates add to the initial disproportion in investigation rates, which are themselves 4.4 times higher for First Nations children at a population level. Both are helpful indicators, with disproportionate population incidence rates pointing to population-based risk, such as poverty, and protective factors, such as access to prevention services. The disparity is also possible due reporting bias, while service-related factors, such as decision biases and lack of access to culturally-appropriate services, are more likely to explain the second.

As with other the methodological issues discussed in this chapter, the choice of methods for calculating rates is another example of the importance of working closely with agency administrators in developing service and population health indicators. As we will see in the next section making comparisons between agencies requires consideration of socio-economic and service access factors that affect the general population, best understood in reference to incidence rates in the general population, and specific agency practices and programs that become more apparent in comparing service rates.

25.2.7 Understanding Differences Between Agencies

Comparative analysis of population- and service-level indicators between jurisdictions potentially provides rich information about the relative efficacy of different programs and service delivery models. In fact, in a field with limited capacity to engage in experimental studies, such comparisons are critical to developing a much-needed evidence base. However, given the limited tradition in child welfare data reporting of using service and population indicators, these indicators are not understood well enough to be used in comparative analyses, which requires a clear and systematic approach to ensure that conclusions drawn are as robust as possible. This is particularly important in working with child welfare agencies that have limited experience in analyzing their own data, and even less experience in being compared to other agencies. To minimize the risk of misuse or misinterpretation of such comparisons, we use five sequential questions that appear to resonate well with the organizations we have been working with, by asking if differences can be explained by: (1) methodological differences, (2) population differences, (3) differences in availability of primary or tertiary services, (4) differences in service models, and (5) differences in service delivery efficacy. Each of these differences will be explained in greater detail in the subsections to follow.

25.2.8 Methodological Differences

More often than not, the first few iterations involving comparative analyses will reveal variations that can be partly explained by methodological differences. As noted earlier, comparative analyses require developing a codebook that includes taking into consideration variations in maltreatment coding between jurisdictions and over time. Some definitional differences, especially those reflecting different interpretations of the same nominal criteria might only emerge and the comparative analytic stage. For instance, we found that recurrence of maltreatment (defined broadly as any new investigation within 12 months of case closure) yields a relative difference of over 50% in the proportion of recurrence reflecting jurisdictional differences in investigation practices, as well as tolerance of risk. However, narrowing the definition of recurrence to children receiving child protection services within 12 months of case closure focuses on urgent protection cases rather than chronic need cases, reducing jurisdictional variations in recurrence.

Other potential methodological problems include: rates and treatment of missing data, differences in inclusion and exclusion criteria in defining denominators, and use of "other" catch-all categories. The later has been a problem in comparisons in permanency outcomes that we have been trying to examine across Quebec. As shown in Fig. 25.2, the rate of children placed in out-of-home care who return home within 36 months varies across Quebec from a low of 34.2% to a high of 65.0%. In discussing this variation with staff from several jurisdictions it became clear that the problem was that faced with a list of over 40 placement termination codes, many workers opted for the convenient "other" category to refer to family reunifications where the "family" to which a child is reunified may have a different composition than the family of origin. This code, therefore, obscures the service outcome, making it difficult to evaluate the efficacy of the specific service interventions used in each case. The list has been reduced to a more manageable number of codes (23) and the "other" response category has been removed.

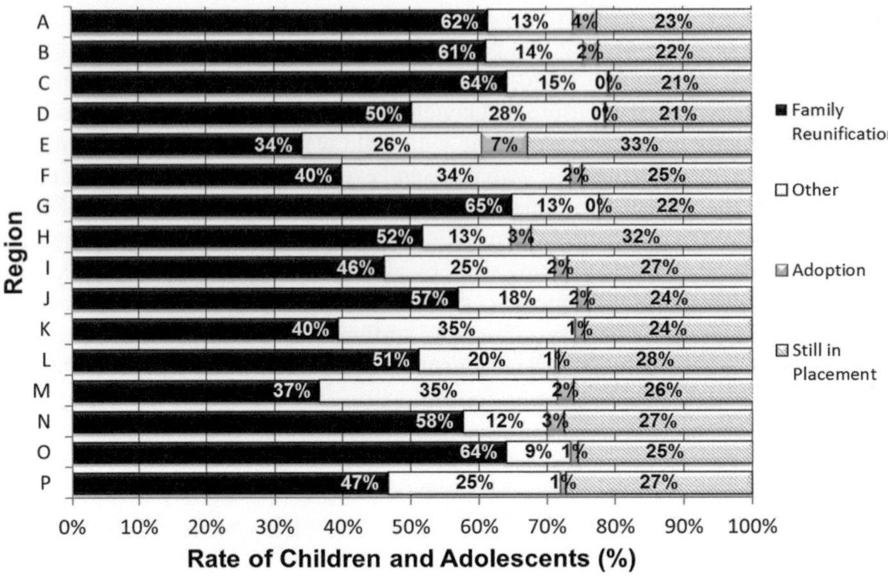

Fig. 25.2 Rates of reunification, adoption, or long-term placement by region across Quebec after 36 months. (Reproduced from Esposito et al. (2017b))

25.2.8.1 Population Differences

Once methodological reasons for the differences in results between agencies are ruled out, the second question to explore in comparing jurisdictions is whether variations in service indicators reflect differences in the populations served. These differences could be explained by poverty and other socio-demographic factors, such as health and social care, and education. Combined, the presence of these risk factors creates greater socio-economic vulnerabilities that may impede family functioning and lead to child welfare service engagement. Jurisdictional placement rates in any given year, for example, vary significantly across Quebec from a 9-year average low of 2.2 per 1000 to a 9-year average high of 9.7 per 1000, reflecting more than a four-fold difference in jurisdictional placement rates. Previous population-based longitudinal research in Quebec by Esposito and associates (2017a) showed that poverty, controlling for health and social services spending, account for 57.1% of the variation in jurisdictional placement for younger children less than 5 years of age, and 38.1% for children age 5–11 years. Indicators such as poverty, health and social care, and educational attainment of a population could explain differences in service outcomes for agencies across jurisdictions.

25.2.8.2 Differences in Availability of Primary and Tertiary Services

Third in the set of questions is the availability and accessibility of prevention and treatment services outside of the child welfare system. This is most particularly an issue in cases that are considered to involve neglect, where child welfare intervention is mediated by access to support programs (e.g., parenting classes, addiction, or mental health treatment), community services (e.g., food banks, employment and skills development programs) and housing quality or security (Choi and Ryan 2007; Shdaimah 2009). In poorly resourced jurisdictions, child welfare services can become the default service for families experiencing a range of difficulties (Delaye and Sinha 2017; Margolis et al. 2001). The 12-fold overrepresentation of First Nations children in child welfare in Canada is attributed in part to differential access to primary and tertiary services, and in particular a failure to fund on-reserve family services other than out-of-home child welfare placement (Sinha et al. 2011; Wien et al. 2007).

25.2.8.3 Differences in Service Models

Once methodological, population and service access differences between agencies have been examined, or if present, statistically controlled for to reduce their influence, the full potential of comparative analyses becomes apparent. In such instances the fourth in our sequence of questions is whether variations in service outcomes reflect different service models or at least different approaches to service delivery. Comparing rates of case re-opening and duration of services across Quebec, for example, we find that recurrence and duration of services are inversely correlated ($r = -.55$, $p < .01$), such that agencies that tend to keep cases open longer have lower rates of case re-openings (Esposito et al. 2017b). In examining differences in approaches in providing shorter- versus longer-term services, the use of case-reopening rates as an outcome measure has to be interpreted with caution. For example, a short-term service agency may in fact be using an intervention model that encourages families facing chronic difficulties to return for services in the face of new difficulties, rather than keep cases open longer than they would consider necessary. In Ontario, we are starting to examine outcomes relative to differences in the organizations' investigation functions (Smith et al. 2018). Although most agencies rely on specialized teams of investigation and assessment social workers who then pass on-going cases on to family service teams, others use a generalist model where family service teams take turns doing investigations, and if a case is kept open for on-going services, the same person who did the investigation continues on as the on-going family service worker. Differences in service models can influence the disparity in outcomes among agencies, knowing the outcomes of service models provides insight into what is working, and what isn't.

25.2.8.4 Differences in the Efficacy of Service Delivery

If service delivery models are comparable, differences in population needs, as well as access to services have been ruled out, the fifth final and rich potential for understanding differences in service outcomes is the relative efficacy of one organization compared to another; or within organizations, the efficacy of one team over another. Empirical, qualitative, and mixed-methods approaches to topics such as variations in caseloads (Yamatani et al. 2009); agency capacity/resources, organization and workplace culture (Glisson 2010; Glisson and Green 2006); worker characteristics and turnover rates (Ellett et al. 2007; Ryan et al. 2006); worker buy-in (Aarons and Palinkas 2007); implementation fidelity (Mildon and Shlonsky 2011); as well as parental engagement with services (Dumbrill 2006a; Kemp et al. 2009) can identify agency-level characteristics and delivery mechanisms that explain differences in service outcomes. In principle, these issues are best examined through implementation evaluation studies to ensure that differences in outcomes can indeed be attributed to implementation efficacy rather than differences in service models. In practice, far more comparative and evaluation research are needed before the distinction between variations in models and implementation efficacy can be teased out. As we note further, comparative analysis of child welfare administrative data is not sufficiently developed to form a valid basis to measure agency 'performance'.

25.2.9 Going Public

In a field with a limited tradition of sharing data about its services, in particular in sharing comparable data, senior administrators and government policy makers approach the public release of data with caution. This hesitancy is shaped in part by the fact that agencies are very careful to protect any potentially identifying information about children and families. Media coverage of child welfare services focus on the most tragic cases (Saint-Jacques et al. 2012; Thomlison and Blome 2012) where agencies feel criticized for either being too interventionist or for failing to intervene (Dumbrill 2006b). Despite this tendency to assume that "no news in good news", our experience in practice is that service statistics, especially when analyzed in terms of service trajectories, usually paint a far more positive picture of child welfare services compared to public and even agency staff perceptions.

Notwithstanding public perception of child welfare services as being focused primarily on child removal, the vast majority of children served never come into care, and the majority of children who come into care return home in less than 6 months. We have developed a number of public and media education information sheets that agencies find very helpful in shifting misleading perceptions about child welfare services (Esposito et al. 2012, 2013, 2017b; Kartusch et al. 2017). A challenge, however, that we had not anticipated was that even when data were made available through publicly released plain language information sheets, there continued to be many errors in the interpretation and presentation of the various indicators that had been developed in partnership. In a field with limited analytic capacity and limited experience in working with longitudinal and population-based data, and health social service reporters with limited numeracy skills, it is easy to confuse cross-sectional and longitudinal counts, or to fail to distinguish between general population and service rates.

25.2.10 Reification and Misinterpretation of Proxy Indicators

While there are many compelling arguments to make better use of administrative data to understand service trajectories, there is growing pressure from government funders to use such data as outcome performance measures before they are fully understood (Barth 2008; Courtney et al. 2004; Tilbury 2004). Service events that are typically documented in administrative data systems are at best proxy indicators of situations that are assumed to be associated with client outcomes. Despite cautionary notes about interpretation, child welfare data is often over-interpreted and de-contextualized (Rubin and Parrish 2007). Recurrence of reports and time in temporary care, for example, are two indicators that can rapidly take on a life of their own and become reified as meaning ‘recidivism’ and ‘permanence’. A high rate of recurrent reports could indeed indicate a concerning pattern of repeated victimization, but it is also partially a function of the status of the case at the time of the new incident since a new incident involving a case that is still open is less likely to be logged as a ‘recurrent report’ (Hélie and Bouchard 2010). As noted earlier, higher rates of recurrent reports could simply reflect a brief service delivery model that encourages re-referrals in the face of new crises.

Time in temporary care is another indicator that is easily over-interpreted. Although keeping children in out-of-home care longer than needed could contribute to a sense of instability and a lack of permanence, there is very little research examining what timeframes are optimal, especially in light of research showing that in some instances returning children too rapidly increases the risk of reunification breakdown (Shaw 2006; Yampolskaya et al. 2007). Most jurisdictions in Canada have set increasingly short time lines for temporary out-of-home placements. Recent changes to the law in Quebec, for instance, set a 12-month limit for children under 2 years of age, an 18-month limit for children from 2 to 5 years of age; and a 24-month limit for children 6 years of age or over (Youth Protection Act 2016). The challenge, however, is that given the paucity of existing data, indicators that track service outcomes are often appropriated as client outcome indicators, usually in the form of a crudely calculated provincial average, before they have been adequately analyzed, understood and contextualized (Trocmé 2017).

25.3 Conclusions

Child welfare administrative data are an underutilized source of rich information that should inform researchers, administrators and policy makers (Brownell and Jutte 2013). Access to–and interpretation of–these data, however, require the development of appropriate tools, infrastructure and an evidence-based culture (Collinscamargo 2007). In a field with a limited tradition of making use of data to develop, plan and evaluate services, the transition to evidence-based decision making requires a significant investment of resources and time to develop a new planning and management culture. Unlike the medical and health services field that have long-established university research partnerships, hospital-based research infrastructures, and government-run surveillance and health data programs, many other sectors, including social services, child care, and education, are at a beginning stage of developing these infrastructures. In expecting too rapid a move to evidence-based practice and evidence-based program development there is a risk that weak or ambiguous evidence ends up being misinterpreted (Barth 2008; Rubin and Parrish 2007). Our experience with the Building Research Capacity initiative and other partnerships with child-welfare organizations points to the importance of taking the time to address basic methodological, conceptual, ethical, and infrastructure related issues to ensure that administrative data are being truly used as evidence to learn from rather than simply becoming another source of 'propaganda' (Gambrill 2010).

Acknowledgment This research was supported by the Social Sciences and Humanities Research Council of Canada.

References

Aarons, G. A., & Palinkas, L. A. (2007). Implementation of evidence-based practice in child welare: Service provider perspectives. *Administration and Policy in Mental Health and Mental Health Services Research, 34*(4), 411–419. https://doi.org/10.1007/s10488-007-0121-3.

Barth, R. P. (2008). The move to evidence-based practice: How well does it fit child welfare services? *Journal of Public Child Welfare, 2*(2), 145–171. https://doi.org/10.1080/15548730802312537.

Barth, R. P., Lloyd, E. C., Green, R. L., James, S., Leslie, L. K., & Landsverk, J. (2007). Predictors of placement moves among children with and without emotional and behavioral disorders. *Journal of Emotional and Behavioral Disorders, 15*(1), 46–55. https://doi.org/10.1177/10634266070150010501.

Boivin, M., & Hertzman, C. (Eds.). (2012). *Early childhood development: Adverse experiences and developmental health*. Royal Society of Canada/Canadian Academy of Health Sciences Expert Panel (with Ronald Barr, Thomas Boyce, Alison Fleming, Harriet MacMillan, Candice Odgers, Marla Sokolowski, & Nico Trocmé). Ottawa: Royal Society of Canada. Retrieved from https://rsc-src.ca/sites/default/files/pdf/ECD%20Report_0.pdf

Brownell, M. D., & Jutte, D. P. (2013). Administrative data linkage as a tool for child maltreatment research. *Child Abuse & Neglect, 37*(2–3), 120–124. https://doi.org/10.1016/j.chiabu.2012.09.013.

Child Welfare Information Gateway. (2016). *Racial disproportionality and disparity in child welfare*. Washington, DC: US Department of Health and Human Services/Children's Bureau. Retrieved from https://www.childwelfare.gov/pubPDFs/racial_disproportionality.pdf

Choi, S., & Ryan, J. P. (2007). Co-occurring problems for substance abusing mothers in child welfare: Matching services to improve family reunification. *Children and Youth Services Review, 29*(11), 1395–1410. https://doi.org/10.1016/j.childyouth.2007.05.013.

Collinscamargo, C. (2007). Administering research and demonstration projects aimed at promoting evidence-based practice in child welfare. *Journal of Evidence-Based Social Work, 4*(3–4), 21–38. https://doi.org/10.1300/J394v04n03_03.

Courtney, M. E., Needell, B., & Wulczyn, F. (2004). Unintended consequences of the push for accountability: The case of national child welfare performance standards. *Children and Youth Services Review, 26*(12), 1141–1154. https://doi.org/10.1016/j.childyouth.2004.05.005.

De La Sablonnière-Griffin, M., Sinha, V., Esposito, T., Chabot, M., & Trocmé, N. (2016). *Trajectories of First Nations youth subject to the Youth Protection Act (Component 3): Analysis of mainstream youth protection agencies administrative data*. Wendake: First Nations of Quebec and Labrador Health and Social Services Commission. Retrieved from https://static1.squarespace.com/static/57320457ab48dea767e5e69f/t/599ce501e6f2e1277db80c78/1503454483817/Analysis+project+on+the+trajectories+-+Component+3+-+eng.pdf

Delaye, A., & Sinha, V. (2017). Community sidelined: The loss of community focus in differential response. *Child & Family Social Work, 22*(3), 1338–1347. https://doi.org/10.1111/cfs.12351.

Dumbrill, G. C. (2006a). Parental experience of child protection intervention: A qualitative study. *Child Abuse & Neglect, 30*(1), 27–37. https://doi.org/10.1016/j.chiabu.2005.08.012.

Dumbrill, G. C. (2006b). Ontario's child welfare transformation: Another swing of the pendulum? *Canadian Social Work Review, 23*(1–2), 5–19.

Ellett, A. J., Ellis, J. I., Westbrook, T. M., & Dews, D. (2007). A qualitative study of 369 child welfare professionals' perspectives about factors contributing to employee retention and turnover. *Children and Youth Services Review, 29*(2), 264–281. https://doi.org/10.1016/j.childyouth.2006.07.005.

Esposito, T., Trocmé, N., Coughlin, L., & Chabot, M. (2012). "Time to permanence": Where do children in out-of-home care end up and how long does it take? *In the Know, 2*(5), 1–2.

Esposito, T., Wegner-Lohin, J., Trocmé, N., & Gallo, S. (2013). Tracking child welfare placement outcomes at BYFC and across Québec. *In the Know, 3*(1), 1–3.

Esposito, T., Chabot, M., Delaye, A., & Trocmé, N. (2015). The stability of residential and family foster care in Quebec, Canada: A propensity weighted analysis. *International Journal of Child and Youth Resilience, 3*(1), 88–100.

Esposito, T., Trocmé, N., Chabot, M., Coughlin, L., Gaumont, C., & Delaye, A. (2016). Better understand to better serve: A province-wide knowledge mobilization initiative in child protection. *Child Indicators Research, 9*(3), 651–661. https://doi.org/10.1007/s12187-015-9335-1.

Esposito, T., Chabot, M., Rothwell, D. W., Trocmé, N., & Delaye, A. (2017a). Out-of-home placement and regional variations in poverty and health and social services spending: A multilevel analysis. *Children and Youth Services Review, 72*, 34–43. https://doi.org/10.1016/j.childyouth.2016.10.013.

Esposito, T., Trocmé, N., Chabot, M., Robichaud, M.-J., Léveillé, S., Desmarais, S., et al. (2017b). *Gestion fondée sur les indicateurs de suivi clinique (GFISC) en protection de la jeunesse: Rapport synthèse*. Institut national d'excellence en santé et en services sociaux (INESSS). Retrieved from https://mcgill.ca/crcf/channels/news/recently-released-gestion-fondee-sur-les-indicateurs-de-suivi-clinique-gfisc-synthesis-report-269155

Fallon, B., Filippelli, J., Black, T., Trocmé, N., & Esposito, T. (2017). How data drive policy and practice in child welfare? Making the link. *International Journal of Environmental Research and Public Health, 14*(10), 1223–1238.

First Nations Centre. (2007). *OCAP: Ownership, control, access and possession*. Ottawa: National Aboriginal Health Organization. Retrieved from http://cahr.uvic.ca/nearbc/documents/2009/FNC-OCAP.pdf

Fluke, J., Jones Harden, B., Jenkins, M., & Ruehrdanz, A. (2010, September). Research synthesis on child welfare disproportionality and disparities. *Disparities and disproportionality in child welfare: Analysis of the research* (2011, December). Papers from a research symposium convened by the Center for the Study of Social Policy and the Annie E. Casey Foundation on behalf of the Alliance for Racial Equity in Child Welfare. Retrieved from https://www.cssp.org/publications/child-welfare/alliance/Disparities-and-Disproportionality-in-Child-Welfare_An-Analysis-of-the-Research-December-2011.pdf

Flynn, R., & Bouchard, D. (2005). Randomized and quasi-experimental evaluations of program impact in child welfare in Canada: A review. *The Canadian Journal of Program Evaluation, 20*(3), 65–100.

Gambrill, E. (2010). Evidence-informed practice: Antidote to propaganda in the helping professions? *Research on Social Work Practice, 20*(3), 302–320. https://doi.org/10.1177/1049731509347879.

Glisson, C. (2010). Organizational climate and service outcomes in child welfare settings. In M. B. Webb, K. Dowd, B. Jones Harden, J. Landsverk, & M. Testa (Eds.), *Child welfare and child wellbeing: New perspectives from the national survey of child and adolescent well-being* (pp. 380–408). New York: Oxford University Press.

Glisson, C., & Green, P. (2006). The effects of organizational culture and climate on the access to mental health care in child welfare and juvenile justice systems. *Administration and Policy in Mental Health and Mental Health Services Research, 33*(4), 433–448. https://doi.org/10.1007/s10488-005-0016-0.

Gough, P. R., Lajoie, J., Shlonsky, A., & Trocmé, N. (2010). Journal watch: An inter-university collaborative learning partnership. *Social Work Education, 29*(1), 18–26. https://doi.org/10.1080/02615470902838752.

Hélie, S., & Bouchard, C. (2010). Recurrent reporting of child maltreatment: State of knowledge and avenues for research. *Children and Youth Services Review, 32*(3), 416–422. https://doi.org/10.1016/j.childyouth.2009.10.013.

Horwitz, S. M., Hurlburt, M. S., Goldhaber-Fiebert, J. D., Palinkas, L. A., Rolls-Reutz, J., Zhang, J., et al. (2014). Exploration and adoption of evidence-based practice by US child welfare agencies. *Children and Youth Services Review, 39*, 147–152. https://doi.org/10.1016/j.childyouth.2013.10.004.

Jones, A., Sinha, V., & Trocmé, N. (2015). *Children and youth in out-of-home care in the Canadian provinces* (Child Welfare Research Portal Information Sheet #167E). Montréal: Centre for Research on Children and Families. Retrieved from http://cwrp.ca/sites/default/files/publications/en/167e.pdf

Jones, C., Taylor, J., MacKay, K., Soliman, F., Clayton, E., Gadda, A. M., et al. (2017). The landscape of UK child protection research 2010 to 2014: A mapping review of substantive topics, maltreatment types and research designs. *Child Abuse Review, 26*(1), 8–18. https://doi.org/10.1002/car.2429.

Kartusch, M., Fallon, B., Trocmé, N., Black, T., Chan, P., & Sawh, P. (2017). *10 answers every child welfare agency should provide*. Resource document. The Children's Aid Society of Stormont, Dundas and Glengarry. Retrieved from https://www.cassdg.ca/images/documents/10_Answers_Every_Child_Welfare_Agency_Should_Provide_English.pdf

Kemp, S. P., Marcenko, M. O., Hoagwood, K., & Vesneski, W. (2009). Engaging parents in child welfare services: Bridging family needs and child welfare mandates. *Child Welfare, 88*(1), 101–126.

Knopf, D. K., Jane Park, M., Brindis, C. D., Mulye, T. P., & Irwin, C. E. (2007). What gets measured gets done: Assessing data availability for adolescent populations. *Maternal and Child Health Journal, 11*(4), 335–345. https://doi.org/10.1007/s10995-007-0179-2.

Lee, B., Fuller-Thomson, E., Trocmé, N., Fallon, B., & Black, T. (2016). Delineating disproportionality and disparity of Asian-Canadian versus White-Canadian families in the child welfare system. *Children and Youth Services Review, 70*, 383–393. https://doi.org/10.1016/j.childyouth.2016.10.023.

MacMillan, H. L., Wathen, C. N., Barlow, J., Fergusson, D. M., Leventhal, J. M., & Taussig, H. N. (2009). Interventions to prevent child maltreatment and associated impairment. *The Lancet, 373*(9659), 250–266. https://doi.org/10.1016/S0140-6736(08)61708-0.

Margolis, P. A., Stevens, R., Bordley, W. C., Stuart, J., Harlan, C., Keyes-Elstein, L., et al. (2001). From concept to application: The impact of a community-wide intervention to improve the delivery of preventive services to children. *Pediatrics, 108*(3), E42.

Mildon, R., & Shlonsky, A. (2011). Bridge over troubled water: Using implementation science to facilitate effective services in child welfare. *Child Abuse and Neglect, 35*(9), 753–756. https://doi.org/10.1016/j.chiabu.2011.07.001.

Pampalon, R., Hamel, D., Gamache, P., Philibert, M. D., Raymond, G., & Simpson, A. (2012). An area-based material and social deprivation index for public health in Québec and Canada. *Canadian Journal of Public Health, 103*(8 Suppl 2), S17–S22.

Price, J. M., Chamberlain, P., Landsverk, J., Reid, J. B., Leve, L. D., & Laurent, H. (2008). Effects of a foster parent training intervention on placement changes of children in foster care. *Child Maltreatment, 13*(1), 64–75. https://doi.org/10.1177/1077559507310612.

Rothwell, D. W., Lach, L., Blumenthal, A., & Akesson, B. (2015). Patterns and trends of Canadian social work doctoral dissertations. *Journal of Teaching in Social Work, 35*(1–2), 46–64. https://doi.org/10.1080/08841233.2014.977988.

Rubin, A., & Parrish, D. (2007). Problematic phrases in the conclusions of published outcome studies. *Research on Social Work Practice, 17*(3), 334–347. https://doi.org/10.1177/1049731506293726.

Ryan, J. P., Garnier, P., Zyphur, M., & Zhai, F. (2006). Investigating the effects of caseworker characteristics in child welfare. *Children and Youth Services Review, 28*(9), 993–1006. https://doi.org/10.1016/j.childyouth.2005.10.013.

Saint-Jacques, M.-C., Villeneuve, P., Turcotte, D., Drapeau, S., & Ivers, H. (2012). The role of media in reporting child abuse. *Journal of Social Service Research, 38*(3), 292–304. https://doi.org/10.1080/01488376.2011.627232.

Shaw, T. V. (2006). Reentry into the foster care system after reunification. *Children and Youth Services Review, 28*(11), 1375–1390. https://doi.org/10.1016/j.childyouth.2009.10.013.

Shdaimah, C. S. (2009). "CPS is not a housing agency"; Housing is a CPS problem: Towards a definition and typology of housing problems in child welfare cases. *Children and Youth Services Review, 31*(2), 211–218. https://doi.org/10.1016/j.childyouth.2008.07.013.

Sinha, V., Trocmé, N., Fallon, B., MacLaurin, B., Fast, E., Thomas Prokop, S., et al. (2011). *Kiskisik Awasisak: Remember the children. Understanding the overrepresentation of First Nations children in the child welfare system*. Ontario: Assembly of First Nations.

Smith, C., Fluke, J., Fallon, B., Mishna, F., & Decker Pierce, B. (2018). Child welfare organizations: Do specialization and service integration impact placement decisions? *Child Abuse & Neglect, 76*, 57–582. https://doi.org/10.1016/j.chiabu.2017.09.032.

Thomlison, B., & Blome, W. W. (2012). Hold the presses: A commentary on the effects of media coverage of fatalities on the child welfare system. *Journal of Public Child Welfare, 6*(3), 243–254. https://doi.org/10.1080/15548732.2012.683327.

Thyer, B. A., Babcock, P., & Tutweiler, M. (2017). Locating research-supported interventions for child welfare practice. *Child and Adolescent Social Work Journal, 34*(2), 85–94. https://doi.org/10.1007/s10560-016-0478-9.

Tilbury, C. (2004). The influence of performance measurement on child welfare policy and practice. *The British Journal of Social Work, 34*(2), 225–241. https://doi.org/10.1093/bjsw/bch023.

Trocmé, N. (2017, June). *Between Scylla and Charybdis: Navigating the stormy seas of proxy indicators morphing into performance measures*. ISCI 2017: 6th conference of the International Society for Child Indicators. Montreal, QC.

Trocmé, N., MacLaurin, B., & Fallon, B. (2000). Canadian child welfare outcomes indicator matrix. In S. Ward & D. Finkelhor (Eds.), *Program evaluation & family violence research* (pp. 165–190). New York: Haworth Press.

Trocmé, N., MacLaurin, B., Fallon, B., Daciuk, J., Billingsley, D., Tourigny, M., et al. (2001). *Canadian incidence study of reported child abuse and neglect: Final report*. Ottawa: Minister of Public Works and Government Services Canada.

Trocmé, N., Fallon, B., MacLaurin, B., Daciuk, J., Felstiner, C., Black, T., et al. (2005). *Canadian incidence study of reported child abuse and neglect – 2003: Major findings*. Ottawa: Minister of Public Works and Government Services Canada.

Trocmé, N., MacLaurin, B., Fallon, B., Shlonsky, A., Mulcahy, M., & Esposito, T. (2009). *National child welfare outcomes indicator matrix (NOM)*. Montreal: McGill University/Centre for Research on Children and Families. Retrieved from https://www.mcgill.ca/crcf/files/crcf/NOM_09Final.pdf

Trocmé, N., Fallon, B., MacLaurin, B., Sinha, V., Black, T., Fast, E., et al. (2010). *Canadian Incidence Study of Reported Child Abuse and Neglect – 2008: Major findings*. Ottawa: Public Health Agency of Canada.

Trocmé, N., Milne, L., Esposito, T., Laurendeau, C., & Gervais, M.-J. (2014). Supporting evidence-based management in child welfare: A Canadian university-agency collaboration. In A. Shlonsky & R. Benbenishty (Eds.), *From evidence to outcomes in child welfare: An international reader* (pp. 171–188). Oxford: Oxford University Press.

Trocmé, N., Roy, C., & Esposito, T. (2016). Building research capacity in child welfare in Canada. *Child and Adolescent Psychiatry and Mental Health, 10*(16), 1–8. https://doi.org/10.1186/s13034-016-0103-x.

Unrau, Y. A., Seita, J. R., & Putney, K. S. (2008). Former foster youth remember multiple placement moves: A journey of loss and hope. *Children and Youth Services Review, 30*(11), 1256–1266. https://doi.org/10.1016/j.childyouth.2008.03.010.

Wien, F., Blackstock, C., Loxley, J., & Trocmé, N. (2007). Keeping first nations children at home: A few Federal policy changes could make a big difference. *First Peoples Child & Family Review, 3*(1), 10–14.

Wulczyn, F., Alpert, L., Monahan-Price, K., Huhr, S., Palinkas, L. A., & Pinsoneault, L. (2015). Research evidence use in the child welfare system. *Child Welfare, 94*(2), 141–165.

Yamatani, H., Engel, R., & Spjeldnes, S. (2009). Child welfare worker caseload: What's just right? *Social Work, 54*(4), 361–368. https://doi.org/10.1093/sw/54.4.361.

Yampolskaya, S., Armstrong, M. I., & Vargo, A. C. (2007). Factors associated with exiting and reentry into out-of-home care under Community-Based Care in Florida. *Children and Youth Services Review, 29*(10), 1352–1367. https://doi.org/10.1016/j.childyouth.2007.05.010.

Youth Protection Act, CQLR. (2016). c P-34.1, s 53.0.1 (CanLII). Retrieved from http://canlii.ca/t/52t55

Chapter 26
Combining Public Health Approaches with Increased Focus on Risk and Safety: A Norwegian Experience

Bente Heggem Kojan, Edgar Marthinsen, and Graham Clifford

26.1 Introduction

This chapter discusses child welfare and child protection policies in relation to public health in Norway, and especially the move within child protection towards risk-assessment models in thinking, reporting and assessing based on an individual focus on families and children. The aims and policies may reach towards a public health model, but what about the measures at play within the population, especially towards meeting needs and building capabilities among vulnerable populations?

26.2 Child Protection and Public Health

Ideas and ideology about knowledge that may promote well-being and welfare may be found in both child protection and public health policies (Davies 2015; Sunstein and Thaler 2009). The idea of a decent future as a paramount goal for investment in children and child protection has been embedded in the Norwegian child protection discourse since early nineties. During the last 30 years we have seen an inflation in the use of 'family' – and parenting investment technologies in welfare. The aims of the plans that were made statutory in work with children and families have to a large extent expressed expectations about the development of personal capabilities that would help the children becoming respectable and successful - at least to some normative extent as well as preventing ill health and burdensome lives (Egelund 1997; Marthinsen 2003; Parton et al. 1997).

B. H. Kojan (✉) · E. Marthinsen · G. Clifford
Department of Social Work, Norwegian University of Science and Technology (NTNU), Trondheim, Norway
e-mail: bente.h.kojan@ntnu.no; edgar.marthinsen@ntnu.no

B. Lonne et al. (eds.), *Re-Visioning Public Health Approaches for Protecting Children*, Child Maltreatment 9, https://doi.org/10.1007/978-3-030-05858-6_26

In different ways we find arguments for why, and how, to do better work or to support the evolution of a more sustainable world for children with a special role for social work. Kamali and Joensson (2018), McDonald (2006), Ferguson (2008) and Rogowski (2010) referred to a wider discourse on social work as challenged by neoliberalist policies. Davies and Duckett (2008), Lonne et al. (2009), Garrett (2009); Featherstone et al. (2014) and Parton (2014) all communicated intentions and directions for change with titles that included phrases like *Transforming social work practice – proactive child protection, Reforming child protection, Transforming childrens services?, Re-imagining child protection – towards humane social work with families* and *… future directions.* Child protection has moved into a wider mandate and its development reflects late modern societies' focus on social investments. According to Paes de Barros (2009 in White and Wastell 2015), the idea of equal opportunity may be seen as a matter of fairness for the left and a matter of personal effort for the right. The term child protection (*barnevern* in Norwegian which means caring for and protecting) may have changed its reference from saving children from harm and serious abuse to concern about failing parenting practices and failing lives (Christiansen and Hollekim 2018).

During the 1970–80s, the discourse on welfare, social democracy and social planning included much of the same arguments and thinking as we now include and relate to public health, although the ideology behind this may be somewhat different. Making a better society for all during the golden age of welfare and equality was regarded as a political aim in itself (Brante 2014; Lorentz 2006). The new social investment policies are based on the idea of increasing wealth and social capital in order to make the country efficient and give our markets an edge, the cost of welfare may be reduced if individuals make better (Cottam 2018), and economy is paramount to all arguments, not pride and respect. The state is not responsible for the individual, but to allocate necessary resources to enable people to take responsibility for their own lives (Lorentz 2006). The public concern related to placements seem to shift from a discussion of costs versus early help and family politics, and to the fact that children placed seem to end up as marginalized as adults. Their lives (more often than children not placed) tend to include drug addiction, criminal activity, drop out and low education, low paid jobs, early parenthood and an increased chance of having their own children removed (Backe-Hansen et al. 2014; See also Chaps. 2 and 3).

The child protection discourse evolved into a discourse on risk and moral order (Parton et al. 1997). Yet child protection operates with myths as well as limited knowledge about what is best for the child – it may in fact often choose between the lesser of evils rather than good. Growing up in 'liquid modernity' means having a childhood of choice rather than stereotypes, but still there is a widespread longing for success leading to stress in ways not experienced earlier. Public health has recently moved into the area of self-care in ways never experienced earlier. High schools have established classes in how to cope with the stress related to self-presentation and the need for critical responses to excess expectations concerning living a life. Norway, as with many other countries, experiences inflationary numbers in psychiatric diagnoses and problems coping with self-esteem and self-presentation, mostly among teenage girls but also large numbers of boys. Public health investments thus have to be regarded in a social context.

Although ideas based on developmental psychology and psychoanalysis heavily influenced social work during the earlier part of the last century, the dominant discourse was medicine and natural science. Marxist views on the influence of the living conditions and material world also had some influence, especially on the need for decent housing, healthy food, dental care, education and redistributive measures based on a strong idea of equity. The discourse on abuse and maltreatment entered politics and created suspicion about how safe a place a home might, and ought, to be. Some even suggested social workers should have unlimited authority to enter every home with children (Marthinsen 1991). In Norway, the 1992 child protection laws introduced managerial standards and deadlines aimed at safeguarding children, with the possibility of prosecuting services and managers not complying with regulations. During the 'clean up' installed by a new government in the early 1990s there were 'queued' children created by large demands for service assessment, but hardly any children seemed to have suffered due to the social workers' routines of giving priority to serious cases. There was no significant increase in out-of-home-care (Marthinsen 2004). There was no proof that the preventive measures reduced the number of children placed, and serious incidents of abuse and child death often came as a surprise to the services. Yet, the assessment and practices in general were heavily influenced by the idea of risk and safety as phenomena to be controlled (Clifford et al. 2015; Haug 2018; Parton 2014).

Gilbert et al. (2011) discussed promotion of child welfare as a significant political and social challenge in modern democratic states. How do you protect (other) adult's children without intruding upon their privacy beyond reasonable argumentation? Children are ascribed individual rights and states have chosen different levels of public responsibility to safeguard them. States that have chosen a narrow range of responsibility tend to focus on protection from harm, while others take a broader view and tend to protect from a wider range of risks found in sometimes challenging childhoods.

No matter what kind of responsibility states may choose, the number of children reported have tended to increase during the last decades. Concern seems to be rising independent of responses. What started as an increase interpreted as child abuse and neglect seems to have continued into a social space of concern for children's lives in general, and especially those who may be regarded as in need or at risk. Gilbert and colleagues divided the reporting systems into two categories, those focusing on child protection and the other on a family service orientation. Child protection may be expected to deal with "degenerative relatives" while family services may conceive the situation in a language of "family conflict" or "dysfunction" (Gilbert et al. 2011, p. 3). The responses following the different outsets may be regarded as investigation of deviance in a highly legalistic way or as a service oriented therapeutic response to needs and the need to assess those. Gilbert et al. assumed that the US and Canadian child welfare future may cement the residual model under development, putting pressure on family and community to show concern for children, while the state will use its swift hand to hit hard on abuse and violence. This is followed by an increasingly intensive surveillance and investigation of mostly poor and working class families (Fauske et al. 2018).

26.3 A Brief History of Child Protection in Norway

In Norway, the first law concerning child protection was passed in 1896 aimed at socializing "unruly children". Stang Dahl (1992) argued that this move was more about protecting society than children and related to the idea that education would help to make citizens of a modern world. The institutions established to treat these children – often on remote islands – later led to disclosure of scandals of maltreatment and abuse. The child protection act of 1953 was based on a broader idea of support to children and families in need, but practice remained focussed on removal of children from unfit parents – based on abuse and maltreatment as well as moral disgust over single motherhood. Social welfare and policies linked to developing practices changed during the last part of the twentieth century with policies increasingly linked to scientific progress and ideas of social planning. This shift from moral approaches to knowledge based ones led to professionalization throughout Norway. The whole northern European area was also heavily influenced by American aid to educating social workers and establishment of several institutions based on scientific ideas about changing people's attitudes, minds and ways of being concerning their social context and health. Practices of rehabilitation and habilitation were introduced and linked to social rights and support. Educated women replaced decent citizens, often laymen but also clergy and teachers who were in charge of the child protection systems (Satka 1996).

A new Child Protection Act was passed in 1992. Ericsson (2000) pointed out the fact that in the preparation for this act it was the intention that child protection/welfare should be able to impose children's interests in all planning sections of society where their safety may be at risk such as roads, power lines, residential planning etc. This would have strengthened the public health perspective in working with children, but the law ended up narrowing rather than expanding the power to intervene in society leaving child protection to intervene in the family (Ericsson 2000, p. 20).

One of the latest changes is the state takeover of out-of-home-care responsibilities regarding institutions and professional teams to counsel municipal work with placement and other demanding tasks. This was earlier on a county level (19 units) and is now organized in five national districts corresponding to the organization of hospitals and other special treatment units. To cope with the challenge of demand and priorities of who to work with and by whom, many larger offices in cities have reorganized into purchaser-provider models and all systems are controlled and monitored by goal attainment measures, deadlines and performance indicators. The unintended result of this is a growing concern about bureaucratization and concern with the delivery of indicators upwards in management rather than focusing upon servicing clients.

Still, there is a paramount interest in developing best practices, evidence-based work models and risk assessment to serve the right child with the right service at the right time. The system is thus flourishing with innovative ideas and projects. These are supported by an increasing investment in building infrastructure for knowledge production and dissemination. During the early 1990s the state established four centres for research and development in child protection, now integrated into major universities. The social work education programs in universities are undergoing thorough reforms and are under scrutiny to increase the competence to meet new demands for applied knowledge. This aims at assessment capabilities, risk management, as well as paying respect to clients, involving users (parents and children alike), and acting according to legal demands. Institutions in child protection have a dubious history of control and care, but professionalization and inspection may have secured children better against abuse, but the prize paid for better working conditions and safety for children seems to be fractured relationships caused by all those working shifts. One of the latest claims from user involvement seem to be the questioning of love and passion in working with children (Thrana 2016).

26.4 Child Protection and Public Health Thinking in Norway

Norway is typically considered to be a social democratic and strong welfare regime (Esping-Andersen 1990). This has been evident through redistributive economies rooted in solidarity, high tax levels and de-commodification. Citizens' welfare has to a high degree been secured by universal services provided by the state. However, neo-liberal politics have since the mid-1980s been introduced in Norway (Kamali and Joensson 2018). Despite recent decades of neo-liberalization, the Norwegian welfare state remains bounded with legal frames for providing universal health and social services, and legal frames for meeting the needs of children and families. At the same time, child welfare policies are moving slightly from population based and universal family services towards a more individualized and isolated framework. Earlier the concern was on the social, social policy and social planning, but the rhetoric has changed to individual capability (Cottam 2018), and different forms of capital related to the individual and public health. The degree of social inequality is increasing in Norway as the population becomes more ethnically and culturally diverse. In 2015, about 10% of children living in Norway had lived at low-incomes for more than three years (Bufdir 2017).

The question of whether a public health perspective might enrich or even provide a better framework for thinking about child welfare and protection has not been raised explicitly in Norway. Which is not to say that thinking usually characteristic of health services has not been consistently adopted over a considerable period of time. Health services in Norway has been concerned with the overall organisation of complex and logistically demanding services in what is a small country whose population is regionally dispersed. Though certain specialist health services (in particular child psychiatry) have often been seen as the main source of expertise that could support local authority child welfare, there have been considerable problems in obtaining adequate coordination of local authority and specialist health service contributions to child welfare. The users of child welfare, including those parents who experience considerable difficulty in caring for their children, have little confidence in (and indeed little comprehension of) the kind of help that health services either at community or specialist level set out to provide. They provide child welfare with its social work staffing and (relatively speaking) greater accessibility even in situations where child welfare has placed children outside the family, or is concerned about the quality of care parents provide (Clifford et al. 2015).

As elsewhere, massive efforts have been made to regulate child welfare in the last two-three three decades. Child welfare has to meet deadlines in investigating cases in which the wellbeing or safety of children is supposed to be at issue, but (again as elsewhere) far more families are investigated than could ever be justified in terms of objective risk that children are exposed to. The technology of assessment has gradually been developed to embrace tools that embody psychological approaches to possible deprivations of care or risk of mental health problems. This can be thought of as maybe appropriate in terms of the presenting problems of around 10–15% of families referred to child welfare. Any broader use of systematic screening in the child welfare service would seem to risk an unregulated transition to a child welfare service *preoccupied with assessment and unable to provide ongoing support and follow-up for vulnerable families.* These trends have emerged clearly enough in recent work (Clifford et al. 2015).

After the mid-1990s Norwegian health policies gradually changed to accommodate a more clearly defined notion of personal responsibility for health. The notion of lifestyle-influenced risks to good health gained a good deal of ground. Obesity, the importance of keeping fit, and reducing smoking and alcohol consumption were all issues in this connection. The fundamental assumption behind official campaigning on these issues and the growth of what might be termed 'health propaganda' is that rationale behaviour to promote one's own or family health can be encouraged. However, the question of whether such persuasive strategies could be applied to issues of upbringing or parental care has scarcely been discussed. It seems that the issues that might be relevant for helping families that struggle to provide adequate care for children are not explicit but, rather, part of child welfare´s (undisclosed) repertoire of criteria for what constitutes proper care (Ericsson 1996). If this is indeed so, the notion of a child welfare consonant with modern public health thinking scarcely seems valid. Instead, objective health risks in Norway, as elsewhere, vary very greatly according to social class, and that recruitment of children and families to child welfare displays the same kind of class bias. The prospects for an inclusive user-aligned child welfare that might enlist parents in efforts to achieve better care for children, might seem rather poor.

26.4.1 Increasing Use of Services

Norway, as many other Western countries, has experienced increasing use of services over the last three decades. During the 1970–80s, the suspicion of hidden maltreatment was still part of the discourse and expanding services were expected to reveal more of the dark side of family life. This is similar to the moral panic we have seen in other countries (Parton 2014). Rather than resulting in more child rescue, the expansion of services have increased the range of services into families who may be regarded as marginalized and lacking necessary resources to promote decent and sustainable childhoods (Marthinsen 2003). With a 20% population growth during the last 50 years, child protection is serving tenfold (to nearly 56,000 children in 2017) – with an additional 58,580 children being reported, of which less than half will receive any services (Statistics Norway 2018). Assistance to children living with their parents became the most used action in 1982 and has increased most since a new children act was introduced 1991. Of those receiving services, only two out of ten cases are forcefully removed from their parents compared to almost all in the 1960s. Other services like pedagogic and psychological assistance for children with learning disabilities and behaviour problems have also increased. There was also a 100% increase in the number of social assistance cases (economic support) during the 1980s where about half were long term receivers (>6 months). These numbers have plateaued but, rather than moving into a career in the work force, many end up as disability pensioners based on diffuse psychosocial and psychiatric diagnoses. Some move in and out of jobs, often low paid and precarious ones with need for supplementary economic support in between – a growing precariat.

Likewise other countries, there are correlations between socioeconomic inequality and child welfare intervention rates in Norway. Children living in poor families, and sometimes also in poorer areas are much more likely to end up in child protection. There are clear regional and local differences of living conditions in Norway. Analysis of national child protection register data shows that there is a relatively strong connection between instances of child welfare intervention and living conditions on a municipal level (Lichtwarck and Clifford 2010). Families where parents have low education, are without employment or have blue-collar jobs are overrepresented in child welfare (Andenæs 2004; Clausen and Kristofersen 2008; Fauske et al. 2018). Single mothers count for more than four out of ten children served by the child protection system (Storhaug et al. 2012). Immigrants also have great difficulties integrating into the work force and are also overrepresented in child welfare (Paulsen et al. 2014). Immigrant families are not overrepresented when it comes to placing children outside the home (Statistics Norway 2016). However, these families are overrepresented when it comes to other forms of supportive interventions in the home (Berg et al. 2017).

The public health model is presented in official policy documents as concerned about the distribution of wealth and possibilities to enhance decent lives, with a sustainable income, fair living conditions and safeguarding. The public health law of 2011 stated that *public health* concerns the health condition and distribution of health in the whole population, whereas *public health work* concerns society's direct or indirect investment to promote health and well-being, prevent mental and bodily illness, harm or suffering, protect against threat and work towards a more equal distribution of factors that may affect health. Not mentioned in the law, but found in departmental is the claim that the most efficient action against social inequality should be directed towards the whole population combined with targeting the most vulnerable.

Distribution of wealth is considered one of the main factors affecting public health in general, but there is no longer any public policy with this goal in practice. Only political parties on the left seem concerned about redistribution, but politics are dominated by parties promoting neo-liberal values putting the fate of the individual in their own hands. In child protection, early intervention and well-being is mostly based on enhancing the agency of parents.

26.4.2 A Case Study of a Possible Public Health Approach

The research program, 'The new child protection' *(Det nye barnevernet),* was designed and carried out in cooperation with the local child protection services with some of the social workers participating in parts of the research, with the whole service involved over several years as informants in the follow up and longitudinal part of the study. A structured interview was carried out by experienced social workers and researchers who met parents at home or at other places they agreed to meet. In addition to the parent interview, services provided formal data regarding measures and their own categorizations used for general statistical purposes. A selection of 100 parents recorded with multiple challenges or stress factors were chosen for a 2-year follow up starting with a life history interview and a later interview about service provision and change, and an update of the survey two years later. About 20 of the children of this selection were also interviewed during the 2-year period, giving children a voice and possibility to identify social work intervention in their lives.

Overall 715 parents were interviewed, using the survey with some open questions, but mostly scales based on social and social work research while much of the data concerning the social and individual capabilities for parents and children where based on a version of common assessment forms used in child protection. The parent data was supplied with data from the services based on their categorizations of child protection and journal text as well as memory recall from social workers. Data were recoded to create categories of burdens versus resources, to rate parents and children in order to make a selection of 70–100 parents and children/families with "heaviest burdens" to follow up for two to three years to see how their needs were met by services and how their lives might change during the time observed. Data were collected through life course interviews with parents and some children, interviews to assess and evaluate social work as seen from the parents, and a repetition of some of the survey to update at the end of the time followed. Several social workers were interviewed during the course of the research and data from the survey and later interviews were presented at teaching/seminars with the services involved. The research program was a continuation of a couple of decades of research on service provision and practice research involving many of those services that participated.

A large survey had not previously been conducted that was able to penetrate into the individual experience of the clients allowing for a more subjective view of their lifeworld and parenthood. This allowed us to ask the question that if a public health model was in operation, we would expect those with complex needs to have these met thoroughly by services aiming at making a better world for children as well as parents. We should have expected an innovative service always looking for better ways to cope with the challenges of wasted or threatened lives.

26.4.3 Main Findings from 'the New Child Protection'

The most deprived children and families were those least likely provided useful assistance from child welfare, as our own recent research has shown (Clifford et al. 2015). We saw that those families in difficulty that had greater resources and higher status much more often obtained useful help from child welfare, perhaps partly because they were judged better able to benefit from the demands imposed by rigorous evidence based interventions. At all events the de facto bias against low income, multi-problem, 'struggling' families were very evident. This appears unacceptable in view of the established aims of Norwegian child welfare policy, which have emphasised the importance of parental choice, participation and empowerment as well as empirically-grounded methods in efforts to reduce risk of inadequate care, and abuse or neglect of children. This policy profile was described in government documents in 2001–2002. In our study The New Child Welfare, we detected clear signs of parents´ willingness to share responsibility with child welfare, but only occasionally a sense of being empowered; very many parents, and not only those from the most severely deprived families, felt unable to deal with the difficulties that affected their children. This was particularly in evidence when children had mental health problems, and in those many instances where children had difficulty in school.

As we saw it, there was a need to reframe child welfare´s approach to the most deprived families by examining the needs of the family as a unit. This seemed to be appropriate because child welfare and the specialist health services most often think in terms of forms of family functioning that can lead to deprivation for children. We also reasoned that since parents very often see children´s situation in terms of risk (for example risk due to their own poor mental health, the children´s poor integration in school, and the risk of malign peer group influences) there would be little likelihood that parents would be alienated by such an approach. But our work with focus groups of child welfare workers and their leaders showed that assessment of risk focussed upon children was seen as the right approach. Parents were much less in focus even though they were so often seen as the real cause of children´s problems.

26.5 Discussion

According to the terminology and the explanations given to the term public health (approaches/model) in this book, much of the policies regarding children and child protection have always had that kind of focus in Scandinavia. Understanding and acknowledging a problem, developing an insight into the phenomena at play, inventing and evaluating measures, and innovating and adapting to new ideas is a sound process. Under what conditions children will thrive relate to standards of living as well as moral aspects.

The public health approach may be regarded along a continuum from social policies (work, housing, food, health and education etc.) to a scientifically and morally informed discourse on lifestyles and living. The first is a project referring to the ideas behind the welfare state and the second to the neo-liberal idea of a social investment state. The movement from one to the other as the dominant discourses have gradually evolved, influencing social work practice from the expert participating in social planning as well as working with clients, to the consultant and adviser who assists in self-development and empowerment understood as personal symbolic capital investments. Within child protection, this may be one of the factors explaining the colonization of the life world of marginalized families and families with children that challenge parenting in different ways. Part of the difficulty we encounter in seeing child welfare in a health or public health perspective seems to be that there is scarce room for long-term investment in marginalized and/or families in need. The combined data from the research program 'The New Child Protection' illustrates this.

We found that there is a clear conflict implicit in the contrast between the preferences on the part of child welfare, and our empirical findings, which suggests that parents in child welfare families more often than children have severe difficulties, which in the long term tend to adversely affect parental care. The desirability of early intervention to offset disadvantages due to risk factors in early and middle childhood, has in Norway mainly been seen as a matter of useful intervention early in children´s development, as being more effective and therefore likely to prevent chronic problems and mental health difficulties. The emphasis is upon the psychopathology or perceived conformity to expectations of the individual child, rather than upon the social context and the family. Early intervention as an overriding service strategy, however, was developed in the USA and advocated by the Surgeon General, because social deprivations affecting children in the more disadvantaged social groups, must be addressed by services offered to families and children at an early stage. Early intervention of the kind adopted in Norway requires access to specialist expertise "locked" away in the specialist health and education services, access that may be difficult to allocate. The importance of addressing parent's difficulties is underlined by a central finding in the NCW survey. Families reported to child welfare and investigated were most often reported due to concern about parents; children´s problems were much less in evidence as a basis for investigation.

Critics of modern child welfare (Clifford et al. 2015; Garrett 2009; Parton 2014) have suggested that an increasing emphasis on risk assessment with a forensic basis has altered the way in which child welfare staff (predominantly social workers) approach families. Little is offered in the way of useful help, instead, parents must master their situation themselves. Parents are disqualified if they do not respond to advice and supervision offered by child welfare staff. Parton argued that risk assessment, despite its apparent objectivity, masks a comprehensive bias; child welfare 'sees' children at risk rather than families in difficulty. An overly investigative frame of mind in child welfare merely reinforces the multiple disadvantages many families suffer. Ferguson (2008) argued that risk is a frame of mind. The risks children are exposed to today are no greater than they have been throughout the modern epoch, but risk is now engrained in professional thinking to such an extent that the procedural apparatus set up to process child welfare reports, investigations and interventions inhibits any broader thinking about families´ predicament and ways of dealing with multiple problem situations. These are, of course, very broad and disturbing conclusions about child welfare.

We saw very clearly that parents had very considerable confidence in child welfare, indeed a degree of trust. This confidence was only expressed toward child welfare and most definitely did not include child psychiatry, school or the health services. Whether these findings reflect the prevalence of some form of institutional trust of the kind discussed in welfare studies is an interesting question. We have concluded that a basis for partnership between child welfare and parents does seem to be present, though it is likely to be eroded if a risk-assessment approach in child welfare work is thoroughly applied. At present, this seems a likely scenario for developments in Norwegian child welfare. Recent legislative changes appear to lay the groundwork for this (Ot. prp. 142 (2013–2014), and the arguments deployed in (NOU 2012, p. 5) have provided a general, if not wholly convincing supporting rationale.

The NOU advances arguments that seem dubious indeed in view of the fact that child welfare is least likely to provide support for those families that are affected by multiple disadvantages, families in which many children must be presumed to be at risk. Apart from the fact that approaches rooted in attachment theory or mentalisation are scarcely feasible (few child welfare workers have anything approaching a satisfactory competence in these areas to be able to apply them, and the availability of expert assistance is severely restricted), the ethical dilemmas inherent in using psychological theories as a basis for non-voluntary interventions on a broad scale in child welfare are very evident. This, like the recent political willingness to impose compulsory orders on parents in respect of interventions that up to now have been voluntary, seems to betray a measure of desperation, if not a dangerous tendency to exclude those who are deemed to fail as parents.

26.5.1 Is it Possible to Promote Investment in Those Who Are Most Marginalised?

Based on the fact that families with multiple challenges and aggregation of stress factors (symbolic burdens) received less services than those with fewer challenges, and especially not services regarding their expressed needs, we wanted to have a closer look at the possibility of change in this practice. Could it be possible to use this acknowledgement of need for better services (in a public health approach model) to promote more investment in marginalized lives? We designed a study involving families with similar traits as those we had followed earlier, from four different services taking part in our earlier research. The social workers would be supported by an 'innovative team' who could be a discussion partner in developing new practices in reassessing and working with the selection of families with complex needs. They were also offered to attend a year master course (20ect) focussing on innovative, research-based and reflexive practices.

The idea of an innovative, competent practice using evidence based-knowledge is generally supported by politicians as well as managers throughout the system. The interest in research supported practices seem to be increasing and there is a discussion about moving social work in the direction of medicine with university clinics – the model has been tested in social services (Austin and Johannessen 2015). Our experience is that according to a public health model we should expect work to be focussed on improving practices that support life time change and secure access to symbolic capital ranging from economic to cultural and social, reducing the amount of symbolic burdens weighing on parents and children. It should also lead positively to evolvement of ever more sustainable services. Do we see this happening? Inspired by the initial research mentioned with the large survey and the longitudinal study following, we managed to have funding for a three-year experiment based on supporting the same services where lacking good social work strategies for troubled families had been identified. Some of the social workers attended a special master course over a year focussing on innovative new practices. The lecturers were highly qualified researchers and practitioners in social work, child work and psychology and the same people were available as previously.

Soon the problems of everyday practice presented themselves with the innovative and research-based work. The services involved were managed after a purchaser-provider model and many of the workers participating in the original research were not in charge of the whole follow up process. Managers and social workers changed due to high turnover. Participants in the master course also changed creating difficulties with catching up on earlier lessons. Based on teaching about complexity theory they learned to view their competing demands in a language allowing them to analyse why things turned out the way they did. We analysed their writings and discussions, and could see how managerial demands related to performance indicators and time limits competed with professional values related to seeing clients at home, engaging in building relationships to adults and children, working in collaborative teams etc., and having a long-term social investment view on practice. Most of the professional values were not monitored by computer systems checked by management and inspection, and suffered when they had to give priority. The logics of practice seemed to mirror a *model of alert*, controlling risk and avoiding safety breaches putting children to harm. Only one project managed to develop positively, since the social workers were reorganized in a special team working only with a few selected families with hardly any bureaucracy involved and no managerial control except qualitative evaluation at long-term intervals (Davidson et al. 2017).

Some of this also fits with critique of new assessment and monitoring practices in the UK moving the attention from clients to systems leaving social work stuck in between (Munro 2011). Critical social work research very often enhances both the structural and operational flaws in systems on several levels (societal as well as on a local and individual level) and this is seldom compatible with ideal aims in politics based on myths about the phenomena at play, which certainly will be undressed by social research.

26.6 Conclusion

This chapter has shown that the public health ideals about promoting enhanced living conditions as well as good health and happiness, has not been realized as a practice within the Norwegian child welfare and protection system, despite its long tradition of a social democratic system orientation. The reasons are certainly complex, however, we have emphasized how child protection may be guarding themselves as a managerial system against accusations of not acting to save children who are in danger or face risk of serious maltreatment. This may be seen as a system being alert to possible dangers, monitoring everyday life in families, but not developing a sustainable social investment practice to enhance the capability as parents or citizens in general.

Welfare society thinking does rest on the premise that users of services are rational agents who will be able to serve their or their dependents´ best interests by exercising choice, listening to advice, and representing themselves. If we look at the transformation of public health thinking that has occurred in Norway since 1990, we see that welfare society thinking reigns there too. Government actively promotes and distributes health advice. The assumption is that rational citizens will follow it. Without discussing the effectiveness of such policies (and there have been apparent successes) it is evident that notions of individual responsibility for one's own health have been massively promoted, extending (with the assistance of the media and internet) to a complex lifestyle discourse. What should we eat? How should we keep fit? A 'Public Health Model' in this context is not only a rational policy based on evidence and sound judgement. It is transformational in the sense that the discourse unleashed by the notion of personal responsibility for health affects daily life, habits and consumer preferences, and notions of what is proper in a profound way. It can of course lead to exclusion or labelling, as possibly has been the case in media discussion of adult and childhood obesity.

References

Andenæs, A. (2004). Hvorfor ser vi ikke fattigdommen? Fra en undersøkelse av barn som blir plassert utenfor hjemmet. *Nordisk Sosialt Arbeid, 24*(1), 19–33.

Austin, M. J., & Johannessen, A. (2015). Introduction. *Journal of Evidence-Informed Social Work, 12*(1), 1–6.

Backe-Hansen, E., Madsen, C., Kristofersen, L. B., & Hvinden, B. (Red.) (2014). *Barnevern i Norge, 1990–2010. En longitudinell studie*. NOVA Rapport 9/2014.

Berg, B., Paulsen, V., Midjo, T., Haugen, G. M., Garvik, M., & Tøssebro, J. (2017). *Myter og realiteter – innvandreres møte med barnevernet.* Rapport. NTNU Samfunnsforskning.

Brante, T. (2014). *Den professionella logiken. Hur vetenskap och praktik förenas i det moderna kunskapssamhället*. Stockholm: Liber.

Bufdir. (2017). *Oppvektsrapporten 2017. Økte forskjeller – gjør det noe?* Oslo: Bufdir.

Christiansen, Ø. & Hollekim, R. (2018). In-home services: A rights-based professional practice meets Children's and families' needs. 10, sider 185–208. In A. Falch-Eriksen, A. & E. Backe-Hansen, *Human Rights in Child Protection Implications for Professional Practice and Policy.* UK, Palgrave Macmillan.

Clausen, S-E., & Kristofersen, L. B. (2008). *Barnevernsklienter i Norge 1990–2005. En longitudinell studie.* NOVA Rapport nr. 03, Oslo.

Clifford, G., Fauske, H., Lichtwarck, W., & Marthinsen, E. (2015). *Minst hjelp til dem som trenger det mest? Sluttrapport fra forsknings- og utviklingsprosjektet «Det nye barnevernet».* NF-rapport nr. 6/2015.

Cottam, H. (2018). *Radical help. How we can remake the relationships between us and revolutionize the welfare state*. London: Virago.

Davidson, B., Bredmar, M., Hellberg, K., Lichtwarck, W. & Petersson, G. (2017). Förändrade arbetsmetoder i det sociala arbetet med familjer med sammansatta behov. En utvärdering av projektet Familjelotsen – utveckling i samverkan i Linköpings kommun. Linköping, FoU-centrum.

Davies, L., & Duckett, N. (2008). *Proactive child protection and social work.* Exeter: Learning Matters.

Davies, W. (2015). *The happiness industry: How the government and big business sold us well-being*. London: Verso.

Egelund, T. (1997). *Beskyttelse af barndommen. Socialforvaltningers risikovurdering og indgreb.* Copenhagen: Hans Reitzels forlag.

Ericsson, K. (1996). *Barnevern som samfunnsspeil.* Oslo: Pax Forlag.

Ericsson, K. (2000). Social control and emancipation – Ambiguities in child welfare. *Journal of Scandinavian Studies in Criminology and Crime Prevention, 1*(1), 16–26. https://doi.org/10.1080/140438500501l6237.

Esping-Andersen, G. (1990). *The three worlds of welfare capitalism.* Princeton: Princeton University Press.

Fauske, H., Kojan, B. H., & Storhaug, A. S. (2018). Social class and child welfare: Intertwining issues of redistribution and recognition. *Social Science, 7*(9), 143. https://doi.org/10.3390/socsci7090143.

Featherstone, B., White, S., & Morris, K. (2014). *Reimagining child protection: Towards humane social work with families*. Bristol: Policy Press.

Ferguson, I. (2008). *Reclaiming social work*. London: Sage.

Garrett, P. M. (2009). *'Transforming' children's services? Social work, neoliberalism and the 'modern' world.* Maidenhead: McGraw Hill/Open University.

Gilbert, N., Parton, N., & Skivenes, M. (Eds.). (2011). *Child protection systems: International trends and orientations*. Oxford: Oxford University Press.

Haug, V. (2018). Haug, Veronica. Barn i risiko og risikable foreldre. En analyse av risikoforståelser i barnevernets institusjonelle praksis. PhD-thesis. Oslomet, Norway.

Kamali, M., & Joensson, J. H. (2018). *Neoliberalism, Nordic welfare states and social work current and future challenges*. UK: Routledge.

Lichtwarck, W., & Clifford, G. (2010). *Modernisering i barnevernet. Ideologi, kontekst og kompetanse*. Oslo: Universitetsforlaget.
Lonne, B., Parton, N., Thomson, J., & Harries, M. (2009). *Reforming child protection*. London: Routledge Taylor and Francis Group.
Lorentz, W. (2006). *Perspectives on European social work. From the birth of the nation state tothe impact of globalization*. Opladen/Farmington Hills: Barbara Budrich Publishers.
McDonald, C. (2006). *Challenging social work: The context of practice*. Basingstoke: Palgrave Macmillan.
Marthinsen, E. (1991). *Fra ide til reform: reformer som reetablering av makt og tilpasning til ideologiske føringer*. Sosialt arbeids rapportserie; 3. Universitetet i Trondheim: Institutt for sosialt arbeid, NTNU.
Marthinsen, E. (2003). *Sosialt arbeid og symbolsk kapital i et senmoderne barnevern*. PhD-thesis. Trondheim: Norwegian University of Science and Technology.
Marthinsen, E. (2004). En radikal analyse av barnevernet. *Norges Barnevern, 2*, 3–12.
Munro, Eileen (2011). *The Munro review of child protection: Final report – A child-centred system*. London: TSO (The Stationery Office).
NOU. (2012). *Bedre beskyttelse av barns utvikling*. Oslo: BLD.
Parton, N., Thorpe, D. H., & Wattam, C. (1997). *Child protection: Risk and the moral order*. Basingstoke: Macmillan.
Parton, N. (2014). *The politics of child protection – Contemporary developments and future directions*. Basingstoke: Palgrave Macmillan.
Paulsen, V., Thorshaug, K., & Berg, B. (2014). *Møter mellom innvandrere og barnevernet: Kunnskapsstatus*. Trondheim: NTNU Samfunnsforskning.
Rogowski, S. (2010). *Social work, the rise and fall of a profession*. New York: Polity Press.
Satka, M. (1996). *Making social citizenship. Conceptual practices from the Finnish poor law to professional social work*. University of Jyväskylä: SoPhi.
Sunstein, C. R., & Thaler, H. T. (2009). *Nudge: Improving decisions about health, wealth and happiness*. New Haven: Penguin Books.
Stang Dahl, T. (1992). *Barnevern og samfunnsvern: om stat, vitenskap og profesjoner under barnevernets oppkomst i Norge*. Oslo: Pax Forlag.
Statistics Norway. (2016). *Delen innvandrarbarn undersøkte av barnevernet aukar med alderen*. Retrieved from https://www.ssb.no/sosiale-forhold-og-kriminalitet/artikler-og-publikasjoner/delen-innvandrarbarn-undersokte-av-barnevernet-aukar-med-alderen
Statistics Norway. (2018). *Child welfare*. Retrieved from https://www.ssb.no/en/sosiale-forhold-og-kriminalitet/statistikker/barneverng/aar
Storhaug, A. S., Kojan, B. H., & Kvaran, I. (2012). Enslige mødre i kontakt med barnevernet. *Fontene forskning, 5*(2), 4–17.
Thrana, H. M. (2016). Love: Recognising relationship in work with vulnerable youth. Joint Special Issue, Love in professional practice. *Scottish Journal of Residential Child Care, 15*(3) and *International Journal of Social* Pedagogy, 5(1), 71–89. https://doi.org/10.14324/111.444.ijsp.2017.06.
White, S., & Wastell, D. (2015). The rise and rise of prevention science in UK family welfare: surveillance gets under the skin. *Families, Relationships and Societies, 6*(3), 427–445.

Part IV
Trends and Future Directions

Chapter 27
Child Maltreatment as Social Harm

Nigel Parton

27.1 Introduction

A major prompt for the growing interest in public health approaches to child maltreatment has been the recognition over many years of the major problems in the operation of traditional child protection systems, particularly in North America, Australia and the UK (see for example Lonne et al. 2009; Waldfogel 1998). Attempts to reform such systems are invariably premised on the apparent evidence that they are being subject to overload such that they are unable to successfully carry out the tasks expected of them.

However, while child protection systems have been extended, revised and updated on many occasions since the early 1970s there have been two major problems with such systems from the outset. As Melton (2005) has argued, the original designers of modern child protection systems made two interconnected and fundamental errors – the *scope* and the *complexity* of the problem of child abuse and neglect were underestimated.

> The assumption early in the history of the modern child protection system was that the problem of child maltreatment was reducible to 'syndromes' – in effect, that abusive and neglectful parents were either very sick or very evil and that they could thus be appropriately characterised as 'those people' who were fundamentally different from ourselves … Although such cases do occur, they are relatively rare. Most cases involve neglect … further, searches for distinctive behavioural syndromes have proven elusive (Melton 2005, p. 11).

The idea that child maltreatment is an individual problem caused by particularly malevolent parents is one projected very strongly in the media and by many politicians. Such ideas are reinforced when most of the public and political discussion of

N. Parton (✉)
School of Human and Health Sciences, University of Huddersfield, Huddersfield, UK
e-mail: n.parton@hud.ac.uk

B. Lonne et al. (eds.), *Re-Visioning Public Health Approaches for Protecting Children*, Child Maltreatment 9, https://doi.org/10.1007/978-3-030-05858-6_27

the problem takes place in a context of a high profile and tragic child death. Even though such scandals have increasingly been seen as evidence of systemic failure, and not just individual failure on the part of workers and managers, the scandal-driven politics of child protection still encourages a narrow view of what is at stake in policy making. In the process the 'failures' of child protection are seen to result from problems in the design and operation of the systems and the decisions of certain professionals, particularly social workers (Gainsborough 2010; Warner 2015).

Through the lens of scandal, discussions about child protection are largely disconnected from any wider appreciation of what harms children, how their welfare might be improved and how such issues are related to wider social and economic processes and structures. Such an appreciation should begin by focussing on what we know about the prevalence of child maltreatment and what some of the prime causes might be. Once we are clearer about that we would then be in a much better position to develop and implement appropriate policies, systems and practices.

27.2 The Prevalence of Child Maltreatment

An authoritative review of research on the prevalence of child maltreatment in 'high-income countries' published in *The Lancet* in 2009 (Gilbert et al. 2009) concluded that every year between 4% and 16% of children were physically abused and one in ten were neglected or psychologically abused. During childhood, between 5% and 10% of girls and up to 5% of boys were exposed to penetrative sexual abuse and up to three times that number were exposed to some form of sexual abuse. The review concluded that the numbers of cases of substantiated child maltreatment known to the official agencies only accounted for a tenth of this total. In addition, exposure to multiple types and repeated episodes of maltreatment was also associated with increased risks of severe maltreatment and psychological consequences. Child maltreatment was found to substantially contribute to child mortality and morbidity and had long-lasting effects on mental health, drug and alcohol misuse (especially in girls), risky sexual behaviour, obesity and criminal behaviour, which persisted into adulthood. The review suggested that neglect was at least as damaging as physical or sexual abuse.

A review of global research published on prevalence between January 1980 and January 2008 (Stoltenborgh et al. 2015) identified 244 publications covering 551 prevalence rates. The overall estimated prevalence rates for self-report studies (mainly assessing maltreatment during childhood) were 127/1000 for sexual abuse, 226/1000 for physical abuse, 363/1000 for emotional abuse, 163/1000 for physical neglect and 184/1000 for emotional neglect. In contrast the studies which analysed the rates where victims had made their abuse known to official agencies were just four per thousand for sexual abuse and a three per thousand for both physical and emotional abuse. The authors concluded that 'child maltreatment in all its forms is a global phenomenon of considerable extent, touching the lives of millions of children' (Stoltenborgh et al. 2015, p. 48) but that much of this is hidden from official view.

Research has consistently demonstrated that only a small number of incidents are ever reported to any agency (Sidebotham and The ACSPAC Study Team 2000; Reece 2016) and that such cases are often described as 'the tip of the iceberg' (Creighton 2004). Crucially there is very little evidence to suggest that those children who are harmed and injured would tell anyone and even less likely they would tell an official agency (see for example Tucker 2011; Wattam and Woodward 1996).

The most comprehensive research on the prevalence of child maltreatment in the UK was funded by the NSPCC and published in 2000 and 2011. The first study (Cawson et al. 2000) was based on a sample of 2689 18–24 year olds who were interviewed in 1998 about their childhood experiences in the late 1970s, 1980s and 1990s. The second study carried out 11 years later (Radford et al. 2011) involved randomly selected households across the UK. While the focus was children and young people aged 0–17, the sample also included 1761 young adults 18–24 to allow for comparison with the findings of the earlier survey by Cawson et al. (2000). For the 2160 children aged 0–10, parents or caregivers were interviewed as proxy reporters. 2275 children and young people aged 11–17 were also interviewed directly, together with a primary caregiver. The interviews were carried out in 2009. Because the 2000 and 2011 studies both excluded young people living in residential care, hostels or in custody, and parental consent was required for all those interviewed under 18, the findings almost certainly underestimated the amount of child abuse and neglect experienced. Even so, severe child maltreatment was reported as an experience for a substantial minority amounting to 25.3% of all the children, young people and young adults at some point in their lives (Radford et al. 2011) and included:

- Physical assault by an adult caregiver – 1.2% of under 11 year olds; 6.9% of 11–17 year olds; 11.5% of 18–24 year olds;
- Neglect – 5% of under 11 year olds; 13.3% of 11–17 year olds; 16% of 18–24 year olds;
- Contact sexual abuse as defined by the criminal law – 0.5% of under 11 year olds; 4.8% of 11–17 year olds; and 11.3% of 18–24 year olds;
- Sexual abuse which included non-contact offences was experienced by 1.2% of under 11 year olds; 16.5% of 11–17 year olds; 24.1% of 18–24 year olds; and
- Under the broad category of emotional abuse:
  - Exposure to domestic violence – 12% of under 11 year olds; 17.5% of 11–17 year olds; 23.7% of 18–24 year olds;
  - Other aspects of emotional abuse: 3.6% of under 11 year olds; 6.8% of 11–17 year olds; 6.9% of 18–24 year olds.

Radford et al. (2011) concluded that:

- There is a substantial minority of children and young people today who are severely maltreated and are experiencing abuse at home, in school and in the community, from adults and from peers. Almost 1 in 5 11-17s (18.6%), 1 in 4 18-24s (25.3%) and 1 in 17 (5.9%) under 11s had experienced severe maltreatment during their childhood (p. 118).

These figures compare with a total number 42,850 who were the subject of a child protection plan on 31 March 2012 (what in other jurisdictions may be called 'substantiated' cases) or 0.42% of the child population under the age of 18. The research by Radford et al. (2011) clearly confirms what Gilbert et al. (2009) and Stoltenborgh et al. (2015) established in their reviews of research that only a small proportion of abuse ever becomes known to official agencies and therefore is included in official statistics.

Another important finding from the research was that it was clear that child abuse did not only arise because of the actions of parents. In particular sexual abuse was perpetrated in a wide range of relationships and in a variety of different contexts but was usually perpetrated by those, usually men, who were known to the child or young person. 65.9% of the contact sexual abuse reported by the children and young people aged 0–17 was perpetrated by other children and young people under the age of 18. In fact it became clear, as was first demonstrated in the earlier research by Cawson et al. (2000), that victimisation by peers was a significant problem and was experienced by 28% of the children aged under 11, by 59.5% of the 11–17 year olds and by 63.2% of the 18–24 year olds. It seems that a high proportion of both physical assault and sexually harmful behaviour was being carried out by peers and siblings and may be seen in terms of bullying. Since children identify relationships with peers as equally as important as those with their families, bullying can have similar consequences to child maltreatment and bullying is widespread (James 2010).

The study by Radford et al. (2011) also underlined the important links between child maltreatment and certain social divisions, particularly in relation to gender and social class. While mothers/mother figures were responsible for marginally more abuse to under 11 s and slightly less abuse of 11–17 s than were fathers/father figures, males were the vast majority of perpetrators of domestic violence against another parent. Gender differences were also evident for severely maltreated young adults. Female 18–24 s reported significantly higher rates of severe maltreatment by a parent or guardian, with 17.5% having experienced this in childhood, compared to 11.6% of male 18–24 s. For specific types of maltreatment, males were the most frequently reported perpetrators and this was most evident for severe physical and contact sexual abuse. For those who reported severe physical violence by a parent or guardian, males were perpetrators in 86.4% of cases reported for the under 11 s, in 72.9% for 11–17 s, and 64.7% for 18–24 s. For those who reported having experienced contact sexual abuse by a parent or guardian around two-thirds of respondents reported a male as being the perpetrator. Gender clearly had a significant but far from straightforward relationship with child maltreatment.

Similarly social class was a complex but important factor in child maltreatment. For example, while 8.1% of those in social classes A-C2 reported neglect, 16% in social classes in D-E did so; 5.2% A-C2 reported regular verbal aggression compared to 8.6% D-E; 9% A-C2 any physical violence compared to 13.1 D-E; and 4.3% A-C2 coercive sexual acts compared to 7.2 D-E. While the prevalence of all forms of abuse seemed significantly greater in the lower social classes, the picture was complex. The 2000 prevalence study (Cawson et al. 2000) suggested there was a clear relationship between social group and physical discipline and abuse, with absence of care and with the more serious absence of supervision being evident, particularly being out all night at a young age. Absence of supervision at the less serious levels, however, were not particularly linked with socio-economic status and appeared to be an equal issue for all social groups. Sexual abuse and emotional abuse showed little differentiation between socio-economic groups.

Finally, while the amount of child abuse known to official agencies increased considerably from 1998 to 2009, a comparison of the two prevalence studies suggested there was an overall reduction in prevalence. The findings from the two representative samples of young adults aged 18–24 showed a decrease in reports of certain types of physical abuse (from 13.1% in 1998 to 9.8% in 2009), sexual abuse (6.8–5%), and verbal abuse (14.5–6%). There were no significant changes found in the prevalence of neglect (Radford et al. 2011).

Radford et al. concluded that the overall findings paint an optimistic picture, with a general decline in reported experiences of harsh and physical punishment by parents and caregivers, and also in the experiences of physical violence between 1998 and 2009. Furthermore, improvements for socially disadvantaged children had matched those for the rest of the population. They suggested that the improvements had arisen because of a number of factors, including: the impact of positive economic changes; public health measures, such as early intervention policies; and, more generally, changes in parental attitudes and behaviour, including a decline in the use of physical punishment of children and young people (Nuffield Foundation 2009). But clearly, child maltreatment was still experienced by a sizeable minority of children and these improvements had taken place in the 11 years prior to the economic crisis of 2008 and the major cutbacks in public expenditure from 2010 onwards in the UK.

Prevalence studies provide considerable insights into the nature and characteristics of child maltreatment and in the process have provided an important demographic picture of who in the population might be most at risk of both experiencing and perpetrating the problem. In the process the importance of developing public health approaches to child maltreatment is underlined.

27.3 A Public Health Approach

Gilbert et al. explicitly located their review of research in a public health approach:

> Maltreatment of children by their parents or other caregivers is a major public-health and social-welfare problem in high-income countries. It is common and can cause death, serious injury and long-term consequences that affect the child's life into adulthood, their family and society in general (Gilbert et al. 2009, p. 7).

The researchers were clearly highly sceptical of the ability of existing child protection systems to overcome child maltreatment, reinforced by the fact that there was absolutely no evidence that existing child protection systems made any impact on any of the child maltreatment indicators in six jurisdictions over a 30 year period

(Gilbert et al. 2012a, b). As with the study by Radford et al. (2011), Gilbert et al. based their approach on the 2006 World Health Organisation report on the prevention of child maltreatment (Butchart et al. 2006) which defined child maltreatment as:

> All forms of physical and/or emotional ill treatment, sexual abuse, neglect or negligent treatment or commercial or other exploitation, resulting in actual or potential harm to the child's health, survival development or dignity in the context of a relationship of responsibility, trust or power (Butchart et al. 2006, p. 9).

There are a number of key assumptions which inform a public health approach.

- First, epidemiology is seen as crucial as attempts to collect and analyse data on prevalence are seen as central to identify the factors which might differentiate geographical areas, social classes, ethnic groups, age groups, and other social divisions;
- Second, it is important to identify some of the key indicators and proxies for children's well-being so that these can be monitored and measured over time;
- Third, there is an emphasis on primary prevention and 'minimally sufficient' interventions which need to be available to all members of the community, in order to reduce risk and optimise the well-being of the total population of children and young people. It is assumed that a substantial percentage of the population will show signs of risk at some level and at some point in their life and that there is therefore a continuum of risk, along which a child's position may change over time;
- Fourth, the provision of universal primary prevention services potentially available to everyone is key but that these can be topped up for those in greater need as required; and
- Fifth, there is an important role for research and evaluation to: identify patterns including risk and protective factors; measure effectiveness; and aid the process of implementation.

As is evident in many of the chapters in this book the approach has received considerable international support in recent years and has increasingly come to inform policy and practice strategies in different countries. I also drew on a public health approach in *The Politics of Child Protection* (Parton 2014) for trying to develop the principals for overcoming the problems with the child protection system in England. However, I was also aware of some of the major problems and challenges of such approaches, particularly as these were implemented via the *Every Child Matters (ECM)* programme (Chief Secretary to the Treasury 2003) and which I have discussed further in Chap. 5 in this volume.

In particular, in emphasising the importance of intervening in problems early, integrating services and stressing the importance of professionals sharing a range of information the rights of both parents and children can be put at risk and there can be a considerable increase in state surveillance. There is a real danger that the focus becomes strengthening secondary and tertiary services and there can be a failure to recognise the importance of primary universal services and the central emphasis which needs to be given to 'minimally sufficient' interventions. I would argue that these are absolutely central issues for any serious attempts to develop public health policies and practices.

27.4 Social Harms and Structural Inequalities

In *The politics of child protection* (Parton 2014) I argued that to address these potential challenges it was important to recognise that the way child maltreatment is defined is central to the way it is recognised, managed and prevented and that most approaches are defined in terms of the physical, emotional and sexual violence or neglect perpetrated by individual adults, usually parents or those in a position of trust. Professional and societal responses are framed in terms of the protection of the child from adult perpetrators. In the process, such approaches do not permit any recognition of the collective harm and exploitation that can be caused by institutions, harmful policies and laws, conflicts, failure of governance and social disruption.

For many years I have been sympathetic to the definition developed over 40 years ago by David Gil in the light of his comprehensive demographic research carried out in 1967/68 of over 12,000 cases of children who had been physically abused and their parents in the USA. A sub-sample of 1380 of the parents was analysed for more detailed socio-economic data. Not only did the research demonstrate an over representation of those from a low socio-economic background, particularly from non-white families, but there were clear links between individual cases and wider social and economic structures (Gil 1970). Gil defined child maltreatment as:

> The inflicted gaps or deficits between the circumstances of living which would facilitate the optimum development of children, to which they should be entitled, and to their actual circumstances, irrespective of the sources or agents of the deficit (Gil 1975, p. 349).

As I argued in *The politics of child abuse*:

> Any act of commission or omission by individuals, institutions or the whole society, together with their resultant conditions, which deprive children of equal rights and liberties, and/or interfere with their optimal development, constitute, by definition, abuse or neglectful acts or conditions (Parton 1985, pp. 167–168).

Child maltreatment can therefore be manifested at both the institutional and societal levels as well as within families and with individuals. In the process the activities of certain institutions, such as schools, the church, processes of racial discrimination, social class exploitation, gender violence, and the role of government and global corporations are all potentially implicated. Of course since 1985 the issue of abuse in a variety of institutions has become well known.

A similarly wide and inclusive definition was adopted by *Childhood Matters: the Report of the National Commission of Inquiry into the Prevention of Child Abuse* in 1996:

> Child abuse consists of anything which individuals, institutions, or processes do or fail to do which directly or indirectly harms children or damages their prospects of safe and healthy development into adulthood (Childhood Matters 1996, para. 1.4).

UNICEF has promoted a children's rights approach to protecting children from 'all forms of violence' (UNICEF 2005) and the definition chosen for the UN's study of violence against children (Pinheiro 2006) follows article 19 of the UNCRC that includes "all forms of physical or mental violence, injury and abuse, neglect or negligent treatment, maltreatment or exploitation, including sexual abuse". It bases its understanding of physical violence on the definition in the world report on violence and health:

> The intentional use of physical force or power, threatened or actual, against a child, by an individual or group, that either results in or has a high likelihood of resulting in actual or potential harm to the child's health, survival, development or dignity' (Krug et al. 2002, p. 5).

Such approaches are clearly consistent with a view that violations of basic human rights constitute 'social harms'. These can be made up of physical, financial/economic, emotional, psychological and sexual harms. It includes the idea of 'cultural safety' which encompasses notions of autonomy, development and growth, and access to cultural, intellectual and information resources generally available in any given society (see Chap. 20 in this volume).

Such ideas have been furthered in recent years with emergence of a new field of study called *zemiology* (derived from the Greek word for harm – *xemia*) which has as its focus the study of *social harm* (Hillyard et al. 2004; Dorling et al. 2008; Roberts 2009; Yar 2012; Pemberton 2015). Where:

> Social harm acts as shorthand to reflect the relations, processes, flows, practices, discourse, actions, and inactions that constitute the fabric of our societies which serve to compromise the fulfilment of human needs and in doing so result in identifiable harms (Pemberton 2015, p. 24).

Crucially such harms are considered to encompass *avoidable* events; they are *preventable* insofar as they are potentially subject to organised human control and grounded in alterable social relations.

A *social harm* perspective takes into account corporate and collective responsibility, together with the activities of the state and focuses on structures of inequality, exploitation and vulnerability. It has a particular concern with trying to produce greater social justice. For example, Wild and others (Wild 2013) have argued that corporate exploitation of children and childhood in terms of a whole variety of unhealthy mass produced and massively advertised products, such as unhealthy foods, material goods, and pornography, have created new forms of child abuse.

A good example of a 'social harms' approach is the research carried out by Danny Dorling who analysed the 13,000 murders committed in Britain between January 1981 and December 2000 (Dorling 2004). He treated murder as a Durkheimian social fact and, therefore, much more than a series of individual acts and related the data to social structures and social change. He demonstrated that the majority of murders were concentrated in the poor parts of Britain. He showed that in the 5 years 1981–85, people living in the poorest 10% of wards in Britain were four and a half times more likely to be murdered than those living in the least poor 10%. This differential increased further in each successive 5-year period, as poverty and, crucially, inequality increased. As a consequence despite the national doubling of the murder rate by 1996–2000, people living in the least poor 20% of the country saw their already low rate of murder fall further. The increase in murder was concentrated almost exclusively in the poorer parts of Britain and most strongly in the poorest tenth of wards – and it was knives, broken glass/bottles and fights which were most important.

It was amongst men born in 1965 and after where the murder rate increased the most with age. As Dorling pointed out, most of these men left school in the summer of 1981, which was the first summer for over 40 years that a young man living in a poor area would find work or training very scarce. The situation got steadily worse as the then Conservative government pursued a neoliberal economic agenda, which decimated the manufacturing sector in Britain. He argued that "murders are placed at the tip of this pyramid of social harm and their changing numbers and distributions provide one of the key clues as to where harm is most and least distributed" (Dorling 2004, p. 191).

The work of Richard Wilkinson (1996, 2005) writing with Kate Pickett (Pickett and Wilkinson 2007; Wilkinson and Pickett 2009) is particularly important in helping us understand the impact of inequality on health and violence in society and why societies that have become more unequal also have the poorest relative levels of child well-being (UNICEF 2007; Mapp 2011). They accumulated a range of evidence to demonstrate that it is material inequality rather than poverty *per se* which is the key factor in understanding the differences in health and violence in society, including how these are reflected in children's well-being. Societies which are poorer but more egalitarian have relatively high levels of good health and less violence because of a higher degree of social cohesion. The *relative* distribution of income, wealth and lifestyle were identified as central factors in influencing an individual's sense of worth and whether they felt valued together with the key mediating role of *social capital* (Szreter and Woolcock 2003). Societies that were becoming wealthier but more unequal, for example the USA and the UK, performed poorly as a result.

Wilkinson and Pickett (2009) argued that in more equal societies:

- There were stronger bonds between people;
- Public space was treated more as social space;
- There was more involvement in social and voluntary activities outside the home and in civic society more generally;
- There was less aggressive behaviour;
- There was evidence of higher self-esteem; and
- There was less stress, insecurity and depression.

The countries which have consistently performed the best in terms of the regular UNICEF assessments of inequality in child well-being in rich countries are from the more social democratically organised countries of Scandinavia – particularly Denmark, Finland and Norway (UNICEF 2016).

There is also clear evidence of a cultural shift towards an emphasis on competitive individualism in many societies which clearly contributes to a poor sense of well-being amongst children and young people (Layard and Dunn 2009; Utting 2009) and where social inequality and its negative impact has increased over the last 30 years (Lansley 2012; OECD 2011). For example, it is now well established that intergenerational social mobility is much reduced by greater levels of inequality (Krueger 2012; Social Mobility Commission 2017).

More specifically in relation to child maltreatment, there is a substantial body of evidence demonstrating a strong association between family poverty and the likelihood of a child experiencing child maltreatment, though clearly this is neither a necessary nor a sufficient factor on its own. As Pelton concluded in a review of over 30 years of studies 'there is overwhelming evidence that poverty and low income are strongly related to child abuse and neglect as well as to the severity of maltreatment' (Pelton 2015, p. 30). Just as in child health and education (Donkin et al. 2014) there is a social gradient in child maltreatment so that at each incremental increase in family socio-economic disadvantage there is a disproportionate increase in the chances of a child experiencing maltreatment (Beimers and Coulton 2011; Berger and Waldfogel 2011; Bywaters et al. 2016; McDaniel and Slack 2005).

While there is considerable evidence of a clear relationship between inequality and the levels of violence in society the issue of how inequality is generated is also important (Ray 2011). For example, Savolainen (2000) and Messner et al. (2008) argued that the effect of economic inequality on the level of lethal violence is limited to nations characterised by relatively weak collective institutions of social protection such as welfare states. It is argued that societies in which the economic market is dominant increases social marginalisation and violence, loss of social bonds, egoistic individualism, loss of empathy and high risk taking – all of which are conducive to higher levels of violence. Such arguments support Pembeeton's contention (2015) that *solidaristic societies* – based on a social democratic state model where there are high levels of public services, high levels of trust are exhibited and there are low levels of inequality – offer the best protections against *social harms*. Whereas neoliberal regimes, characterised by deregulated markets, residual welfare systems and highly individualised and fragmented societies offer the least protections against *social harms*. However, we cannot assume that such an approach is appropriate for all dimensions of child maltreatment – particularly sexual abuse. Keith Pringle (2005, 2010) has argued that while Nordic welfare systems may have a positive impact on forms of child maltreatment associated with poverty and class inequality, via their more collectivist/solidaristic approach, this is not necessarily appropriate for other forms of maltreatment. Such systems are much less concerned with what Pringle (2005, 2010) calls 'bodily integrity or citizenship' where issues associated with sexual violence are central.

27.5 Conclusions

What I am arguing is that a public health approach which is serious about addressing *social harms* provides the most positive framework for developing policy and practice. In doing so we need to recognise that child maltreatment has cultural, institutional and structural dimensions as well as individual ones and that these must be taken seriously and addressed. Similarly it is also vital that approaches informed by a public health model are not simply imposed from above. It is important to recognise the key role of a whole variety of community-based and user-led groups and initiatives (see for example Colclough et al. 1999; Pasura et al. 2013), and that local communities are actively involved in the development of policies and services (Jack and Gill 2010) in the way promoted by Freymond and Cameron (2006).

What this analysis suggests is that the way society is *organised* is the essential ingredient for minimising *social harms* and thereby addressing the *social problem* of child maltreatment. The success of any public health approach is crucially dependent on the broad range of social policies in which it is located and the nature of the welfare regime in which it operates.

References

Beimers, D., & Coulton, C. (2011). Do employment and type of exit influence child maltreatment among families leaving temporary assistance for needy families. *Children and Youth Services Review, 33*(7), 1112–1119.

Berger, L. M., & Waldfogel, J. (2011). *Economic determinants and consequences of child maltreatment.* OECD Social, employment and migration working paper no. 111. Washington: OECD Publishing.

Butchart, A., Kahane, T., Phinney Harvey, A., & World Health Organization. (2006). *Preventing child maltreatment: A guide to taking action and generating evidence*. Geneva: WHO/ International Society for the Prevention of Child Abuse and Neglect.

Bywaters, P., Bunting, L., Davidson, G., Hanratty, J., Mason, W., McCarten, C., & Steils, N. (2016). *The relationship between poverty, child abuse and neglect, an evidence review*. York: Joseph Rowntree Foundation.

Cawson, P., Wattam, C., Brooker, S., & Kelly, G. (2000). *Child maltreatment in the UK: A study of the prevalence of child abuse and neglect*. London: NSPCC.

Chief Secretary to the Treasury. (2003). *Every child matters*. Cm. 5860. London: Stationary Office.

Childhood Matters: Report of the National Commission of Inquiry into the Prevention of Child Abuse. (1996). Volumes 1 and 2. London: The Stationery Office.

Colclough, L., Parton, N., & Anslow, M. (1999). Family support. In N. Parton & C. Wattam (Eds.), *Child sexual abuse: Responding to the experiences of children*. Chichester: Wiley/NSPCC.

Creighton, S. (2004). *Prevalence and incidence of child abuse: International comparisons.* London: NSPCC.

Donkin, A., Roberts, J., Tedstone, A., & Marmot, M. (2014). Family socio-economic status and young children's outcomes. *Journal of Children's Services, 9*(2), 83–95.

Dorling, D. (2004). Prime suspect: Murder in Britain. In P. Hillyard, C. Pantazis, S. Tombs, & D. Gordon (Eds.), *Beyond criminology: Taking harm seriously*. London: Pluto Press.

Dorling, D., Gordon, D., Hillyard, P., Pantazis, C., Pemberton, S., & Tombs, S. (2008). *Criminal obsessions: Why harm matters more than crime* (2nd ed.). London: Centre for Crime and Justice Studies, King's College.

Freymond, N., & Cameron, C. (Eds.). (2006). *Towards positive systems of child and family welfare: International comparisons of child protection, family service and community caring*. Toronto: University of Toronto Press.

Gainsborough, J. F. (2010). *Scandalous politics: Child welfare politics in the states*. Washington DC: Georgetown University Press.

Gil, D. (1970). *Violence against children*. Cambridge: Harvard University Press.

Gil, D. (1975). Unravelling child abuse. *American Journal of Orthopsychiatry, 45*(3), 346–356.

Gilbert, R., Widom, C. P., Browne, K., Ferguson, D., Webb, E., & Janson, S. (2009). Burden and consequences of child maltreatment in high-income countries. *The Lancet, 373*(9657), 68–81.

Gilbert, R., Woodman, J., & Logan, S. (2012a). Developing services for a public health approach to child maltreatment. *International Journal of Children's Rights, 20*(3), 323–343.

Gilbert, R., Fluke, J., O'Donnell, M., Gonzallez-Izquierdo, A., Brownell, M., Gulliver, P., Jansen, S., & Sidebotham, P. (2012b). Child maltreatment: Variation in trends in six developed countries. *The Lancet, 379*(9817), 758–772.

Hillyard, P., Panazasis, C., Tombs, S., & Gordon, D. (Eds.). (2004). *Beyond criminology: Taking crime seriously*. London: Pluto Press.

Jack, G., & Gill, O. (2010). The role of communities in safeguarding children and young people. *Child Abuse Review, 19*(2), 82–96.

James, A. (2010). *School bullying: Research briefing*. London: NSPCC.

Krueger, A. (2012). *The economic report of the president and the annual report of economic advisors*. Washington, DC: US Government Printing Office.

Krug, E. J., Dahlberg, L. L., & Mercy, J. A. (2002). *World report on violence and health*. Geneva: WHO.

Lansley, S. (2012). *The cost of inequality: Why equality is essential*. London: Gibson Square.

Layard, R., & Dunn, J. (2009). *A good childhood: Searching for values in a competitive age*. London: Children's Society/Penguin.

Lonne, B., Parton, N., Thomson, J., & Harries, M. (2009). *Reforming child protection*. London: Routledge.

Mapp, S. C. (2011). *Global child welfare and well-being*. New York: Oxford University Press.

McDaniel, M., & Slack, K. S. (2005). Major life events and the risk of child maltreatment investigation. *Children and Youth Services Review, 27*(2), 171–195.

Melton, G. (2005). Mandated reporting: A policy without a reason. *Child Abuse and Neglect, 25*(1), 9–18.

Messner, S. F., Thome, H., & Rosenfeld, R. (2008). Institutions, anomie and violent crime: Clarifying and elaborating institutional-anomie theory. *International Journal of Conflict and Violence, 2*(2), 163–181.

Nuffield Foundation. (2009). *Time trends in parenting and outcomes for young people*. London: Nuffield Foundation.

OECD. (2011). *Divided we stand: Why inequality keeps rising*. Paris: OECD.

Parton, N. (1985). *The politics of child abuse*. Basingstoke: Palgrave/Macmillan.

Parton, N. (2014). *The politics of child protection: Contemporary developments and future directions*. Basingstoke: Palgrave/Macmillan.

Pasura, D., Jones, A., & Da Breo, H. (2013). IMPACT: Interventions and mitigations to prevent the abuse of children – it's time. A public health oriented systems model for change. In A. Jones (Ed.), *Understanding child sexual abuse: Perspectives from the Caribbean*. Basingstoke: Palgrave/Macmillan.

Pelton, L. (2015). The continuing role of material factors in child maltreatment and placement. *Child Abuse and Neglect, 41*(1), 30–39.

Pemberton, S. (2015). *Harmful societies: Understanding social harm*. Bristol: Policy Press.

Pickett, K., & Wilkinson, R. G. (2007). Child wellbeing and income inequality in rich societies: Ecological cross sectional study. *British Medical Journal, 335*(7629), 1080–1087.

Pinheiro, P. S. (2006). *World report on violence against children*. Geneva: UN.
Pringle, K. (2005). Neglected issues in Swedish child protection policy and practice: Age, ethnicity and gender. In M. Erikson, M. Hester, S. Keskinen, & K. Pringle (Eds.), *Tackling men's violence in families: Nordic issues and dilemmas*. Bristol: Policy Press.
Pringle, K. (2010). Epilogue: On developing empowering child welfare systems and the welfare research needed to create them. In H. Forsberg & T. Kroger (Eds.), *Social work and child welfare politics: Through Nordic lenses*. Bristol: Policy Press.
Radford, L., Corral, S., Bradley, C., Fisher, H., Bassett, C., Howat, N., & Collishaw, S. (2011). *Child abuse and neglect in the UK today*. London: NSPCC.
Ray, L. (2011). *Violence and society*. London: Sage.
Reece, G. (2016). Child maltreatment. In J. Bradshaw (Ed.), *The Well-being of children in the UK* (4th ed.). Bristol: Policy Press.
Roberts, D. (2009). *Social harm and crime at a global level*. London: Centre for Crime and Justice Studies.
Savolainen, J. (2000). Inequality, welfare state and homicide: Further support for the institutional anomie theory. *Criminology, 38*(4), 1021–1042.
Sidebotham, P., & The ACSPAC Study Team. (2000). Patterns of child abuse in early childhood: A cohort study of the 'children of the nineties'. *Child Abuse Review, 9*(5), 311–320.
Social Mobility Commission. (2017). *Time for change: An assessment of government policies on social mobility 1997–2017*. London: The Social Mobility Commission.
Stoltenborgh, M., Bakermns-Kranenburg, M. J., Alink, L. R. A., & van Ijzendoorn, M. H. (2015). The prevalence of child maltreatment across the globe: Review of a series of meta-analyses. *Child Abuse Review, 24*(1), 37–50.
Szreter, S., & Woolcock, M. (2003). Health by association? Social capital, social theory and the political economy of public health. *International Journal of Epidemiology, 33*, 1–18.
Tucker, S. (2011). Listening and believing: An examination of young people's perceptions of why they are not believed by professionals when they report abuse and neglect. *Children and Society, 25*(6), 458–469.
UNICEF. (2005). *Council of Europe actions to promote children's rights to protection from all forms of violence*. Florence: UNICEF Innocenti Research Centre.
UNICEF. (2007). *Child poverty in perspective: An overview of child-wellbeing in rich countries,* Innocenti report card 7. Florence: Innocenti Research Centre.
UNICEF. (2016). *Fairness for children: A league table of inequality in child-wellbeing in rich countries*. Innocenti report card 13. Children in the developed world. Florence: UNICEF.
Utting, D. (Ed.). (2009). *Contemporary social evils*. Bristol: Policy Press/Joseph Rowntree Foundation.
Waldfogel, J. (1998). *The future of child protection: How to break the cycle of abuse and neglect*. Cambridge, MA: Harvard University Press.
Warner, J. (2015). *The emotional politics of social work and child protection*. Bristol: Policy Press.
Wattam, C., & Woodward, C. (1996) '… And do I abuse my children? No! Learning about prevention from people who have experienced child abuse. *Childhood matters: Report of the National Commission of inquiry into the prevention of child abuse*. Vol. 2: Background papers. London: TSO.
Wild, J. (Ed.). (2013). *Exploiting childhood: How fast food, material obsession and porn culture are creating new forms of child abuse*. London: Jessica Kingsley.
Wilkinson, R. G. (1996). *Unhealthy societies: The afflictions of inequality*. London: Routledge.
Wilkinson, R. G. (2005). *The impact of inequality: How to make sick societies healthy*. London: Routledge.
Wilkinson, R. G., & Pickett, K. (2009). *The spirit level: Why more equal societies almost always do better*. London: Allen Lane.
Yar, M. (2012). Critical criminology, critical theory and social harm. In S. Hall & S. Winlow (Eds.), *New directions in criminological theory*. London: Routledge.

Chapter 28
New Directions for Public Health Approaches: Key Themes and Issues

Todd I. Herrenkohl, Bob Lonne, Debbie Scott, and Daryl Higgins

28.1 Introduction

Authors in this volume call for reform of child protection (CP) systems that refocuses services on prevention and early intervention grounded in a public health framework. The goal is to reach families in need of support well before problems worsen and potentially become intractable and resistant to change. The public health model stresses the importance of universal, 'whole-of population' level efforts (Higgins et al. Chap. 1 in this volume) that seek to lessen risk factors for child maltreatment and to promote protective factors that enhance the well-being of all children, including those who are more vulnerable to child maltreatment and associated outcomes because of the effects of poverty (see Klevens and Metzler Chap. 13 and Bywaters Chap. 17 in this volume).

The public health model calls for comprehensive reform of an outdated CP system that increasingly stigmatizes and punishes families who require assistance from public agencies. Authors argue that reform across a broad scale can reduce

T. I. Herrenkohl (✉)
University of Michigan School of Social Work, Ann Arbor, MI, USA
e-mail: tih@umich.edu

B. Lonne
School of Health, University of New England, Armidale, NSW, Australia
e-mail: blonne@une.edu.au

D. Scott
Monash University, Richmond, VIC, Australia
e-mail: debbie.scott@monash.edu

D. Higgins
Institute of Child Protection Studies, Australian Catholic University, Melbourne, VIC, Australia
e-mail: daryl.higgins@acu.edu.au

B. Lonne et al. (eds.), *Re-Visioning Public Health Approaches for Protecting Children*, Child Maltreatment 9, https://doi.org/10.1007/978-3-030-05858-6_28

disproportionality and systemic marginalization and racism, which has been well-documented in CP internationally. There are significant issues with regard to the ethics of current risk-saturated and avoidant policy and practice frameworks that drive CP and fall disproportionally upon particular groups who have long been overrepresented in contact with these systems and who show the intergenerational impacts of this (see Duthie and colleagues Chap. 20 in this volume).

Arguably, public health approaches provide a critical way to reform and re-calibrate CP approaches, particularly regarding the humane treatment of families who are marginalized and struggling, and with respect to children in out-of-home care whose issues are highlighted in Chaps. 2 and 3 in this volume. Featherstone et al. (2014), and Lonne et al. (2016) have highlighted how the (mis)use of power with vulnerable groups and families reflects on many levels the individual focus of child protection that allocates almost total responsibility to parents and downplays or ignores the structural factors at play, and the neoliberal underpinnings of many contemporary social welfare policies. Families who often have significant issues with alcohol and drug abuse, family and domestic violence, disability and poverty can find that the interventions they receive do not readily provide tangible assistance and support to address these. Rather, they can find themselves immobilized by forceful directions to provide a level of care that appears out of reach in the short time frames demanded by the interveners. Removal of children in these situations, while providing immediate safety, can result in their permanent separation and many years in out-of-home care which sometimes entails numerous placements and poor life outcomes. Unfortunately this can end up as a state intervention that leaves no one better off.

28.2 The Limitations of Child Protection

The history of CP shows that many groups who are overrepresented have high support needs and require longer intervention periods to address the significant life issues they encounter in their daily lives. Yet, regrettably, much of CP uses case management approaches that embrace very short-term intervention timeframes, with removal seen as the option when families are hostile toward ongoing involvement with state authorities.

Current policies and practices within CP disadvantage Indigenous children and children of color, who are both overrepresented and underserved. Responding to child maltreatment within a public health paradigm requires actions to address how economic, social and environmental factors influence not only the incidence of maltreatment but also the inequitable distribution of maltreatment (see for example Chaps. 13 and 17 in this volume). Because proportionally more Indigenous children and children of color involved with CP also live in poverty, their needs are complex and systems that include CP are poorly equipped to respond in turn (see Chaps. 2 and 12 in this volume). Further, authors (e.g., Duthie et al. Chap. 20) note that Indigenous and First-Nations families are disproportionately impacted by a CP system that is "founded in European or Western worldviews," which they and others believe perpetuate racist and discriminatory practices and policies that add to the burden of risk encountered by Indigenous peoples. It is important to recognize that inter-generational trauma is present for many of these groups, and that continual removal of their children by the state perpetuates this trauma cycle. Different approaches are therefore needed. Unsurprisingly, there is evidence that CP approaches have led to distrust within Aboriginalcommunities and fear of statutory protective interventions (Newton 2017).

As noted by Higgins et al. (Chap. 1), CP has become narrow in its mission and limited in its approach, primarily managing the highest risk families to avoid serious harm befalling vulnerable children. CP involvement comes too late to address the factors that impinge on the functioning of families. Instead, services are, as Higgins et al. suggest, forensically oriented – meaning that the focus is mainly on investigating and prosecuting crimes of mistreatment. Recent noteworthy incidents of children who are harmed while under the watchful eye of CP workers have highlighted notable gaps and oversights in case planning that have degraded trust in the system and have led to outcries by the public to hold CP workers accountable. It is an understandable reaction to a tragic series of events. However, CP workers are also victims of a system in decline and disarray (see for example Chaps. 2 and 15 in this volume). According to Higgins et al., "Statutory child protection services are overwhelmed, and have over-grown their intended purpose, and many would argue are at risk of failing to deliver well enough on the aims they have espoused."

In Part I, the authors address in detail the significant shortcomings that befall contemporary child protection systems, with many service users not experiencing satisfactory outcomes. Buckley and colleagues (Chap. 2) have drawn on numerous studies to highlight that many service users including parents and children, as well as staff, can find that the relationships they experience with others in the system are not facilitative toward change, and their experiences are stigmatizing and blaming. Conley Wright and Kaltner (Chap. 3) closely examine out-of-home care and conclude that public health approaches offer much potential in evaluating the outcomes for children in more systematic ways whereas at present this is haphazard. Parton and Williams (Chap. 4) use their recent research to understand how community members conceptualise neglect. They critically examine the implications for public education strategies and community mobilization approaches to enlist the support and assistance of citizens to assist vulnerable families and children in need.

A 2015 Springer publication *Mandatory reporting laws and the identification of severe child abuse and neglect* evidenced how mandatory reporting is a contested policy and one which has some intended consequences (identification, quantification and protection of children at risk of harm) as well as some unintended and unwelcome ones (fear of seeking help by some families and net widening, along with mistrust in system responses by mandated reporters) (see also Sedlack and Ellis 2014). Importantly, in regard to the development of public health approaches, the institutional success of mandatory reporting can place hindrances upon the propensity of key stakeholders within health, education, and other systems, to embrace active referral processes for community-based supports for struggling families. Yet, a public health system for protecting children from maltreatment relies upon an ability of various professionals and organizations being able to refer and pass on information so that families and children can receive the help they need when they need it, and in ways that encourage them to access assistance free from stigmatization. Hence, the policy framework of public health needs to resolve the practice and legal tensions that currently exist in CP particularly with respect to human rights of various parties (see Bross and Mathews Chap. 18 in this volume). Differential responses appear to have a particular relevance with regard to these vexed issues and may well provide a set of institutional and organizational arrangements that can provide targeted assistance (See Merkel-Holguin et al. Chap. 12) in combination with universal services that underpin a public health approach (see Daro and Karter Chap. 8).

Costs of maintaining CP services, as they are, are unsustainable. Because children who enter the CP system stay in care longer, fewer children are served but costs are problematically high – and they are climbing higher. At the same time, it is unknown whether children who enter CP actually benefit beyond being extracted from an unsafe home environment. CP lacks a robust infrastructure for evaluation and it has been slow to embrace the use of evidence-based programs and practices (Jonson-Reid and Chiang Chap. 21), leading to accusations that the system is wasteful and ineffective. This seems to be a critical issue with respect to moving toward a public health approach, which embraces as foundational the embedding of robust data systems and evaluations of intervention efficacy (see Runyan and Runyan Chap. 6, and Scott and Faulkner Chap. 16). Trocmé and colleagues (see Chap. 25) have highlighted the complexities and difficulties inherent when trying to implant research and evaluation methodologies within existing child protection administrative data systems. Yet, it seems inexplicable that, given the huge social investments, there is little by way of robust program or system evaluation of CP systems that have been around for decades, and seem to continually introduce new programs of intervention and services for ameliorating risk of harm, but without much evidence of effectiveness or success. Within this context for CP systems, Merkel-Holguin et al. (Chap. 12) highlight that hostile debates around extending differential responses have been unhelpful to overall system development, and may indeed hinder the development of innovation for public health approaches.

28.3 Promoting Systems Change/Reforming the System

With concerns as heightened as they are, it is surprising that changes within CP have not come about more rapidly. Authors touch on several reasons why. One reason is financial; there is simply too little money made available by government agencies to bring about reform that will change the system as we know it. Added to that are the politics around government 'intrusion' on the privacy of families (see Higgins et al. Chap. 9). Efforts at reform have been slowed or blocked altogether by strong and prevailing beliefs about the privacy of families and hard resistance to the idea of having government agencies become even more involved in the care of children. The use of evermore sophisticated ICT to expand social surveillance, particularly for 'troublesome' groups and communities has fostered broader concerns about the role of the state and its data collection systems in combatting child maltreatment (see Parton Chap. 5 and Gray and Schubert Chap. 14). Further, some believe that the current system preserves a deeply rooted model of Colonization and domination that has historically advantaged the needs of some over others (Duthie et al. Chap. 20).

Gray and Schubert (Chap. 14) outline that there are a number of limitations and challenges with public health approaches to preventing child maltreatment. For example, they highlight that public health approaches utilise conceptualizations of risk in order to target interventions at various levels, yet for impoverished communities this may well entail or be perceived as increased social surveillance of people who are highly vulnerable and in desperate need of assistance. They question the extent to which public health approaches that utilize whole of population strategies can be truly effective in providing necessary social and emotional supports to groups who perceive themselves to be 'targeted' by risk-saturated and punitive CP systems that must be a part of a system-wide reform and re-calibration. In Chap. 5 Parton notes the criticality of having the social determinants of health as central to public health approaches but notes how conceptions of risk have altered over time to become dominant within the context of increasingly neoliberal policy frameworks that emphasize individual rather than collective responsibilities.

In Chap. 28 Parton argues that where public health approaches have been introduced they have often not addressed the key social and structural dimensions to the problem of child maltreatment and its associations with poverty and inequality (see also Klevens and Metzler Chap. 13 and Bywaters Chap. 17). He posits that children's well-being and overall social capital will be improved in public health approaches by integrating a children's rights perspective within them that attends to the "wide-spread *social harms* to children." Hence, public health approaches should not be seen as a panacea but, rather, an important development in the quest to eradicate child maltreatment and do so with ethical measures and practice.

28.4 Public Health Model

The public health model positions services along a continuum, with universal programs as the first level of engagement. The model supports an 'upstream' approach that locates evidence-based prevention programs and practices centrally. Primary prevention focuses on eradicating risk factors for child maltreatment before they enter the child welfare system and relies on "universal" strategies that reach all segments of a population. These are foundational to a public health model, yet they often remain under resourced by governments despite their established benefits (See Daro and Karter Chap. 8). Secondary prevention focuses on reducing risk levels in segments of a population that are more vulnerable and at higher risk for child maltreatment. And, tertiary prevention involves strategies to lessen the recurrence of abuse and neglect among child victims. The current structure of CP is more aligned to tertiary approaches than to primary or secondary prevention, but a public health model is reliant for its success upon the integration of all three levels of response.

Adopting a public health model helps to address the limitations of the current system because it fundamentally changes how services are conceptualized and delivered. Embracing Bronfenbrenner's (1979) ecological systems theory, public health approaches conceptualise societies and communities, and the citizens within them, as being deeply relational and interconnected. Different system levels function using rules, norms and roles to enable people to meet their various needs from a variety of sources, with support being fashioned in accessible and timely ways. Whereas the goal of a reactive system is to protect children at the last possible point before removal is imminent, a primary prevention focus turns attention to upstream approaches that engage families far earlier, before children are in danger. The model supports proactive strategies over reactive measures and places an emphasis on universal programs, followed by those geared to subgroups of the population in need of more intensive intervention (Herrenkohl et al. 2015). Because universal programs apply to all families, there is less stigma attached to services that are received, and there are more ways to help families rebound and return to a higher level of functioning (see Daro and Karter Chap. 8), but nonetheless there are major issues faced in trying to build cohesive systems where universal services are well integrated with secondary and tertiary ones – this remains as a critical obstacle to the introduction of effective public health approaches (see Harries and O'Donnell Chap. 15).

Authors draw on different aspects of the public health model in Chaps. 5–22. They discuss how a public health model can better serve the needs of children and families – and also the obstacles that stand in the way of reforming CP to align with the model. The key elements are a population perspective, a focus on primary prevention, and interventions that rely on evidence and attempt to solve the root causes of problems through large-scale social change, all underpinned by a embedding evaluation of approaches so that service responses are evidence-based. Runyan and Runyan (Chap. 6) propose the use of an injury prevention model, Haddon's Matrix, to clearly articulate primary, secondary and tertiary responses, and which enables well conceptualized and clearly targeted programmatic responses to be delivered and integrated within the whole system. Herrenkohl and Klika posit that the study of risk and protective factors are central to increasing capability of services to adequately response to the polyvictimization that many maltreated children experience (see Chap. 7).

Moreover, because of its multi-pronged capabilities, a public health model provides opportunities for a variety of innovative intervention approaches. For example, Quadara (Chap. 10), Walsh (Chap. 22), and Kaufman and colleagues (Chap. 11) outline population-level strategies for preventing child sexual abuse as well as organizational and situation prevention programs to protect children from egregious sexual assaults and other maltreatment that impacts their well-being. Taussig and Weigler (Chaps. 19) extend these sorts of innovative approaches further and focus upon mentoring for youth in foster care, arguing that, done well, these evidence-based programs have much to offer regarding prevention of the sometimes poor outcomes for alumni of the care system.

Merkel-Holguin et al. (Chap. 12) introduce the idea of 'differential response' (DR), an approach that allows discretion in the provision of services when allegations of child abuse and neglect are made. The authors argue that DR can serve the goal of advancing public health prevention by placing resources in services focused on low and moderate risk families, while also attending to the needs of those at higher levels of risks. DR grew out of a concern about the growing number of cases reported to CPS and the awareness that many reports do not require the resources of a full investigation. DR is thought to increase transparency in CPS decisions, prioritizing support of families over punishment. The authors suggest that DR "embodies" principles of early intervention that align with a public health model, including an emphasis on social support and providing non-stigmatizing services to help parents succeed in their caregiving responsibilities. Importantly they argue that DR provides an evidence-based approach that can be foundational to rolling out a broader preventive and early intervention system, and that this can provide an institutional basis for service delivery that enables CP organizations to operate as a residual program for high-risk cases rather than diverting its focus on investigating matters that do not require a statutory forensically-oriented intervention.

Daro and Karter (Chap. 8) argue for a strategy that strongly emphasizes universal services, noting that targeted interventions for families at high risk have not always worked well, and have generally failed to establish conclusive efficacy. This strategy of universalism should, according to the authors, focus on "raising awareness around a common need or shared concern and providing a mechanism to ensure families are provided access to the level of support they require." This theme is also built upon by Bross and Mathews (Chap. 18) who detail the success of historical public health approaches and detail its application in the area of child maltreatment, and how legal foundations are necessary for ongoing system reform.

Moving to a universal model will improve outcomes for families, contain costs, and reduce stigma for those who are served. Indeed, universal service systems are the bedrock upon which public health approaches are founded. This approach assumes that all children can benefit from a stronger and more deliberate engagement of the community in their care and well-being. As we have noted elsewhere, this appears to be a largely undeveloped aspect of public health approaches, yet there is growing empirical evidence of how informal helping networks can provide robust, timely and non-stigmatizing support to families and children in need (Holland 2014; Molnar and Beardslee 2015; Scott et al. 2016).

Harries and O'Donnell (Chap. 15) emphasize the need for coordination across service sectors to align with a vision for public health prevention. This, according to these authors, will require a "culture shift" in service planning that engages families differently. Here, government agencies and community organization work collaboratively to design and implement services that meet the needs of families locally. They explain that an overhaul of the child welfare system requires organizational changes that re-orient services to this new model and also a restructuring of roles that allow for a more integrated system oriented to universal approaches. Klevens and Metzler (Chap. 13) propose a more radical approach that targets the "conditions and contexts" that increase child maltreatment. The authors encourage a dual emphasis on increasing prevention efforts while also working to make systems more responsive and dedicated to the needs of vulnerable children and families. They view community organizing and partnerships between public health and grassroots organizations as helping to further this cause.

Drawing on data from the UK, Bywaters (Chap. 17) focuses on a similar set of issues. He attends to neighbourhood structural and social factors that drive disparities and undermine the functioning of poor families. He calls for a focus on primary, secondary and tertiary prevention, while also underscoring the need for more research that differentiates cause from correlation so that programs can target the most salient risks. His work here attests to the history of CP and its non-use of available data to identify the salient and underpinning associations of maltreatment within impoverished communities in England. However, this point also applies to many other jurisdictions where the social determinants of health data and analysis is typically given scant attention when developing programs and services aimed at reducing maltreatment prevalence and incidence.

Within the latter chapters in Part III, a number of countries' initiatives are outlined, including Australia, Canada and Ireland (see Chaps. 15, 24 and 23). Norway's situation is also outlined, (see Chap. 26) albeit from the perspective of a country that has a very well-developed early intervention and prevention approach. Norway is trying to attend to the limitations of this by putting increased emphasis upon statutory capacity to ensure that family environments that pose significant risk for children are addressed within a framework that provides necessary protective measures, particularly for adolescent children. Canavan and colleagues (Chap. 23 in this volume) provide a detailed outline of Ireland's major reforms towards an early intervention and prevention system, but also describe the challenges in addressing system and community complexity and how developing an overarching data collection and evaluation framework is fraught within a dynamic and evolving policy environment.

From a different cultural and social perspective Barraclough et al. (Chap. 24) describe the reform of Alberta's CP system to incorporate a range of different approaches that promote community-based programs to deliver support and assistance, including practice models that enable CP staff to work collaboratively within Indigenous communities. Their account illustrates a central principle of this book: That each jurisdiction has its own unique history, cultural, social, institutional and political environment and that public health systems, and for that matter CP systems, must be congruent with the local context. But still, there are some common elements as Trocmé and colleagues show (Chap. 25) with their sharing of how embedding a culture of data collection, evaluation and utilisation of the available evidence is quite difficult, and takes time to develop. Although their chapter concerns their longstanding work in Canada including the Canadian Incidence Study, the issues they highlight could also be found in many other jurisdictions. Their chapter portends to the very real and practical challenges to be faced in operationalizing public health approaches to improve protective system outcomes for children and families.

28.5 Challenges to Overcome

Gray and Schubert (Chap. 14) highlight "tensions" and barriers to change, as they relate to the public health model, both theoretically and operationally. These include competing priorities related to "control" and "care" in systems that are difficult to align, as well as the difficulties that come with trying to implement a model that current systems are not prepared to support. In many jurisdictions there is very little system integration or organizational communication, collaboration or conflict resolution that are necessary for inter-professional and inter-organizational practice to be reliable and effective. For decades CP has been hamstrung by a lack of buy-in to calls for children's protection to be "everybody's business," and this has particularly been evidenced by adult services' and programs' reluctance to recognize or operationalize a remit to embrace policies and practices that meet children's needs for protection. Rather, many organizations have used narrow foci upon their own clients' interests and privacy as their priority. Indeed, there currently is no infrastructure for the rollout of a large scale universal strategy that supports primary prevention, nor are there agreed upon models for promoting cross-institutional coordination, communication, and collaboration that will enable the implementation of integrated system responses characteristic of a public health approach.

Recent efforts at reform have focused on professional sources of help and there does not yet seem to be a clear set of strategies for community participation in prevention and early intervention. Relatedly, there is a need for workforce development to accompany public health initiatives so that staff have the requisite skills, understandings, and knowledge to work in prevention and early intervention.

Another significant challenge has to do with evidence and the use of evidence-based programs. As noted above, there currently is little information about which interventions are best suited to a public health approach and limited evidence for their effectiveness—in part because programs have often gone untested (see for example Chaps. 21 and 25 in this volume). Relatedly, there is no systemic culture of evidence-based practice underpinning CP systems. This will need to change for reform efforts to move forward. As they do, there attention will also need to focus on developing robust evaluative data systems that can measure multi-dimensional change in processes, outcomes and program/service efficacy. Linkages between system stakeholders and universities/research institutes need to be strengthened and funded to ensure that there is increased capacity for robust foundational research and program evaluation.

Foundational research is required with respect to the associations between indicators of social and economic disadvantage and prevalence of maltreatment, community and family needs, contact with CP, and development of service responses that foster community social capital and social care capacity (see Scott and Faulkner Chap. and 16 Bywaters Chap. 17). There is as yet an under focus on the development of models for service user and community involvement in the ongoing system reform processes (see Chap. 15), but there is clear evidence of the centrality of local, bottom-up community-led engagement in building community social capital and collective approaches that nurture and protect children and foster their socialisation (Jack and Gill 2010; Melton 2014; Melton and Anderson 2008; Molnar et al. 2016). But all too often present reforms tend to supplant grass roots involvement and leadership with a professionalised model of intervention. Is this because CP system reform processes that accompany public health initiatives seem to be fraught and unable/unwilling to let go power unless there is strong leadership?

Perhaps the most daunting challenge is overcoming political resistance to having public agencies engage with families, particularly at a time when some are calling for scaling back services organized centrally in favor of more localized control and oversight of child welfare programs. Public health approaches offer encouraging approaches to address the over-representation of Indigenous children (see Chap. 20), but the bigger issues that remain largely ignored are the over-representation of dominant CP rescue discourses that are not culturally safe and bypass recognition of the intergenerational impacts of Colonisation, trauma and inequity/inequality. To succeed in reforming the CP system, there will need to be political and institutional/administrative support that is steadfast and has a vision for the new system, as well as community willingness to institute reforms. Scandals and tragedies that have undermined trust in CP will have to be addressed and repaired.

Despite the many real and significant challenges, a number of jurisdictions are demonstrating success in smaller scale reform efforts. In fact, there is growing evidence internationally of the promise of public health approaches in Ireland, Australia, Canada and some parts of Europe and USA, many of which are captured in chapters in this volume (see for example Chaps. 23 and 24). Each is being done in within particular ideological, political and institutional, and organisational contexts and it is impossible to portray this as a single 'model' of intervention – a lot of diversity is evident. Much can be learned from these examples and translated into goals to be scaled.

But judicious appraisal is required rather than slavish adherence to a notion that even evidence-based programs can easily or successfully be transplanted into environments that are quite different from the contexts in which their program or service efficacy was established. Unfortunately, in some jurisdictions the imperatives of system reform have oft translated into what *Yes Minister's* Sir Humphrey Appleby once described as the 'politician's syllogism'; "something needs to happen", "this is something", therefore "we should do this". Political exigency should not supplant the requirement for careful consideration of the context and how the evidence-based interventions might best be applied in light of the local circumstances.

As Barraclough and colleagues illustrate (Chap. 24), plans for reform do not have to be all laid out at the front, but the principles and broad architecture, including the portals and processes for the community accessing help when they need it, do need to be articulated. However, shifting beliefs and norms to normalize outside engagement with families; strengthening data systems; and building capacity for more progressive models by linking and reforming systems are all required to realize this vision for more universal care.

28.6 Conclusions

This volume has involved researchers and authors from many countries and, despite the jurisdictional diversity and variations in the social, political and institutional environments, there are nonetheless some key points and principles made that are applicable across the board. First, CP approaches are critical to addressing the needs of children at risk of significant harm and need to be a core part of every protective system, and a public health model includes these as part of the tertiary level responses. CP is, however, subject to a variety of significant limitations that have been outlined here, particularly in Part I of this volume. For example, many families and children find the forensically- and risk-oriented interventions deeply stigmatizing. Further, the life course outcomes of many children in out-of-home care are unacceptable – there is far more required for these children and their families than mere 'child rescue'. The disproportionality that is found amongst those in contact with these systems is also unacceptable. As Parton notes, (in Chap. 27), CP does not really address the underlying social and structural inequities that are associated with much child maltreatment. But nor was CP designed to do so.

A public health model, on the other hand, is designed to do so, with multiple strategies and formal interventions across the primary, secondary and tertiary levels, and a focus upon addressing the social determinants of health and, thereby, reducing the prevalence of child maltreatment. This is necessary if we are to address the inequities and resulting inequalities that are found associated with all forms of child maltreatment, but particularly neglect which is the 'big kid on the block'. Using data to provide the information to target interventions to where they are most needed and likely to have the greatest preventive effects is essential. But this is not value free, and community concern about intrusive state interventions is an important consideration when designing and implementing system responses. Gray and Schubert (Chap. 14) point out that the use of data mining and predictive risk modelling remains contentious and must be done within an ethical framework, and that public health models entail a risk of ever-expanding social surveillance by the state.

Trocmé and colleagues (Chap. 25) and Scott and Faulkner (Chap. 16) highlight how developing robust data collection systems and analytical frameworks is fraught, takes many years of hard work to accomplish, and yet is ongoing with the job never quite coming to completion. Using data to establish program and service efficacy is not a 'magic wand' for resolving these system issues which hinder the operationalization of public health approaches (see Chap. 21). The reality is that establishing the 'right' models for specific jurisdictions and then implementing change processes to bring about improved system processes and outcomes is very difficult indeed, and requires inter-organizational collaborations and system integration which hitherto have proved to be major obstacles to successful reform and improved system outcomes for children, families and communities (see Chaps. 8, 12, 15, 23 and 24).

But despite these impediments there is a groundswell trend across many nations toward the implementation of public health models for preventing child maltreatment. This is a new direction in many jurisdictions, but has also been a 'slow train coming'. These new directions entail the key themes outlined in this volume, such as employing epidemiological approaches, and building in system capability for the expanded use of a diverse information systems as a foundation to determining program and system efficacy beyond the often narrow outcomes measured within current CP approaches.

An important aspect of reform noted by many authors here has been the importance of community-based and -led responses that utilise informal neighbourhood and community relationships and connections to build webs of care for vulnerable children and families, who are often struggling to get by within impoverished communities that involve significant hardships and inequality. Public health initiatives need to supplement these informal caring networks, not supplant them. We endorse these approaches as important alternatives to 'power over' professional interventions that do not yet properly utilise the strengths and resilience of these communities and their citizens. Future responses to the plight of many Indigenous peoples and their child rearing needs must embrace approaches that no longer utilize discourses that over-represent western world viewpoints and attitudes steeped in colonising perspectives. Public health approaches offer much to combat such negative and unjust belief systems and interventions, and instead promote community led and controlled services that entail embedded culturally-safe practices and attitudes.

Parton's emphasis upon system reforms steeped in a child rights framework and the concept of the social harm caused by maltreatment (see Chap. 27) are noted as being congruent with a public health model, not least because they provide an overarching understanding that children's well-being entails far more than just the prevention of maltreatment. Public health approaches and strategies provide us with the conceptual and operational wherewithal to tackle the pernicious effects of deeply imbedded social inequities that result in the profound inequalities associated with higher likelihoods of children being abused and neglected. This volume provides much of value to enable us to re-vision public health approaches for protecting children and supporting their families and communities, and thereby to reduce the prevalence of maltreatment. In doing so it provides a mind map and practical guidance for the sorts of system reforms and innovations that can help make the world a better place for all children, their parents, families, friends and communities.

References

Bronfenbrenner, U. (1979). *The ecology of human development: Experiments by nature and design*. Cambridge, MA: Harvard University Press.

Featherstone, B., White, S., & Morris, K. (2014). *Reimagining child protection: Towards humane social work with families*. Bristol: Policy Press.

Herrenkohl, T. I., Higgins, D. J., Merrick, M. T., & Leeb, R. T. (2015). Positioning a public health framework at the intersection of child maltreatment and intimate partner violence. *Child Abuse & Neglect, 48*, 22–28. https://doi.org/10.1016/j.chiabu.2015.04.013.

Holland, S. (2014). Trust in the community: Understanding the relationships between formal, semi-formal and informal child safeguarding in a local neighbourhood. *British Journal of Social Work, 44*, 384–400.

Jack, G., & Gill, O. (2010). The role of communities in safeguarding children and young people. *Child Abuse Review, 19*, 82–96.

Lonne, B., Harries, M., Featherstone, B., & Gray, M. (2016). *Working ethically in child protection*. London: Routledge (Taylor & Francis).

Melton, G. B. (2014). Strong communities for children: A community-wide approach to prevention of child maltreatment. In J. Korbin & R. D. Krugman (Eds.), *Handbook of child maltreatment* (pp. 329–339). New York: Springer.

Melton, G. B., & Anderson, D. (2008). From safe sanctuaries to strong communities: The role of communities of faith in child protection. *Family & Community Health, 31*(2), 173–185.

Molnar, B., & Beardslee, W. (2015). Community-level prevention of child maltreatment. In J. Korbin & R. Krugman (Eds.), *Handbook of child maltreatment* (pp. 301–316). Dordrecht: Springer.

Molnar, B., Goerge, R., Gilsanz, P., Hill, A., Subramanian, S. V., Holton, J., Duncan, D., Beatriz, E., & Beardslee, W. (2016). Neighborhood-level social processes and substantiated cases of child maltreatment. *Child Abuse & Neglect, 51*, 41.

Newton, B. J. (2017). An Aboriginal community's perceptions and experiences of child neglect in a rural town. *Australian Journal of Social Issues, 52*, 262–277. https://doi.org/10.1002/ajs4.18.

Scott, D., Lonne, B., & Higgins, D. (2016). Public health models for preventing child maltreatment: Applications from the field of injury prevention. *Trauma, Violence, & Abuse, 17*(4), 408–419. https://doi.org/10.1177/1524838016658877.

Sedlack, A., & Ellis, R. (2014). Trends in child abuse reporting. In J. Korbin & R. Krugman (Eds.), *Handbook of child maltreatment* (pp. 3–26). Dordrecht: Springer.

Index

B. Lonne et al. (eds.), *Re-Visioning Public Health Approaches for Protecting Children*, Child Maltreatment 9, https://doi.org/10.1007/978-3-030-05858-6

MIX
Papier aus verantwortungsvollen Quellen
Paper from responsible sources
FSC® C105338

If you have any concerns about our products,
you can contact us on
ProductSafety@springernature.com

In case Publisher is established outside the EU,
the EU authorized representative is:
Springer Nature Customer Service Center GmbH
Europaplatz 3, 69115 Heidelberg, Germany

Printed by Libri Plureos GmbH
in Hamburg, Germany